Speech Sound Disorders

Speech Sound Disorders

Shelley Lynn Velleman, PhD, CCC-SLP
Chair and Professor
Communication Sciences and Disorders
University of Vermont
Burlington, Vermont

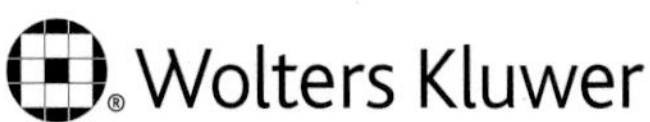

Philadelphia • Baltimore • New York • London
Buenos Aires • Hong Kong • Sydney • Tokyo

Acquisitions Editor: Michael Nobel
Product Development Editor: Staci Wolfson
Editorial Assistant: Tish Rogers
Marketing Manager: Leah Thomson
Production Project Manager: Marian Bellus
Design Coordinator: Joan Wendt
Artist/Illustrator: Jennifer Clements and Integra
Manufacturing Coordinator: Margie Orzech
Prepress Vendor: SPi Global

9 8 7 6 5 4 3 2 1

Printed in China

Library of Congress Cataloging-in-Publication Data
Velleman, Shelley Lynne, author.
Speech sound disorders / Shelley Lynne Velleman. — First edition.
p. ; cm.
Includes bibliographical references.
ISBN 978-1-4963-1624-0
I. Title.
[DNLM: 1. Speech Disorders. 2. Language Development Disorders. 3. Phonetics. 4. Speech Therapy. WL 340.2]
RC423
616.85'5—dc23
2015025336

LWW.com

CCS0915

This book is dedicated to my sisters, Debby Roth, AvtarKaurKhalsa, Jocelyn Melanson, and Stephanie Button, with gratitude for all your love and support.

REVIEWERS

Ruth Crutchfield, SLPD, CCC-SLP
Assistant Professor
Communication Sciences and Disorders
University of Texas-Pan American
Edinburg, Texas

Karen Czarnik, PhD, CCC-SLP/L
Associate Professor
Communication Sciences and Disorders
Saint Xavier University
Chicago, Illinois

Janet Dodd, PhD, CCC-SLP
Assistant Professor
Communications Sciences and Disorders
Chapman University–Orange
Orange, California

Kellie Ellis, CCC-SLP
Assistant Professor
Department of Communication Disorders
Eastern Kentucky University
Richmond, Kentucky

Regina Enwefa, PhD, CCC-SLP, ND
Professor
Speech Language and Pathology
Southern University and A&M College
Baton Rouge, Louisiana

Heidi Harbers, PhD, CCC-SLP
Associate Professor
Communication Sciences and Disorders
Illinois State University
Normal, Illinois

Alice Henton, CCC-SLP
Assistant Professor
Communication Sciences and Disorders
Harding University
Searcy, Arkansas

Iris Johnson, PhD, CCC-SLP
Associate Professor
Speech Pathology and Audiology
Tennessee State University Nashville
Nashville, Tennessee

Carol Koch, EdD, CCC-SLP
Associate Professor
Communication Sciences and Disorders
Samford University
Homewood, Alabama

M. Gay Masters, PhD, CCC-SLP
Assistant Professor
Speech-Language Pathology
University of Louisville
Louisville, Kentucky

Angela McLeod, PhD
Clinical Assistant Professor
Communication Sciences and Disorders
University of South Carolina
Columbia, South Carolina

Benjamin Munson, PhD
Professor
Speech Language Hearing Sciences
University of Minnesota
St. Paul, Minnesota

Barbara Oppenheimer, CCC-SLP
Clinical Associate Professor
Speech, Language and Hearing Sciences
Boston University
Boston, Massachusetts

Carol Tessel, PhD, CCC-SLP
Assistant Professor
Communication Sciences and Disorders
Florida Atlantic University
Boca Raton, Florida

Maggie Watson, PhD, CCC-SLP
Professor
School of Communicative Disorders
University of Wisconsin–Stevens Point
Stevens Point, Wisconsin

PREFACE

One of the main purposes of this book is to illustrate key relationships within pairs of factors that some might see as opposites. The first of these apparently contradictory concepts is the concrete usefulness of theories. Although many people think of theory and practice as opposing forces, as Lewin (1951) said:

> Nothing is as practical as a good theory to enable you to make choices confidently and consistently, and to explain or defend why you are making the choices you make (p. 169, as quoted by Larson & McKinley, 1995, p. 32).

As a person who followed a PhD in linguistics with a masters degree in speech-language pathology and many years of hands-on clinical experience, I know acutely well that it is impossible to present in any book or course every possible profile of communication disorder that a speech-language pathologist (SLP) will encounter. Every client or patient is a unique case study for whom we call upon the integrated benefits of knowledge, experience, and skills. In the face of a confusing combination of history and symptoms, the SLP must rely on evidence-based concepts to craft a hypothesis about the profile of the individual child and to make evaluation and intervention plans based upon that hypothesis. Therefore, current theories of phonology, motor speech, development, disorder, delay, evaluation, and intervention are thoroughly explained in this book. In every case, the applications of the theories are not only stated but illustrated using actual data and practiced via review problems, essay questions, and case study assignments. Theory and practice are interwoven throughout every chapter. Videos available on thePoint illustrate many of these concepts and provide the basis for additional assignments.

The second surprising linkage is how universals of human language and the characteristics of individual languages interact to impact the process of development and the manifestations of delay and disorder. For this reason, every chapter includes information not only about English speech sound development, delay, and disorder but also about speech development, delay, and disorder in a variety of different languages. This information is critical to every practicing SLP in our increasingly diverse world.

The third set of interacting opposites is composed of standardized tests, which provide normed relational data that allow us to determine severity and official eligibility for services, and informal analysis procedures, which facilitate consideration of the functionality and typicality of the child's phonological system and thereby deepen and broaden our understanding of the true nature of the problem. The relative contributions of both of these approaches to evaluation are fully presented with respect to each aspect of phonology, including easy-to-use worksheets for less formal, more in-depth analysis of many of these aspects. Suggestions are provided for how to balance and integrate these findings in order to develop a comprehensive speech sound profile and intervention goals that will result in maximal therapy outcomes.

Another innovation of this book is its organization. In my many years of teaching speech sound disorders and discussing teaching with colleagues, I have found that evaluation and intervention often get short shrift because those chapters come at the end of most textbooks, where they are presented in a rush at the end of the semester. Students complain that they haven't learned enough practical information to know what to do in the clinic. In this book, precursors to speech production and general principles of evaluation and intervention are covered first. Then, every aspect of phonology—phones and phonemes, phonotactics, error patterns, and prosody—is addressed thoroughly, including typical development, delays/disorders, evaluation strategies, and intervention approaches. In this way, assessment and treatment approaches appropriate to each aspect of deficit are presented in the same chapter as that type of deficit itself, while the related concepts are fresh. For speech-language pathology departments in which students begin clinical work while taking related courses, this has the advantage that students are exposed to diagnostic and therapy principles and techniques from early in the semester.

Another teaching challenge for professors of speech sound disorders is the wide range of knowledge bases that graduate students bring to our courses. Some have a thorough knowledge of both phonetics and phonology; others barely recognize the IPA symbols used for broad transcription. For this reason, Chapter 2 provides a thorough review of the phonetics and phonology material that we wish all of our students brought to graduate school. This chapter—and the accompanying review activities—can be assigned as independent work for those students who need it, covered in class to whatever extent the instructor so chooses, and/or used as a resource for an undergraduate phonetics or phonology class.

The motivation and inspiration for this book—and for most of my scholarly activities—comes from the many children who have invited me into their lives to support them as they developed into successful communicators, as well as the SLPs and other professionals with whom I've collaborated on these cases. I am especially grateful to the families who have been willing to allow me to share their children's videos so that future generations of SLPs will use their deeper understanding of speech sound development and disorders to assist children with communication disorders to find and use their unique voices.

Thank you all!

Shelley Velleman

Larson, V. L., & McKinley, N. (1995). *Language disorders in older students: Preadolescents and adolescents.* Eau Claire, WI: Thinking Publications.

Lewin, K. (1951). *Field theory in social science: Selected theoretical papers.* New York, NY: Harper & Row.

ACKNOWLEDGMENTS

I am very grateful to the many people who have made this book possible. The most important is, of course, my husband Dan, who has supported and encouraged me throughout. Many students and several anonymous reviewers have provided invaluable feedback on several different drafts of this work. Prita Kottaveetil enthusiastically double-checked the references, compiled the first draft of the glossary, and helped identify useful video clips. Bobby Coutu provided further invaluable assistance with the video clips and the associated case study assignments. Many colleagues, especially Babs Davis, Carol Stoel-Gammon, Marilyn Vihman, Mary Andrianopoulos, Vani Rupela, Myra Huffman, Carolyn Mervis, Larry Shriberg, Lise Menn, Elena Zaretsky, Kristine Strand, Diane Forman Judd, and Sharon Gretz, have supported me both directly and indirectly in many ways for many years by sharing their ideas, their clinical conundrums, and their research findings and by raising the really hard questions that push our field forward. I have been further inspired and motivated by the thoughtful, rigorous work of far too many other colleagues to list here. Barry Guitar not only encouraged and commiserated with me but also sent me in the direction of Wolters Kluwer Health, where I have received excellent support, advice, and editing from Staci Wolfson and Michael Nobel. At a more basic level, Kathy Dunn and many other remarkable writers in her Amherst Writers and Artists group have helped me thrive as a writer for decades.

CONTENTS

CHAPTER 3
Precursors to Speech

CHAPTER 4
Basic Principles for Speech Sound Evaluation

CHAPTER 5
Basic Treatment Principles

CHAPTER 6
Beginnings: Pre-Speech and First Words

CHAPTER 7
Phones and Phonemes

CHAPTER 8
The Phonological Framework

CHAPTER 9
Phonological Patterns

CHAPTER 10
Prosody

LIST OF FORMS

CHAPTER 1

Perspectives on Speech Sound Development and Disorders

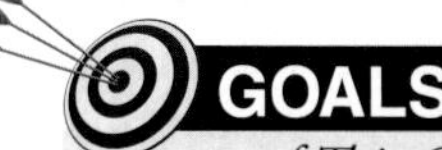

GOALS of This Chapter

1. Review the physiologic bases for speech and speech processing.
2. Explore the concept of a phonology as a system.
3. Describe the components of phonological systems.

INTRODUCTION

"Susie has a **functional phonological disorder**." What does that mean, both literally and in terms of appropriate assessment and intervention strategies? This is not an easy question. The rest of this book will be devoted to answering these questions, addressing different types and aspects of childhood speech sound disorders (SSDs), and discussing how such disorders can and should be identified, assessed, and treated. Some brief preliminary answers are provided here.

First, what is meant by "phonological?" A **phonology** is a system for using human anatomic structures (typically, but not exclusively, the vocal tract) to communicate by producing speech sounds. These are combined into a set of **syllable** and word shapes, which are in turn grouped into phrases and sentences using pitch, pauses, and other prosodic features. All of these processes are carried out as specified by the language(s) of the speaker and the listener. In this book, the term "phonological" will be used as a cover term to encompass all aspects of speech sound processing and production—including motor planning and execution as well as speech perception and everything in between. The reason for this is that it is very difficult to draw a clear line between motoric and cognitive/linguistic aspects of child SSDs. Dividing SSDs into those that are purely articulatory versus those that are purely phonological is extremely difficult and often misleading, as discussed in greater detail below. Therefore, the term "phonology" will be used here to refer to the entire system that is responsible for all aspects of the perception, production, processing, and awareness of speech sounds. The reader should be aware, however, that other authors may use this term in other ways.

Secondly, what is meant by a "functional" disorder? Speech-language pathologists (SLPs) use the term "functional phonological disorders" to refer to SSDs with no known physiologic or neurologic basis. It does not mean that the child is functioning typically. Rather, it means that—as far as can be determined—the child's speech sound dysfunction has no anatomic or physiologic source. That is, the problem is with the function, not with the structure, of the system. It is also not intended to imply that children whose SSDs do have a known cause are more or less functional than are children with "garden variety" SSDs. An established neurodevelopmental diagnosis (such as **Williams syndrome**) may have a mild impact on speech; a functional phonological disorder may be severe. In practice, we find many overlaps between the speech sound characteristics of children whose disorders result from known causes versus those for which we don't yet know how to identify the source. Furthermore, all children with SSDs are at higher risk of reading and spelling deficits through the school ages and into adulthood (Lewis, Freebairn, Hansen, Iyengar, & Taylor, 2004) with negative consequences for academic performance and even long-term impacts on relationships and employment (McCormack, McLeod, McAllister, & Harrison, 2009). Thus, SSDs have important implications for key human social, academic, and eventually professional functions.

Unfortunately, the meaning of the term "functional disorder" in the sense of a **non-functioning** phonological system has had less effect upon approaches to remediation than it should. It is easy to get caught up in developmental norms, competing theories, and commercial therapy materials, thereby forgetting that the true goal is actually a very simple one: function. That is, the purpose of evaluation and intervention is to make the person's speech system more functional—both for oral communication and as the foundation of more abstract phonologically based skills such as reading and spelling. The many different analysis techniques and therapy packages available to us as SLPs for identifying and treating phonological malfunctions are convenient tools that can be used. The heart of the matter is that Susie's phonology is functionally disordered. That is, it is not working properly at its job of transmitting messages via sound. Our job is to figure out what is not working about her current system and what types of change can be facilitated in order to make it more functional.

Physiologic Bases for Speech and Speech Processing

All human beings—whether adults or children—have certain physiologic, neurologic, and cognitive limitations that have profound effects on human phonologies. As speakers, we cannot communicate only via thoughts, so we typically use our mouths and ears.[1] There are limits to our fine motor coordination, so the sounds we attempt must not be too difficult to produce consistently or too similar to one another articulatorily. We have to breathe occasionally, so there are limits on the number of words we produce without a pause, and so on.

As listeners, we have neither unlimited memory nor unlimited attention, so the speaker must occasionally pause to let us reflect upon what we are hearing. Our mammalian perception is fine-tuned to detect certain types of differences far better than others, so certain pairs or sets of speech sounds can be discriminated from each other much more easily than others. We cannot pay attention to more than a certain number of acoustic details at once, so the speaker must produce speech sounds as predictably as possible under the circumstances.

Such limitations, the characteristics of the language being learned by the child, the specific patterns of the speakers to whom the child is exposed (e.g., dialects, favorite expressions, characteristic tones of voice), and the child's own preferences

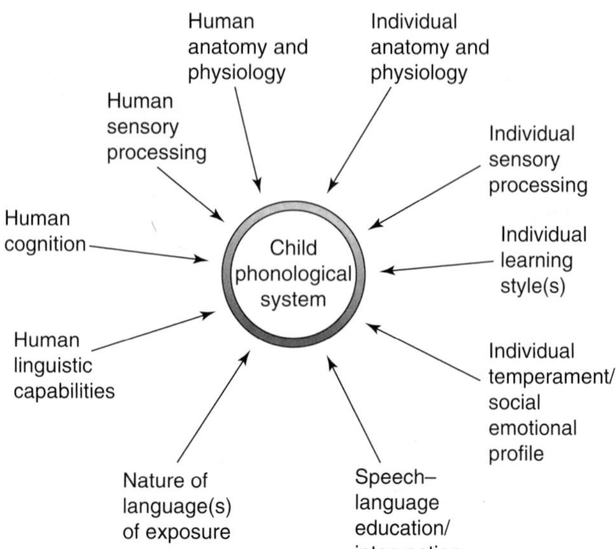

FIGURE 1-1. Factors impacting a child's phonological system.

and learning style will combine to determine a particular learner's **phonological patterns**. There are only a limited number of types of phonological patterns that the combination of these factors makes available to any human being. Therefore, the phonological systems of all languages and all people must share the same components (consonant and vowel repertoires, word and syllable shape patterns, prosodic contours, etc.), and these components tend to interact within these linguistic systems in certain, often predictable ways.

The factors that are most likely to impact the phonological systems of children are illustrated in Figure 1-1.

The similarities among the phonologies of different children—and of different languages—are far greater than the differences. There are many causes for a child's speech to lack functionality, including cognitive limitations, motor speech disorders (such as **Childhood Apraxia of Speech** or **dysarthria**), and anatomic/physiologic differences that range from subtle (e.g., slightly low **muscle tone**) to obvious (e.g., **cleft lip and palate**). However, in many cases, there is no identifiable physiologic or cognitive basis for the disorder. Such children are said to have functional phonological disorders.

However, any type of disorder that interferes with the oral transmission of ideas will incur similar challenges. For example, a child with a cleft palate has some different physiologic limitations to overcome in developing her phonology, but the phonology that she develops must include the same components (e.g., consonants and vowels combined into syllables and words with an overarching prosodic envelope that organizes them into grammatical units), which must interact with each other in basically the same ways—as if she were physically intact. The deaf typically cannot use oral-aural communication as efficiently as the hearing can, so they often use sign languages, which have their own manual phonological systems based upon hand shapes and hand movements rather than oral

[1] Of course, many people use manual communication—in this country, typically American Sign Language. As noted below, sign languages, like oral languages, have phonological systems. However, the phonology of sign language is beyond the scope of this book.

articulatory positions and movements of the oral articulators. Nonetheless, sign language phonologies parallel oral phonologies quite closely in many ways. The components of these phonologies are basically the same as those of oral phonologies—a repertoire of articulatory positions (places of articulation) formed in specific ways (manners of articulation) and combined into larger units (syllables, words, phrases, etc.). Most of the differences are actually superficial ones that are induced by the change in perceptual modalities (vision versus hearing) and in articulators (hands and to some extent, faces rather than oral structures). Although such cases have not been documented extensively, it is this author's assumption that the phonologies of children who are learning a manual language can be non-functional in ways that parallel the non-functional oral phonologies that are the focus of this book. It is the functionality of these adjustments in the face of human limitations that interests us and that is of far more relevance in this context than are the non-phonological causes of such limitations.

RATIONALE FOR STUDYING PHONOLOGICAL SYSTEMS IN GENERAL

In order to truly understand what a functional phonology is, it is necessary to explore many phonological systems and discuss how they work, including both functional and non-functional phonologies of adults and children from a variety of language backgrounds. To understand the many different ways in which a phonology can properly function, one must consider the phonologies of other languages. Knowledge of phonological tendencies among the languages of the world can be extremely helpful to the SLP for the following reasons:

- It is becoming less and less possible for an SLP anywhere in the English-speaking world to work with only monolingual, monodialectal clients. Ideally, bi/multilingual or bi/multidialectal children should be treated by SLPs with similar linguistic backgrounds, but this too is currently usually impossible. As of 2013, only 7% of American Speech-Language-Hearing Association (ASHA) members reported belonging to racial and ethnic minority groups (in comparison to 37% of the U.S. population, as estimated by the U.S. Census Bureau in 2014). Only 4.6% identified as Hispanic or Latino (in comparison to 16.9% of the U.S. population, per the U.S. Census Bureau in 2014). From 2008 to 2011, 12.9% of U.S. residents were immigrants (i.e., not born in the United States; U.S. Census Bureau, 2014); this percentage is expected to rise. About half of these immigrants reported not speaking English "very well" (Ryan, 2013). Thus, the people we are serving professionally are much more racially, ethnically, and linguistically diverse than we are as a collective profession. Therefore, those of us who have the misfortune of being monolingual, monodialectal speakers of General American English (GAE) must learn as much as possible about other linguistic systems in general as well as about specifics of other languages, dialects, and cultures in order to best serve our clients.
- Those sounds and sound patterns that are most universal (such as consonant-vowel "CV" syllables, stop consonants, etc.) tend to be perceptually or articulatorily (or both) easier than those that are rare. They can therefore be assumed to be good targets for early remediation in many cases.
- Children may use word shapes, sounds, or phonological patterns that are not typically found in English but that do occur in other languages. In some of these cases, the pattern chosen by the child may actually be more common within universal phonology than the pattern that happens to be used in English. Presumably, children who use patterns that are used in some languages have a better prognosis for improvement than do those who use deviant patterns (i.e., patterns that are not found in any languages).
- By understanding what makes a phonology tick (i.e., what the critical components of the system are and how they interact), one can get a better understanding of what has gone wrong in a particular child's phonological system. Because all components of a child's system are developing at the same time, these interactions are sometimes more difficult to discern in children's systems than they are in adult phonologies. By exploring the components of adult phonologies, it is easier to identify the types of interactions that may be present in those of children.

Schwartz and Leonard (1982) demonstrated that individual children are more likely to attempt new words if the words fit within their existing phonological systems. The children imitated and learned to say these "in" words more quickly than they imitated and/or learned "out" words that did not fit their current systems. Understanding which words are in and out of a child's phonology necessitates a thorough intuitive grasp of what a phonology is. Although many different types of possible phonological patterns will be discussed in this book, an effort will also be made to step back often, to remember the big picture whenever possible in order to feel less overwhelmed by these details, and to re-focus on the ultimate goal—functional communication.

GOALS

These are the goals of this book:

1. To take phonology apart into its various components, to understand each component and its physiologic and cognitive bases, and to describe how these components interact in order to analyze what a functioning phonological system is
2. To present methods and practice opportunities for assessing the functioning of those components both separately and in combination
3. To illustrate how to put the puzzle back together so that any impaired pieces that have an impact on the

functioning of the system as a whole can be easily identified and targeted in therapy

4. To provide practice opportunities for writing goals and objectives that address non-functional pieces of the system in an integrative manner
5. To describe, compare, and contrast strategies and methods for treating the various aspects of a non-functional phonological system

Once the functioning—and malfunctioning—aspects of a child's phonological system have been identified, it is far easier to determine which of these must be targeted in remediation in order to improve that child's communicative effectiveness. It's easy to get caught up in the procedural details of a particular system of phonological analysis and to forget the phonological system as a system. Stepping back from the details to say "What's the real problem here?" yields a deeper understanding of the nature of the communication disorder. Once a more general pattern of malfunction has been identified, phonological analysis becomes a tool rather than an additional source of confusion, and the clinician can see more clearly what to do about the problem and how to do it.

THE COMPONENTS OF PHONOLOGICAL SYSTEMS

In thinking about how any mechanical system is built, one tends to think first about its parts—switches, gears, cranks, wires, nuts, and bolts. But at least as important to the proper functioning of the system are several other factors: how the parts are connected to one another to form functional subcomponents; how each part's function contributes to the ultimate outcome; the mechanical process, or how each part's function interacts with the functions of others and how each subcomponent's function contributes to the final outcome; and, finally, the rate and intensity of the work done by the system.

Like any other functional system, phonological systems include basic elements (e.g., **features**, such as "**stop**" and "**velar**," which combine to form **phones**) with assigned roles (e.g., **phonemes** providing **lexical** contrast) that are combined in specific ways into larger units (the syllables, words, and sentences). All of these elements interact in certain ways (as exemplified by patterns referred to as **processes** or **constraints**, among other terms) at specified frequencies, rates, and **intensity** levels (the **prosody**) in order to achieve the final result, spoken language (**discourse**). All of these elements, levels, and interactions can be defined in terms of the questions they answer about the phonological system:

- The **phonetic repertoire**: What sounds are available to be combined into syllable and word shapes? What features or **articulatory gestures** are combined to form these phones? What types of phonetic/articulatory "slop" are allowed in the final pronunciations of words and utterances in fast or casual speech? This component clearly depends upon the person's motoric capabilities as well as the person's understanding of the linguistic rules that govern word formation in his or her language (e.g., which sounds occur in which positions).
- The **phonemic repertoire**: What is each sound's role in the language? More specifically, how do the sounds contrast to yield distinctive words? This component depends upon the child's speech perception—his or her bottom-up linguistic processing of the sounds of speech—as well as upon his or her top-down linguistic expectations about the sounds produced by others based upon the organization of his or her linguistic system.
- The **phonotactic repertoire**: What syllable and word shapes are available for use? That is, how can the elements be combined into larger units?
- **Phonological patterns** (processes, constraints): How do the syllable, word, and phrase shapes interact with the sounds and contrasts to yield the final pronunciation of the utterance? What systematic modifications in the target forms can be identified (processes)? What patterns in the outcomes can be detected with respect to favorite sounds and forms or avoided sounds and forms (constraints)? What influence does the **morphology** of the language have on the pronunciation of different types of words and endings?
- **Suprasegmental patterns**, or prosody: What are the rhythms and melodies of the language? Is **stress** marked by the loudness, the pitch, and/or the duration of the segments? Are relatively unstressed syllables timed about equally, or do they follow some other rhythmic pattern? What other purposes do loudness, pitch, and/or duration serve in the language? How does the morphology of the language influence the prosody?

The relationships of all of these components to each other are illustrated in Figure 1-2.

As noted by Fee (1995), all levels of phonological organization are simplified in child phonology, but all are relevant. Unless all of these subcomponents and how they interact with each other are considered, therapists will be agonizing needlessly over intervention priorities. Including all aspects of the phonological system in assessment and planning sounds like extra work, but it will in fact simplify goal-setting and assessment of progress to a remarkable degree, and it can often be done fairly simply and quickly.

As noted above, some people are careful to make a distinction between "articulation impairments" and "phonological impairments." The former phrase is used to refer to SSDs for which there is a clear-cut anatomic or motoric basis (as in cleft palate) or a clear lack of a cognitive basis (as in a "simple" distortion of a single sound, such as /ɹ/[2] [English "r"] or /s/). A phonological impairment might be defined as "a conceptual or linguistic difficulty with the organization and use of phonemes to signal meaning" (Baker & McLeod, 2011, p. 105).

[2][ɹ] is the proper IPA symbol for the American English consonantal "r" sound, as in the word "rat." Many American linguists and SLPs use [r], but this symbol actually represents the trilled "rr" of Spanish, as in the word "perro."

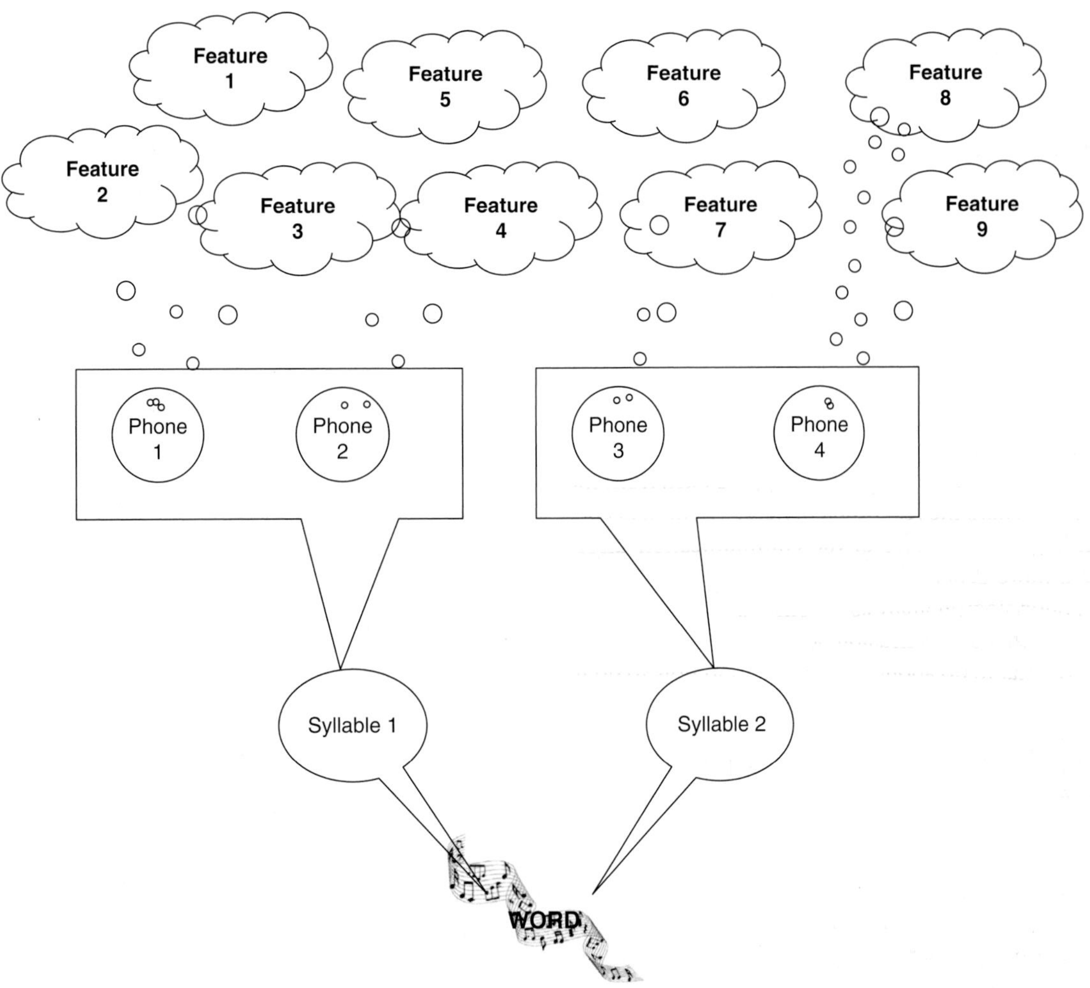

FIGURE 1-2. Elements combining into larger wholes.

However, it is often very difficult to distinguish between these two in practice. Many children display characteristics of general motor or motor speech deficits (e.g., low tone, poor coordination affecting the whole body or the oral structures only) but also demonstrate an apparent lack of understanding of the **phonological rules** of the language(s) to which they have been exposed. Children with Childhood Apraxia of Speech (CAS), for example, a disorder of motor speech planning, are at increased risk for literacy disorders, which have a clear cognitive basis (ASHA, 2007). Furthermore, children with SSDs that appear to have a cognitive-linguistic basis often display subtle motoric deficits nonetheless. For this reason, many scholars in the field have resorted to the label "SSDs" as a means of avoiding this distinction and embracing all types of deficits that impact the production of speech sounds. One drawback of this new phrase is that it implies that the disorder impacts only the production of individual sounds, whereas some of the patterns that have the most significant impact on intelligibility relate to the misproduction of speech structures, such as final consonants, consonant clusters, and multisyllabic words. Another is that some speech sound errors reflect the child's misperception of speech sounds rather than an inability to actually produce them. In this book, the terms "SSDs" and "phonological disorders" are used interchangeably. If a purely motoric impairment or a purely **cognitive-linguistic impairment** is intended, that will be made clear.

SUMMARY

"Phonology" will be used here as a cover term to refer to a child's or a language's phones, phonemes, allophones, syllable and word shapes, the production and perception of these, and the patterning of these in rules or processes. Any strategy that a child uses to convey meaning by sound, including strategies that are inspired by physiologic limitations (such as cleft palate), will be considered to be part of that child's phonology. A phonology (child or adult; functional or non-functional) has several components, each of which can function in various ways by itself and in interaction with other components. Each of these depends on various combinations of elements. However, phonologies also must be considered in their entireties. We cannot look at any one component alone and draw adequate conclusions about phonological malfunction without considering every other aspect of the child's phonology as well.

A phonology is a functioning system. Children begin the language acquisition process without such a system; they learn their first words as unrelated wholes. Children who are normally developing, however, quickly begin to systematize.

In order to efficiently assess a child's phonology, it must be viewed as a system that may or may not be functioning adequately for the child's communication needs at that time. For this reason, it is critical to consider the effectiveness of the system as such (**independent analysis**) as well as to compare it to the adult norm (**relational analysis**); both perspectives contribute key information for effective goal-setting.

All of these concepts will be revisited, in most cases multiple times, throughout the remainder of this book.

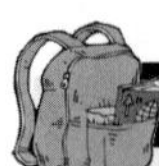

KEY TAKE-HOME MESSAGES

1. A phonology is a system composed of components at many different levels.
2. Conceptualizing phonology as a system helps us to understand the sources and impacts of non-functional components.

References

ASHA. (2007). *Childhood apraxia of speech [Technical report]* (No. TR2007-00278). Rockville Pike, MD: American Speech-Language-Hearing Association.

ASHA. (2013). *Highlights and trends: Member and affiliate counts, Year end 2013*. Rockville Pike, MD: American Speech-Language Hearing Association.

Baker, E., & McLeod, S. (2011). Evidence-based practice for children with speech sound disorders: Part 1 narrative review. *Language, Speech, and Hearing Services in Schools, 42*, 102–139.

Fee, E. J. (1995). Segments and syllables in early language acquisition. In J. Archibald (Ed.), *Phonological acquisition and phonological theory* (pp. 43–61). Hillsdale, NJ: Lawrence Erlbaum Associates.

Lewis, B. A., Freebairn, L. A., Hansen, A. J., Iyengar, S. K., & Taylor, H. G. (2004). School-age follow-up of children with Childhood Apraxia of Speech. *Language, Speech, and, Hearing Services in Schools, 35*(2), 122–140.

McCormack, J., McLeod, S., McAllister, L., & Harrison, L. J. (2009). A systematic review of the association between childhood speech impairment and participation across the lifespan. *International Journal of Speech-Language Pathology, 11*(2), 155–170.

Ryan, C. (2013). *Language Use in the United States: 2011*. Retrieved June 9, 2014, from http://www.census.gov/prod/2013pubs/acs-22.pdf

Schwartz, R. G., & Leonard, L. B. (1982). Do children pick and choose? An examination of phonological selection and avoidance in early lexical acquisition. *Journal of Child Language, 9*, 319–336.

U.S. Census Bureau. (2014). USA Quick Facts. Retrieved June 9, 2014, from http://quickfacts.census.gov/qfd/states/00000.html

CHAPTER 2

Review of Phonetics and Phonology

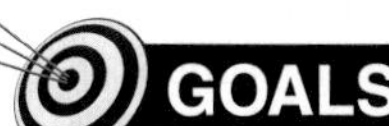

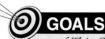

GOALS *of This Chapter*

1. Review speech sounds, phonetic universals, phonetic features, and the contrastive roles of phonemes.
2. Review concepts from phonology that are key to understanding speech sound development, disorders, evaluation, and intervention.
3. Compare and contrast phonological theories with important implications for speech sound development, disorders, evaluation, and intervention.

Many concepts from linguistics are key to understanding child phonological development, delay, and disorders. Some of these terms have different uses and even different definitions within various theories. Furthermore, students come to graduate courses in speech sound disorders with extremely varied backgrounds. For some, the majority of the concepts in this chapter will be review; for others, many may be new. This chapter is provided in an attempt to put all readers on an equal footing, so that these concepts can be only briefly reviewed in later chapters.

PHONOLOGY

The most important term to define, for obvious reasons, is phonology. Crystal (1991) defines phonology as:

> *a branch of linguistics which studies the sound systems of languages. ... Putting this another way, phonology is concerned with the range and function of sounds in specific languages ... and with the rules which can be written to show the types of phonetic relationships that relate and contrast words and other linguistic units. (p. 261)*

As Crystal points out, this term is often used in different ways by different phonologists. In many models, some of the components that will be described here—especially the phonetic repertoire and the optional **fast speech rules** (casual speech patterns)—are omitted from the phonology proper. In this book, however, "phonology" will be used to encompass all actions, patterns, elements, and linguistic structures relating to the use of sound in speech production and perception. This term will also be used to include the compensatory strategies used by children with physiologic, cognitive, neurologic, perceptual, or articulatory limitations. Thus, in this context, the often-asked question, "Is this a phonological disorder or is it an articulation disorder?" can be a misleading one. *The critical question to ask about a child's phonology is "What aspects of this system are interfering the most with its effective functioning?"* In some cases, the answer will clearly lie in the motor system or even the anatomy itself. In some cases, the answer will clearly lie in the child's incomplete learning of the sound contrasts (phonemes) or the patterns (rules, processes, or constraints) that operate in the ambient language. But in many other cases, the answer will lie in the interaction among multiple systems. Furthermore, just because the child's speech sound disorder presents as motoric at one age does not mean that the speech-language pathologist (SLP) should cease to attend to the other aspects of that youngster's phonological system.

"Cognitive–linguistic," "motor speech," and "articulation" disorders are distinct. Yet, delays and disorders rarely fall exclusively into one domain or another. For this reason, the use of the term "speech sound disorders" has recently come into popularity, as it encompasses all of these. The definition of phonology given above encompasses the physiologic (motor and perceptual) as well as the cognitive aspects of oral communication. Therefore, in this book, the terms "speech sound disorder (or delay)" (henceforth abbreviated "SSD") and "phonological disorder (or delay)" will be used synonymously; no distinction is implied by the use of one or the other. However, other phrases will be used with more specificity. "Cognitive–linguistic disorder" (or delay) will be the term used to refer to speech sound deficits reflecting incomplete linguistic knowledge on the part of the learner. "**Motor speech disorder**" will be used to refer to conditions affecting motor planning or programming (as in Childhood Apraxia of Speech) or motor execution (as in childhood dysarthria). "**Articulation disorder**" will refer to difficulty accurately producing specific speech sounds, in the absence of a motor speech disorder, even though the child is aware of their roles in the language. For example, a child might know that /s/ is distinct from /θ/ and that "sing" and "thing" are not homonyms despite the fact that he produces [s] in a more fronted position than is appropriate for English. "**Mixed speech sound disorder**" will refer to some combination of the above.

Phonology has both input and output components, as well as a central organizational component. Learning the phonological system of a language requires far more than merely hearing a speech sound and repeating it. As children struggle to make sense of this complexity, some aspects of adult phonology may not be perceived as important. Children with deficits in phonological memory, language skills, attention, social awareness, or other precursors to successful speech-language acquisition (all of which are thoroughly discussed in Chapter 3) may be especially vulnerable to errors of this sort. Youngsters with one or more of these weaknesses may therefore screen out some key phonological aspects of words as they are storing or retrieving them, resulting in a cognitive–linguistic speech sound disorder. This can occur even if the child is perfectly capable from an auditory point of view of hearing every phonological distinction and even articulatorily capable of producing them in certain contexts. Under these circumstances, the child may not be attempting to produce a word as adult speakers of the language expect it to be produced; his production goal may be different or simply indistinct. For this reason, although the word "target" will be used to refer to the adult production of the word, this should *not* be construed as implying that the adult production of the word actually is the child's current target; it is *the therapist's* eventual intervention target on behalf of the child.

PHONETIC CONCEPTS

Phonological Elements

Some of the elements that are relevant to phonology include the following:

Words

In order to define other phonological elements, it is often necessary to refer to "the word," so this term must be defined first. Crystal (1991) explains that words are "the most stable of all linguistic units" (p. 380). The subcomponents of each particular word have a fixed order. The parts of the word "rearrangement" cannot be rearranged into, for example, "mentarrangere" and still retain the identity of the word. Words are typically not interrupted by pauses within the flow of speech, unless the speaker stutters or revises the utterance. In order to be considered a word, a unit of meaning must be able to express that meaning on its own. Thus, "is" is a word, but "-ist" is not, since it only has meaning when it is added to another unit of meaning (such as "commun-"). All of these meaning units are called **morphemes,** whether they can stand on their own (as a word) or not. In many cases, a word is composed of multiple morphemes that also are single words themselves. The word "lighthousekeeper," for instance, is composed of three **free morphemes** that can each stand on their own as a word, plus one **bound morpheme** ("-er") that cannot be used independently.

Words come in all different shapes and sizes, depending upon the number of meaning units (morphemes) they contain, the number of **syllables** they contain, and the consonants and vowels that make up these smaller elements. As used in this book, a one-syllable word is **monosyllabic**, a two-syllable word is **disyllabic**, and a word with three or more syllables is **multisyllabic**.

Syllables

But what is a syllable? The syllable is a very difficult entity to define, despite the fact that native speakers of any language are usually very good at counting the syllables in their own words. There is no one definition of the syllable that is agreed upon by all linguists, but most focus on a key component, often in the middle of the syllable, that is very **sonorous** (resonant) and is produced with a relatively open vocal tract—typically a vowel (Blevins, 1995). This is called its **nucleus**. The edges of most syllables are less sonorous and are produced with a more closed vocal tract (such as a consonant). The first consonant (or set of consonants) at the beginning of a syllable, if any, is referred to as the **onset**. The final consonant (or set of consonants), if any, is called the **coda**. The nucleus and coda together form the **rhyme**. The onset and nucleus together form the **body** (Share & Blum, 2005). This syllabic organization is displayed in Figure 2-1.

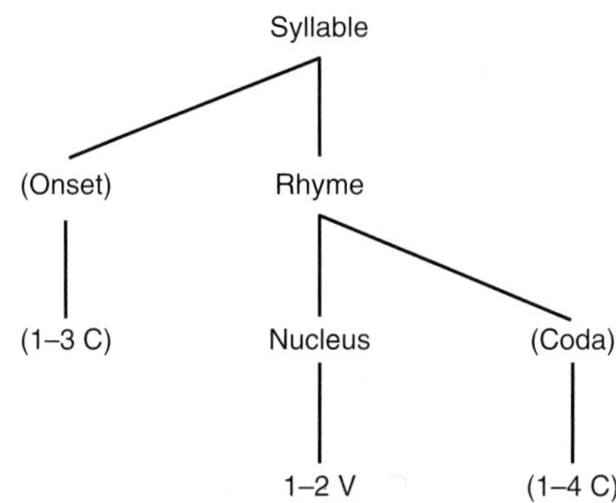

FIGURE 2-1. Components of the syllable.

Phones

Phones are speech sounds that are used by speakers in some language, regardless of whether they are used contrastively or not and regardless of whether any particular language uses them. Thus, any sound that is used for speech in any language is a phone. Phones are enclosed in square brackets: [m], [f], [u],[1] etc. The adjective used to refer to phones or analyses of phones is **phonetic**. The set of sounds that are available within a particular speaker's phonological system is that person's phonetic repertoire.

Phonetic Universals

Human **ease of perception** and **ease of production** as well as some organizational principles together yield **phonetic universals** (see later section). These are statements that can be made about tendencies within the sound systems of all languages; they are assumed to result primarily from human physiologic restrictions. Universals have been collected and/or described by Greenberg (1978), Maddieson (1984), Maddieson and Precoda (1989), and Lindblom and Maddieson (1988). Such universals are important to an understanding of child phonology because all children are affected by human physiologic restrictions in important ways, especially in early phonologies and in children whose SSDs have a motor or perceptual component. Sounds that are universally preferred are typically acquired early. Those that are rare among the languages of the world are usually acquired later (Locke, 1983), although the language that the child is learning can influence this (de Boysson-Bardies & Vihman, 1991; de Boysson-Bardies et al., 1992; Vihman 1996). The universals that are most relevant to phonological development in English are given in the sections below (from Maddieson [1984] unless otherwise specified[2]).

[1]IPA symbols whose pronunciations differ from the pronunciations of English orthography are given and exemplified in Appendix A, as are the phonetic diacritics used in this book.

Vowels

Vowels are speech sounds that are formed by shaping the articulators rather than using them to constrict the oral and pharyngeal cavities. They play the important role of serving as the nucleus of a syllable, carrying most of the loudness, pitch, and voice quality variations that communicate stress, tone, tone of voice, and the like. Vowel universals include the following:

1. All languages have at least three vowels.
2. The most common number of vowels in a language is five.
3. Of all languages, 86% have vowel systems with vowels that are articulatorily evenly spaced; that is, their places of articulation are distributed evenly throughout the oral cavity. Another 10% have nearly even spacing.
4. About two-thirds of the languages in the world have diphthongs. Of these, about 75% have [ɑɪ] (or something similar), and 65% have [ɑʊ] (or something similar; Ladefoged & Maddieson, 1996).

Stops

Stops are consonants that result from enough constriction to completely close off the vocal tract, interrupting the airflow. Air pressure builds up behind the constriction and is then released. Depending on the timing of the release versus the onset of voicing, the release may be audible (**aspiration**). Universals include the following:

5. All languages have stops.
6. If a language has two stop series, the two will differ in voicing (as do the two English series [p, t, k] and [b, d, g]). It is important to note in this connection that what English speakers tend to think of as **voiced** stops are actually voiceless unaspirated. Among the languages in the world, there are three types of voicing:
   - **Voiceless aspirated**: long lag (delay) between consonant release and beginning of voicing, so that we perceive the puff of air being released with the consonant, as in English word-initial /p, t, k/ in the words "pea," "tea," and "key:" [pʰi], [tʰi], [kʰi].
   - **Voiceless unaspirated**: short or no lag between consonant release and beginning of voicing, exemplified by English so-called voiced consonants such as those in the words "bow," "dough," "go," which are usually transcribed by English speakers as [bo], [do], and [go]. Because the burst and the voicing begin at roughly the same time and the voicing is louder, the

[2]Note that Maddieson (1984) is actually reporting on sounds that are presumed to be phonemes in these languages. In this section of the chapter, the phone–phoneme distinction is being ignored. It is possible that the data reported here would be slightly different if all phones had been counted (allophones as well as phonemes), but the differences in proportions of occurrence would likely be very small.

burst is not heard. The same sounds also occur as English voiceless stops in s- clusters, such as "speed," "steep," and "ski," usually transcribed as [spid], [stip], and [ski]. English speakers typically think of these two sets of sounds (/b, d, g/ in initial position and /p, t, k/ following [s]) as being different, but they are in fact acoustically very similar.

- Voiced or **prevoiced**: voicing begins before consonant release—before the burst, thus making it inaudible. This typically does not occur in English except in the oral communication of deaf speakers. It is a voicing option that is used by many other languages such as Spanish, French, and Chinese, however.

In a language with two stop series, each of those two series is likely to fall in a different one of the three categories listed above.

In keeping with common practice in the English-speaking world, voiceless unaspirated stops will be referred to as voiced ("b, d, g") and voiceless aspirated stops as "voiceless" ("p, t, k") throughout the remainder of this book except where the distinctions noted above are critical to understanding some concept (e.g., when comparing English to other languages).

7. Most languages (98%) include stops at bilabial, dental or alveolar (i.e., **coronal**), and velar places of articulation.
8. If a language has [p] then it has [k], and if it has [k] then it has [t] (dental or alveolar voiceless stop). In other words, [t] is most commonly followed by [k] and then [p].
9. If a language has [g] then it has [d] (dental or alveolar voiced stop), and if it has [d] then it has [b]. In other words, [b] is most commonly followed by [d] and then [g]. (Note that the order of this **implicational universal** [universal that specifies the likelihood of one sound or structure based on the presence of another] is different with respect to place of articulation from the order for the voiceless stop series. The aerodynamic reasons for this are beyond the scope of this book.)

Nasals

Nasals are considered to be noncontinuant consonants, like stops, because the airflow is interrupted within the oral cavity. In fact, they are sometimes referred to as nasal stops. However, the velopharynx is open, so the air does flow continuously into and through the nasal cavity. Therefore, voicing energy resonates in that large cavity and out through the nose. Universals include the following:

1. Most languages (97%) have at least one nasal.
2. Most nasals (93%) are voiced (as are English nasals, except when following /s/).
3. If a language has any nasals at all, it will have [n].
4. If a language has a nasal at a certain place of articulation, it will have a non-nasal obstruent (stop, affricate, or fricative) at that same place of articulation ([m] and [b]; [n] and [t], etc.).

Liquids

Liquids, like vowels, depend upon shaping the articulators. There is more constriction than for vowels, but the oral cavity is still fairly open. Liquids differ from each other with respect to the way the articulators are shaped (e.g., tongue tip up versus down) and the location of the area of constriction. Universals include the following:

1. Most languages (96%) have at least one liquid.
2. Languages with only one liquid most often (99%) have a lateral liquid (such as [l]).
3. Languages with two or more liquids usually (86%) include one lateral (such as [l]) and one non-lateral (such as [ɹ]).

Fricatives

Fricatives are hissing sounds that result from using the articulators to form a narrow constriction in the oral cavity. Because the air is constricted but not completely blocked (as in a stop), the sound is continuous; in other words, it can be prolonged. Universals include the following:

1. Of all languages, 93% have at least one fricative.
2. If a language has only one fricative, it is [s] (dental or alveolar voiceless sibilant).
3. If a language has only two fricatives, it is most likely to have [s] and [f], though other pairs also occur. Languages with only two fricatives avoid pairs that differ in voicing only (e.g., [s], [z]).
4. The most common fricatives are [s], [f], and [ʃ].
5. Voiced fricatives are far less common than voiceless ones (for aerodynamic reasons). Languages with any voiced fricatives usually have an entire set of voiced–voiceless fricative pairs. (That is, if a language has any voiced fricatives at all, it will have as many or more voiceless fricatives as voiced ones.) If any one voiced–voiceless pair in the language is incomplete, it is likely to be [ʃ]–[ʒ] (as was the case for American English until repeated exposure to French led to the gradual introduction of [ʒ] in a small set of words).

Glides

Glides are sounds that are formed with a slight constriction—more than for a vowel, but less than for a liquid. The articulators are shaped to influence the resonance, as for vowels and liquids. The distinctive quality of these "semivowels" results from the fact that they glide from an initial partially constricted state to a more open vowel-like state. Thus, glides are on the boundary between consonants and vowels; they are neither consonantal nor vocalic. Universals include the following:

1. Of all languages, 86% have at least one glide.
2. Languages with only one glide are more likely to have [j].
3. Most languages (71%) that have [w] also have [j].

Markedness/Defaults

Any linguistic patterns that are present but uncommon in the languages of the world (or in a specific language) are referred to as **marked.** For instance, 75% of the languages of the world use either SVO (subject–verb–object) or SOV (subject–object–verb) word order in sentences. These word order choices are therefore considered to be **unmarked**. Object-first word orders (OSV and OVS) are the least common—in other words, the most marked (Crystal, 1987), and they sound very alien to many of us (as when the *Return of the Jedi* character Yoda says, "Your father he is" and "When 900 years you reach, look as good you will not").

The notion of markedness can also be applied to the semantics of a particular language, using the term unmarked to refer to the more general or expected element of a pair. For example, we use "tall," not "short," when we ask about a person's height, unless we are intentionally insulting them: "How short are you?" Therefore, "tall" is considered to be the unmarked and "short" the marked element of this pair of opposites. Similarly, in English morphology, adding "-s" is the usual (unmarked) way to indicate plural in English. Therefore, voicing changes (e.g., "elf" to "elves") and vowel changes ("woman" to "women") are considered to be marked morphologic patterns (Crystal, 1991).

Speech sounds and features can also be unmarked, either because they are easy to pronounce (e.g., stops) or easy to perceive (e.g., [s]). Interdental fricatives such as [θ] and [ð], for example, are rare in the languages of the world due to their low perceptual **salience** and are therefore considered to be marked phones. In contrast, [s] is extremely common and is therefore in the universally unmarked category.

The markedness of sounds can also be language-specific. For instance, many languages have a **default** vowel that tends to be used whenever a vowel needs to be **epenthesized** (inserted). In French, [ə] is used in songs and poetry, in hyperformal speech, and in some contexts to separate two consonants. For example, "Arc de Triomphe" may be pronounced as [ˈaʁk**ə** də triˈɔ̃f] (Hyman, 1975) to separate the [k] and [d] sounds, or even (if someone is being very snobby) as [ˈaʁk**ə** də triˈɔ̃f**ə**]. In Japanese, [u] is the default vowel. It is used via **epenthesis** (insertion) to break up disfavored consonant clusters and also to avoid ending words with certain types of (nonnasal) consonants. This [u]-epenthesis is demonstrated when a Japanese speaker tries to pronounce an English loan word. For instance, "public" would be pronounced [pab**u**rikk**u**] and "pulse" would sound like [par**usu**] (Hyman, 1975).

Very young children and those with phonological disorders may have defaults—favorite vowels, consonants, syllables, etc.—as well. If so, that sound or structure is unmarked for that child. It is important to be aware of markedness in individual children's sound systems as well as in different languages, as this is a factor that should be taken into account in selecting therapy goals.

EXERCISE 2-1

IPA Review

Summary

Oral languages are made up of words, syllables, and sounds. Speech sounds are referred to as phones. As well as being more or less frequent in a particular language, particular phones or groups of phones are generally especially frequent or infrequent in the languages of the world. Those that are used most commonly, the unmarked speech sounds, are generally physiologically easier to produce. They also occur earlier, more frequently, and with greater accuracy in the speech of young children and those with SSDs.

CONTRAST

The most critical function of a phonological system is that of differentiating messages. If all words sounded the same or the differences between them were random, then we could not communicate. If the number of contrasts in a given language were reduced, its vocabulary would be reduced, and the effectiveness of that language would be compromised.

Phonemes

Phonemes are those sounds that are used contrastively with each other by speakers of a specific language (or by a specific speaker). That is, they help us to differentiate one word from another. A phoneme in one language may not be a phoneme in another. Thus, it doesn't make any sense to ask whether a certain phone is a phoneme without specifying the language to which you are referring. For example, the fact that the English language includes the words "bat," "hat," "cat," "fat," "mat," "gnat," "sat," "rat," "vat" and that each of these words has a different meaning tells us that the consonant sounds [b], [h], [k], [f], [m], [n], [s], [ɹ], [v] are each separate phonemes in this language. In some other languages (such as French, for example), some of these same phones (in this case, [h] and [ɹ]) may not have the same function; they may not be phonemes. Phonemes are enclosed in slashes: /b/, /h/, /k/, /f/, /m/, /n/, /s/, /ɹ/, /v/.

Another way to think about the difference between phonemes and phones is that we think in phonemes: when we recall a word from memory in order to produce it (or while reading it), what we recall is the phonemes in the word (as well as the meaning, of course). But in the process of production, the sounds in the word influence each other (via coarticulation); they are also affected by many other factors, such as the state of the person's articulators (e.g., eating while talking, affected by novocaine), attention and fatigue levels, and so on. For these reasons, it's not possible to speak in phonemes. The sounds that come out of our mouths and into our listeners' ears are phones. If we communicate successfully, the listeners will figure out the correspondences between the

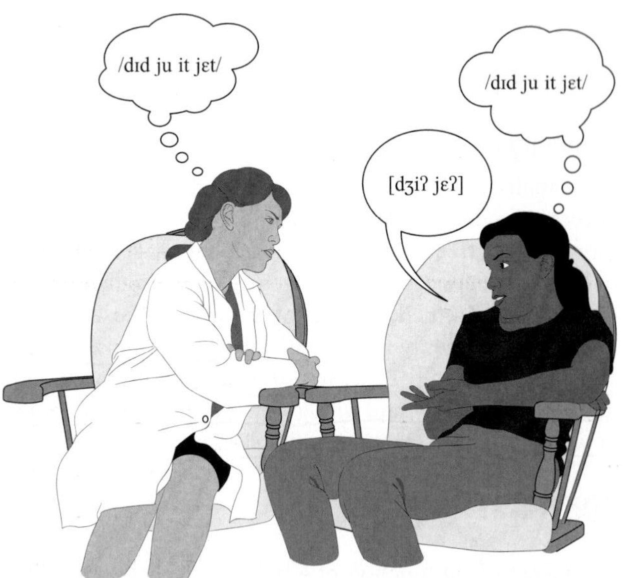

FIGURE 2-2. Phones–phonemes illustration.

phones we spoke and the phonemes we intended. Thus, they will perceive phonemes. This idea is illustrated in Figure 2-2. The girl is thinking in phonemes ("Did you eat yet?:" /dɪd ju it jɛt/) but producing the corresponding phones ("Jeet yet?:" [dʒiʔ jɛʔ]). The nurse is hearing those phones, but perceiving the intended phonemes.

Phonemes can be identified through the use of **minimal pairs**. These are pairs of words with different meanings that differ by only one sound. Rhyming words, in which the initial phonemes (the onsets) contrast, are one type of minimal pair that comes easily to mind: "goat/coat, seat/sheet, man/pan, national/rational," etc. But the phoneme contrast within a minimal pair can also occur in other positions of the word: "goat/got," "seat/sit," "mat/map," "batter/battle," "better/beggar," "ridicule/reticule," "formicate/fornicate," and so on. The presence versus absence of one sound can also be critical to a minimal contrast: "preference/reference," "blouse/louse," "bolster/boaster," "tent/ten," "peat/pea," "peat/eat," etc. Word pairs that are spelled similarly but that don't sound almost the same, of course, do not count as phonological minimal pairs (e.g., "bead/dead," "breath/break," "cone/gone"). Nor do homonyms ("reed/read," "bow/bough") count as phonological minimal pairs because they sound identical rather than differing in one phoneme.

What minimal pairs tell us is that the sounds that differ from one member of the pair to the other change the meanings of the words and that they are therefore contrastive phones, or phonemes, within the language. A sound that changes the meaning of a word when it is substituted for another sound (e.g., /t/ and /ɹ/ in "tent/rent") is a phoneme in that language. Each language has its own set of phonemes as well as other speech sounds that occur in the language but without a contrastive function. Multiple minimal pairs within a set, such as "mat," "hat," "pat," "tat," "cat," "rat," "sat," "that," "bat," "fat," "gnat," "vat," give us the highest level of confidence that we have indeed identified the appropriate phonemes. Typically, the phonemes correspond for the most part to those sounds of the language that are represented by an alphabetic writing system (if the language has one) and to those sounds of which the speakers are consciously aware. (Can you think of some exceptions from our alphabet?)

The phonemes of some other languages represent contrasts that lack lexical function in English. Voiced versus voiceless nasals, for instance, are contrastive phonemes in Burmese; [nɑ] means "pain" but [n̥ɑ][3] means "nostril;" [ŋɑ] means "fish" but [ŋ̊ɑ] means "rent" (Hyman, 1975). There are no such minimal pairs in our language. If an English speaker used voiceless nasals throughout her speech, SLPs might question her velopharyngeal status and send her to an ENT. Despite her apparent vocal deviance, however, listeners would most likely have no trouble understanding what this person was saying. Voiceless nasals do not contrast with voiced nasals in English.

Homonymic Clash

The need to preserve contrast is clearly evident in the histories of languages. Phonological change often appears to operate without regard for its potentially major impact on the lexicon of the language (Bynon, 1977). However, if phonological changes occur that reduce the potential for contrast, further changes—whether phonological or not—often arise in order to restore the potential for contrast in some other way. The most challenging phonological changes are those that lead to **homonymy** (the presence of homonyms), which is a lexical loss of contrast (i.e., a loss of contrast in the vocabulary of the language). This is not a problem unless the two words that have become homonymous are used in similar contexts. For instance, if someone says, "I'm going to read this book," the fact that "read" and "reed" are homonyms causes no problems whatsoever.

American back vowels are a current real-life example of the potentially benign consequences of pronunciation changes that cause words to become homonyms. In many parts of the United States, the distinction between [ɑ] and [ɔ] is becoming more and more **neutralized** (lost). "Law" ([lɔ]) and "la" ([lɑ]), "caught" ([kɔt]) and "cot" ([kɑt]), "naught" ([nɔt]) and "not" ([nɑt]), etc. are now homonyms in those regions. In some areas of the country (e.g., California), all of these words are pronounced with [ɑ] and in others (e.g., the greater New York metropolitan area), with [ɔ]. Most people seem to be unaware of this change, and they do not appear to be compensating in any way for this loss of contrast, probably because there are few pairs of homonyms that actually cause confusion.

Similarly, in parts of the northeastern United States the [æ] sound is raised (produced with a higher tongue position) before nasals to the extent that, in some **dialects** of Boston, the names "Anne" and "Ian" sound identical. Again, however, the neutralization of this high/low vowel contrast does not yet appear to have triggered any compensatory mechanisms.

[3]The circle under the [n] indicates voicelessness.

When a conflict does result from loss of contrast, called a **homonymic clash,** it is usually resolved lexically. Put simply, people change their word use in order to make their meanings clear. In Texas English, for instance, where [ɛ] is raised before nasals, "pen" and "pin" are pronounced the same way: [pĩn]. To reduce the resulting confusion, Texans talk about "ink pins" ([ĩŋk pĩnz]) when they wish to refer to such writing implements.

Another example of homonymic clash from older English is provided by the word "ass," pronounced [as] or [ɐs] in British. Originally, this word was used only to refer to donkeys. However, a similar word, "arse," was used to refer to the buttocks. As the language changed and many dialects became "r-less" (similar to the "Hahvad yahd" accent), the contrast between [aɚ] and [a] was neutralized. As a result, the words "ass" and "arse" came to resemble each other more and more. Through guilt by association, "ass" lost its popular use, and the far safer word "donkey" largely replaced it (Funk, 1978).

Sometimes the solution to a homonymic clash is phonological, rather than lexical. In modern-day American English, medial alveolar stops (/t, d/) are flapped or tapped, with the tongue just briefly touching the alveolar ridge. This creates a sound ([ɾ]) that is actually quite close to the Spanish singleton "r" sound (as in "para"). As a result, the contrast between words such as "writer" and "rider" could be lost, since the medial /d/s and /t/s are both flapped. Although the final consonants in "write" and "ride" still sound different, there is no longer any difference between the medial consonants in the two words when "er" is added. In other words, /t/ and /d/ are neutralized in medial position following a stressed vowel. However, the contrast is maintained by the duration of the vowel before the consonant. Even in "ride/write" the vowel is prolonged (as indicated in International Phonetic Alphabet [IPA] by a colon) before the voiced /d/ and shortened before the voiceless /t/: [ɹɑɪːd] versus [ɹɑɪt]. The vowel length is not needed to distinguish the verbs, but it is the only way to tell the nouns apart: [ɹɑɪːɾɚ] (someone on a horse) versus [ɹɑɪɾɚ] (a novelist, poet, etc.). Vowel duration is not usually phonemic (contrastive) in English, but it serves a contrastive function in this case to compensate for the neutralization of the original contrast.

Homonymic clash is a source of great frustration for many children with SSD, not to mention for their parents. A child who says "I want [bɑ]" in the presence of a ball, a bottle, a balloon, and other b-initial words may initiate a prolonged, exasperating guessing game. Therefore, reducing homonymy is an important functional goal of intervention for many of our clients.

Allophones

Although voiceless nasals are not separate phonemes in English (as they are in Burmese), they do occur in clusters with [s] in casual speech in our language. The /m/ in "small," for example, is usually pronounced as a partially devoiced [m̥] ([sm̥ɔl]), because the [m] begins before the vocal folds have come fully together to vibrate. In contrast, the /m/ in "mall" is fully voiced ([mɔl]). Although [smɔl] and [sm̥ɔl] are acoustically different, they have exactly the same meaning in our language, so no lexical confusion could result if a speaker failed to devoice the [m] as the fast speech rules indicate. In this case then, [m] and [m̥] are **allophones** of the English phoneme /m/. Allophones are variants of phonemes that do not change word meanings.

Another example of English allophones is the fact that the way Americans pronounce the /t/ in "hot" differs depending upon the situation. In casual speech, it may be produced either very slightly ([hɑt˺][4]) or as a glottal stop ([hɑʔ]). In more formal speech, it is pronounced completely, usually with aspiration, a noticeable puff of air ([hɑtʰ]). The different pronunciations do not change the meaning of the word in any way. Thus, these pronunciations are all allophones of the phoneme /t/. Allophones are enclosed in square brackets, as they are a special kind of phone: [m̥], [tʰ]. They represent the way we actually pronounce words, not the way we represent words in our mental lexicons (phonemes).

Because the [m̥] and [m] allophones of the English phoneme /m/ are predictable based on context, they are considered to be allophones in **complementary distribution**. Native speakers produce and expect each allophone in a certain context: the voiceless allophone comes after [s]; the voiced one occurs elsewhere. This occurs because it is articulatorily easier to produce a voiceless nasal right after the voiceless [s]. No one would be confused by a speaker who used the wrong nasal allophone in a particular word position, but it would take some extra effort on the speaker's part to do so, and some people might think that that person had an accent (or possibly velopharyngeal insufficiency).

Another example of complementary distribution from English relates to the so-called **dark [l]** allophone, [ɫ]. In English, the articulatory gesture for [l] consists of both retracting (pulling back) and lowering the tongue dorsum (the back of the tongue) and raising the tip of the tongue toward the alveolar ridge. In final position and before velars, the lowering and retracting is earlier and more extreme, yielding a velarized [ɫ]. The contrast is evident in producing pairs such as "milk" versus "lick;" the [ɫ] in "milk" both feels and sounds less consonant-like. This dark [ɫ] is made with less tongue contact because the tongue is retracted and lowered in the mouth. For these reasons, [ɫ] is actually more vowel-like than other [l] allophones (Sproat & Fujimura, 1993). However, most speakers are totally unaware of the difference. They produce [ɫ] in final position and before velars, but they think they are producing a light [l] all of the time. If someone actually did produce a light [l] in these dark [ɫ] contexts, it would have very little impact on listeners' perceptions, although it might sound as though the person were speaking somewhat carefully. This fact, that listeners would be unlikely to notice a light [l] substituted for a [ɫ], is due to the fact that light and dark /l/ are allophones of the same phoneme and are therefore not important for perceiving the speaker's message.

[4] The diacritic on the [t˺] indicates that this sound is unreleased; in other words, the tongue moves into position for the [t], but there is no audible release of air.

The predictable patterning of light and dark [l] may account for the fact that children often vowelize [l] in just those positions in which it is dark in adult speech: in final position and before velars (e.g., [mɪʊk] for "milk"). Children may be hearing dark [l]s, recognizing their vowel-like nature, and assuming that a vowel goes there (e.g., they may assume that the word actually is /mɪʊk/). However, unlike the substitution of a light [l] for a dark [ɫ], which is a substitution of one allophone for another, vowelized /l/s—those that are pronounced as [ʊ]—are usually noticed. This is because /l/ and /ʊ/ are different, contrastive phonemes. Even though dark [ɫ] and [ʊ] are no more different than light and dark /l/, the impact on the listener of the former is much more negative than the impact of the latter. However, in therapy, we should be teaching children to produce dark /l/, not light /l/ in these contexts (i.e., they should not be told to put their tongues on their alveolar ridges when producing the /l/ in "milk" or "middle"). Producing allophones correctly is important for sounding like a native speaker of the language.

Similarly, the use of [tʰ] versus [ʔ] (e.g., [hɑtʰ] versus [hɑʔ] for "hot") in final position changes the sounds of the words but does not change their meanings. Because of the type of alternation that they exhibit, these two sounds ([t] and [ʔ]) are also allophones, but not in complementary distribution. These allophones are in **free variation** in final position.[5] That is, either one may occur in the final position of a word without changing the meaning of that word. The speaker's decision whether to use a fully released [tʰ] versus [ʔ] (or something in between) at the end of the word "mat" is a social one, not a phonological one. If the conversation is informal and the listener has no hearing or comprehension problems, glottal stop will likely be chosen. If the situation is formal or ease of perception is a paramount concern, a fully released [tʰ] will be used. In the intermediate situation, the speaker may opt for an unreleased but supraglottal [t˺].

Figure 2-3 may be helpful in illustrating the decision-making process for determining whether two sounds are distinct phonemes, allophones in complementary distribution, or allophones in free variation in a given language.

Sometimes a pair of sounds or **sound classes** may be in contrast (phonemic) in some word positions, but allophonic (i.e., neutralized) in others. One example of this comes from German. German does have a voicing contrast in initial and medial position. For example, [gɑbəl] ("Gabel[6]"—"fork") and [kɑbəl] ("Kabel"—"cable") are a minimal pair, as are [klɪŋɪn] ("klingen"—"to clink or tinkle") and [klɪnkɪn] ("klinken"—"to operate a latch"). However, the contrast is neutralized in final position, where all stops are pronounced as voiceless, as in [ʃlʌk] ("schlug"—"struck") and [ʃlʌk] ("Schluck"—"a gulp, a sip").

Thus, just as the distinction between voiced and voiceless alveolar stops (/t, d/) is lost in medial position in English, the distinction between all voiced and voiceless stops is neutralized in final position in German. Fortunately, the numbers of word pairs that are affected by these neutralizations are small, and context usually helps to differentiate them.

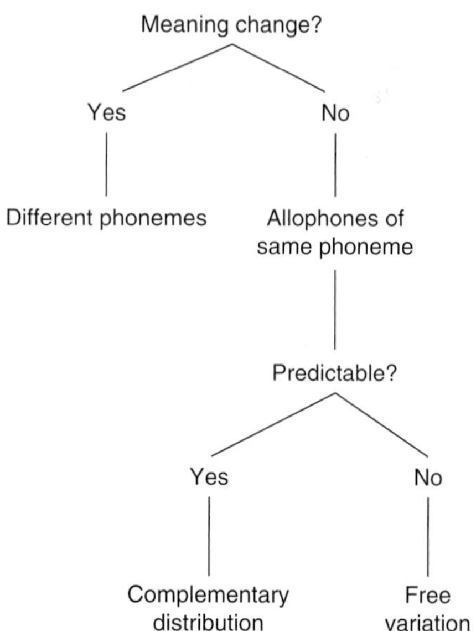

FIGURE 2-3. Phoneme/allophone tree.

Summary

Speech sounds may be contrastive (i.e., they may function to differentiate words [minimal pairs] in a specific language). In this case, they are phonemes in that language. Phonemes are most easily identified using minimal pairs—pairs of words that differ by a single phoneme. This contrastive function is crucial to successful communication. When pronunciations change and homonymic clashes occur, the speakers of the language typically compensate in some way. Children with SSD are often unable to differentiate enough phones in the language to preserve an appropriate level of contrast. As a result, they have many homonyms, and typically they also lack compensatory strategies. This reduces their communicative effectiveness and not surprisingly raises not only their own frustration levels but those of their communication partners as well.

EXERCISE 2-2

Identifying Allophones Versus Phonemes

Distinctive Features

Features are articulatory/perceptual characteristics of phones that differentiate them from each other, such as **voicing** (e.g., [s] versus [z]), **aspiration** (e.g., [tʰ] in "top" versus [t] in "stop"), **rounding** ([o] versus [e]), and so on. One of the critical tasks of a child mastering his native language is to identify those phonetic features to which he has to attend in order to understand the words of that language. This is not a trivial problem, given the huge amount of variation that

[5]These two allophones are not in completely free variation, of course, as [ʔ] does not occur in initial position or in most consonant clusters.

[6]Note that, in German, nouns are capitalized.

occurs in every person's speech from word to word and from time to time. Only certain aspects of that variation are linguistically important in any given language.

Those features—those phonetic characteristics—that serve to help distinguish phonemes from each other are often referred to as **distinctive features**. For example, voicing is a distinctive feature of English because it differentiates phonemes and therefore it differentiates words, such as /d/ versus /t/ in "dot" versus "tot," /b/ versus /p/ in "cab" versus "cap," and so on. An important task for the child learning a language is to identify which features are distinctive and which are not; in other words, he has to determine which distinctions are important for communicating effectively and learn to make those distinctions in a native manner.

A thorough familiarity with features is critical to being able to describe children's speech errors. For example, the production of [b] for /p/, [d] for /t/, and [g] for /k/, which many young children exhibit in initial position, are all errors involving the feature voice. Similarly, the production of [p] for /f/, [t] for /s/, and so on are errors involving the feature continuant, which differentiates consonants produced with continuous airflow (including fricatives) from those during which the air is stopped (including stops). Without knowing the features, one would not know that these errors are related to each other.

Phones or phonemes are sometimes labeled with features using "+" or "–" to indicate whether or not that feature is present. For example, the phonemes /d/ and /t/ could be differentiated with distinctive features as follows:

$$/d/: \begin{bmatrix} \text{C} \\ \text{+alveolar} \\ \text{+voice} \end{bmatrix}$$

$$/t/: \begin{bmatrix} \text{C} \\ \text{+alveolar} \\ \text{–voice} \end{bmatrix}$$

The consonant phone [d] is a stop produced with the tongue tip elevated to the alveolar ridge and with voicing; the consonant phone [t] is articulated similarly but is produced without voicing.

Sounds are grouped into sets by their articulatory, auditory, and/or phonological characteristics. Those speech sounds that share features form sound classes (e.g., the stops, the rounded vowels, etc.). These are sometimes referred to as **natural classes** of sounds. Members of natural classes typically undergo similar changes in speakers' productions. For example, voiceless stops are aspirated in initial position in English; neither voiced stops nor voiceless fricatives are produced in this way in this context. A given consonant or vowel may belong to several natural classes. For example, /d/ falls within the class of alveolar stops (with /t/) but also within the class of voiced stops (with /b/ and /d/). Similarly, children's speech errors often affect entire classes of sounds (e.g., producing all fricatives as stops). Thus, it is useful to think of speech sounds with respect to the natural phonetic feature classes to which they belong as well as with regard to their individual combinations of features.

Many feature classification systems have been proposed. However, since the purpose here is not to take a theoretical stand on which classification system is better, the feature terminology of Chomsky and Halle's (1968) *The Sound Pattern of English,* which is familiar to most SLPs, will be used whenever possible. Tables 2-1 through 2-4 display the application of these feature terms to English consonants and vowels. Table 2-1 shows the distinctive features of American English consonants, and Table 2-2 does so for our vowels. Tables 2-3 and 2-4 are perhaps more familiar displays of English consonants and vowels (respectively) by place and **manner of articulation**, which make it easier to identify natural classes of phones.

Feature terms will be defined throughout this chapter and this book as needed. A key to the IPA and to the diacritic symbols used in this book is provided in Appendix A.

TABLE 2-1 Feature Specifications for American English Consonants

	p	b	f	v	m	t	d	θ	ð	n	s	z	tʃ	dʒ	ʃ	ʒ	k	g	ŋ	ɹ	l	h	w	j
Syllabic	–	–	–	–	–	–	–	–	–	–	–	–	–	–	–	–	–	–	–	–	–	–	–	–
Consonantal	+	+	+	+	+	+	+	+	+	+	+	+	+	+	+	+	+	+	+	+	+	+	–	–
Sonorant	–	–	–	–	+	–	–	–	–	+	–	–	–	–	–	–	–	–	+	+	+	–	+	+
Nasal	–	–	–	–	+	–	–	–	–	+	–	–	–	–	–	–	–	–	+	–	–	–	–	–
Continuant	–	–	+	+	–	–	–	+	+	–	+	+	–/+	–/+	+	+	–	–	–	+	+	+	+	+
Anterior	+	+	+	+	+	+	+	+	+	+	+	+	–	–	–	–	–	–	–	–	+	–	+	–
Coronal	–	–	–	–	–	+	+	+	+	+	+	+	+	+	+	+	–	–	–	+	+	–	–	+
Strident	–	–	–	–	–	–	–	–	–	–	+	+	+	+	+	+	–	–	–	–	–	–	–	–
Back	–	–	–	–	–	–	–	–	–	–	–	–	–	–	–	–	+	+	+	–	–	–	+	–
High	–	–	–	–	–	–	–	–	–	–	–	–	+	+	+	+	+	+	+	+	–	–	+	+
Low	–	–	–	–	–	–	–	–	–	–	–	–	–	–	–	–	–	–	–	–	–	+	–	–
Voice	–	+	–	+	+	–	+	–	+	+	–	+	–	+	–	+	–	+	+	+	+	–	+	+

TABLE 2-2 Feature Specifications for American English Vowels

	i	ɪ	e	ɛ	æ	ʌ/ə	u	ʊ	o	ɔ	ɑ
Syllabic	+	+	+	+	+	+	+	+	+	+	+
Consonantal	–	–	–	–	–	–	–	–	–	–	–
Sonorant	+	+	+	+	+	+	+	+	+	+	+
Tense	+	–	+	–	–	–	+	–	+	–	–
High	+	+	–	–	–	–	+	+	–	–	–
Low	–	–	–	–	+	–	–	–	–	–	+
Front	+	+	+	+	+	–	–	–	–	–	–
Back	–	–	–	–	–	–	+	+	+	+	+
Round	–	–	–	–	–	–	+	+	+	+	–

Based on Chomsky, N., & Halle, M. (1968). The sound pattern of English. New York, NY: Harper & Row.

TABLE 2-3 American English Consonants by Place and Manner of Articulation

MANNER	PLACE / VOICING	Bilabial	Labiodental	(Inter)Dental	Alveolar	(Alveo)Palatal	Velar	Glottal
Stop	**Voiced**	b			d		g	
	Voiceless	p			t		k	ʔ
Nasal	**Voiced**	m			n		ŋ	
Glide	**Voiced**	w				j		
Fricative	**Voiced**		v	ð	z	ʒ		
	Voiceless		f	θ	s	ʃ		h
Affricate	**Voiced**					dʒ		
	Voiceless					tʃ		
Liquid	**Voiced**				l	ɹ		

The primary feature distinctions that must be made within any classification scheme are those that differentiate among consonants, vowels, and those sounds (such as glides) that have some of the characteristics of both consonants and vowels. The features **consonantal** and **syllabic** differentiate consonants ([+consonantal, –syllabic]) from vowels ([–consonantal, +syllabic]). Recall that glides are considered to be in between, "neither here nor there" ([–consonantal, –syllabic]). Similarly, the feature sonorant differentiates resonant sounds, such as liquids and nasals, which are ([+sonorant]), from non-resonant sounds such as stops and fricatives, which are ([–sonorant]).

TABLE 2-4 American English Vowels by Place and Manner of Articulation

	Front	Central	Back
High			
Tense	i		u
Lax	ɪ		ʊ
Mid			
Tense	e		o
Lax	ɛ	ʌ,ə	ɔ
Low			
	æ		ɑ

The other major consonant feature distinctions that are made are those of **place of articulation** (**anterior**, etc.), **manner of articulation** (**continuant**, nasal, etc.), and voice (voiced or voiceless). Each consonant must be able to be distinctly described using these features. Some feature terms that are used for this purpose are not always taught in phonetics classes. These include coronal, which refers to consonants produced by placing the tongue tip or blade on or near the hard palate. Thus, the feature [+coronal] encompasses sounds as far front as the interdental [θ] and [ð] as well as those as far back as the (alveo–)palatals such as [ʃ], [dʒ], and [ɹ]. As such, the feature coronal differentiates, for instance, anterior labial stops (/p/ and /b/, which are [–coronal]) from anterior alveolar or dental stops (such as [t, d]), which are [+coronal]).

In another subdivision of the class of consonants by manner of articulation, the feature **strident** differentiates the louder fricatives that are produced with a narrow groove, such as [s, ʃ, z, ʒ], from those quieter sounds that are produced with a flatter constriction, such as [f, v, θ, ð].[7] Thus, for example, [s] is

$$\begin{bmatrix} \text{+consonantal} \\ \text{+continuant} \\ \text{+anterior} \\ \text{+coronal} \\ \text{−voice} \\ \text{+strident} \end{bmatrix}$$

while [θ] is

$$\begin{bmatrix} \text{+consonantal} \\ \text{+continuant} \\ \text{+anterior} \\ \text{+coronal} \\ \text{−voice} \\ \text{−strident} \end{bmatrix}$$

Delayed release, in which a stop is released slowly as the air is squeezed out in a fricative, is a feature used to differentiate affricates from simpler consonants: [t] is [−delayed release] (i.e., the air is released quickly) while the affricate [tʃ] is [+delayed release]. Another way to differentiate stops and fricatives from affricates is to specify that while stops are [−continuant] (the air flow is stopped) and fricatives are [+continuant] (the air flows continuously), affricates are both: ([−/+ continuant]); in other words, the air is stopped briefly and then allowed to flow.

Other consonant distinctive features, such as **palatalization** or **glottalization** of consonants with other primary places of articulation (e.g., glottalization of an alveolar), are used in other languages. Many American SLPs will encounter non-English features or combinations of features, both in their work with the diverse populations that are coming to characterize our nation more and more and in their work with children and adults with SSDs, who may use features that are not expected in English even though they are native speakers of English.

Vowels are differentiated amongst themselves with respect to two aspects of place of articulation: height (high, low—e.g., [u] versus [ɑ]) and front/back (e.g., [i] versus [u]). Other vowel features include tense/lax ([i] versus [ɪ]), which corresponds roughly to the "long" and "short" vowels we learned about in elementary school, and round/unround (also exemplified by [i] versus [u]).

When distinctive features are used to differentiate two phonemes, only the most major features that are absolutely necessary to differentiate them are used. For example, /i/ and /o/ differ in many respects, including roundness. But the fact that /i/ is [+front] implies that it is not [+round] because no front vowel is round in English. It also goes without saying that /o/ must be [+round] because it is [+back] and [−low]; all back vowels that are not low are round in English. So, there is no need to specify that these two also differ with respect to roundness: saying that /i/ is front and high and /o/ is back and not low is sufficient to differentiate them. However, roundness plays a more important role in some other languages, as do more "exotic" vowel distinctive features, such as "ATR," which stands for **advanced tongue root** or the moving forward of the root of the tongue, resulting in an expansion of the pharynx.

[7]Note that the Hodson Assessment of Phonological Processes includes the labiodental fricatives [f, v] within the strident class, excluding only the interdentals [θ, ð]. This is unusual.

Surface and Underlying Representations

When a word is actually pronounced, each phone may be affected in some way by the other phones within the word. If there is a nasal nearby, it may be slightly nasalized; if there is a velar, it may be somewhat backed; if there is a rounded vowel, it may be slightly rounded; and so on. The production of each phone may also be affected by its position in the word without any meaning change. As mentioned above, for example, /t/ is often produced as [ʔ] in word-final position in English.

In this sense, a speaker cannot produce a phoneme in its pure, unadulterated state within a word. The phoneme itself is an abstract mental concept, representing the speech sound that the speaker intends to produce. The sound that is actually produced is some allophone (whether in free variation or in complementary distribution) of that phoneme.

Because phonemes are viewed as abstract units that can't actually be produced, the phonemes in a word are sometimes referred to as the **underlying representation** of the word: the word in its conceptual state before the phonological rules and the vagaries of speech performance become involved. The word as it is actually pronounced—using allophones of the intended phonemes—is referred to as the **surface representation**.

Summary

Speech sounds, or phones, are represented by articulatory features that allow SLPs to be both more specific and more general in their characterizations of SSDs. Using these features, each phoneme of the language can be uniquely specified using those language-specific contrastive (distinctive) features that differentiate them. At the same time, classes of sounds that share certain features can be grouped in this way (e.g., all stops, all coronals, all back vowels), allowing generalizations about the production of such natural sound classes (e.g., all fricatives are produced as voiceless in final position). These concepts are key to identifying error patterns in the speech of children, both those who are typically developing and those with SSDs.

The abstract mental representation of a word—its phonemes—is sometimes referred to as the underlying representation of the word. The phones/allophones as they are actually produced and heard, in contrast, are referred to as the surface representation. Again, as will be explained in great depth later in this book, these concepts facilitate the identification, assessment, and remediation of speech sound development and disorders.

EXERCISE 2-3

Distinctive Features

THE FUNCTIONING OF A PHONOLOGICAL SYSTEM

Ease of Perception and Production

If one were to enumerate all of the possible combinations of speech sound features or of articulatory configurations, the number of potential speech sounds would be far higher than the numbers that are actually used. Nonetheless, the IPA includes well over 100 phones that are incorporated in various languages throughout the world; no language uses anywhere near this number of sounds. Each language selects some subset of those consonants and vowels for use in its words. These subsets are by no means random. At least two major forces work together to determine a subset of possible sounds that will be functional for the language: ease of perception and ease of production.

Ease of perception requires that the set of sounds in a given language be easily perceptible and different enough from each other that the listener can tell which sound is intended by the speaker. This is why [θ] is not a popular sound among the languages of the world; it has very low acoustic energy and is therefore hard to hear. Although [f] is also difficult to perceive auditorily, it has the benefit of easy visual identification and is therefore far more common than [θ].

Other sounds may be easy enough to hear but auditorily too close to each other to be easily discriminated. Phones that are acoustically too similar (e.g., the voiceless labiodental fricative [f] and the voiceless bilabial fricative [ɸ]) are not used contrastively within a single language (Maddieson, 1984). English, for instance, includes the auditorily salient (noticeable; prominent) alveolar ([s]) and palato-alveolar ([ʃ]) voiceless fricatives as well as the less salient interdental ([θ]). Already this is quite a large set of voiceless coronal fricatives. Sometimes listening conditions (e.g., telephone) or speaking conditions (e.g., drunkenness) make these three difficult to differentiate. Some languages include a retroflex voiceless fricative, which is made in a manner similar to [s], but with the tongue tip curled back ([ʂ]). Other languages include a lateral voiceless fricative ([ɬ]), which is also made in a manner similar to [s], but with a flatter tongue, making the frication noise "slushier" sounding. These languages do not include the English interdental fricative sounds as well; too much confusion would result. Similarly, if such sounds were to be added to the English sound repertoire, ease of perception could be seriously compromised. Speakers would confuse these other fricatives quite often with [s], [ʃ], and/or [θ].[8]

Ease of production requires that most of the sounds in the language be fairly easy to produce in an appropriate number of combinations with each other to create a reasonably sized, pronounceable vocabulary. Stops and nasals, for example, are among the simplest to produce and to combine. Therefore, they are very common in the languages of the world. Some sounds, such as the English retroflex [ɹ], are more difficult to produce accurately. Such sounds are less commonly used by languages of the world and are typically learned later by children. Other sounds may be easy to produce but difficult to combine into syllables. Raspberries ("lingua-labial trills"), for example, are not hard to do, but try substituting them in words that have the [b] or [p] sound in them—not very efficient! (Try "ru**bb**er **b**a**b**y **b**uggy **b**um**p**ers" three times with raspberries in place of "b" and "p," then see how long it takes to untangle your tongue!) Your tongue and your jaw have to protrude so far to make a good juicy raspberry that it takes much too long to get them back into an appropriate position for making a vowel.[9]

The phonemes in a language should ideally be easy to pronounce yet also easily differentiated from one another. Ease of perception and ease of production compete with each other in many cases. For instance, [s] is one of the trickiest sounds to produce accurately. We know this not only from acquisition data but also from studies of speakers who become deaf, whose trigeminal nerves are anesthetized (Borden & Harris, 1980), who are drunk (Lester & Skousen, 1974), or who are subjected to delayed auditory feedback (Smith, 1962). Under all of these conditions, [s] is one of the first sounds to be distorted in production. The fact that English includes both /θ/ and /ʃ/ as well as /s/ places a heavier burden on speakers. We have to produce /s/ very accurately so that it is not misperceived as either of these close neighbors. Despite these challenges, [s] is very popular among the languages of the world because it is such a high-intensity sound that it is very easy to perceive, even at a distance. Velleman (1988) has demonstrated that children who misproduce /s/ typically can discriminate it perceptually (i.e., hear the difference) from their substitution sound ([θ], [ʃ], etc.). In contrast, children who misproduce [θ], which is much less acoustically salient, often do not appear to be aware of distinctions between this sound and its substitutes ([f], etc.).

Ease of perception and ease of production, then, exert a major influence on the sound repertoires of a language. They also exert influences on each other. Sounds that occur close together in a word may affect each other, as when a vowel becomes nasalized before a nasal consonant (e.g., [hæ̃nd]) or an [l] is devoiced following an [s] ([sl̥ɪp]) because the [s] is voiceless. Many people assume that these types of coarticulation are merely a low-level

[8] In fact, we do use a retroflex voiceless fricative immediately before [ɹ] in words such as "shrub." However, this sound is never in contrast with [s] or [ʃ]. It is merely a predictable allophone (of either /s/ or /ʃ/, depending on which linguist you ask) in complementary distribution; confusion is avoided.

[9] Note that more controlled labio-lingual trills are used in some languages, however.

motoric phenomenon, occurring because we are too lazy to produce each speech sound concisely and independently. It's also often assumed that coarticulation makes the listener's task more difficult. These are both misconceptions. Coarticulation actually facilitates speech perception in native speakers of the language, even when the speaker has dysarthria (Tjaden & Sussman, 2006). Furthermore, coarticulation differs from language to language and therefore must be learned (Kingston & Diehl, 1994)—for both receptive and expressive purposes. For example, languages with more vowels permit less vowel coarticulation in order to prevent confusion among them (Manuel, 1990). Thus, this phenomenon is far more complex than mere motoric sloppiness would yield.

Functional Load

Not every phoneme is as useful to the language as every other. Some phonemes, such as stops in English, are included in many words and involved in many contrasts; they have high **functional loads.** Others, such as [ʒ], play a minor role in the language as they differentiate only a small set of words; they have a low functional load.

Functional load is of course related to ease of perception and ease of production. (Isn't everything?) Those phonemes that are easily articulated and perceptually salient tend to have higher functional loads for the same reasons that they are more commonly found in the languages of the world, in babbling, and in early child vocabulary. If two phonemes within a language are perceptually similar, at least one of them is likely to have a low functional load. In English, for instance, both /f/ and /θ/ are phonemes despite the fact that they are easily perceptually confused (Velleman, 1988). The language has protected itself by giving /θ/ a low functional load (i.e., including few f-θ minimal pair words). Those pairs that do exist typically include at least one word that is either uncommon, archaic, or slang (e.g., "fie/thigh," "fink/think") or they include words from different parts of speech (e.g., "thin"/"fin"). This doesn't eliminate all possible confusions,[10] but it does minimize them.

It's important to note that although functional load is related to the frequency of occurrence of a phoneme, the two may be very different. For example, /ð/ is an extremely frequent phoneme in English, but it is used almost exclusively in articles and other fairly redundant function words ("the," "that," "there," etc.). Thus, its frequency of use is quite high, but its functional load is quite low. Although it may be noticeable, it's rarely confusing when a non-native speaker substitutes [z] or [v] for /ð/ as in "Zee cat is on zee roof."

[10] This author once thought that she was discussing *death* counseling with her sister for 15 to 20 minutes in a noisy subway car before her sister finally made a comment about sign language and she thereby discovered that her sister had been talking about *deaf* counseling all that time!

Inventories

Because of ease of production and perception, sound *systems* of languages (and of typically developing children) are not random; they are usually quite predictable. Rice and Avery (1995) state that small consonant inventories, in particular, tend to be similar, including mostly the least marked (i.e., the most common articulatorily and/or acoustically easiest) segments. As the phonetic inventories of some languages expand over time, different languages may elaborate different aspects of the initial repertoire. Each language tends to use the new sound features that it has adopted in as many combinations with other features as possible, making maximum use of the available features (Lindblom & Engstrand, 1989). These facts are quite often true of children's developing sound inventories as well.

Consonant Inventories

The set of stops used by English, which follows the universals given above for stops in that it includes a voicing contrast and three places of articulation, is an example of an inventory that makes full use of all of the relevant distinctive features as shown in Table 2-5. There are no holes in this table; every place of articulation is used in combination with both values of the feature [voice]. Our set of fricatives, shown in Table 2-6, is similar with the exception of [h].[11]

Word shapes that follow the rules of the language but just don't happen to occur, such as "blick" in English, are called lexical **accidental gaps** (Hyman, 1975). The same term can be used for holes in sound classes: phones composed only of features that are used in the language but don't happen to occur in that particular combination in the language. Accidental gaps that occur in sound systems are believed to be easier to fill in (i.e., to learn or to borrow from another language) than sounds that do not fit an existing pattern. For example, French previously included three-member sets of voiced and voiceless stops (/b, d, g; p, t, k/) but only two nasals (/m, n/). Thus, [ŋ] was an accidental gap in its system: velar (a.k.a. **dorsal**), noncontinuant (stop), and nasal were all active features in the language, but they did not occur together. Eventually, this missing sound was borrowed from English in words such as "dancing" and "smoking," which are now French nouns corresponding

TABLE 2-5 English Stops

	Labial	Alveolar	Velar
Voiced	b	d	g
Voiceless	p	t	k

[11] In fact, a voiced "h"—transcribed as [ɦ] in IPA—does occur in English, but it is an allophone, not a phoneme. It occurs only before [ju] as in "huge" [ɦjudʒ].

TABLE 2-6 English Fricatives

	Labiodental	Interdental	Alveolar	Palatal	Glottal
Voiced	v	ð	z	ʒ	
Voiceless	f	θ	s	ʃ	h

to "dance hall" and "smoking jacket" in American English (Bynon, 1977[12]).

Similarly, [ʒ] has not been used in English for long, especially in final and initial position as illustrated by the small number of words that incorporate this sound as well as the exotic sound of some of them ("gara**ge**," "mira**ge**," "rou**ge**," "**g**enre," "**Zs**a **Zs**a," etc.). In fact, some American dialects still have not added this phoneme in final position, and therefore speakers of these dialects pronounce "garage," for instance, as [gəˈɹɑdʒ] instead of [gəˈɹɑʒ]. This phone was an accidental gap because English already had an almost-full set of voiced and voiceless fricatives, including a voiceless palatal ([ʃ]). It was added to the English sound repertoire gradually, through contact with other languages (especially French) (Bynon, 1977). Adding a voiced palatal to complete the series of voiced fricatives in English was far more natural than it would be to add a voiced palatal fricative to a language with no other voiced fricatives or no other palatal fricatives.

This latter type of case, in which an entire sound class is missing, is called a **systematic gap**. For instance, a systematic gap in English is its lack of click consonants, such as those that occur in some African languages. We also lack front round vowels like those that are quite frequent in French (as in "tu"—"you" and "noeud"—"knot").

Languages do resist additions to their sound repertoires but are usually far less resistant if the sound in question is an accidental gap than if it is a systematic gap. Lindblom, Krull, and Stark (1993) have hypothesized that an economic phonological system with no gaps is learned more quickly than a disorganized collection of sounds would be. Of course, adding a new sound to a repertoire is not effortless; as Menn and Vihman (2011) point out, despite having both velars and fricatives in their native language, English speakers learning German might still have difficulty learning the velar fricative [x], just as Arabic speakers struggle to distinguish English /b/ and /p/ even though there are other voiced–voiceless stop phoneme pairs in their language (e.g., /d/ and /t/). These concepts may apply to child speech sound development as well.

Vowel Inventories

Like consonant inventories, vowel inventories also may be more receptive to new members that will make them more symmetrical. In some of the German dialects spoken in northeastern Switzerland, for example, both back- and front-rounded vowels occur, but there is one accidental gap, marked by a question mark in Table 2-7. This accidental gap, of a low front-rounded vowel, has been filled in some dialects, such as that spoken in the town of Kesswil (Bynon, 1977).

Vowel systems are so commonly patterned that predictions can be made about which vowels a language will have based upon how many vowels it has. For instance, most languages with only three vowels have exactly those three vowels that make up the so-called **vowel triangle**: [i, ɑ, u]. These three vowels are perceptually and articulatorily quite distinctive yet do not require extreme effort to produce. Because of their articulatory positions toward the extremes of the vowel space, they are often referred to as **corner vowels**. Like the sink, stove, and refrigerator of the much-acclaimed kitchen work triangle, they are each easy to get to yet do not interfere with one another's function. In addition, Stevens (1972, 1989) has proposed that the acoustic qualities of these vowels are less affected by slight changes in articulation than are the acoustic qualities of more central vowels. Thus, speakers can be articulatorily sloppier when producing these corner vowels yet still be clearly understood.

However, languages with three-vowel systems make up less than 6% of the languages of the world. The most common size for a vowel system is five vowels; approximately 21% of the world's languages have opted for such a system (Maddieson, 1984). These five vowels are almost always spaced in such a way as to maximize articulatory and perceptual distinctiveness, leaving as few gaps as possible. The most common configuration for a five-vowel system is also a triangle. Over 90% of the five-vowel systems studied by Maddieson and Precoda (1989) had the set of vowels illustrated in Table 2-8.

The English vowel system includes far more elements, but it also forms a slightly flattened triangular shape, as shown previously in Table 2-4. In English, the non-low (i.e., high and mid) vowels ([i, ɪ, e, ɛ, u, ʊ, o, ɔ]) pattern together, and the low

TABLE 2-7 Swiss German Vowels

	Front-Rounded	Back-Rounded
High	y	u
Mid	ø	o
Low	?	ɔ

From Bynon, T. (1977). *Historical linguistics.* Cambridge, UK: Cambridge University Press.

[12]For instance, "Il va au dancing" = "He is going to the dance hall;" "Il met son smoking" = "He puts on his smoking jacket;" the words "parking," "camping," and "skiing" have been adapted as nouns in similar ways.

TABLE 2-8 **Five-Vowel System**

	Front	Central	Back
High	i		u
Mid	e		o
Low		a	

From Maddieson, I., & Precoda, K. (1989). Updating UPSID. *The Journal of the Acoustical Society of America*, 86, S19.

vowels ([æ, ɑ]) pattern together. For example, the non-low front vowels are all unrounded and they occur in tense–lax pairs ([i] - [ɪ], etc.). The non-low back vowels are all rounded and they also occur in tense–lax pairs ([u] - [ʊ], etc.). None of the low vowels are either rounded or paired in a tense–lax set.

Summary

Sound systems most commonly incorporate phonemes that contribute to both ease of perception and ease of production. Those sounds that are the least challenging to perceive and produce tend to have the highest functional loads in the language. However, sound systems are not random collections of articulatorily or perceptually easy sounds. Each language tends to maximize the use of the features that it has selected by incorporating sounds with all possible combinations of those features. Combinations that could but do not happen to occur in that language's phonology are called accidental gaps, and these are more likely to be borrowed from other languages. Entire sound classes that are not present in a particular phonology are termed systematic gaps and are far less subject to borrowing.

Presumably, these same principles apply to child phonological systems: those phonetic repertoires that are more systematic are less disordered, even if some gaps are present. Accidental gaps—phones composed of features the child has already mastered in different combinations—should be easier to teach than systematic gaps, entire sound classes that are missing. However, remediating systematic gaps may have more impact on intelligibility and therefore on communicative function. These clinical hypotheses have yet to be tested empirically.

PHONOLOGICAL PATTERNS

One goal of any theoretical proposal about phonological features must be that the feature system makes it easy to generalize about the production (or perception) of the sounds described by the feature system. Whatever feature system is used, sounds that are articulatorily and/or acoustically similar—either in place or manner of articulation or in voicing—tend to behave in similar ways. It is not a surprise to any clinician, for example, to find that a child who stops one fricative may stop others, that a child who glides /l/ may also glide /ɹ/, or that a child who voices initial /p/ and /t/ may also voice initial /k/. This is the basic insight behind theories of phonological patterns (rules, processes, or constraints). Knowledge of the features that are relevant to the sound repertoire of a particular language—such as those displayed in previous Tables 2-1 through 2-4 for English—enables us to recognize such patterns.

There are three primary theoretical models that have been developed to characterize and classify phonological patterns: rules, processes, and constraints. All three allow the phonologist or the SLP to detect, analyze, and—in the case of the SLP—remediate speech patterns more efficiently and effectively. They will be described below in the order in which they were developed, since each led to the next over time.

Phonological Rules

Phonological rules are statements about relationships among phonological elements at different phonological levels. The assumption is that the underlying mental representation of a word—the way the person thinks about it sounding—is changed in the process of being planned and pronounced. Some of these alterations are assumed to be phonetically based. In other words, they are seen as articulatory (physiologic) rather than phonological (cognitive). In this sense, they are sometimes referred to as surface rules. Other rules are viewed as more abstract linguistic patterns that each language may or may not choose to implement. Some of these patterns reflect interactions between the phonology and the grammar (especially the morphology) of the language. Although English is a fairly morphology-poor language (i.e., we have relatively few bound morphemes), morphology–phonology interactions can be identified even in our language. For example, English speakers routinely match the voicing of certain morphologic endings with the consonants that come before them, such as plural ([kæts] "cats" versus [kɪdz] "kids"); third person singular ([kɪks] "kicks" versus [dʒɔgz] "jogs"); possessive ([pɑps] "Pop's" versus [bɑbz] "Bob's"); and past tense ([kɪst] "kissed" versus [bʌzd] "buzzed"), although these voicing differences are not reflected in our spelling.

The information included in any phonological rule must include the element that will change, the change that it will undergo, and the **environment** (context) in which this change will occur. The element is typically a phoneme or a class of phonemes (e.g., stops). The change may be an alteration in the feature specifications of the phoneme, such as [+voice] becoming [−voice]. In other cases, the change involves deletion, insertion (epenthesis), or even movement of an element. The environment typically includes the syllable or word position of the element in question (e.g., initial position), or the neighboring segments (e.g., between vowels, before [p], etc.). Thus, a typical rule might state that stops (the elements) become unaspirated (the change) following a word-initial [s] (the environment) (e.g., the /t/ in /stɑp/ is pronounced without aspiration, as [st⁼ɑp]).

These pieces of information are typically expressed using features and phonological symbols whenever possible in order to capture phonological generalizations. Decomposing segments into features allows us to be both more specific and more general. It is more specific in the sense that only those features that are critical to the operation of the rule are specified. If all fricatives are pronounced as stops without any other changes, there is no reason to specify that voiceless fricatives are pronounced as voiceless stops and voiced fricatives are pronounced as voiced stops. Voicing is an irrelevant feature; only continuance (whether or not the air is flowing throughout the sound) matters.

The use of features allows us to be more general in the sense that we can expect any segment with the relevant feature (or features) to be subject to that rule in the right environment. If voiceless stops are aspirated in initial position, then we don't have to specify that this impacts each voiceless stop (/p, t, k/). All members of the sound class (voiceless stops) change in the same way, in the relevant context (beginning of the word).

Generative phonological rules are written as formulas using special symbols. For example, "#" marks the edge of a word and "__" marks a position. Therefore, "#__" indicates initial position and "__#" indicates final position. "V__V" refers to an **intervocalic position** (between two vowels). Remembering that stops are consonants that are [−continuant] (the airflow is stopped) and [−nasal], we can write:

$$\begin{bmatrix} +\text{consonantal} \\ -\text{continuant} \\ -\text{nasal} \\ -\text{voice} \end{bmatrix} \rightarrow \left[+\text{aspiration}\right] / \#\_\_\_\_$$

In other words, noncontinuant, non-nasal, unvoiced consonants (voiceless stops) are aspirated (released with a puff of air) in initial position (the beginning of the word).

Similarly:

$$\begin{bmatrix} +\text{consonantal} \\ -\text{continuant} \\ -\text{nasal} \end{bmatrix} \rightarrow \left[-\text{aspiration}\right] / \#\text{s}\_\_\_\_ + \text{consonantal}$$

That is, stops are unaspirated after a word-initial [s].

Considering the features that are affected and the ways and contexts in which they are affected often provides important insights. For example, in the dialect of this author, [s] is often pronounced as [ʃ] before [ɹ]. Thus, "groceries" is pronounced [gɹoʃɹiz], "nursery" as [nɝʃɹi], and so on. This is palatal assimilation; the alveolar sibilant (underlyingly, /s/) is palatalized before the palatal [ɹ]:

/s/→[ʃ]/__[ɹ]

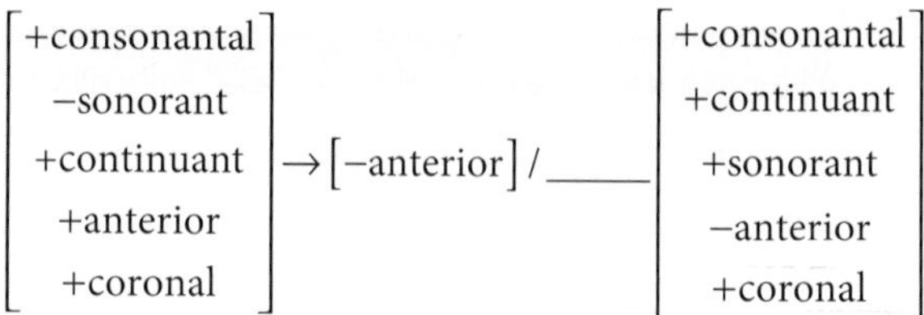

$$\begin{bmatrix} +\text{consonantal} \\ -\text{sonorant} \\ +\text{continuant} \\ +\text{anterior} \\ +\text{coronal} \end{bmatrix} \rightarrow \left[-\text{anterior}\right] / \_\_\_\_ \begin{bmatrix} +\text{consonantal} \\ +\text{continuant} \\ +\text{sonorant} \\ -\text{anterior} \\ +\text{coronal} \end{bmatrix}$$

This occurs because [ɹ] is produced with the tongue raised toward the palate (as it is for [ʃ]) rather than toward or on the alveolar ridge (as it would be for [s]). The rule shows the reason for the change: the place of articulation of the fricative is changing to match the place of articulation of the liquid.

In fact, this rule is actually more general; it's an example of the fact that palatals affect preceding alveolars. For instance, the /t/ in "mattress" and the /t/ in "train" are pronounced as [tʃ] in the same dialect ([mætʃrɪs], [tʃɹeɪn])—they are palatalized in assimilation with the following [ɹ]s. In other words, all anterior coronals lose their anteriority (i.e., are pronounced farther back in the palatal area) in anticipation of the palatal liquid, [ɹ]. Thus, we can drop the manner of articulation (stop versus fricative; i.e., continuance) specification on the "input" side of the rule. However, in this dialect, the change in place of articulation does not show up before other palatals (such as [j]), so the manner features that indicate liquids must remain as follows:

$$\begin{bmatrix} +\text{anterior} \\ +\text{coronal} \end{bmatrix} \rightarrow \left[-\text{anterior}\right] / \_\_\_\_ \begin{bmatrix} +\text{consonantal} \\ +\text{continuant} \\ +\text{sonorant} \\ -\text{anterior} \\ +\text{coronal} \end{bmatrix}$$

Although phonological rules are no longer used clinically, the exercise of thinking about pronunciation changes that are caused by certain aspects of the context—that is, coarticulation—is an excellent practice for problem-solving unusual speech sound errors. Often, even very unexpected phonological changes and errors can be found to have some articulatory basis when the features of the target are compared to those of the context and those of the actual production. Some examples of this sort will be provided in the exercises and later in the book.

Generative phonologists have also demonstrated that in many languages, phonology and morphology interact. We have seen that English speakers routinely assimilate the voicing of certain morphologic endings, such as plural, third person singular, possessive, and past tense, though the assimilation is not reflected in our spelling. Similarly, the various forms of the prefix "in-" (roughly meaning "not") are **phonologically conditioned**. That is, the morpheme changes to match the surrounding phones. The nasal assimilates to match the place of articulation—and sometimes even the manner of articulation—of the following consonant, and we spell the words as we say them to the extent that our alphabet allows. This yields words such as "**in**ept," "**im**possible," "**in**delible," "**il**legal," and "**ir**reverent."[13]

EXERCISE 2-4

Generative Phonological Rules

Phonological Processes

Phonological processes are another way to describe systematic differences between the targeted sound and the sound that the client produces. They are based on the theory of **natural phonology**, which was an attempt by Stampe and Donegan (e.g., Stampe, 1972; Donegan & Stampe, 1979) to emphasize the universal phonetic foundation of phonology. They proposed that all phonological patterns have their basis in human physiologic limitations on speech production. Such limitations were described as **natural processes**. For example, the physical difficulty of producing three consonants within a cluster leads to the tendency among humans to reduce such lengthy clusters. This natural process of **cluster reduction** is seen in the speech of young children. But those who are learning languages such as German and English must cease to use this pattern by the time they are adults because consonant clusters have a contrastive function in these languages (e.g., "please/peas" is a minimal pair). In some languages, such as Japanese, cluster reduction is always allowed because this language excludes consonant sequences altogether. Every language must allow some difficult syllables or word shapes, however. Thus, different languages require speakers to overcome different limitations. Or, in Stampe's (1972) terms, different languages allow different processes to apply to different extents. For example, cluster reduction is given free rein in Japanese, but syllable reduction is not.

Overcoming a physiologic limitation in order to produce the sound patterns of a language is referred to as **suppression** of a natural process. An infant does not know how to overcome her physiologic limitations in order to produce speech sounds. The child's mission, then, is to learn to **suppress** those processes that are not permitted to apply in her language—in other words, to learn to produce the difficult sounds and sequences required by the language. If the language has many clusters (e.g., German), she must suppress the process of cluster reduction. If the language has many multisyllabic words (e.g., Japanese), she must suppress syllable deletion and so on.

Importantly, many processes are neither totally suppressed nor totally applied in a language. In American English, for example, we may neglect to pronounce word-final [t] as such. It is often substituted by [ʔ] (e.g., "I've [gɑʔ] a [koʔ]," rather than "I've [gɑtʰ] a [kotʰ]"). When this occurs typically depends upon sociolinguistic factors, such as the formality of the situation and the status and dialect of the speaker. The glottal stop [ʔ] also routinely substitutes for [t] in the medial position of certain words with a stressed–unstressed stress pattern and a final nasal consonant, such as "curtain" ([ˈkɝʔn̩]) and "button" ([ˈbʌʔn̩]), except in very formal speech or citation contexts (e.g., reading a word list). Stops from other places of articulation, however, are rarely replaced with glottals. The voiced alveolar /d/ may be replaced by a glottal stop in final position in African American English (AAE) (e.g., [mæʔ] for "mad"), but this is not allowed in General American English. Thus, the natural process of glottalization is permitted to apply in certain English phonological contexts (e.g., word-finally and word-medially under certain circumstances) to certain English phonemes (/t/ and sometimes /d/) under certain sociolinguistic circumstances. In cases that do not meet these criteria, the process is suppressed.

It is important to note that process theory is strongly grounded in phonetic reality. Therefore, phonological patterns that do not have a clear physiologic basis or that are not well attested (relatively frequent) among the languages of the world are not considered to be natural. They are sometimes referred to as **deviant processes**.

Phonological processes were adopted more easily into speech-language pathology than phonological rules because they are easier to state. Typically, the name of the process is a description of the feature change that is occurring. For example, a child who produces [pɪt] for "fish" is **stopping**, producing fricatives (/f, ʃ/) as stops ([p, t]). Thus, phonological processes refer to changes in the articulatory or perceptual features of the target sounds. For example, voicing is the production of a voiceless ("[−voice]") consonant with voice ("[+voice]"). Similarly, **fronting** involves producing a consonant that is typically produced in the back of the oral cavity (e.g., a velar) as a more front consonant (e.g., an alveolar). The place of articulation feature has changed from back ("[−anterior]" and/or "[+dorsal]," depending on the phonetic feature system one uses) to front ("[+anterior]"). Stopping involves producing a consonant that should be produced with a continuous flow of air ("[+continuant]"), such as a fricative, as a noncontinuous ("[−continuant]," stopped) sound. Thus, whenever an SLP refers to the processes that young children or children with speech sound delays or disorders are using, she is referring to the articulatory or perceptual features of the sounds that they are actually producing. Unfortunately, many SLPs use process names too generally, such as using the term "fronting" to refer to both producing velars as alveolars and producing interdentals (/θ, ð/) as labiodentals ([f, v]) without specifying which the child is doing. Often the context (e.g., word position) is omitted from the description as well. This overgeneral manner of using process names causes much confusion. If a diagnostic report

[13]Writing this rule in generative phonological notation involves levels of complication and notation that go beyond the scope of this book.

states only that a child is fronting, for instance, another SLP cannot be certain what the author meant.

Phonological Avoidance: Constraints

The idea of phonological constraints was actually included within generative phonology (e.g., Branigan, 1976; Kenstowicz & Kisseberth, 1977), though it gained little attention at the time. This approach is also similar in some ways to the basic principles of natural phonology. Constraints reflect the same patterns as rules or processes, but from the perspective of preferences and avoidances rather than of changes. For example, rather than saying that in Japanese all consonant clusters are reduced to single consonants, it can be said that Japanese has a strong constraint against consonant clusters. In other words, clusters are not allowed in this language; they are highly marked in Japanese. This is written with an asterisk to indicate a non-preferred pattern or **markedness constraint**[14]:

$$^*[+\text{consonantal}][+\text{consonantal}]$$

or

$$^*\text{CC}$$

Japanese also highly ranks the markedness constraint against non-nasal final consonants. In other words, only nasal consonants can occur in final position. Using "#" to indicate a word boundary (in this case, the end of the word), this is written as follows:

$$^*\begin{bmatrix}-\text{nasal}\\+\text{consonantal}\end{bmatrix}\#$$

In other words, a consonant that is not nasal may not occur in final position.

Similarly, in English [ŋ] does not occur in word-initial position. This markedness constraint may be written as follows:

$$^*\#\text{ŋ}$$

or

$$^*\#\begin{bmatrix}+\text{nasal}\\-\text{anterior}\\-\text{coronal}\end{bmatrix}$$

This constraint states that the dorsal (velar; non-anterior, non-coronal) nasal may not appear immediately after a word boundary (i.e., at the beginning of a word). In fact, [ŋ] is not even allowed at the beginning of a syllable in English, a fact that may be represented using "$" to represent a syllable boundary:

$$^*\$\text{ŋ}$$

The voiced palatal fricative [ʒ] is also prohibited from initial position, except in foreign names. Similar markedness constraints prohibit [j] and [w] from final position in English. There is also a restriction on which vowels can occur in open syllables word-finally in our language. English [ɪ] and [ɛ] are not permitted in word-final position, while [i] ("knee") and [e] ("neigh") are allowed. The low front vowel [æ] is marginal; it occurs mostly in slang/colloquial and **baby talk** contexts, such as "yeah" for "yes," "nah" for "no," "dada" for "daddy," etc. This constraint against word-final front lax vowels can be written as follows[15]:

$$^*\begin{bmatrix}+\text{vocalic}\\+\text{front}\\-\text{tense}\end{bmatrix}\#$$

Spanish provides an example of a highly ranked initial consonant cluster markedness constraint. This language does not allow *initial* sequences of [s] + stop, although it does allow them in medial position (where the [s] may close one syllable while the stop opens the next). That is, words such as "steak," "scare," and even "Spanish" are not allowed, but words like "Español" ("Spanish"), in which the /s/ and the stop are in different syllables, are fine. The constraint may be written as follows:

$$^*\#[\text{s}]\begin{bmatrix}+\text{consonantal}\\-\text{continuant}\end{bmatrix}$$

As in natural process theory, constraints are not seen as all-or-nothing patterns. All constraints are viewed as existing in all languages. In each language, some are absolute, while others are much weaker (lower ranked). Within constraint theory (also known as "optimality theory"), the language's (or the speaker's) set of constraints is seen as a ranked list of preferences. Certain ones are frequently violated, and others are violated only when the situation requires it. Those at the top of the ranking (a.k.a., the **constraint hierarchy**) are very strong and rarely or never violated. The lower the constraint is in the hierarchy, the more likely the speakers of the language are to violate it when this is called for in order to avoid violating a more highly ranked constraint.

For example, the Japanese very highly ranked constraint against consonant clusters is never violated. English, on the other hand, may be said to have a very weak markedness constraint against consonant clusters. English speakers slightly prefer not to use clusters and will reduce them when

[14]The constraint labels and other jargon associated with Optimality Theory are deliberately avoided here to the extent possible. This should not be seen as the author's attempt to rename common constraints, nor to develop her own constraint system. Rather, it is an attempt to explain the basic concepts as simply as possible without immersing the reader in the complications of competing sets of theoretical labels.

[15]The actual constraint is a bit more complicated, as [ʊ] (as in "book") is also disallowed, but [ɔ] (as in "law") is permitted. Note also that there is some disagreement in the field as to whether [æ] is lax or tense.

the linguistic or social situation allows (e.g., in casual speech in a redundant context, such as leaving out the [d] in "sandwich" or one of the [st] sequences in "next stop" [nɛk stɑp] when speaking quickly with friends), or when the physiologic situation requires (e.g., when very tired, drunk, etc.). However, this constraint is violated frequently in English. That is, English speakers most often produce most or all of the consonants within a cluster; clusters are not very marked.

Constraints may also represent preferences with respect to the available strategies for avoiding a certain sound or structure. These **faithfulness constraints** specify what types of repairs are preferred. For example, Japanese speakers are far more likely to use epenthesis to avoid a cluster (e.g., pronouncing "public" as [pabuɹiku] when using this word borrowed from English, as described by Hyman, 1975) rather than to use deletion ([pʌbɪk]). Thus, in Japanese, the faithfulness constraint against deletion ("Keep what's there") is higher-ranked than the constraint against epenthesis ("Don't add new stuff"). English speakers, however, are far more likely to use deletion (e.g., pronouncing "library" as [ˈlɑɪbɛɹi] or "next stop" as [nɛk stɑp]) than to use epenthesis ([ˈlɑɪbəɹɛɹi]). Thus, our ranking of these **repair strategies** is the opposite of theirs; the faithfulness constraint against epenthesis is higher ranked in English than the faithfulness constraint against deletion while the reverse is true for Japanese.

There are at least three clinical benefits of describing phonological patterns in terms of constraints rather than as rules or processes. The first is that the constraint is typically the *reason* for the rule or process; therefore, it provides greater insight about the person's patterns. For example, a Japanese person learning English is likely to demonstrate the processes of epenthesis and cluster reduction because of his constraint against clusters. The constraint is the *cause*; the processes are the *effect*. Secondly, in many cases (as in this one), multiple processes may operate as a result of the same constraint. A child who has a constraint against initial /s/, for instance, may stop it ([ti] for "see"), glide it ([wup] for "soup"), move it to word-final position ([puns] for "spoon"), and delete it [twit] for "street") depending on the details of the context. These multiple processes all reflect one simple constraint: *#s—no [s] in initial position. Analyzing that child's speech with respect to processes yields four individual goals with no apparent connection: to teach the child to decrease stopping, gliding, movement, and deletion. Analyzing it with respect to constraints yields one goal: to teach him to produce word-initial /s/.

Finally, identifying a child's preferred strategies can be helpful when selecting intervention exemplars and approaches. For instance, a child with a history of consonant **harmony** (e.g., saying [gɔg] for "dog") who no longer uses harmony in short words may nonetheless master multisyllabic words more easily if words with harmonized consonants are attempted first (e.g., "bumblebee," "lullaby," "memory").

EXERCISE 2-5

Phonological Constraints

Summary

There are three primary models of phonological patterns: generative rules, natural processes, and constraints. Rules and processes focus on the phoneme or word shape target and the way it may be pronounced in a given context (e.g., clusters are reduced in final position) by speakers of a language or by a client with a SSD. Markedness constraints focus on identifying the sounds or structures that are dispreferred (e.g., clusters). In this sense, the rules and processes are the symptoms, and the markedness constraints are the causes: the language (or the child) alters the pronunciation of the word in a certain way in order to avoid a segment or a structure that is challenging. Faithfulness constraints, which specify the language's or the person's preferred strategies for dealing with difficult sounds or structures (e.g., deletion, epenthesis), parallel the rules and processes in the sense of identifying the chosen remedies for the difficulty.

Specific Types of Phonological Patterns

Phonological patterns can be broken down into two primary types: those that affect the features of a consonant or vowel (substitution patterns) and those that affect the structure of the syllable or the word (phonotactic patterns). It is also not unusual, however, for patterns to reflect both the features and the structure of the affected word.

Substitution Patterns

Substitution patterns occur when the features of a segment change, typically because the person has a constraint against certain speech sound features. Consonant substitution

COMMON Confusion

When we talk about substitutions, the preposition that is used is very important. Poor preposition choices often cause confusion, especially if the writer is not careful about using / / for phonemes (targets) versus [ ] for phones/allophones (substitutes). For example, if the child is attempting to produce the phoneme /X/ but he actually produces the phone [y], we can say:

Substitute first:

He substitutes/produces [y] **for** /X/

He produces [y] **instead of** /X/

Target first:

He produces /X/ **as** [y]

He replaces/substitutes /X/ **with** [y]

/X/ is replaced **by** [y]

patterns can be grouped into three major categories: place substitutions, manner substitutions, and voicing substitutions.

Place Substitutions

Place substitutions occur when there are constraints against certain places of articulation—that is, those places of articulation have not been mastered. Common patterns among both young children and children with SSDs include, for example, velar fronting. This is the production of velars as alveolars (e.g., "okay" produced as [oteɪ]) due to a constraint against the velar (a.k.a., dorsal) place of articulation. The converse of velar fronting, backing of alveolars to a velar place of articulation (e.g., "toad" produced as [kog]), is fairly rare among even the youngest typically developing children. The coronal place of articulation (which includes dental, alveolar, palatal, and points between) is very common universally. Substitution of the unmarked feature (coronal) with the marked feature (dorsal) is considered unnatural; constraints against dorsal are far more common than are those against coronal in the languages of the world and in children's phonologies.

Manner Substitutions

Manner substitutions occur when a consonant is produced with the wrong manner due to a constraint against the target manner. A common example is the production of target fricatives (/f, v, θ, ð, s, z, ʃ, ʒ/) as the stops from the same or the closest place of articulation ([p, b, t, d]), called stopping, due to a constraint against fricatives. Again, the reverse is less common. However, frication of stops does occur, especially in children with muscle weakness (as may occur in dysarthria); they may be unable to make and hold complete closures so some air leaks through the constriction, yielding the perception of a fricative.

Voicing Substitutions

Voicing substitutions are most often positional. Typically, voice is constrained in final position and voicelessness is constrained in initial (and medial) position. Therefore, initial voiceless consonants are substituted with voiced ones ("voicing"), and final voiced consonants are substituted with voiceless ones ("devoicing"). Intervocalic medial voiceless consonants may also be voiced in assimilation with the surrounding vowels.

Phonotactic Patterns

As we have seen, words come in all different shapes and sizes. The major components of any word are its syllables, which may range in number from one to over 20. Syllables can also be of different shapes and sizes. These structural options, like phonemes, provide opportunities for contrast in the language while simultaneously adding to the challenges of speaking it. For instance, singletons are easier to produce than clusters, but singletons alone may not yield sufficient contrast. Simple V and CV syllables are easier to produce than syllables with diphthongs and complex clusters. Yet, a constraint that allows only these simple syllable shapes forces the language to compensate somehow, for example, by including a wide variety of consonants and vowels or many long words.

The shapes and sizes of syllables and words are determined by each language's (or each person's) **phonotactic constraints**. These patterns can be based upon a variety of different factors, including the following:

- the numbers of syllables that tend to occur in each word;
- the presence or absence of initial consonants;
- the role of the vowel as the nucleus of the syllable
- the presence or absence of diphthongs or long vowels;
- the presence or absence of final consonants (open versus closed syllables);
- the syllable weights that are allowed;
- the numbers, types, locations, and features of consonants in clusters;
- the amount of **variety** that is permitted within a syllable or word (i.e., the presence of harmony/assimilation patterns, in which consonants or vowels within a word become more similar to each other); and
- **phrase-level effects**, which change the pronunciations of sounds in phrases and sentences.

Different languages have different phonotactic patterns, but there must always be a certain amount of phonotactic freedom within the language. There is a trade-off among the patterns that are allowed by the language. If the language is more restrictive in some ways, it must be less restrictive in others. Without a certain amount of flexibility, the vocabulary of the language would either be very limited or composed of nothing but homonyms. Overall, languages are about equal in difficulty, with each one balancing perceptual distinctiveness with production difficulty in its own ways.

Many adult and child phonological patterns (processes, rules, or constraints) appear to operate at the syllable or word level, rather than affecting particular segments in isolation. For this reason, phonotactic constraints are important in the analysis of delayed or disordered phonology. Many children with non-functional phonologies have too many phonotactic constraints for the number of meanings they would like to express. As a result, they must restrict their vocabularies, produce many homonyms, and/or supplement their oral words with gestures and non-speech sounds in order to communicate. Their phonotactic constraints may also be developmentally inappropriate or unusual.

A person's phonotactic repertoire can often be described using notation that is not sound-specific, such as "CV" to represent an open consonant (C)–vowel (V) syllable (e.g., [gu]), or "#CC" to represent a word-initial consonant cluster (e.g., "st-;" recall that "#" represents a word boundary—either the beginning or the ending edge of a word). However, phonotactic patterns also include effects of one part of the word on the other, such as harmony, assimilation, and **reduplication**. Descriptions of these phonotactic patterns often require us to refer to sound classes or even to specific sounds. For example, many young children demonstrate consonant harmony in which the initial consonant may take on some feature of the final consonant (e.g., [gɔg] for "dog") or vice versa (e.g., [dɔd] for "dog").

Phonotactic patterns are far from random. They are based, at least in part, upon human speech production constraints. In order to communicate, each language must incorporate some components (such as complex clusters or lengthy multisyllabic words) that are articulatorily more difficult. But every language has a limited number of more challenging production patterns. The overall difficulty level of every language is still manageable by its speakers. If the language becomes too difficult to speak, it must either change or die. Furthermore, the most frequent words in the language will be the shorter, simpler ones. Longer or more complex words that come into frequent use will be simplified (as "television" has been reduced to "TV" or "telly" in different dialects of English).

Phonotactic patterns are of major importance in our judgments (usually subconscious) of which words are or are not acceptable in our language. Often, we are perfectly capable of saying the sounds in a foreign word—it is made up of phones that approximate English phones—but it doesn't sound right to us because of its shape. For example, a chain of sub shops was named "Jreck," using the owners' initials. This name is composed of English sounds so it is pronounceable, but these sounds are not in a typical order, so it seems very strange to native English speakers.

In many cases, English speakers will mispronounce such impossible words, especially those that are borrowed from foreign languages, in ways that fit our language's phonotactic patterns more closely. For example, the name "Schwarzkopf" is usually pronounced by Americans without the penultimate "p" sound: [ʃwɑɚtskɔf]. Most Americans actually have no trouble pronouncing a final -pf cluster. We even use this sequence of consonants medially in some words (e.g., "capful"). But it is a cluster that is not allowed in English in final position, so we are not comfortable saying it in that position, and we simplify it to make it a better fit with our ideas of Englishness.

The above are all feature-specific examples. Such feature-specific restrictions are one type of **distribution requirement**. Distribution requirements, in general, are constraints on which types of sounds or syllables can occur in which positions in the word.

Languages (and children) have constraints at more basic levels as well. Both young typically developing children and those with SSDs struggle with the more phonotactically complex structures of their languages. As SLPs, we must understand both the nature of these phonotactic challenges and the strategies that are available to languages and to children for coping with them. Adult languages with phonotactic constraints provide examples of these types of phenomena. Japanese, for instance, avoids consonant clusters in any position and also most final consonants. When Japanese speakers attempt to produce English words with clusters or codas in them, they epenthesize (insert) extra vowels (such as [u]) to make the words conform to Japanese phonotactic restrictions. In some words, this may double or even triple the number of syllables in the word (Hyman, 1975). Thus, Japanese who practice singing American songs by [fʌɹæŋku sinataɹa san] (Frank Sinatra) in their [karaoke baksu] (karaoke practice rooms or "boxes") sing their own version of "Smoke Gets in Your Eyes:"

"..*and [sʌmʌdeɪ] you'll [faɪnʌdo]*
(and someday you'll find)
All true love is [bʌlaɪnʌdo]...
(all true love is blind)"
(Reid, NPR, 1992).

Our phonotactic constraints are so ingrained in us that we almost never violate them, although most people are not consciously aware of what the constraints are. Even in slips of the tongue these rules are rarely broken. We might interchange phonemes (as in "You hissed all my mystery lectures"), or even occasionally features (as in the anticipation of nasality and the preservation of labial in "mang the mail" instead of "bang the nail;" example from Crystal, 1987). But Shattuck-Hufnagel and Klatt (1979), among others, have demonstrated that we rarely produce errors that result in illegal word or syllable shapes. When a phoneme moves to another place within a word or phrase, its landing site will almost always be one that is allowed by English phonotactic restrictions. For instance, "maying prantis" for "praying mantis" is a typical error. Errors such as [pɹeɪjɪm ŋæntɪs] or "paying mrantis" would be highly unexpected slips of the tongue because mr- is not a possible consonant cluster, and [ŋ] is not allowed in syllable-initial position in English. Similarly, a Japanese person would be highly unlikely to produce a slip of the tongue that resulted in an initial or final consonant cluster.

Below, we review some of the phonotactic restrictions that are most commonly found in the languages of the world and in the speech of young children and/or children with SSDs.

Word Length

While no language has a specific upper limit on the number of possible syllables in a word, some languages (such as Japanese and Hawaiian) tend to have far more multisyllabic words than others (possibly to compensate for other phonotactic restrictions). Other languages, such as English, tend to have shorter words *on the average,* many of which are composed of only one syllable. In contrast, some languages (such as Kannada, spoken in India) have very few monosyllabic words. Generally, the number of syllables in a word is inversely proportional to its frequency of occurrence.

In other words, the most commonly used words in any language are the monosyllabic or disyllabic ones (Crystal, 1987).

Inclusion of Consonant Onset

All languages allow a syllable to begin with a consonant (i.e., to have an onset). Many languages do not allow syllables that lack an onset; that is, syllables may not begin with a vowel (Prince & Smolensky, 2004). According to Blevins (1995), however, languages that allow vowel-initial syllables are more common than languages that do not. Adult languages that do not allow them use various strategies for avoiding onsetless syllables that occur as the result of morphologic changes, in borrowed words, etc. These strategies include epenthesis—adding an initial consonant to the syllable. In casual English, in fact, we often epenthesize a glide to the beginning of a vowel-onset word when the previous word ends in a vowel, saying, for example, [hu **w**ɑɚ ju] for "Who are you?" or [wɑɪ **j**ɑɚ ju hiɚ] for "Why are you here?" A final consonant may also serve as onset to a following vowel-initial word in casual speech, as exploited in the old childhood game of saying, "oh wah ta goo sigh yam" (*Oh what a goose I am)* many times fast. These examples illustrate that English has a weak phonotactic constraint against vowel-initial syllables. When this same process occurs in French, it is called "liaison," such as the use of the final [n] from "bon" as the onset of the second syllable in the phrase "bon ami" [bõ nami].

Vowel as Syllable Nucleus

Many languages require a vowel at the heart (nucleus) of each syllable. English is one of the exceptions to this; our language does allow a nasal or a liquid to carry an entire syllable in words like "butt*on*" [ˈbʌʔn̩][16] or "bott*le*" ([ˈbɑdl̩]). Consonants that serve in this role are called **syllabic consonants**. Berber (a Moroccan language) goes even further in this direction than English does, allowing words such as [tl̩tl̩kʷ] ("swallow") and [g.p̩.g̩.hup] ("skin irritation") in which more than one syllable per word may have syllabic consonants as nuclei and in which the nuclei of some syllables are fricatives or even stops (Bagemihl, 1991). This level of permissiveness is rare, however.

Inclusion of Sequences of Vowels

About one-third of the languages of the world include diphthongs. Numerous languages also include long versus short vowels (Ladefoged & Maddieson, 1996). Languages that do not permit two vowels to occur in a row (called **hiatus**) typically use either deletion or epenthesis to eliminate or separate the vowels when morphology or borrowed words would otherwise result in such a sequence. Deletion of one vowel from a sequence often occurs in English phrases. This is the basis for several contractions, such as "I'm," "you're," and "he's." Similar reductions occur in French, including "j'ai" ("I have"), "l'air" ("the air"), etc. (Clark & Yallop, 1995) and also in Spanish (Hammond, 2001). In casual speech, Americans often delete one vowel or merge the two vowels in phrases such as "go away" ([goweɪ]) and "try again" ([tɹɑɪgɛn]; Crystal, 1987). As noted above, we also insert glides to separate two vowels when they occur in a phrase ([go wɑn] for "go on"). In contrast, Spanish speakers tend to substitute one of the vowels with a glide (e.g., [lwɛstima] for "lo estima," "I value it" [Hammond, 2001]). These patterns reveal weak phonotactic constraints against hiatus in these languages with a variety of strategies to avoid this occurrence. Children must learn these rules about if and when vowel reductions are allowed in their own languages.

[16]The line under the [n] indicates that this consonant is syllabic.

Open Versus Closed Syllables

Another basic markedness constraint that some languages place on their phonologies is a prohibition against closed syllables, which are those with one or more final consonants. Such a phonology would have no VC or CVC syllables. All languages have CV syllables (Crystal, 1991); very few have no VCs or CVCs because of the severe limitations that such a restriction places on word shapes. But such languages do exist. Hawaiian, for instance, only permits V and CV syllables; no syllable may have more than one consonant, and some have none. As a result, this language has only 162 possible syllables. Thai, in contrast, has 23,638 possible syllables (Crystal, 1987). Hawaiian compensates for its limited syllable variety with extremely long words. Children who produce only a small number of different syllable shapes are often also unable to produce long words, which puts them at a serious communicative disadvantage in most languages.

Syllable Weight

Many languages have constraints on the "weight" of syllables. Typically, weight depends on the number of vowels within the syllable, as well as on whether or not the syllable is closed. Thus, a syllable such as [wɑɪt] would be much heavier than one such as [wɑ]. Light syllables may not be allowed to appear in a stressed position; heavy ones may not be allowed in unstressed contexts. In English, for example, the vowels [ɪ], [ʊ], and [ɛ] are not allowed in final position (except as components of diphthongs).

Cluster Constraints

Languages—and children—may differ in the number of consecutive consonants they allow in various word positions as well as in the ordering of consonant types within clusters. These reflect **sonority**—the relative openness of the consonant (see below)—as well as the *number* of consecutive consonants that the language will permit.

Some languages, such as Japanese, are far more constrained than English with respect to sequences of consonants. Japanese has almost no consonant clusters and allows only one specific type of consonant (nasals) in final position.

Like Hawaiian, this language compensates for these limits by having many very long multisyllabic words. The syllables themselves are much simpler than in some other languages (such as English), but there are many more of them per word. Many common words that are monosyllabic in English are bisyllabic or trisyllabic in Japanese, such as [kokoɹo] for "heart" and [ʔotoko] for "man" (Hyman, 1975).

Languages such as Japanese, Hawaiian, and Yawelmani (a native American language from the west coast of the United States) have entire sets of rules or processes, such as deletion and epenthesis, that work together to prevent the occurrence of clusters because of their constraints against them. Deletion simplifies the cluster and/or epenthesis separates the consonants with an intervening vowel. For example, Hawaiians trying to pronounce the English word "flour" say "p<u>a</u>looa," and they pronounce "velvet" as "wel<u>e</u>weka" (Archangeli, 1997).

In English, a wide variety of clusters are allowed. However, English speakers tend to use deletion in order to simplify clusters in casual or fast speech: "facts" may be pronounced without the [t] ([fæks]), "fifths" without either the second [f] or the [θ] ([fɪθs] or [fɪfs]), or "library" without the first [ɹ] ([ˈlɑɪbɛɹi]) (Clark & Yallop, 1995). Long clusters that are created by adjoining two words into a phrase may also be simplified. Americans rarely pronounce all of the medial consonants in a phrase such as, "mashed potatoes," "stopped speaking" (Crystal, 1987), or "next stop."

Coalescence is also used in English at times, also in more casual speech. For example, the historical [d] and the [j] of the medial cluster in "soldier" (/ˈsoldjɚ/) are merged into an affricate in most dialects, yielding [ˈsoʊl**dʒ**ɚ] (Clark & Yallop, 1995). Sometimes even whole words can be coalesced within a phrase. The most often-cited example of this is the coalesced version of "Did you eat yet?" ([dʒiʔ jɛʔ]), to which the standard reply is the also-coalesced, "No, did you?" ([noʊ dʒu]), as illustrated in Figure 2-2.

Clusters are examples of cases in which phonetic constraints and phonotactic constraints may interact. That is, there are constraints on which consonants may co-occur as well as on how many consonants may occur in a sequence. For example, skw- is allowed in English, but spw- and stw- are not. In fact, one of the most common examples given of cluster constraints (i.e., distribution requirements that affect clusters) in English is that of initial triple-consonant clusters. If three consonants occur in sequence at the beginning of a word in English, the first one must be [s], the second one must be a voiceless stop ([p, t, k]), and the third must be a liquid or a glide ([ɹ, l, j, w]). Actually, the rule is even more specific than that, as there are restrictions on which liquids and which glides can follow which voiceless stops in such a cluster, shown in Table 2-9. Akmajian, Demers, and Harnish (1984) point out that if the second consonant is [t], the third must be [ɹ], since #stl- and #stw- are not permitted (in some dialects #stj- is allowed, as in "stew" [stju]). This particular part of the rule is especially interesting for three reasons. First, #tw- is permitted at the beginning of a word, but #stw- is not ("twin" is allowed but not "*stwin"). Second, this -stw- cluster is permitted in medial position where two morphemes adjoin, as in "westward." Finally, many children appear to violate this restriction by producing #stw- clusters (e.g., in [stwɪŋ] for "string"). Whether the first two factors may influence children to assume at some point in their phonological development that #stw- should be an approved cluster is an open question.

TABLE 2-9 English Allowable Three-Element Initial Consonant Clusters

First Consonant: /s/	Second Consonant: Stop	Third Consonant: Liquid or Glide
s	p	l, ɹ j
s	t	ɹ j (British)
s	k	l (rare), ɹ j, w

Other languages have very different phonotactic constraints (distribution requirements) for initial consonant clusters. Spanish, for example, does not allow initial [s] + stop clusters of the sort described above but does allow them in medial position. This is why Spanish speakers tend to epenthesize a vowel before these clusters when they speak English, making the clusters medial instead of initial. This leads to stereotypical productions such as "I a-speak a-Spanish" ([ɑɪ əspik əspænɪʃ]; Hyman, 1975). German, on the other hand, allows different types of clusters than English, such as the ʃw- and -pf clusters (as in "Schwarzkopf") mentioned earlier.

Clusters that are similar to allowed clusters often make their way into our language, but they still sound funny, and may be more likely to be adopted with humorous meanings. This may account, for instance, for the Yiddish words that have and have not been assimilated into American culture. For instance, [ʃ] is not allowed in an initial cluster in standard English with either the sonorant [m] or the obstruent [v], but it (or a very similar retroflex fricative) is allowed before the sonorant [ɹ], as in "shrub." Also, sm- is allowed in initial position, but sv- is not. Thus, ʃm- is similar to allowed clusters (ʃr- and sm-), but ʃv- is somewhat more distant. This may explain, at least in part, why words like "shmooze" and "schmaltzy" have been adopted into colloquial English while other words such as "shver" (difficult), "shviger" ("mother-in-law"), and "shvitz" ("sweat") have not. Many Yiddish words with similar borderline clusters and humorous meanings have been adopted into American slang (e.g., "schlock, shlemiel, shlep, shnook, shnoz"). The shm- cluster has also been adopted as a marker of sarcasm, as in "Cluster, shmuster!"

Words that have clusters that are farther out and words that are not humorous are rejected (e.g., "shtuss," "shtarker," "shmaktes," "shlaff," etc.; see Naiman [1981] for definitions and a humorous introduction to Yiddish English).

Dialects within the same language may also differ with respect to the clusters that they allow. Some speakers of southern American dialects, for example, avoid the -kl- cluster, and may use various strategies to simplify this. The best-known instance of this is the pronunciation of "nuclear" as [nukjəlɚ] rather than [nuklijɚ] in some dialects. Some speakers of AAE dialects avoid -sk-, and tend to **metathesize** (reverse the order of) the [s] and the [k] to yield a preferable cluster, as in [æks] for "ask."

Several phonologists have proposed that the order of consonants in clusters (and indeed, the positioning of all sounds within words) is dependent, at least in part, on a **sonority hierarchy**. Sonority is the "degree of opening of the vocal apparatus during production, or the relative amount of energy produced during the sound" (Goldsmith, 1990, p. 110). The most sonorant segments (e.g., vowels) occur in the middle of the word, with segments of decreasing sonority toward the edges, so that the least sonorant segments (e.g., stops) are at word boundaries. The order of sonority from most to least is roughly as follows:

Most sonorant:	vowels
	glides
	liquids
	nasals
	fricatives
	affricates
Least sonorant:	stops

If clusters were bound by this hierarchy, then initial clusters such as pl- and sm- and final clusters such as -rk, and -nt would be allowed, but clusters such as initial lt- or final -pm would not. In fact, these statements are true of English and many other languages. However, [s] breaks the rules in English (and some other languages); clusters such as initial sp-, st-, sk- and final –ps, –ts, –ks should not occur, since [s] is more sonorous than the stops and should therefore be closer to the middle of the syllable. Similarly, [ʃ] breaks the rules in German; clusters such as ʃp-, ʃt-, ʃk- are allowed in that language. However, the sonority hierarchy does explain many of the cluster patterns observed around the world, and phonologists continue to tinker with it in hopes of getting it exactly right (Goldsmith, 1990).

Variety Constraints: Harmony/Assimilation/Reduplication Patterns

Harmony, assimilation, and reduplication are among the phonological patterns that are the most difficult to describe without referring to an entire syllable or word. They all require one element—a consonant, a vowel, or even a whole syllable—to peek ahead or back at another segment in order to resemble it more closely. Consider a child who pronounces "doggie" as [ˈgɔgi] but "donut" with appropriate alveolar consonants ([ˈdonʌt]). It is simply incorrect to say that this child is using a backing process. The child's velar and alveolar production patterns clearly depend upon the phonology of the entire word, not simply upon substitution of one phone for another.

Technically, assimilation refers to *adjacent* elements becoming more alike, such as vowels becoming nasal before a nasal consonant (e.g., [bæ̃ŋ] for "bang"). By definition, harmony refers to units that are more distant becoming more alike. In the "doggie" example, for instance, the /d/ and /g/ are separated by a vowel, but the /d/ harmonizes with the /g/ "across" the /ɔ/. This harmony "at a distance" is relatively rare in adult languages (Cruttenden, 1978) but common in the speech of young children. Despite their technical definitions, in practice the terms "assimilation" and "harmony" are often used interchangeably to refer to segments anywhere within a word that come to resemble each other more closely.

Due to ease of production, Americans (and speakers of many other languages, as well) tend to assimilate some clusters in casual speech. This phenomenon is partly responsible for the pronunciation of "sandwich" as [sæmwɪtʃ] in some dialects, for example. In this case, the [d] is deleted to simplify the cluster, and then the nasal /n/ is labialized in anticipation of the labio–velar [w]. The assimilation continues the process of making a somewhat difficult medial cluster more manageable. This is easier because [m] and [w] share a place of articulation, while -nd- and [w] do not. Similarly, it's easier to say two palatals in a row than an alveolar (such as [t] or [s]) followed by a palatal (such as [ɹ]), so some of us pronounce "train" as [tʃɹeɪn] and "groceries" as [groʃɹiz], as described above.

Some English assimilation patterns are morphologic. For instance, recall that English speakers routinely assimilate the voicing of certain morphologic endings, such as plural, although the assimilation is not reflected in our spelling. Other English morphologic assimilations have become so standard that they actually are spelled in their assimilated forms. The nasal in the negative morpheme "in-," for example, assimilates to match the place of articulation—and sometimes even the manner of articulation—of any following consonant. The words are spelled as we say them to the extent that our alphabet allows,[17] as in "impossible," "illegal," and "irresponsible." The morpheme retains its default form, [ɪn], before vowels and also before alveolars since [n] is also alveolar (e.g., "inadequate," "indeterminate"). Nasals that assimilate to the following (or preceding) consonant are often referred to as **homorganic** in reference to the fact that they are articulatorily ("organically") similar to the neighboring segment.

When consonants and vowels that are adjacent become more alike in adult languages or in child speech, this is

[17]We have no orthographic symbol for [ŋ] (as in [ɪŋkrɛdəbl̩]), so this is spelled with "n."

consonant–vowel assimilation. The most familiar example from English is the nasalization of vowels before nasal consonants (e.g., "hand" [hæ̃nd]). Consonant–vowel assimilation also results in the palatalization of many alveolars in English, especially in casual speech. The palatal place of articulation of vowels such as [i, u] may spread to the preceding consonant (as anticipatory assimilation, in other words, assimilation in which the articulators prepare ahead of time for an upcoming sound), causing this consonant to become palatal as well, as in [tɪʃu] for "tissue" /tɪsju/.

Vowel harmony constraints prohibit vowels that are too different from each other occurring within the same word. Therefore, they require that certain vowels in certain types of words or syllables must share certain features. For instance, in some languages, vowels that occur in the same word must agree by having the same height (e.g., [i] and [ɑ] cannot occur in the same word), the same backness (e.g., [i] and [u] cannot occur in the same word), or the same roundness (e.g., [o] and [ɑ] cannot occur in the same word). If some morphologic circumstance or the borrowing of a word from another language might force the speakers into saying a word that would violate these constraints, they would apply a harmony process to make the two vowels more similar (resulting in, for instance, lowering, raising, or rounding).

In a sense, reduplication is a combination of vowel and consonant harmony. Multisyllabic words are formed by repeating one syllable of the base word so that all consonants and vowels are the same. This pattern is found in baby talk **register** (**motherese** or **child-directed speech**) in some languages, including English ("dada," "mama," "baba," "boo-boo," "no-no," "nigh'-nigh'," etc.).[18] Although English speakers may think of it as a silly type of phonological rule, to be used only with very young children, some languages use reduplication grammatically in their everyday words. In Warlpiri (a language spoken in Australia), for instance, the plurals of some nouns referring to human beings are made by total reduplication. That is, the entire word is repeated to indicate plurality, even if it's a multisyllabic word. Thus, "mardukuja" means "woman" and "mardukujamardukuja" means "women" (Marantz, 1982).

Summary

Languages, young children, and children with SSDs use a variety of strategies to achieve ease of production (i.e., to produce challenging segments and structures). These include feature substitutions based on the manner, place, or voicing of a consonant, or on the height, advancement, tension, or rounding of a vowel. Other patterns are phonotactic, including deletions of initial or final consonants or syllables, simplification of clusters via deletion or coalescence, and harmony or assimilation to reduce the variety within a given structure.

EXERCISE 2-6

Specific Pattern Types

INTRODUCTORY CONCEPTS: PROSODY

Prosody is often thought of as the musical aspect of language: it comprises the beat and the melody of speech. The three primary components of prosody are loudness, duration, and pitch. These three characteristics are used together to form the precepts we call **intonation** and stress.

Loudness

Loudness, more technically referred to as intensity, relates to the amount of energy in the speech signal. Intensity in and of itself does not play a role in the linguistic system, but it does have some important functions in conjunction with other aspects of prosody, as described below.

Duration

Duration refers to the lengths, in time, of linguistic units. The average rate of speech is approximately five to five and a half syllables per second. Many factors influence this. One of these is the **inherent relative durations** of different speech sounds. In general, vowels last longer than consonants with tense vowels longer than lax ones and diphthongs longer than simple vowels. The durations of segments are also influenced by context at various levels. All segments have shorter durations when we speak more quickly. Less obviously, in English, vowels are prolonged in stressed syllables and before voiced consonants. Both the nucleus (vowel) and the final consonant (if any) of a syllable are prolonged at the end of a phrase or sentence in a process called **phrase-final lengthening** (Behne & Nygaard, 1993).

These types of lengthening are possible in English (and similar languages) because segment length is not contrastive. However, in languages such as Finnish and Japanese, the length of a vowel or a consonant can change the meaning of the word. In Japanese, for example, /kaite/ means "buyer," while /kaite:/ (with a prolonged final vowel) means "seabed" (Kato, Tajima, & Akhane-Yamada, 2001). In such languages, segment lengths cannot be subject to contextual influences such as phrase-final lengthening, or meaning will be jeopardized.

Another aspect of duration is the lengths of pauses (called **junctures**; marked with a vertical line "|") in connected speech. Typically, speakers pause at the ends of grammatical units. This aids listeners in parsing the sentences. The ambiguities and confusions that can be caused by misplaced junctures are exemplified by the following minimal pair sentences:

1. He ate | a donut hole.
2. He ate a donut | whole.

[18]Baby talk (motherese or child-directed speech) rules are considered to be a special subset of the phonological rules of a language that one learns as one learns the language. Even preschool children demonstrate knowledge of this register by using it with younger siblings.

3. Her toes were examined | by seven | foot doctors.
4. Her toes were examined | by seven-foot | doctors.

How do pauses change the meaning of the following sentence?

Woman without her man is nothing.[19]

Pitch

Pitch refers to the **fundamental frequency** of the speaker's voice. In some languages, pitch has a lexical function. That is, different **tones** (pitches) change the meanings of words. For example, in Thai, [na:] has many different meanings depending on the tone that is used, as shown in Table 2-10. Tone languages seem very exotic to many English speakers, but they are actually more common than intonation languages. In some tone languages, only single tones change semantic meaning; in others, combinations of pitches (e.g., high–low; low rising) also provide contrast.

In intonation languages, such as English, pitch has the grammatical function of indicating a yes-or-no question (rising pitch) versus a wh-question or a statement (falling pitch). Intonation also demarcates the last element of a list; the pitch rises on each item listed until it falls on the last one. Pitch can also express affect, such as surprise, boredom, excitement, and a range of other emotions. In intonation languages, also, **phrase-final pitch declination**, in which the pitch tends to fall toward the end of the utterance for physiologic reasons, is typical. This signals the end of a phrase or sentence. Of course, this declination is counteracted by the rises that accompany yes-or-no questions.

Stress

In English, duration, pitch, and intensity work together to create the percept of stress. Despite the fact that it is an overlaid function, stress is critical to listener comprehension and judgments of intelligibility (van Rees, Ballard, McCabe, Macdonald-D'Silva, & Arciuli, 2012). Speakers integrate the use of these three features of stress. If one aspect of stress that they are attempting to convey appears to be impaired (e.g., if their perceptions are altered so it sounds like they are not producing higher pitch on stressed words), they will not only exaggerate that feature but also increase their use of the other features to ensure their own communicative success (Patel, Niziolek, Reilly, & Guenther, 2011).

Stress may apply at the phrase or sentence level ("phrasal stress") to express emphasis or contrast (e.g., "I want the BLUE one, not the RED one") or at the syllable level ("word stress," for example, "MIssiSSIppi"). Stressed syllables within words are referred to as **strong** and unstressed syllables as **weak.** Words or phrases with stress on the first syllable ("PAper" [ˈpeɪpɚ]) are called **trochaic**, while weak-syllable-initial words ("reDUCE" [ɹiˈdus]) are **iambic**. In English, words are most often—though by no means always—trochaic, while phrases are most often iambic. This fact helps us to distinguish between compound words (trochaic, like "HOTdog" and "GREENhouse") and phrases (iambic, like "hot DOG" and "green HOUSE").

TABLE 2-10 Thai Tones

Word	Tone	Meaning
nàa	Low falling	A nickname
naa	Mid falling	Field
náa	High rising	Aunt
nâa	High falling	Face
nǎa	Low falling-rising	Thick

Adapted from Ladefoged, P. (2011). *A course in phonetics.* Retrieved February 19, 2011, from http://www.phonetics.ucla.edu/course/chapter10/thai/thai.html.

Word stress in English is quite complex, with a variety of stress patterns, and not in a completely predictable rule-based system. (See examples in Appendix B, Chapter 10.) The syllables of a word tend to roughly alternate between strong and weak ("SUperCAliFRAgiLISticEXpiAliDOcious"—SWSWSWSWSWSWSW), though many words violate this pattern, some extremely (e.g., "indefatigable" [ɪndəˈfæɾɪgəbl̩], which is WWSWWW). Furthermore, heavy syllables (those containing diphthongs, tense vowels, or codas) are more likely to be stressed and vice versa; the vowels of unstressed syllables tend to be reduced to schwa. (Compare, for example, the pronunciation of the second vowel in "COllege" [ˈkɑlədʒ] versus that in "colLEgial" [kəˈlidʒəl].) Nouns and adjectives tend to be trochaic (as in "PREsent" [ˈpɹɛzənt] and "REcord" [ˈɹɛkɚd]) and verbs tend to be iambic (as in "preSENT" [pɹiˈzɛnt] and "reCORD" [ɹəˈkɔɚd]). However, there are many exceptions to these rules.

In some languages, stress has other grammatical roles, such as differentiating tenses (e.g., in Russian: uznaJU [uznaˈju] = "I find out;" uzNAju [uzˈnaju] = "I will find out"). It may also have an active lexical function, differentiating words from each other (e.g., in Russian: MUka [ˈmuka] = "torment;" muKA [muˈka] = "flour"). There are very few word pairs that are even close to being stress minimal pairs in English, in part because stress changes vowel qualities (e.g., "desert" [ˈdɛzɚt]; "dessert" [dəˈzɝt]).

In other languages, stress may be far more predictable. For example, in French, word stress always falls on the final syllable of the word and phrase stress always on the final syllable of the phrase. As a result, stress plays no role in differentiating meaning in French, and monolingual speakers of this language have no reason to pay attention to it. Peperkamp and Dupoux (2002) have described them as being "stress deaf."

Pitch cannot play a role in stress in a tone language, nor can duration contribute to stress in a language in which duration is phonemic. Such dual roles of pitch or duration would result in too many confusing cues. In other cases, pitch, duration, and/or loudness may work together to convey stress but without all falling on the same stressed

[19]"Woman without her man | is nothing" versus "Woman | without her | man is nothing."

syllable. Welsh, for instance, has a very complex system in which the stressed syllable is louder (as in English), but pitch is higher on the syllable after the stressed one, the consonant after the stressed vowel is lengthened, and the stressed vowel is shorter—not longer—than are those in neighboring syllables (Williams, 1999; Watkins, 1993 as cited by Vihman, Nakai, DePaolis, & Halle, 2004). It's almost as confusing to a non-native speaker as trying to figure out which syllable should be stressed in English words!

Stress patterns play an important role in an even larger domain of prosody within the languages of the world: the domain of rhythm or meter. In some languages (called "mora-timed"), rhythm is based upon the contents of the syllable. Recall that a CVV or a CVC syllable is heavier than a CV syllable. In mora-timed languages, every vowel and every coda have equal duration, so a CVV or a CVC syllable would last roughly 1.3 times as long as a CV syllable. In other languages called "syllable-timed" languages, each syllable lasts the same amount of time as every other syllable, even if one syllable includes more segments than another (e.g., CV [pu] versus CCVCC [pʁust).

The third type of rhythm found in some languages—including English—is stress timing. The original simplistic view of this type was that in languages with stress-timed rhythm, there is an equal amount of time between each stressed syllable, even if there is more content in between two stressed syllables than in between two others. In the sentence, "The BIG boy MADE a satisFACtory readJUSTment," for example, the duration of "boy" would be the same as the duration of "a satis" and "tory re-ad." This simplistic view of stress timing appears not to be precisely correct in all respects, but the basic insight remains valid. Vowel reduction, as found in English, is one of the hallmarks of stress-timed languages (Nazzi, Bertoncini, & Mehler, 1998).

Despite the fact that these distinctions are not as clear-cut as originally conceived, rhythm is nonetheless an important aspect of language. For example, newborn infants already discriminate between languages from these three timing categories, but not between languages within the same rhythm group, such as Spanish and Italian or English and Dutch (Nazzi, Bertoncini, & Mehler, 1998).

Summary: Prosody

Prosody is comprised of loudness, duration, and pitch. Although it does convey emotional meaning, this is by no means its only function. These three prosodic features also serve to differentiate words from each other, compound words from phrases, questions from statements, and items in the middle of a list from those at the end of the list. In addition, it can signal the boundary of a word or phrase, thereby assisting the listener in parsing the utterance. Finally, it impacts the basic rhythmic structure of a language, which is one of the first aspects infants recognize of their native languages.

EXERCISE 2-7

Prosody

CHAPTER SUMMARY

"Phonology" will be used in this book as a cover term to refer to a child's or a language's phones, phonemes, allophones, syllable and word shapes, intonation, and the patterning of these in rules or processes. Any strategy that a person uses to convey meaning via sounds emerging from the vocal tract, including strategies that are inspired by physiologic limitations (such as cleft palate), will be considered to be part of that person's phonology. A phonology (child or adult) has several components, each of which can function in various ways by itself and in interaction with other components. However, phonologies also must be considered in their entireties. We cannot look at any one component alone and draw adequate conclusions about phonological malfunction without considering every other aspect of the child's speech sound system as well.

Segmental contrast is achieved via phones that signal meaning contrasts within a language. Not every phone is contrastive; sets of phones that alternate with each other without changing meanings are individually called allophones. Collectively, the allophones from each set represent the outward manifestation of one phoneme. Allophones may be in free variation or in complementary distribution with each other. Phoneme contrasts may be neutralized in certain contexts. The frequency of occurrence of a phoneme is less important than its contrastive value within the language, known as its functional load.

Contrast is also achieved via phonotactics and prosody. Various aspects of syllable and word structure—such as the inclusion of onsets, codas, diphthongs, and clusters, as permitted in particular languages—differentiate words from each other. Duration, loudness, pitch, and combinations of these used to form stress patterns are key to intelligible, effective communication at the word level and well beyond.

In order to efficiently assess a child's phonology, it must be viewed as a system that may or may not be functioning adequately for the child's communication needs at that time. All of these concepts will be revisited, in some cases multiple times, throughout the remainder of this book.

KEY TAKE-HOME MESSAGES

1. Phones are any speech sounds, from any language. Phonemes have language-specific contrastive functions.
2. Phonetic universals reflect ease of production and ease of perception and help us understand developmental patterns.
3. Phonological elements combine into structures and interact in systematic ways that differ from language to language.
4. Generative rules and phonological processes describe patterns in the way speech sounds are used in the languages of the world.
5. Prosody knits sounds, words, phrases, and sentences together into rhythmic, melodic communications.

CHAPTER 2

Phonetics Review

Exercise 2-1: IPA Review[21]

1. IPA Warm Up: Translate into regular spelling:

   aɪ tek ɪt ju ɔlˈɹɛdi noʊ |
   ʌv tʌf | ænd baʊ | ænd kɔf | ænd doʊ ||
   ˈʌðɚz meɪ ˈstʌmbəl | bʌt nɑt ju |
   ɑn ˈhɪkʌp | ˈθʊɹoʊ | læf | ænd θɹu ||
   wɛl dʌn | ænd naʊ ju wɪʃ | pɚˈhæps |
   tu lɝn ʌv lɛs fəˈmɪljɚ tɹæps ||

(From "Hints on Pronunciation for Foreigners" by T. S. W.)

2. Translate each stanza into IPA. Be careful of vowels!
   a. Beware of heard, a dreadful word,
      That looks like beard and sounds like bird.
      And dead, it's said like bed, not bead —
      For goodness' sake, don't call it "deed!"
      Watch out for meat and great and threat.
      (They rhyme with suite and straight and debt.)
   b. A moth is not a moth in mother,
      Nor both in bother, broth in brother,
      And here is not a match for there
      Nor dear and fear for bear and pear.
      And then there's dose and rose and lose –
      Just look them up – and goose and choose.
   c. And cork and work and card and ward,
      And font and front and word and sword.
      And do and go and thwart and cart –
      Come, come, I've hardly made a start!
      A dreadful language? Man alive!
      I'd mastered it when I was five.
3. Select one correct answer per question.
   a. In this author's view, phonology encompasses **only**:
      ______the cognitive–linguistic aspects of oral communication.
      ______actions, patterns, elements, and linguistic structures relating to speech production and perception.
      ______motor programming, planning, and execution of speech acts.
      ______the central organizational component required for learning the phonological system of a language.
   b. The word "argumentation:"
      ______includes five syllables.
      ______includes five morphemes.
      ______includes free morphemes only.
      ______includes bound morphemes only.
      ______is disyllabic
   c. A typical English syllable includes the following elements in the order given:
      ______coda—body—rhyme
      ______nucleus—coda—onset
      ______rhyme—coda
      ______onset—nucleus—coda
      ______body—nucleus
4. Mark each statement as "true"—a real phonetic universal—or "false"—not a real phonetic universal.
   a. ______All languages have at least five vowels.
   b. ______[n] is the most common nasal.
   c. ______[ɑɪ] is the most common diphthong.
   d. ______A language is more likely to have a glide than a liquid.
   e. ______ Most languages have three stop places of articulation.
   f. ______[s] and [f] are more common than [z] and [v].
   g. ______[p] and [b] are more common than [t] and [d].
5. Number the manners of articulation from least sonorous ("1") to most sonorous ("6").
   a. ______glide
   b. ______stop
   c. ______fricative
   d. ______vowel
   e. ______liquid
   f. ______nasal

Exercise 2-2: Identifying Allophones Versus Phonemes

1. *Fill in the blanks.*

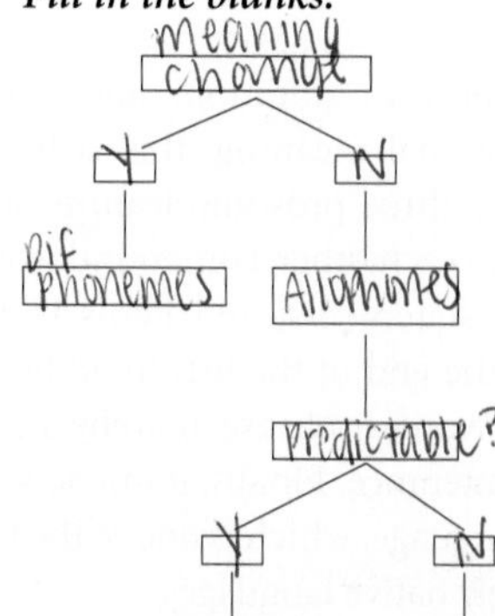

---

[21]NOTES on IPA:

- There are multiple ways to transcribe rhotic diphthongs. Some American transcribers use [ɚ] and some use [ɹ]. Some use tense vowels and some use lax. Some use [ɹ] and some use [r]. Thus,

"ear" can be written: iɚ = ɪɚ = iɹ = ɪɹ = ir = ɪr

"air" can be written: eɚ = ɛɚ = eɹ = ɛɹ = er = ɛr

"oor" can be written: uɚ = ʊɚ = uɹ = ʊɹ = ur = ʊr

"or" can be written: oɚ = ɔɚ = oɹ = ɔɹ = or = ɔr

"are" can be written: ɑɚ = ɑɹ = ɑr

- Recall that [oʊ] and [o] are allophones of the same phoneme (/o/), as are [eɪ] and [e] (of /e/).

2. *Consider the following data from a hypothetical language.*

Pronunciation	Meaning
so	car
sa	flower
su	computer
se	strut
sæ	lemon
ʃi	letter
ʃɪ	friend
oso	candle
asa	shoe
usu	book
æsæ	boat
iʃi	admire
ɪʃɪ	delivery

Answer the following questions:

1. Identify two minimal pairs (two words per pair). How can you tell that they are minimal pairs?
2. Identify at least one vowel and at least one consonant that only occur in certain contexts (i.e., in combination with certain consonants or vowels). Specify the relevant contexts.
3. Use your answer to No. 1 and/or No. 2 to determine whether [s] and [ʃ] are allophones or separate phonemes in this language. Justify your answer.
4. Use your answer to No. 1 and/or No. 2 to determine whether [a] and [æ] are allophones or separate phonemes in this language. Justify your answer.

Exercise 2-3: **Distinctive Features**

Use Tables 2-1 through 2-4 to indicate the feature category or categories (place, manner, and voicing for consonants; height, advancement, tension, and roundness for vowels) and the features that differentiate the two phones:

Example: [f], [s]: *place of articulation: [−coronal] versus [+coronal]; manner of articulation: [−strident] versus [+strident]; voicing: not different*

1. [dʒ], [z]
2. [i], [ʌ]
3. [j], [ɹ]
4. [ɔ], [ɑ]
5. [l], [w]

Exercise 2-4: **Generative Phonological Rules**

1. Interpret the following phonological rules (i.e., restate them in words). Then speculate about why they are natural (i.e., why they make sense articulatorily).

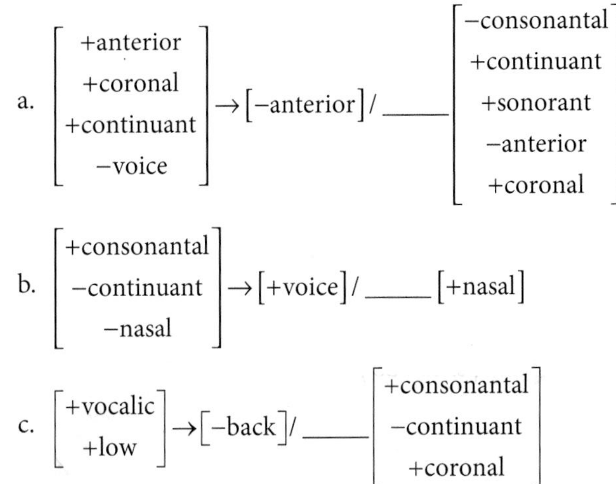

a. $\begin{bmatrix} +\text{anterior} \\ +\text{coronal} \\ +\text{continuant} \\ -\text{voice} \end{bmatrix} \rightarrow [-\text{anterior}] \,/\, \_\_\_ \begin{bmatrix} -\text{consonantal} \\ +\text{continuant} \\ +\text{sonorant} \\ -\text{anterior} \\ +\text{coronal} \end{bmatrix}$

b. $\begin{bmatrix} +\text{consonantal} \\ -\text{continuant} \\ -\text{nasal} \end{bmatrix} \rightarrow [+\text{voice}] \,/\, \_\_\_ [+\text{nasal}]$

c. $\begin{bmatrix} +\text{vocalic} \\ +\text{low} \end{bmatrix} \rightarrow [-\text{back}] \,/\, \_\_\_ \begin{bmatrix} +\text{consonantal} \\ -\text{continuant} \\ +\text{coronal} \end{bmatrix}$

Exercise 2-5: **Phonological Constraints**

1. In a certain language, there is a highly ranked markedness constraint against final consonants. That language's faithfulness constraint against deletion is stronger than the faithfulness constraint against epenthesis. Therefore, speakers of the language would be most likely to produce the word /tip/ as:
   a. [pit]
   b. [tipə]
   c. [ti]
   d. [pipi]
2. Speakers of Dialect A of Language B tend to pronounce the word /bɪto/ as [bito]. This may be due to:
   a. a markedness constraint against having both [+round] and [−round] vowels in the same word.
   b. a markedness constraint against having both [+tense] and [−tense] vowels in the same word.
   c. a markedness constraint against having both [+high] and [+low] vowels in the same word.
   d. a faithfulness constraint against changing vowel quality.
3. *CC means:
   a. no clusters in initial position.
   b. no clusters in final position.
   c. no more than two consonants in a row.
   d. clusters are preferred.

Exercise 2-6: **Specific Pattern Types**

Based upon the phonemic target and the actual phonetic production, fill in the type of change that occurred in the third column.

Substitutions:
MAN = manner
PLC = place
VOI = voicing
RND = vowel rounding
HT = vowel height
ADV = vowel advancement

TNS = vowel tension
Phonotactic:
CDEL = consonant deletion
CRED = cluster reduction
COAL = coalescence
HAR = harmony
ASM = assimilation
RDUP = reduplication

Target	Actual Production	Type of Change
1. /sʌmtɑɪm/	[sʌtɑɪm]	
2. /sʌmtɑɪm/	[sʌpɑɪm]	
3. /θɪsəl/	[sɪsəl]	
4. /θɪsəl/	[fɪsəl]	
5. /pit/	[put]	
6. /pit/	[pɪt]	
7. /fit/	[pit]	
8. /fit/	[vit]	
9. /wægən/	[wæwæ]	

Exercise 2-7: **Prosody**

1. Put the correct letter(s) on the blank to indicate which aspect of prosody achieves this function.
   P: pitch
   D: duration
   L: loudness
   S: stress

   ______ a. differentiates compound words from phrases.
   ______ b. signals the end of a phrase or sentence.
   ______ c. differentiates word meaning in some languages, but not in English.
   ______ d. differentiates questions from statements.
   ______ e. contributes to the percept of stress.
   ______ f. differentiates word meaning in English (and other languages).
   ______ g. differentiates parts of speech (e.g., nouns versus verbs) in English.

References

Akmajian, A., Demers, R. A., & Harnish, R. M. (1984). *Linguistics: An introduction to language communication*. Cambridge, MA: The MIT Press.

Archangeli, D. (1997). Optimality theory: An introduction to linguistics in the 1990s. In D. Archangeli & D. T. Langendoen (Eds.), *Optimality Theory: An overview* (pp. 1–32). Malden, MA: Blackwell.

Bagemihl, B. (1991). Syllable structure in Bella Coola. *Linguistic Inquiry, 22*(4), 589–646.

Behne, D. M., & Nygaard, L. C. (1993). Syllable internal timing: Effects on vowel and consonant duration. *The Journal of the Acoustical Society of America, 93*, 2296.

Blevins, J. (1995). The syllable in phonological theory. In J. Goldsmith (Ed.) *The handbook of phonological theory* (pp. 206–244). Cambridge, MA: Blackwell.

Borden, G. J. & Harris, K. S. (1980). *Speech science primer: Physiology, acoustics, and perception of speech*. Baltimore, MD: Williams & Wilkins.

de Boysson-Bardies, B., & Vihman, M. M. (1991). Adaptation to language: Evidence from babbling and first words in four languages. *Language, 67*, 297–319.

de Boysson-Bardies, B., Vihman, M. M., Roug-Hellichius, L., Durand, C., Landberg, I., & Arao, F. (1992). Material evidence of infant selection from target language: A cross-linguistic phonetic study. In C. Ferguson, L. Menn, & C. Stoel-Gammon (Eds.), *Phonological development: Models, research, implications* (pp. 369–391). Timonium, MD: York Press.

Branigan, G. (1976). Syllabic structure and the acquisition of consonants: The great conspiracy in word formation. *Journal of Psycholinguistics Research, 5*(2), 117–133.

Bynon, T. (1977). *Historical linguistics*. Cambridge, UK: Cambridge University Press.

Clark, J., & Yallop, C. (1995). *An introduction to phonetics and phonology*. Cambridge, MA: Blackwell.

Chomsky, N., & Halle, M. (1968). *The sound pattern of English*. New York, NY: Harper & Row.

Cruttenden, A. (1978). Assimilation in child language and elsewhere. *Journal of Child Language, 5*(2), 376.

Crystal, D. (1987). *The Cambridge encyclopedia of language*. New York, NY: Cambridge University Press.

Crystal, D. (1991). *A dictionary of linguistics and phonetics*. Cambridge, MA: Basil Blackwell, Inc.

Donegan, P. J., & Stampe, D. (1979). The study of natural phonology. In D. A. Dinnsen (Ed.), *Current approaches to phonological theory* (pp. 126–173). Bloomington, IN: Indiana University Press.

Funk, W. (1978). *Word origins and their romantic histories*. New York, NY: Bell.

Goldsmith, J. A. (1990). *Autosegmental and metrical phonology*. Cambridge, MA: Basil Blackwell.

Greenberg, J. (1978). *Universals of language, Volume 2: Phonology*. Stanford, CA: Stanford University Press.

Hammond, R. M. (2001). *The sounds of Spanish: Analysis and application*. Somerville, MA: Cascadilla Press.

Hyman, L. H. (1975). *Phonology: Theory and analysis*. New York, NY: Holt, Rinehart, and Winston.

Kato, H., Tajima, K., & Akhane-Yamada, R. (2001). Native and non-native perception of phonemic length contrasts in Japanese. *The Journal of the Acoustical Society of America, 110*, 2686.

Kenstowicz, M., & Kisseberth, C. (1977). *Topics in phonological theory*. New York, NY: Academic Press.

Kingston, J., & Diehl, R. L. (1994). Phonetic knowledge. *Language, 70*, 419–454.

Ladefoged, P. (2011). *A course in phonetics*. Retrieved February 19, 2011, from http://www.phonetics.ucla.edu/course/chapter10/thai/thai.html.

Ladefoged, P., & Maddieson, I. (1996). *The sounds of the world's languages*. Cambridge, MA: Blackwell.

Lester, L., & Skousen, R. (1974). The phonology of drunkenness. In A. Bruck, R. A. Fox, & M. W. LaGaly (Eds.), *Papers from the parasession on natural phonology* (pp. 233–239). Chicago, IL: Chicago Linguistic Society.

Lindblom, B., & Engstrand, O. (1989). In what sense is speech quantal? *Journal of Phonetics, 17*, 107–121

Lindblom, B., Krull, D., & Stark, J. (1993). Phonetic systems and phonological development. *Developmental Neurocognition: Speech and Face Processing in the First Year of Life. NATO ASI Series, 69*, 399–409.

Lindblom, B., & Maddieson, I. (1988). Phonetic universals in consonant systems. In L. H. Hyman & T. Li (Eds.), *Language, speech and mind: Studies in honor of Victoria Fromkin* (pp. 62–78). London, UK: Routledge.

Locke, J. L. (1983). *Phonological acquisition and change* New York, NY: Academic Press.

Maddieson, I. (1984). *Patterns of sounds.* Cambridge, UK: Cambridge University Press.

Maddieson, I., & Precoda, K. (1989). Updating UPSID. *The Journal of the Acoustical Society of America, 86,* S19.

Manuel, S. Y. (1990). The role of contrast in limiting vowel-to-vowel coarticulation in different languages. *The Journal of the Acoustical Society of America, 88,* 1286–1298.

Marantz, A. (1982). Re reduplication. *Linguistic Inquiry, 13*(3), 435–482.

Menn, L., & Vihman, M. M. (2011). Features in child phonology: Inherent, emergent, or artefacts of analysis? In N. Clements & R. Ridouane (Eds.), *Where do phonological features come from? Cognitive, physical and developmental bases of distinctive speech categories* (pp. 261–301). Amsterdam, the Netherlands: John Benjamins.

Naiman, A. (1981). *Every goy's guide to common Jewish expressions.* Boston, MA: Houghton Mifflin.

Nazzi, T., Bertoncini, J., & Mehler, J. (1998). Language discrimination by newborns: Toward an understanding of the role of rhythm. *Journal of Experimental Psychology: Human Perception and Performance, 24*(3), 756–766.

Patel, R., Niziolek, C., Reilly, K., & Guenther, F. H. (2011). Prosodic adaptations to pitch perturbation in running speech. *Journal of Speech, Language, and Hearing Research, 54,* 1051–1059.

Peperkamp, S., & Dupoux, E. (2002). A typological study of stress "deafness". In C. Gussenhoven, N. Warner, et al. (Eds.), *Laboratory Phonology* (pp. 203–240). Berlin, Germany: Mouton de Gruyter.

Prince, A., & Smolensky, P. (2004). *Optimality theory: Constraint interaction in generative grammar.* Cambridge, MA: Blackwell.

Rice, K., & Avery, P. (1995). Variability in a deterministic model of language acquisition: A theory of segmental elaboration. In J. Archibald (Ed.), *Phonological acquisition and phonological theory* (pp. 23–42). Hillsdale, NJ: Lawrence Erlbaum.

Share, D. L., & Blum, P. (2005). Syllable splitting in literate and preliterate Hebrew speakers: Onsets and rimes or bodies and codas? *Linguistic Constraints on Literacy Development: Journal of Experimental Child Psychology, 92*(2), 182–202.

Shattuck-Hufnagel, S., & Klatt, D. (1979). The limited use of distinctive features and markedness in speech production: Evidence from speech error data. *Journal of Verbal Learning and Verbal Behavior, 18,* 41–55.

Smith, K.U. (1962). *Delayed sensory feedback and behavior.* Philadelphia, PA: W.B. Saunders Co.

Sproat, R., & Fujimura, O. (1993). Allophonic variation in English /l/ and its implications for phonetic implementation. *Journal of Phonetics, 21,* 291–311.

Stampe, D. (1972). *A dissertation on natural phonology* (Doctoral dissertation). Chicago, IL: University of Chicago.

Stevens, K. N. (1972). The quantal nature of speech: Evidence from articulatory-acoustic data. In E. E. David, Jr., & P. B. Denes (Eds.), *Human communication: A unified view* (pp. 51–66). New York, NY: McGraw-Hill.

Stevens, K. N. (1989). On the quantal nature of speech. *Journal of Phonetics, 17,* 3–46.

Tjaden, K., & Sussman, J. (2006). Perception of coarticulatory information in normal speech and dysarthria. *Journal of Speech, Language, and Hearing Research, 49,* 888–902.

van Rees, L. J., Ballard, K. J., McCabe, P., Macdonald-D'Silva, A. G., & Arciuli, J. (2012). Training production of lexical stress in typically developing children using orthographically biased stimuli and principles of motor learning. *American Journal of Speech-Language Pathology, 21,* 197–206.

Velleman, S. L. (1988). The role of linguistic perception in later phonological development. *Journal of Applied Psycholinguistics, 9,* 221–236.

Vihman, M. M. (1996). *Phonological development: The origins of language in the child.* Cambridge, MA: Blackwell Publishers, Inc.

Vihman, M. M., Nakai, S., DePaolis, R. A., & Halle, P. (2004). The role of accentual pattern in early lexical representation. *Journal of Memory and Language, 50,* 336–353.

Watkins, T. A. (1993). Welsh. In M. J. Ball (Ed.), *The Celtic languages* (pp. 289–348). London: Routledge.

Williams, B. (1999). The phonetic manifestation of stress in Welsh. In H. van der Hulst (Ed.), *Word prosodic systems in the languages of Europe* (pp. 311–334). New York, NY: Mouton de Gruyter.

APPENDIX A

International Phonetic Alphabet Symbols and Diacritics Used in This Book

Note: Sounds that have the same sound as in orthographic English (e.g., "b" = [b]) are not listed here.

CONSONANTS

Orthographic Symbol	IPA Symbol	Example Word
ng	ŋ	si**ng**
y	j	**y**ou
th	θ	**th**igh
th	ð	**th**y
sh	ʃ	**sh**y
g	ʒ	bei**g**e, **g**enre
ch	ʧ	**ch**eese
j, g, dg	ʤ	**j**u**dg**e
r	ɹ	**r**ed
t, d (tap/flap allophone) (also Spanish "r")	ɾ	ba**tt**er, bla**dd**er
t (allophone), h	ʔ	uh-oh
h (English voiced glottal fricative allophone)	ɦ	**h**uge
l (English velarized liquid allophone)	ɫ	mi**l**k
m (English voiced labio-dental nasal allophone)	ɱ	co**m**fort
r (French uvular fricative)	ʁ	Pa**r**is
rr (Spanish alveolar trill)	r	pe**rr**o (dog)
f (Japanese voiceless bilabial fricative allophone)	ɸ	**f**uhai (decay)*
b (Spanish voiced bilabial fricative allophone)	β	la**b**io
ch (German voiceless palatal fricative allophone)	ç	ni**ch**t (not)*
ll (Welsh voiceless lateral fricative)	ɬ	**Ll**oyd
ch (German voiceless velar fricative)	x	a**ch** (oh)
g (Spanish voiced velar fricative)	ɣ	a**g**ua (water)
c (Zulu dental click)	ǀ	i**c**i**c**i (earring)*

*Example from en.Wikipedia.org

VOWELS

Orthographic Symbol(s)	IPA Symbol(s)	Example Word
ee, ea, ie, y	i	b**ea**d
i	ɪ	b**i**d
a, ay, ai, a_e, ey	e, eɪ	b**a**d**e**
e	ɛ	b**e**d
a	æ	b**a**d
u, oo, u_e, ew	u	br**oo**d
oo	ʊ	b**oo**k
o, as, o_e, ough, ow	o, oʊ	b**o**d**e**
aw, au, augh, ough	ɔ	b**ough**t
o, a	ɑ	b**o**p
o, a (Boston, British)	a, ɐ	b**o**p, f**a**ther
u	ʌ	b**u**t
any unstressed vowel	ə	**a**bout
er, ir, ur	ɚ (unstressed), ɝ (stressed)	butt**er**, b**ir**d
ow, ough, au	ɑʊ	b**ow**ed
i, i_e, y, uy	ɑɪ	b**i**d**e**
oi, oy	ɔɪ, oɪ	b**oy**
ear, eer, ier	ɪɚ, iɚ, ɪɹ, iɹ	b**ear**d
air, are	ɛɚ, eɚ, ɛɹ, eɹ	b**are**d
oor, ure	ʊɚ, uɚ, ʊɹ, uɹ	p**ure**
or, ore, oar	ɔɚ, oɚ, ɔɹ, oɹ	b**ore**d
ar	ɑɚ, ɑɹ	b**ar**d
u, ü (French, German high front round vowel)	y	v**u**, **ü**ber
eu, ö (French, German mid front round vowel)	ø	peu, sch**ö**n

DIACRITICS		
Acoustic Feature	**IPA Symbol**	**Example Word**
aspirated	h	tʰap (top)
unaspirated	⁼	st⁼ap (stop)
no audible release	˺	tap˺ (top)
nasalized	˜	bõn (bone)
partially devoiced	̥	bæd̥ (bad)
prolonged	ː	bæːd (bad)
labialized	w	sʷu (Sue)
break between syllables	.	bə.næ.nə (ba-na-na)
syllabic (consonant playing role of syllable nucleus)	̩	baɾl̩ (bottle)
retroflex (tongue curled back) *Note: hook added to any symbol*	ʂ	bæʂ (bass with distorted [s])

For further information about these and other IPA symbols, see: International Phonetic Association. (1999). *Handbook of the International Phonetic Association.* Cambridge, UK: Cambridge University Press.
To install an IPA font (Doulos SIL) on your computer, go to: http://scripts.sil.org/cms/scripts/page.php?site id=nrsi&id=doulossil download

CHAPTER 3

Precursors to Speech

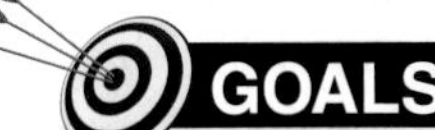

GOALS
of This Chapter

1. Identify the impacts of anatomic, motoric, sensory, cognitive-linguistic, and social precursors on speech development.
2. Describe typical developmental profiles associated with certain conditions (e.g., recurrent otitis media) and neurodevelopmental syndromes (e.g., Down syndrome).
3. Describe influential models of speech production.

Sheila has Down syndrome. At 18 months, she has successfully survived cardiac surgery, including several weeks of hospitalization. Several symptoms typical of Down syndrome remain: low muscle tone, frequent otitis media, an apparently large tongue, and a cognitive impairment. How will these features of her syndrome affect her speech development?

INTRODUCTION TO PHYSIOLOGIC, COGNITIVE, AND SOCIAL BASES FOR PHONOLOGY

From birth or even before, infants' auditory, articulatory, social, and cognitive experiences gradually build the foundation for successful, adult-like oral communication. In this chapter, we review motor, sensory, cognitive, and social precursors to oral communication—some of which have been shown to be prerequisites for speech and some of which have not. In particular, speech motor control appears to develop in parallel with non-speech motor functions, rather than being derived from them (Kent, 2009; Moore & Ruark, 1996; Ruark & Moore, 1997; Steeve, Moore, Green, Reilly, & McMurtrey, 2008; Wilson, Green, Yunusova, & Moore, 2008). Specific disorders that affect each of these precursors will be described briefly as well as general assessment and intervention considerations for children with deficits in these areas.

ANATOMIC AND MOTOR PRECURSORS

In order to produce speech typically, a person must be equipped with musculature within motor systems for respiration, phonation, resonance, and articulation that are relatively intact as well as a relatively intact sensory system. This is not enough, however; one must also have the ability to make, store, and retrieve **motor plans**; to adjust those plans according to the context; to execute those plans smoothly and rapidly; and to monitor the outcomes in order to make further adjustments if needed. This is no small feat. Furthermore, the relationships between motor systems and their functions are neither simple nor unidirectional. Different structures and systems influence each other. It is obvious that physiology affects function. But it is also the case that one's anatomy—including even the bony structures!—is shaped by the uses to which it is put (Bosma, 1975, as cited by Kent, 2009). Relationships between motor control and cognitive and communication skills are also complex. For example, **specific language impairment** and even dyslexia are often accompanied by motor immaturity,

COMMON *Confusion*

PRECURSORS VERSUS PREREQUISITES

The division of this chapter into specific types of **precursors** to speech should not be taken to imply that deficits—in particular, precursors—occur in isolation from each other, that they do not interact in important ways, or on the other hand that one particular precursor predetermines the others. Precursors should not be confused with **prerequisites**. Precursors are conditions that precede others, but they may or may not be required for the (typical) development of other conditions or abilities. For example, Cleland, Wood, Hardcastle, Wishart, and Timmins (2010) demonstrate that although children with **Down syndrome** typically demonstrate deficits in speech, oromotor, language, and cognitive abilities, these typically are not correlated with each other. Although these factors no doubt interact within the individual child's development, each also makes its own contribution to the resulting child-specific communication profile. Prerequisites, on the other hand, are conditions that are required for other aspects of development. For example, Bates (2004) proposes that certain very basic cognitive skills, such as cross-modal perception, are required for the ability to imitate, which is in turn required for communication development.

especially in younger children (Bishop, 2002; Webster, Erdos, Evans, Majnemer, Kehayia, et al., 2006; Zelaznik & Goffman, 2010).

Motor Programming and Planning

What does it mean to make, store, retrieve, adjust, execute, and monitor a motor plan? To speak a word, one must be able to identify the required set of target articulatory configurations (i.e., the oral gestures corresponding to each sound in the word), including their relative sequences, timings, and placements and their relative intensities, durations, and forces. Before beginning to speak, the person must also determine the current state of the articulators and compute the trajectory from there to the first sound in the word as well as determining any other factors that may impact either the listener's needs or her own performance. Only then is she ready to send the appropriate set of signals to the relevant muscles. As the word is produced, she must also monitor the results and adjust the commands as needed if things have gone awry. Motor planning refers to generating that appropriate set of signals to be sent to the muscles. It is the result of a dynamic, complex, context-specific process that includes coarticulation—the **transitions** from one articulatory configuration to the next. Initially, for a new task (e.g., repeating an unfamiliar word), the motor plan will be constructed from scratch. If it is needed a second time, it will be recalled for reuse through motor memory. With repeated productions, the motor plan will be refined.

A **motor program** is an abstract set of motor commands that is "at the ready" to be adapted to a particular task (Maas, Robin, Austermann Hula, Freedman, et al., 2008). The motor program is generalized from the repeated use of a motor plan or a set of similar or related motor plans. In addition, when a series of motor tasks is consistently used to perform a larger motor task, those motor plans are chunked together into an even more abstract generalized motor program (Schmidt & Lee, 2005). Initially, each plan may be specific to an individual action in a unique context because the person (e.g., an infant) may have very few experiences to generalize from and few related plans to chunk together into a less specific program. Over time, the programs will become more and more abstract as the person generalizes and chunks them. At the same time, he will become increasingly expert at adjusting a general motor program to particular circumstances, developing a specific motor plan for that action at that instant in time. This expertise reflects increases in speed, accuracy, and ability to adjust online while developing or carrying out each new motor plan, resulting from his motor memory of many similar tasks. For example, a generalized walking motor program may be invoked each time a person wants to take a step. However, that program will need to be specifically tailored to many factors in any given instance: the terrain, the status of the person's body (barefoot or wearing shoes, healthy or injured, fresh or fatigued, etc.), the intended pace and distance, and so on.

The terms "motor program" and "motor plan" may seem to imply fixed entities, like musical scores; it's important to remember that they refer to complex, dynamic, interactive processes. This imperfect terminology represents an attempt to model the fact that movement skill grows from rigid automatic movement patterns to flexible, dynamic, responses to goals and contexts; from simpler patterns to more complex patterns; and from isolated movements to more integrated movement patterns, as summarized in Figure 3-1.

Thus, a specific motor plan is assembled for the execution of the general task in each particular set of circumstances. Each time the program is used to develop and

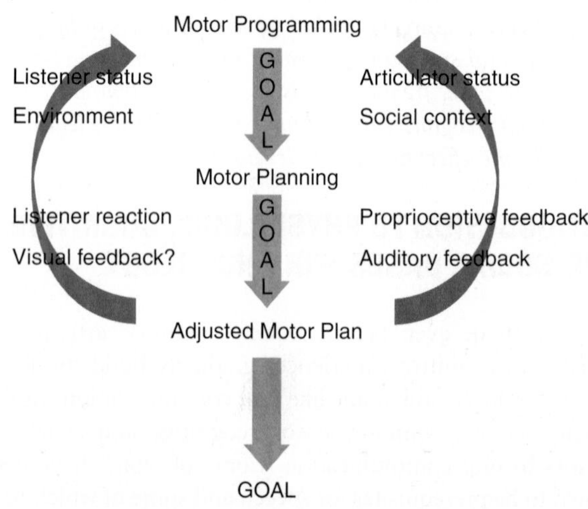

FIGURE 3-1. Motor programming and planning.

implement an instance-specific motor plan, the program may be modified as learning occurs based on the outcome of the action. For example, as a baby learns from reaching for various objects in various types of circumstances, the planning process for reaching will become more flexible and efficient, such that the outcome of his reaches will become more consistent regardless of the various factors that may have to be taken into account. In short, the motor program is general and abstract; the motor plan is specific to a given context. Over time, the child develops both broadly applicable motor programs and the ability to adjust them efficiently and quickly to the particular situation. These adjustments eventually result in high levels of coarticulation, which reflects increased motor efficiency. Recall, however, that coarticulation is language-specific as well as motorically advantageous. Thus, even this very motoric aspect of speech production has a cognitive component.

In addition to limited (but not absent) awareness of the rule-based patterns of their own languages, infants initially have a restricted set of motor options. They typically have little control over their lips and tongues; the lips may not be independent from each other or from their jaws. As a result, their first speech sounds may be dependent upon jaw movement (Davis & MacNeilage, 1995; Green, Moore, Higashikawa, & Steeve, 2000; Wilson & Nip, 2010). In addition, research shows that young children's speech production is highly variable, especially when the target is linguistically complex; motor programs and motor planning processes continue to be perfected through late adolescence (Sadagopan & Smith, 2008; Smith & Zelaznik, 2004).

It is beyond the scope of this book to review the entire anatomy and physiology of the speech and hearing mechanism. Instead, we will focus on a few key systems and their development, referring to some of the **syndromes** and disorders as a result of which these systems are likely to be impaired, as we go along. Then, a few of the most prominent models of the motor speech production system will be reviewed.

Infant Versus Adult Resonatory and Articulatory Anatomy and Physiology

Neonatal respiration differs from that of older infants, children, and adults with respect to the anatomy and physiology of the rib cage and the diaphragm. Neonates' rib cages are softer—primarily composed of cartilage—and angled at almost 90 degrees to the spine, as illustrated in Figure 3-2. Thus, the ribs are rounded and raised, and the diaphragm is relatively flat in comparison to the position that these structures will gradually, naturally assume once the baby begins to sit upright, the ribs stiffen and lower, and the respiratory muscles increase in bulk (Gaultier, 1995).

The position of the larynx also differs at birth; it sits high in the pharynx near the soft palate, protecting the infant

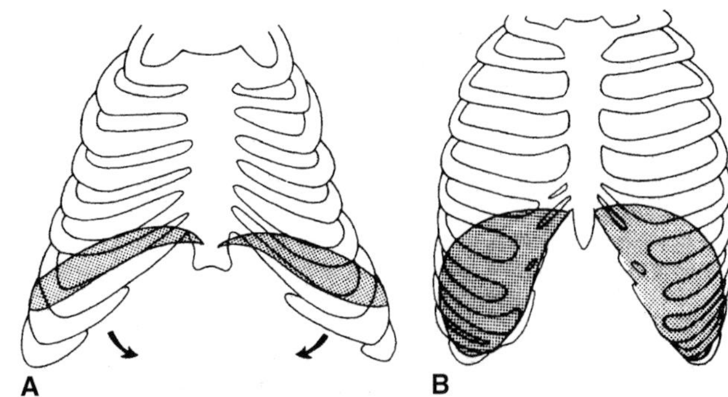

FIGURE 3-2. Infant **(A)** versus adult **(B)** rib cage.

from aspiration and forcing her to breathe nasally. It moves downward slightly when the infant vocalizes to permit oral airflow (German & Palmer, 2006). From infancy, the vocal folds also lengthen. As different portions of the vocal tract grow at varying rates, the relative proportions of the larynx shift (Vorperian, Kent, Lindstrom, Kalina, Gentry, et al., 2005). The larynx gradually descends to its adult location in a process that can take up to the age of 6 years to complete (Crelin, 1987). The infant versus adult resonatory cavities are compared in Figure 3-3.

Similarly, the tongue, which is disproportionately large for the oral area, sits back in the mouth near the velum. In this position, the tongue dorsum (back) is in contact with the short, lower, wider hard palate, facilitating sucking and contributing to the need for nasal breathing (Crelin, 1973). This tongue position accounts for the common perception that young infants say "goo goo;" with the tongue dorsum so close to the velum, a velar-like sound is the only type of **closant** (consonant-like sound) that can be produced and the **vocant** (vowel-like sound) portion is most likely to be similar to a high back vowel. The tongue dorsum also gradually lowers to its adult-like position within the first 6 years of life (Crelin, 1973). The palate increases in width and height to 80% of adult size by the age of 18 months (Vorperian et al., 2005), yielding a larger oral cavity, and the tongue tip elongates while the nerves serving the intrinsic tongue muscles **myelinate** (become covered with an insulating material that causes nerve impulses to travel more quickly). These changes result in greater independence of different portions of the tongue (Gibbon, 1999).

Reflexes

By birth, infants benefit from a set of reflexes that provide automatic responses to a variety of stimuli, including body positioning. The most commonly noted oral reflexes include the following, which foster feeding:

- **Rooting reflex**: As shown in Figure 3-4, the orientation of the head in the direction of a light touch stimulus in the peri-oral area, typically followed or accompanied by mouth opening and sucking or swallowing movements (Sheppard & Mysak, 1984; Woolridge, 1986)

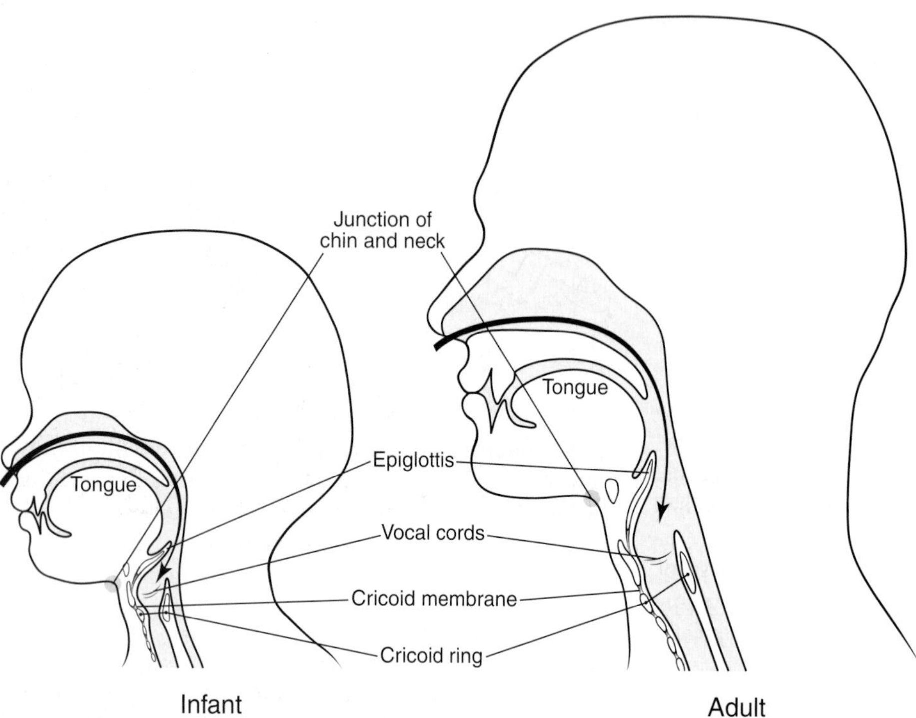

FIGURE 3-3. The infant versus adult airway.

- **Sucking reflex**: As shown in Figure 3-5, sucking movements stimulated by touch on the palate (Woolridge, 1986)
- **Biting reflex**: Mouth closing in response to light touch on the anterior gingiva (gums) (Sheppard & Mysak, 1984)

Normally, many innate reflexes are gradually suppressed, replaced by more mature, often volitional (conscious, deliberate) responses to stimuli. For example, in typically developing children, the rooting and biting reflexes become more difficult to observe after about 5 months of age, yet they persist in more subtle forms up to about 8 months (Sheppard & Mysak, 1984). Some children with neonatal disorders, such as **cerebral palsy**, Down syndrome, and **Angelman syndrome**, may demonstrate increased or decreased reflexes or the persistence of infantile reflexes to much later ages (Arvedson, 2000; Hennequin, Faulks, Veyrune, & Bourdiol, 1999). Differences in the development and expressions of reflexes may even occur in less apparently physiologic disorders, such as autism (Teitelbaum, Teitelbaum, Fryman, & Maurer, 2002).

However, this is not the whole story about reflexes. More recent studies have suggested that some reflex responses—such as the jaw stretch reflex (which is manifested by jaw closing when the area below the lower lip is tapped)—actually increase, then decrease again in the early school years (Smith, 2010). Children with **speech delays** may have less extensive reflex responses to stimulation (Wood & Smith,

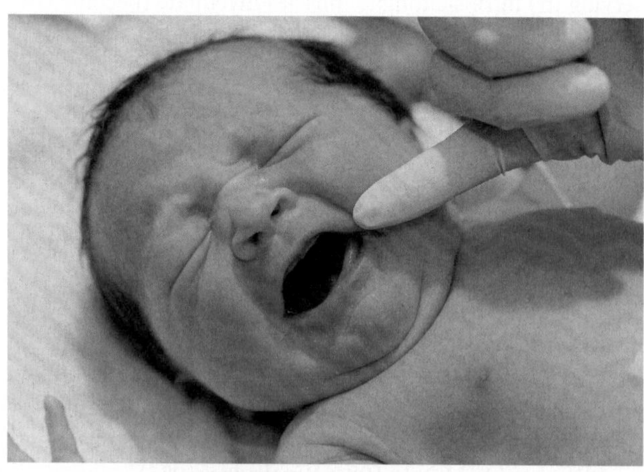

FIGURE 3-4. Rooting reflex.

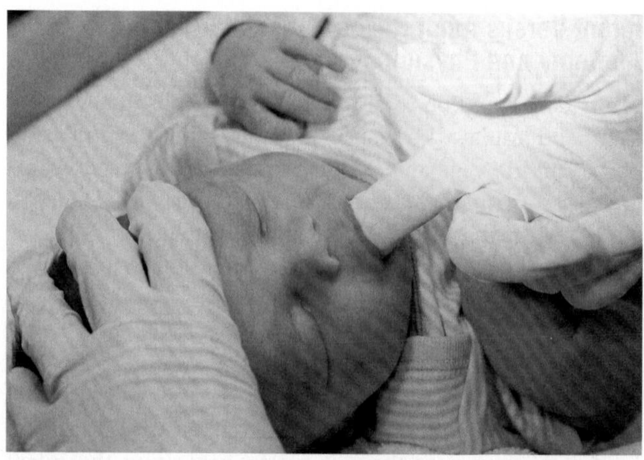

FIGURE 3-5. Sucking reflex.

1992). The exact significance of these findings for speech development is unclear to date.

Muscle Tone

Muscle tone is also key to normal motor function. Through the process of muscle innervation, the muscles are activated by the appropriate motor neurons. Muscle tone refers to the muscles' readiness when they are at rest to respond to these incoming stimuli, a state of partial contraction. If the muscles are either completely lax (i.e., totally uncontracted) or tight (i.e., fully contracted), they will not be able to respond promptly or appropriately to the body's changing needs. Note that muscle tone is not the same as muscle strength, which comes into play when the muscles are actually active. Muscle weakness may be due to either too few muscle fibers (atrophy) or inadequate activation of the muscles (perhaps due to a neuronal disorder or blockage). Low tone (hypotonia), high tone (hypertonia or spasticity), and fluctuating tone are seen in children with various genetic syndromes (e.g., Down syndrome, **achondroplasia, familial dysautonomia, Marfan syndrome, Prader-Willi syndrome, Tay-Sachs disease, Werdnig-Hoffmann disease, muscular dystrophy, Duchenne dystrophy, spinal muscular atrophy**), perinatal trauma (e.g., perinatal stroke, hypoxia; cerebral palsy), or prematurity. In fact, muscle tone abnormalities are also common in children with autism spectrum disorders, especially when they are young (Flanagan, Landa, Bhat, & Bauman, 2012; Ming, Brimacombe, & Wagner, 2007).

Low tone results in muscles that are too "floppy;" they are not ready to perform precise movements with high degrees of accuracy. Features that typically accompany low tone include slow reflexes; a sagging posture with a resultant tendency to lean to help support the body; hyper-flexible joints; "w-sitting" (i.e., sitting flat with the feet bent back at the knees, as shown in Figure 3-6); and drooling with slight tongue protrusion. The overall appearance is of weakness and poorly defined muscles, as shown in Figure 3-7. However, some

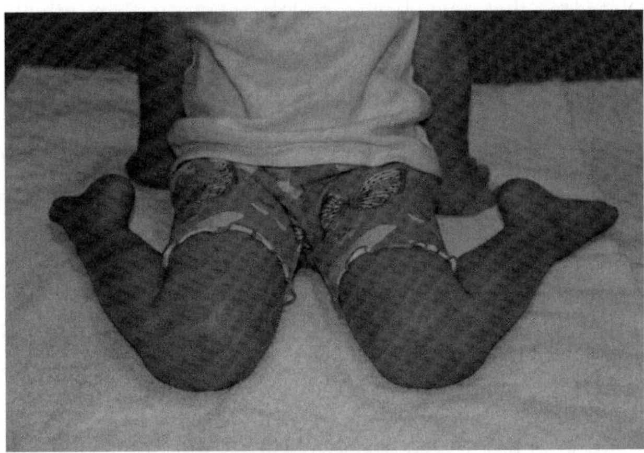

FIGURE 3-6. "W-sitting."

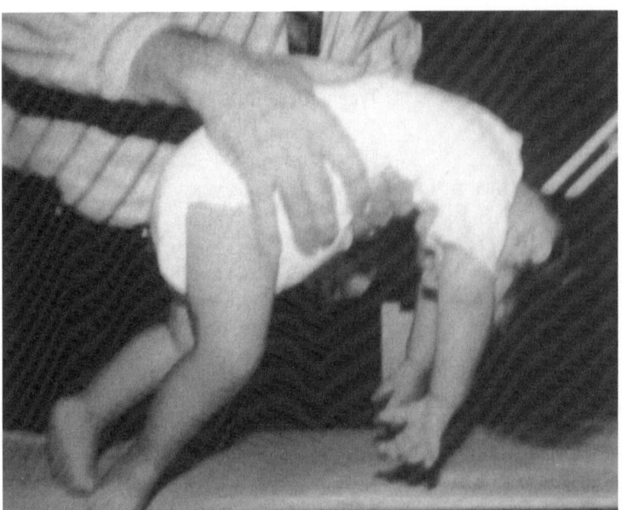

FIGURE 3-7. Hypotonia.

compensatory strategies—such as hiking the shoulders up to support the neck—may be deceptive because they appear to be more effortful than the posture of a child with typical tone. Hypotonia is commonly associated with Down syndrome and Williams syndrome as well as some forms of cerebral palsy.

High tone results in muscles that are tensed at rest, resulting in restricted ranges of movement and decreased flexibility. A person with hypertonia has the appearance of being "tightly wound." Muscles and joints are stiff, and reflexes may be exaggerated. High tone is a defining characteristic of spastic cerebral palsy. Fluctuating tone, a characteristic of **athetoid cerebral palsy** (Kent & Netsell, 1978), is diagnosed when the infant's tone varies unpredictably from low to normal to high over time.

Dysarthria

The motor speech disorders that result from the medical conditions and events mentioned in the "Muscle Tone" section, as well as many other disorders not so listed, are often grouped together as the dysarthrias. Childhood dysarthria is a neurologically based disorder that results in decreased control of speech. It may be caused by brain damage before, during, or after birth through early childhood, and it "affects the tone, power and coordination of any or all of the muscles used for speech" (Pennington, Miller, & Robson, 2010, p. 10). The dysarthrias are characterized by deficits in respiration, phonation, articulation, resonance, and/or prosody as a result of damage or difference in a variety of neuromotor systems, as listed in Table 3-1. As noted in this table, the majority of types of dysarthria result in articulatory imprecision (distortions) and omissions of speech sounds (Pennington et al., 2010), often due to abnormalities in the motor neurons that provide information to the tongue (Chen & Stevens, 2001; Tomik, Krupinski, Glodzik-Sobanska, Bala-Slodowska, Wszolek, Kusiak, et al., 1999). Several types of dysarthria also cause prosody and

TABLE 3-1 **Dysarthrias**

Affected Area	Type of Dysarthria	Respiratory Symptoms	Phonatory Symptoms	Articulatory Symptoms	Resonance, Prosodic Symptoms
Lower motor neuron; cranial nerves	Flaccid (e.g., bulbar palsy)	Breathiness	Breathiness	Imprecise consonants	Hypernasality
Upper motor neuron	Spastic (e.g., pseudobulbar palsy)		Monopitch	Imprecise consonants	Reduced stress; slow rate; hypernasality
Cerebellum	Ataxic		Phonatory insufficiency	Imprecise consonants	Excess–equal stress, irregular articulatory breakdowns
Extrapyramidal system	Hypokinetic (e.g., Parkinson disease)	Monoloudness	Monopitch		Reduced stress
Extrapyramidal system	Hyperkinetic (e.g., chorea, dystonia)		Harsh voice quality	Imprecise consonants, distorted vowels	Variable rate with prolonged intervals
Mixed	Mixed (e.g., amyotrophic lateral sclerosis)		Harsh voice quality	Imprecise consonants	Hypernasality

Adapted from Darley, F., Aronson, A., & Brown, J. (1975). *Motor speech disorders.* Philadelphia, PA: Saunders.

resonance disorders, especially with respect to stress and nasality. Speech rate is often slow or irregular (Laures & Weismer, 1999; Tjaden, Rivera, Wilding, & Turner, 2005), resulting in part from inadequate respiratory volumes (Pennington et al., 2010). Athetoid cerebral palsy, which may result from **bilirubin** abnormalities or **anoxia**, is particularly challenging, given that it is characterized by unbalanced, fluctuating muscle tone. This can lead to persistent reflexes, spasms, and jerky, extreme movements. For these reasons, children with this type of cerebral palsy may have difficulty controlling their jaws, lips, tongues, and velopharynxes, resulting in imprecise, variable, slow speech with inappropriate nasality (Kent & Netsell, 1978). There is a wide range of severity levels of cerebral palsy that may occur, from speech that is slightly slurred and pitch that is atypically low to a complete inability to produce intelligible speech (Pennington et al., 2010).

Spastic cerebral palsy, the most common type, is associated with decreases in motor control but also with decreases in cognitive ability. These two are correlated, but the half of children with CP whose intelligence is within normal limits demonstrate motor control deficits nonetheless. Their speech intelligibility levels may not be directly related to their scores on standardized tests of motor speech skill (Chen, Lin, Chen, Chen, Liu, et al., 2010).

Pennington and colleagues' (2010) study based on a systematic review of the literature suggests that some types of speech-based intervention may result in improved intelligibility and/or vocal clarity and quality, while non-speech exercises appear to have no positive effects on speech. Further in-depth discussion of the specific features of various types of dysarthria or of assessment and treatment approaches and techniques for these disorders is beyond the scope of this book. However, some differentially diagnostic features of the dysarthrias, including appropriate identification or intervention strategies, will be referenced elsewhere as appropriate.

Key Communication-Related Motor Systems and Disorders

The four motor systems that are key to oral communication are respiration, resonance, phonation, and articulation; prosody depends upon the intact functioning of all four of these. As noted above, each of these is immature anatomically, physiologically, or both at birth, rendering adult-like speech physically impossible as well as cognitively out of reach. Certain genetic syndromes, other birth defects, and early-acquired disorders may impact these systems.

Respiratory Disorders

Disorders that may have enough impact on an infant's respiratory function to affect speech include cerebral palsy (Solomon & Charron, 1998) and **broncho-pulmonary dysplasia** (Lewis, Singer, Fulton, Salvator, Short, et al., 2002), a pulmonary disorder that can result from incomplete lung development in infants born prematurely. Many neuromuscular problems, such as **spina bifida** and muscular dystrophy, also affect respiratory function.

Anatomically Based Resonatory and Articulatory Disorders

Cleft Palate

Some children have cleft palate, **submucous clefts**, or **velopharyngeal insufficiency** with the hypernasality that accompanies these physiologic differences, which are

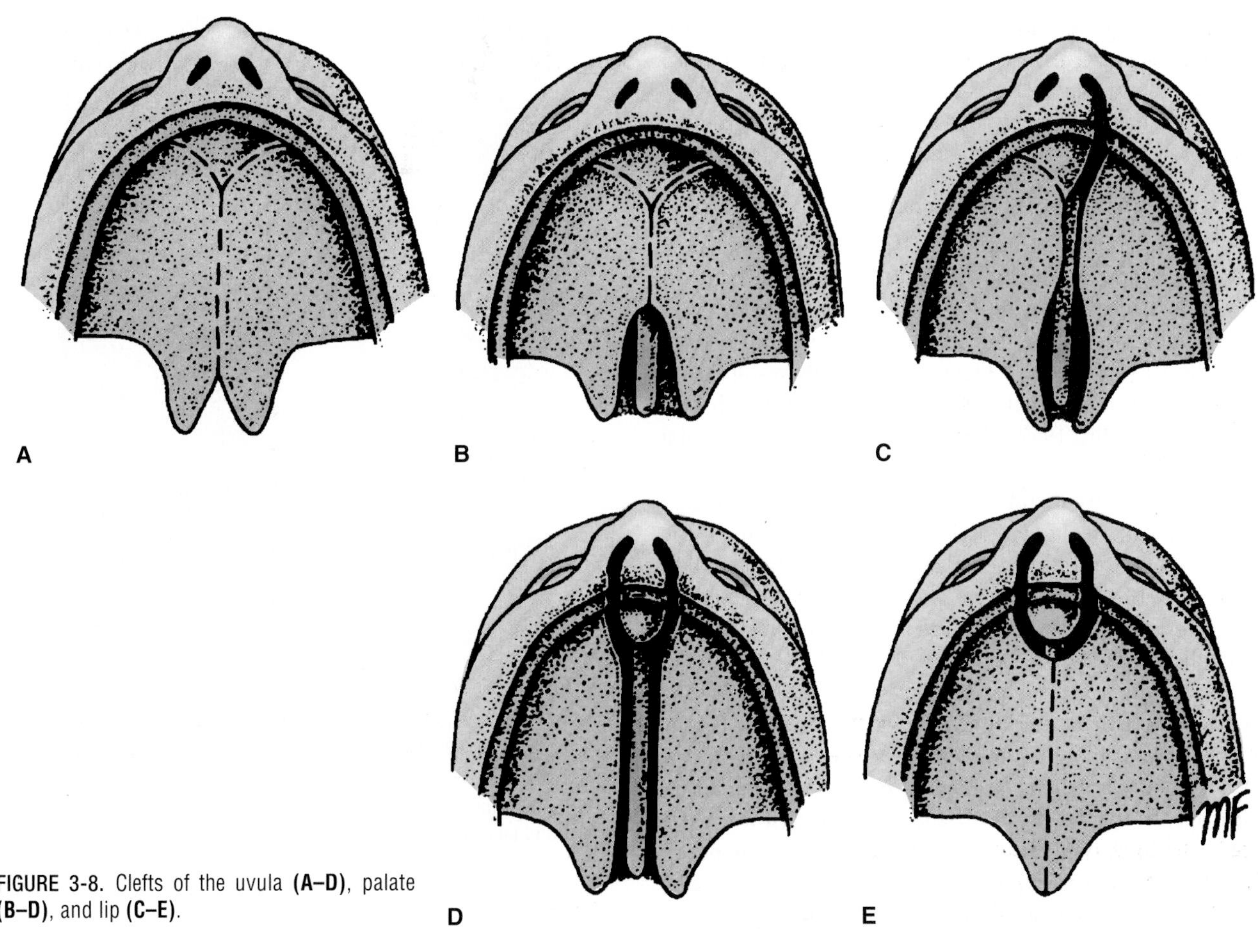

FIGURE 3-8. Clefts of the uvula **(A–D)**, palate **(B–D)**, and lip **(C–E)**.

illustrated in Figure 3-8. This hypernasality results from leakage of air through the nasal cavity because raising the velum does not completely close off this large resonant chamber. The most common, yet often unidentified, cause of hypernasality is **velocardiofacial syndrome (VCF)**, which is caused by a chromosomal deletion at 22q.11 (i.e., from the long arm of the 22nd chromosome). In addition to hypernasality and decreased intra-oral pressure (often leading to difficulties in the production of [s] and [ʃ]), children with VCF often demonstrate compensatory articulatory errors as well as phonological deficits or motor speech disorders (dysarthria, apraxia) not directly attributable to their palatal differences (Carnoel, Marks, & Weik, 1999; Kummer, Lee, Stutz, Maroney, & Brandt, 2007). However, although they do demonstrate decreased nonverbal intelligence, their articulatory deficits do not appear to be related to decreased speech perception skills or decreased ability to learn new words (Baylis, Munson, & Moller, 2008). Thus, although the assessment and treatment of cleft lip and palate per se are well beyond the scope of this book, much of the material included here on SSDs, including motor speech disorders, may be relevant to some children with palatal differences.

The Impact of Palatal Structure on Articulatory Disorders

Children with certain disorders (e.g., Prader-Willi syndrome: Edmonston, 1982; **de Lange syndrome**: Cameron & Kelly, 1988; **Laurence-Moon-Biedl syndrome**: Garstecki, Borton, Stark, & Kennedy, 1972; **Sotos syndrome**: Shuey & Jamison, 1996; **Noonan syndrome**: Hopkins-Acos & Bunker, 1979) or who are intubated for long periods of time immediately after birth may have very high-arched palates. Many of these conditions (e.g., Prader-Willi, de Lange, Laurence-Moon-Biedl, Sotos, and Noonan syndromes) are also associated with speech delay or articulatory impairments. Typical adult speakers compensate for widely varying oral dimensions by adjusting tongue height to palate height (Hasegawa-Johnson, Pizza, Alwan, Cha, & Haker, 2003). However, refinements in tongue–palate contact patterns for anterior (e.g., alveolar) versus non-anterior (e.g., velar) consonants in various coarticulatory contexts continue to be made by children into young adulthood (Cheng, Murdoch, Goozee, & Scott, 2007). It is not known whether or how children with syndromes or prematurity respond physiologically to the presence of a high-arched palate, nor whether or how this affects their speech. However, children with articulatory/phonological disorders have been shown to produce less distinct tongue–palate contact patterns than do children whose speech is developing normally, most likely due to decreased independent control of different portions of the tongue (medial and lateral margins as well as the tip, blade, and body; Gibbon, 1999). Therefore, it is reasonable to assume that children are less adept than adults at compensating for a high-arched palate.

The Articulatory Anatomy of Down Syndrome

Children with Down syndrome (DS) typically have short hard palates and unusually small oral cavities. In contrast to popular belief, however, their tongues (and lower jaws) are normally sized. The perception that their tongues are unusually large, as seen in Figure 3-9, actually results from the sizes of the smaller than typical oral cavities in which they are housed (Crelin, 1987) as well as from their low lingual tone.

The facial musculature of people with Down syndrome is also atypical; one large muscle mass replaces many of the individual muscles in the typical face (Bersu & Opitz, 1980), as Figure 3-10 illustrates. This results in far less flexibility with regard to facial expression and fine motor control of the lips (Miller & Leddy, 1998).

In addition to the size mismatch and the muscle differences, the articulation difficulties of those with DS may also be affected by oral–motor problems, hearing loss, linguistic–cognitive deficits, sequential processing difficulties, motor speech deficits (dysarthria resulting from low muscle tone; sometimes symptoms of Childhood Apraxia of Speech [CAS]), and/or altered parental input resulting from different patterns of infant–toddler responsiveness (Rupela & Manjula, 2007; Swift & Rosin, 1990; Velleman, Mangipudi, & Locke, 1989).

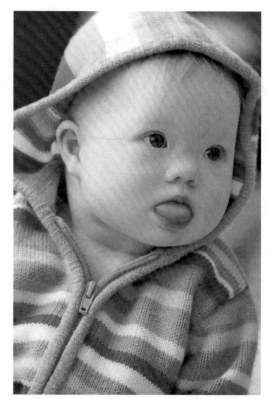

FIGURE 3-9. Down syndrome child. Note the epicanthal folds of the eye, round face, and depressed nasal bridge, all typical features of Down syndrome.

Articulatory Physiology of Moebius Syndrome

Moebius syndrome, which has no consistent genetic basis (National Institutes of Health, N.D.), affects cranial nerves VI and VII, resulting in complete or partial paralysis of the facial nerve, sometimes accompanied by palsy of the ocular (VI), trigeminal (V), vagus (X), or glossopharyngeal (IX) nerves; hypoplasia of the tongue (paralysis of nerve XII); and oral–facial anomalies. Thus, the eyes, lips, tongue, palate, ears, and even the larynx may be affected. These features lead to limitations or inability to move the facial muscles for smiling, frowning, blinking, sucking, and speech (Kumar, 1990). Figure 3-11 shows the face of a child with this syndrome.

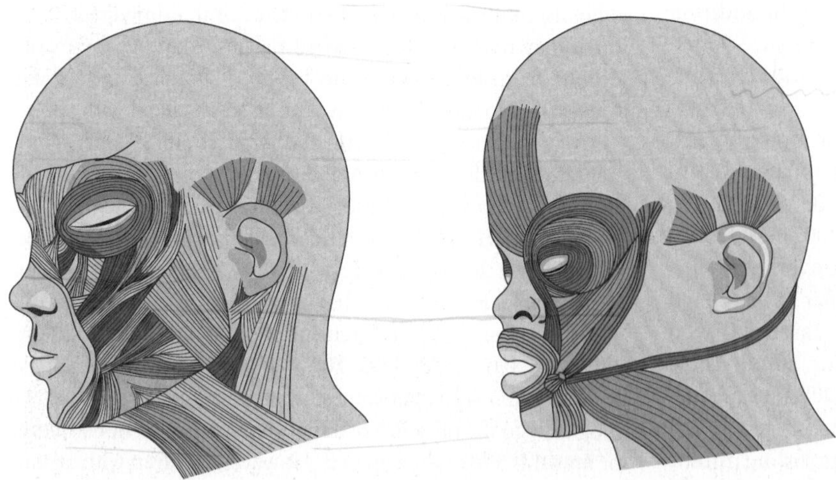

FIGURE 3-10. Typical facial muscles versus facial muscles of person with Down syndrome.

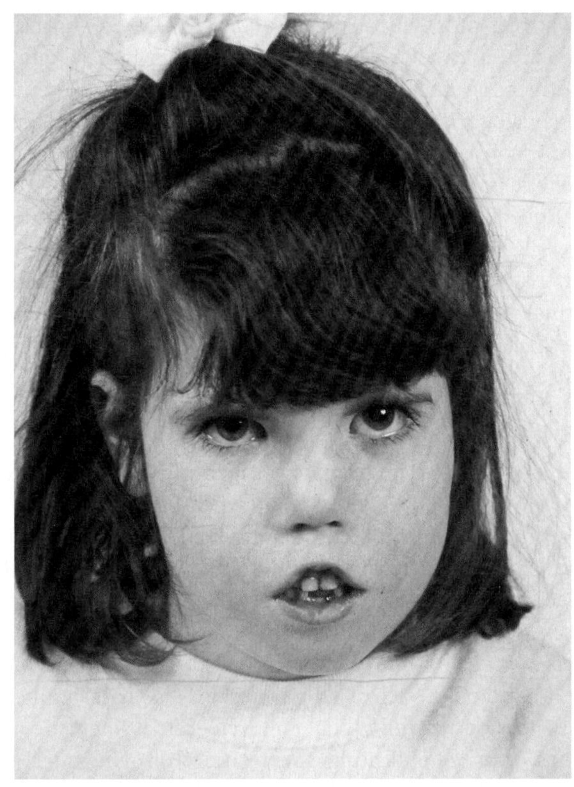

FIGURE 3-11. Moebius syndrome.

Tongue Tie (Ankyloglossia)

"Much entertaining nonsense has been written about tongue-tie" (Wallace, 1963 quoted without page number by Lalakea & Messner, 2003). The surgery used to release tongues restricted by short **lingual frenula** (a.k.a. frenulums), as shown in Figure 3-12, has apparently been in use since biblical times. In the Bible, Mark (7:35) tells us that "... the string of his tongue was loosened and he spoke plain" (King James Version). Tongue tie does affect breast feeding about 25% of the time, but typically does not impede bottle feeding. As of 2000, about 50% of speech-language pathologists believed that ankyloglossia can cause speech production problems. In one recent study, 71% of children with tongue tie did have resulting speech articulation problems, as determined by speech-language pathologists. However, tongue tie did not cause language delay in any cases (Messner & Lalakea, 2002).

In this study, the extent to which the child was able to protrude his or her tongue—sometimes used as a diagnostic measure—was *not* a reliable indicator of whether or not there would be a speech problem. **Interincisal distance**—the distance between the upper and lower teeth when the child opens his mouth as far as possible with the tongue tip on the upper teeth—was more prognostic. Furthermore, the percentage of children whose problems might have resolved without surgery is unclear. Finally, it is important to note that the full effects of clipping the lingual frenulum may not be evident until one to three months after the surgery and that tongue exercises must be performed post-operatively to avoid scarring that may restrict the tongue just as much as the tight frenulum previously did (Messner & Lalakea, 2002).

In short, the decision about whether or not to clip the lingual frenulum is a knotty problem that should not be undertaken lightly. This author's conclusion from her review of the literature (summarized in the paragraph above) is that there is not enough evidence to determine best practice at this time. Until further research is performed, a knowledgeable physician, a lactation expert, and/or an experienced speech-language pathologist (depending upon the age of the child) should be involved in the decision. If clipping is the option of choice, care should be taken to ensure that follow-up exercises are carried out under appropriate supervision.

For information about other genetic syndromes and medical conditions affecting the anatomic and physiologic

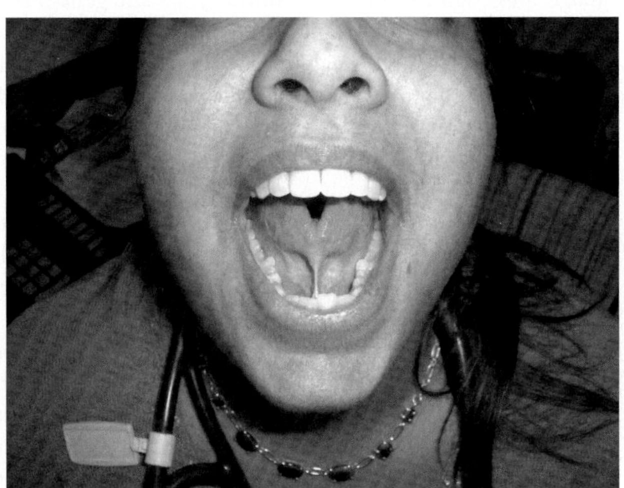

A

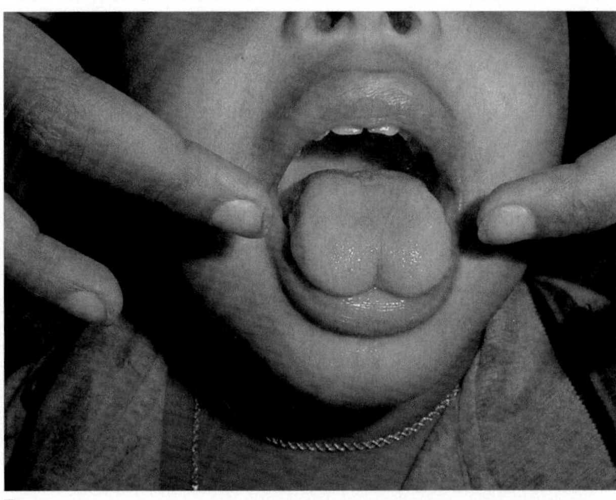

B

FIGURE 3-12. Ankyloglossia: short frenulum **(A)** and restricted tongue tip **(B)**.

underpinnings of speech, readers are encouraged to consult Robin (2008), Shprintzen (2000), and similar references.

Summary

Speech accuracy, fluency, and rate can depend on many factors, including the ability to formulate, refine, and tailor motor programs, implementing and adjusting them (as motor plans) for the specific linguistic, social, and articulatory circumstances. Fluent speech is characterized by high levels of learned coarticulation that listeners use to decompose the intended message. Purely physical/motoric factors that may interfere with the efficient and effective functioning of the motor speech system include age-inappropriate reflexes; reduced or increased muscle tone; impaired cranial nerves; and anatomic differences such as the relative sizes and shapes of various structures (e.g., tongue, jaw, palatal arch) and the configuration of the oral muscles.

EXERCISE 3-1

Anatomy/Physiology and Motor Functions/Differences

Sensory Functioning

Hearing

Clearly, auditory input is crucial for oral speech development. It is extremely difficult to learn to speak a language that one cannot hear (or see, in the case of sign languages). Even decreased hearing levels cause concern if they are ongoing (Ambrose, Berry, Walker, Harrison, Oleson, et al., 2014; Harrison & McLeod, 2010). The idea that **recurrent otitis media** (OM, i.e., ear infections), which results in a fluctuating conductive hearing loss, can impact a child's later speech has been around since 1969 or earlier (Shriberg, Flipsen, Thielke, Kwiatkowski, Kertoy, et al., 2000a). The impacts of OM on linguistic processing are significant but complex.

The effects of OM on speech can be immediate. Rvachew, Slawinski, Williams, and Green (1999b) found that infants with OM before 6 months produced less **canonical babble** (babble composed of consonant + vowel syllables) than do infants who did not experience OM until later. Furthermore, there was a correlation between canonical babble and later expressive vocabulary (at 18 months), indicating that the impact of early OM is far-reaching. This long-term impact of OM has been demonstrated in many studies.

Mody, Schwartz, Gravel, and Ruben (1999) compared 9-year-olds with and without histories of OM and found that those with the condition performed somewhat worse on both speech perception and verbal memory tasks, although both their patterns of errors and the factors that increased their errors (e.g., phonetic similarity) were similar. Likewise, Groenen, Crul, Maassen, and van Bon (1996) reported that 9-year-olds with histories of severe OM demonstrated poorer performance on speech perception tasks requiring identification and discrimination of voicing cues. The children's categorizations of voiced versus voiceless phonemes were inconsistent. The authors concluded that OM affects phonetic processing.

Roberts (1997) noted effects of OM on speech processing as early as 14 to 16 months. He found that despite the fact that the children's hearing was reported to be within normal limits at the time of the study, infants at that age with histories of OM were less able to use the presence of the unstressed article "the" as a cue to an upcoming noun than infants whose hearing had never been compromised.

This early impact of OM on syntactic processing may help elucidate the findings of Shriberg, Friel-Patti, Flipsen, and Brown (2000b) that a child's hearing levels at 12 to 18 months (i.e., decreased or not depending on the occurrence of OM) don't have a simple, direct impact on later speech and language. The effect of OM-induced hearing losses was significant with children with lowered hearing levels being at 16 times greater risk of speech-language delay, but other factors such as language skills also had significant influences on the individual children's actual linguistic outcomes, thus complicating the relationship. Nittrouer and Burton (2005) similarly found that children with chronic OM with effusion (fluid) demonstrated decreases in comprehension of complex sentences as well as poorer phonemic and syllable awareness, immature speech perception, and reduced ability to recall word lists. **Socioeconomic status** (SES) exacerbated the effects of the OM.

Paradise, Dollaghan, Campbell, Feldman, Bernard, and team (2000) reported even more striking effects of income levels than of remediation of OM. Their results indicated no difference between not treating ongoing middle ear effusion versus placement of tubes to relieve OM with respect to improvement in 3-year-olds' speech, language, and cognitive skills. In contrast, SES and gender had striking effects on the participants' performance in these areas. Paradise and colleagues concluded that "In children younger than 3 years of age who have persistent OM, prompt insertion of tympanostomy tubes does not measurably improve developmental outcomes at the age of 3 years" (p. 1179).

Other types of hearing loss have more clear-cut effects than OM. Overall, 70 2-year-olds fitted for hearing aids with mild to severe **sensorineural** or permanent conductive hearing loss (25 to 75 dB HL in the better ear) in a recent study demonstrated delayed but parallel acquisition of consonants in comparison to typically developing peers (Ambrose et al., 2014). However, they were more likely to demonstrate final consonant deletion, indicating that not all aspects of their development were merely delayed. Not surprisingly, age of the hearing aid fitting (the younger the better), gender (with an advantage for females), and pure tone average were positive predictors of speech performance. Both the ages at which they were fitted with hearing aids and their percentages of both consonants and vowels correct at age 2 were predictive of their performance on the same measures at age 3. This indicates that early attention to speech production deficits is vital in children with hearing aids (Ambrose et al., 2014).

In another study, infants with bilateral sensorineural hearing loss (**pure tone average** for better ear 38 to 97 dB; for worse ear 45 to 107 dB) demonstrated delayed consistent canonical babble, smaller consonant inventories, and delays in the development of more mature syllable shapes. They also developed fricatives and affricates more slowly than other children and than would be expected given their other phonological skills (Moeller, Hoover, Putman, Arbataitis, Bohnenkamp, et al., 2007). The phonetic repertoires of such children are typified by labial consonants (which are more visible than others) and neutral vowels (Warner-Czyz, Davis, & Morrison, 2005). Even those who receive hearing aids early on demonstrate these delays to an extent that can be predicted by their unaided pure tone averages (von Hapsburg & Davis, 2006). Twenty-four-month-olds with bilateral sensorineural hearing loss demonstrate smaller expressive vocabularies, including fewer recognizable words. "Early measures of syllable production predicted unique variance in later speech production and vocabulary outcomes" (Moeller et al., 2007, p. 628). That is, reduced babble production in such children presaged deficits in speech and semantic development. However, these children's delays were less extreme than those reported a decade or more ago when sensorineural hearing loss was less likely to be detected at such early ages. This implies that intervention does have a positive impact.

Older children with slight or mild bilateral sensorineural hearing loss exhibit receptive and expressive language skills within normal limits, but their phonological memory and phonological discrimination skills are reduced in comparison to those of normally hearing peers (Wake, Tobin, Cone-Wesson, Dahl, Gillam, et al., 2006). Children between the ages of 6 and 14 who have mild to moderate sensorineural hearing loss also perform less well on frequency discrimination, nonword repetition, and word reading than their normally hearing peers, although word reading may nonetheless fall within normal limits (Halliday & Bishop, 2005).

With the advent of **cochlear implants** (shown in Fig. 3-13), the outcomes of children with more significant hearing loss have significantly improved. These surgically implanted electronic devices replace non-functioning hair cells to provide an altered yet often functional type of hearing to those with severe to profound hearing impairments. Implantation has been shown to improve both children's speech perception (Blamey, Barry, & Jacq, 2001) and language development (Dawson, Blamey, Dettman, Barker, & Clark, 1995; Miyamoto, Svirsky, & Robbins, 1997). Children who undergo this procedure typically begin to babble within two to six months of receiving the implant. Phonetic repertoires gradually diversify over the first several months following implantation, although accuracy may still be quite decreased. After about nine months, vowel accuracy improves (Warner-Czyz et al., 2005), with consonant accuracy gradually increasing thereafter. Children who are implanted at earlier ages develop more quickly (Schwauwers, Taelman, Gillis, & Govaerts, 2006).

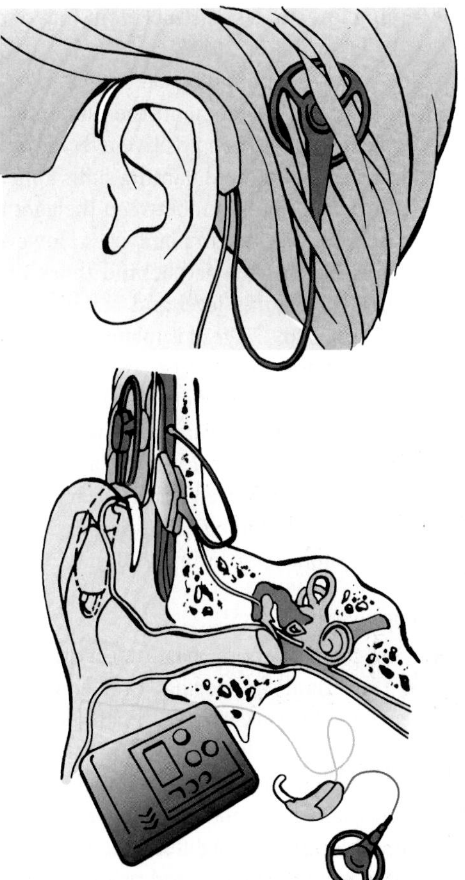

FIGURE 3-13. Cochlear implant.

Even with cochlear implants, hearing loss sometimes has phonological implications similar in type to those of children with hearing aids. The phonetic repertoires of children with implants may be delayed in the preschool to early school years, as are those of children with hearing aids. As noted above, vowel repertoires reach age-appropriate levels before consonant repertoires (Law & So, 2006). Furthermore, the phonological profiles of children with implants may include atypical (nondevelopmental) patterns as well as typical patterns (Flipsen & Parker, 2008; Law & So, 2006). However, their consonant production accuracy tends to be better than that of children with hearing aids (Law & So, 2006). Furthermore, as cochlear implants and the implantation process improve, speech development in these children is quickly becoming less and less distinct from that of children with no hearing loss (Blaiser, 2011).

With respect to those phonological processing skills that are critical for literacy development, the outcomes of children with cochlear implants are positive overall, but mixed. Phonological memory and rapid naming skills appear to fall within normal limits for children between the ages of 7 and 18 with at least four years of implant use. However, their **phonological awareness** skills lag behind those of hearing children matched for reading level and maternal education (Spencer & Tomblin, 2009). Age of implantation has an effect on preliteracy and literacy outcomes, as well as on vocabulary. Children implanted earlier (before age 4) perform better on measures of phonological awareness (awareness of syllables, rhymes, and phonemes), vocabulary, and reading than children implanted later (between 5 and 7 years of age). They also respond better to phonological awareness intervention (James, Rajput, Brinton, & Goswami, 2008).

Speech Perception

Prelinguistic speech perception has a clear important role in preparing the infant for normal oral communication, and its influence begins very early. At birth, typically developing human infants can already discriminate between (1) word-like stimuli based on the number of syllables they contain even when their durations don't differ (Bijeljac-Babic, Bertoncini, & Mehler, 1993); (2) different languages based on rhythm only (i.e., with segmental and prosodic information removed) (Mehler, Jusczyk, Lambertz, Halsted, Bertoncini, et al., 1988; Ramus, 2002); (3) grammatical (function) versus lexical (content) words, probably based on amplitude, duration, and syllable structure (Shi, Werker, & Morgan, 1999); and (4) some vowels (Kuhl & Miller, 1975).

Shortly thereafter (at 1 to 2 months of age), babies can detect changes in pitch and duration (Goodsit, Morse, Ver Hoeve, & Cowan, 1984). They also discriminate between different places, manners, and voicing qualities of consonants if the consonants are presented within syllables; fricatives are most challenging (Eilers, 1977; Eilers & Minifie, 1975; Jusczyk, Murray, & Bayly, 1979; Levitt, Jusczyk, Murray, & Carden, 1988). This discrimination is called **categorical perception** because the perceptual differentiation between categories (e.g., labial versus alveolar, voiced versus voiceless) is very abrupt. That is, there are broad regions where a change seems to make no difference (e.g., somewhat voiced versus very voiced, somewhat voiceless versus very voiceless) separated by narrow areas of change that make a huge difference (e.g., between voiced and voiceless). Infants demonstrate this in experiments involving a procedure termed **high-amplitude sucking**. The infant's sucking patterns indicate whether or not he is habituated to a certain sound (e.g., [ba ba ba ba ba]). If he detects a change in the sound (e.g., to [pa pa pa pa pa], a **critical difference** in the amount of voicing), his sucking pattern will change.

Some of these capacities, especially categorical perception of many consonant contrasts, appear to be common to all mammals. However, other speech perception skills are clearly learned, beginning before birth. For example, neonates already show a preference for their own mothers' voices (DeCasper & Fifer, 1980) and for the prosody of their own languages in conversational speech (Mehler et al., 1988). They also prefer passages that were frequently read aloud by their mothers during the last six weeks of the pregnancy (DeCasper & Spence, 1986). Furthermore, they already recognize which vowels are from their own languages rather than from different languages (Moon, Lagercrantz, & Kuhl, 2013).

Two-month-olds detect differences between syllables presented in trisyllabic chunks (e.g., [badaba] versus [bagaba]) if the trisyllables are presented in baby talk (a.k.a. infant-directed speech [IDS], a.k.a. motherese) (Goodsit et al., 1984). Four-month-olds recognize their own names (Mandel, Jusczyk, & Pisoni, 1995) and discriminate between running speech in baby-talk mode in which pauses are placed between grammatical clauses (e.g., noun phrase and verb phrase), as would occur in natural speech, versus pauses that interrupt grammatical clauses (Hirsh-Pasek, Kemler Nelson, Jusczyk, Wright-Cassidy, Druss, et al., 1987; Kemler Nelson, Hirsh-Pasek, Jusczyk, & Wright-Cassidy, 1989). Six-month-olds show a preference for words as well as conversational speech produced in their own languages (Jusczyk, Friederici, Wessels, Svenkerud, & Jusczyk ,1993b). By 10 months, they are also sensitive to the stress patterns (Jusczyk, Cutler, & Redanz, 1993a; Morgan 1996; Weissenborn, Hohle, Bartels, Herold, & Hofmann 2002), consonants, and sequences of consonants and vowels (Friederici & Wessels, 1993; Gerken & Zamuner, 2004; Jusczyk, Friederici, et al., 1993b; Jusczyk, Luce, & Charles-Luce 1994) that occur in their own languages. Infants of this age also demonstrate awareness of sequences of consonants that are most likely to occur word-medially (e.g., [ŋk] as in "monkey" is more common than [pt] as in "reptile" in English) in their languages (Morgan, 1996). By 11 months, this perceptual learning extends to recognition of particular words (Halle & Boysson-Bardies, 1994; Vihman, Nakai, DePaolis, & Halle, 2004). For English-learning babies, changing the initial consonant blocks recognition; changing other consonants or the stress pattern slows but does not prevent the child from recognizing the word. For French-learning babies, the medial consonant is more important for recognition (Halle & Boysson-Bardies, 1996). Unlike 9-month-olds, by 11 months, babies prefer words that are not interrupted by pauses (Myers, Jusczyk, Kemler Nelson, Charles-Luce, Woodward, et al., 1996).

These findings imply that prelinguistic children can segment running speech into smaller parts: clauses, phrases, and words. This ability has been documented directly by repeatedly exposing infants to a certain word (e.g., "cup"), then playing paragraphs composed of sentences that either do or do not contain that word; even at 7½ months, babies do recognize the words within the passages (Jusczyk & Aslin, 1995). English-speaking babies can do so at that age with two-syllable words only if they are trochaic (stress is on the first syllable); 9-month-olds can do it even for two-syllable iambic words (in which stress is on the second syllable) (Mattys, Jusczyk, Luce, & Morgan, 1999). However, this ability is limited to the infant's own language or languages that are very similar prosodically (e.g., English and Dutch or German; Houston, Jusczyk, Kuijpers, Coolen, & Cutler, 2000; Jusczyk 1998; Polka & Sundara, 2003).

The information that infants could be using to achieve these feats includes **distributional probabilities** (the frequencies with which various elements occur together or in series) and prosody (intonation and rhythm). Both are available in natural speech. Morgan and Saffran (1995), for example, demonstrated that 6-month-olds exposed to English pay attention to syllable stress but not to syllable order. In contrast, 9-month-olds use both to help them learn to identify words.

Attunement to one's native language also involves fine-tuning one's attention to those elements or structures that are important for that language. Thus, 10- to 12-month-olds perform worse on speech discrimination tasks involving non-native contrasts than do younger infants (e.g., Werker & Tees, 1984). This decrease in irrelevant perceptual abilities is gradual, reflecting the frequency of occurrence of various perceptual features in the native language. For example, infants continue to discriminate contrasts in the dorsal (velar, in English) place of articulation even when they no longer discriminate coronal (alveolar or palatal) consonants that do not occur in English. This may be because coronals are more frequent in English, causing the infants to learn more about the specifics of English coronals at an earlier age (Anderson, Morgan, & White, 2003).

Infants learn that two sounds contrast in their language better if the tokens of the two sounds to which they are exposed are more consistently different from each other. Thus, if they are exposed to tokens of two sounds (such as [b] and [p]) that mainly come from the endpoints of the continuum (e.g., very voiced tokens of [b] versus very voiceless tokens of [p]), 8-month-olds discriminate them better (Maye & Weiss, 2003). Repeated exposure to tokens that are indeterminate (e.g., slightly voiced [b], slightly voiceless [p]) can decrease the infants' ability to hear that the two sounds are different (Maye Werker, & Gerken, 2002).

In addition to the speech to which they are exposed, the speech-like sounds that babies themselves produce can also influence their perception. For instance, 1-year-olds listen longer to consonants from their own languages that they themselves do not yet produce frequently than to those consonants that occur often in their own babble (Vihman & Nakai, 2003). Presumably, this increased attention to what remains to be learned is key to ongoing progress in the native languages.

These findings about the speech perception skills of infants are impressive. It is important to note, however, that the ability to discriminate two sounds or recognize a sound pattern in an experiment such as the ones described above does *not* imply that the infant can use the same distinction in a functional linguistic context. A baby may detect the difference between two sounds, yet still fail to recognize that a pair of words that differ only in that very way could have two different meanings. Noticing an auditory change in a context that requires only detection of that change is very different from gleaning meaning in an ongoing communication context; that will come later (Stager & Werker, 1997; Werker & Stager, 2000).

Vision

Hearing is not the only sense involved in speech production and perception, however. Vision has a powerful role to play as well. Lewkowicz and Hansen-Tift (2012) showed that infants shift their visual focus from the speaker's eyes to the mouth starting between 4 and 8 months of age. At 12 months, they return to looking at the eyes when listening to their own native languages, but they still focus on the mouth if the speaker is speaking some other language. This suggests that they are relying on visual information about articulation as they learn to connect the sounds of speech with their own articulatory capabilities. The use of salient visual cues to enhance auditory–visual integration and speech perception continues to improve between the ages of 3 and 4 years (Lalonde & Holt, 2015).

Vision continues to make its contribution to speech perception even after speech has been mastered. For example, due to the **McGurk effect**, older listeners can be deceived into hearing [dadada] when they are shown a video of someone saying [gagaga] accompanied by synchronized audio of [bababa]. Infants "fall for" this audiovisual illusion as well (Desjardins & Werker, 1996). (To try this for yourself, go to http://auditoryneuroscience.com/McGurkEffect or simply search for "McGurk Effect" on the internet.)

Tactile Sensitivity and Proprioception

Some children are hypersensitive or hyposensitive to touch within the oral area, around the outside of it (the peri-oral area), or both. This is common among children diagnosed with autism, for example, and is also found in many children with Childhood Apraxia of Speech. In some cases, it is the result of lack of oral sensory experience, as in infants who are not fed orally during the first few months of life. In others, it may result from negative oral stimulation, as in babies who are intubated for long periods of time. Many children with birth defects, neonatal trauma, or premature birth undergo either or both of these unfortunate, but often life-saving, types of experiences. These tactile sensory differences can result in feeding difficulties and may affect the SLP's ability to use tactile cues in speech therapy. However, it is important to note that research on relationships among oral sensory perception tasks, such as oral pressure detection or discrimination of plastic forms placed within the mouth, and speech production skills has been equivocal. Some studies have demonstrated oral sensory deficits in those with SSDs (e.g., Ringel, House, Burk, Dolinsky, & Scott, 1970), and others have not (e.g., McDonald & Aungst, 1970). It is highly likely that the ability to make conscious decisions about oral sensations is different from the ability to use internal sensory information to subconsciously self-monitor speech production.

Sensory–Motor Connections

Proper motor function depends also upon intact sensory–motor connections. In particular, motor sensory receptors such as **muscle spindles**—sensory fibers that lie parallel to muscle fibers and that are sensitive to the position, velocity, and motion of the muscles in which they are embedded—provide sensory monitoring of motor performance and facilitation of online adjustments as needed via the alpha–gamma motor neuron system depicted in Figure 3-14. The information that they provide is **proprioception**: sensations of movement and orientation in space that are based upon internal stimuli. Proprioception includes **kinesthesis**: the detection of muscle, tendon, or joint movement and of body position and weight. Such **afferent** muscle spindles have been identified in the tongue, the jaw-closing (but not jaw-opening) muscles, the palatoglossus, the tensor veli palatini, and the levator veli palatini (Kuehn, Templeton, & Maynard, 1990; Liss, 1990).

Sensory–motor connections of this sort have increasingly been shown to be important not only for complex tasks but even for behaviors that were previously believed to be purely reflexive. For example, sucking and swallowing are thought to be controlled by **central pattern generators** in the brainstem. However, even these extremely basic motor functions are responsive to subtle changes in sensory input very early in infancy (Smith, 2010).

Motor sensory receptors have been hypothesized to provide **feedforward** (planning) information as well as **feedback** for speech (Kuehn et al., 1990). In order to plan an articulatory gesture, it is necessary to first detect one's starting point: the current positions of the relevant articulators. During the speaking process, the proprioceptive and kinesthetic feedback provided through this afferent system is faster than that provided via auditory self-monitoring. Thus, these muscle spindles, in conjunction with other sensory receptors such as **free nerve endings**, **mucosal receptors**, and **Golgi tendon organs**, "may contribute to the proprioceptive and kinesthetic information necessary for the development of context-dependent sensory-motor patterning of velopharyngeal activity [and other oral muscular activity] for speech" (Liss, 1990, p. 744). Put more simply, "cells that fire together wire together," a commonly used phrase in the neuroscience literature (e.g., Smith, 2010); in other words, sensory and motor neuronal activities that occur during the same action become linked. In this way, connections and expectations are established for very specific contexts (e.g., producing a certain syllable) and are also generalized to similar sensory–motor situations.

Additional powerful sensory–motor connections are made possible as a result of **mirror neurons**, motor neurons that fire when a person observes someone else performing an action that is within her own motor repertoire. This sensory–motor system likely helps infants make connections between the sensory–motor experience of their

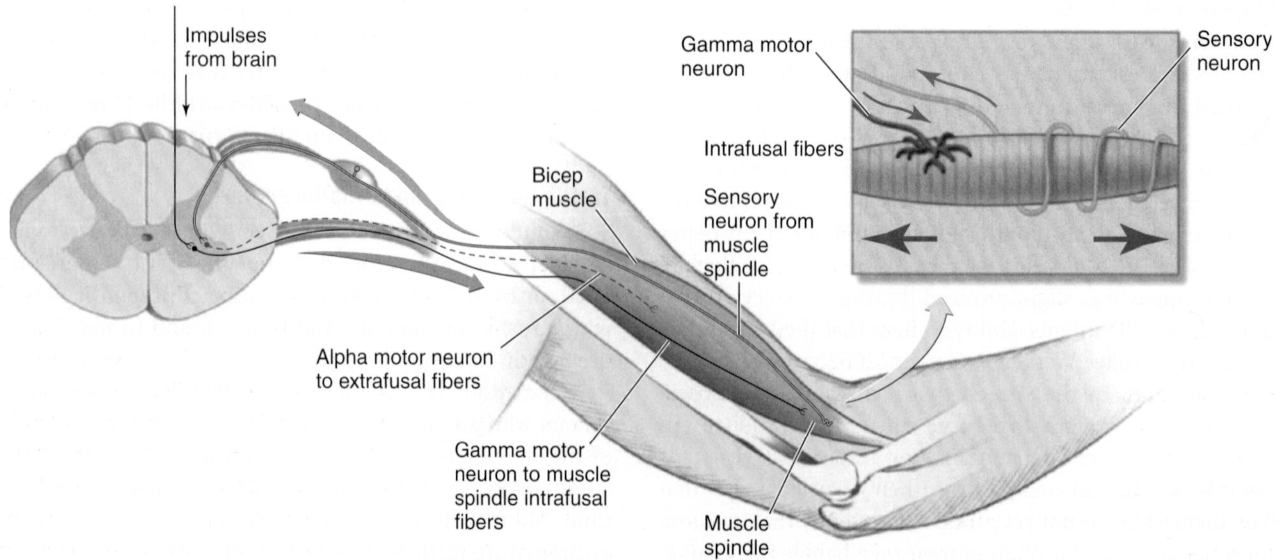

FIGURE 3-14. Alpha–gamma motor neuron system.

own vocalizations and the auditory and visual experience of hearing and watching someone else produce similar vocalizations (Velleman & Vihman, 2007; Vihman, 2002). Indeed, Fadiga, Craighero, Buccino, and Rizzolatti (2002) have demonstrated that motor neurons within a listener's tongue respond when that person hears words spoken that "strongly involve, when pronounced, tongue movements" (p. 399). The corresponding neurons in the Broca area and the premotor cortex fire at the same time (Buccino, Binkofskib, & Riggioa, 2004). However, this system is not engaged when speech is only heard, not visually observed (Sundara, Namasivayam, & Chen, 2001).

Mirror neurons may account for the fact that the extensive speech perception learning described above also impacts the prelinguistic child's vocalizations. Infants from 3 to 4 months old, for example, can imitate their mothers' **pitch contours** if these are exaggerated (Masataka, 1992). At 6 to 12 months old, they produce falling versus rising pitch contours in keeping with the contours most often found in the languages to which they have been exposed (Whalen, Levitt, & Wang, 1991). Similarly, 10-month-olds' **vowel formants** tend to be similar to those of their mother tongues (Boysson-Bardies, Halle, Sagart, & Durand, 1989); the same is true of consonant places of articulation (Boysson-Bardies & Vihman, 1991) and of utterance lengths (monosyllabic versus disyllabic "words;" Boysson-Bardies, Vihman, Roug-Hellichus, Durand, Landberg, et al., 1992).

Summary: Sensory Precursors and Contributions

Vision, hearing, and higher-order auditory processes, such as speech perception, have known impacts on the child's development of spoken language. The roles of tactile and proprioceptive processing are not clear. Sensory–motor relationships are facilitated by neuronal connections provided by the alpha–gamma motor neuron system, among others.

EXERCISE 3-2

Sensory and Sensory–Motor Connections

Speech Production Models

Many models of the early development and/or of the mature functions of speech perception and production have been proposed, though none has been universally accepted. In many ways, they represent complementary rather than opposing viewpoints. It seems likely that at least some components of most of these shed light on the complexities of this process, that is, that some future integrated model that includes aspects from several current theories will gain respect. We review a few key theories here.

Gestural Phonology

The extreme complexity of managing all of the motor systems reviewed above in order to produce a simple syllable has led to the development of several complex models of speech production. One such model, commonly referred to as **gestural phonology** is based on the concept that speech sounds are not produced as single units, one by one, like beads on a string. Because of phonemic awareness, literate people tend to think of words as series of discrete phonemes. From this perspective, it's easy to think of coarticulation as an after-effect, a type of sloppiness that results from speaking at a rapid rate that listeners are forced to cope with in order to understand each other. Hockett (1955) made the analogy of a row of decorated Easter eggs (the phonemes: mental images of the sounds to be produced) traveling along a conveyor belt and through a wringer (the articulators). The eggs are crushed and mushed together; the recipient–listener then has to pick through the mess (the series of speech sounds actually produced) to try to find a message. Hockett was right in the sense that speech cannot be neatly segmented into phoneme-sized units. There is considerable overlap of consonants and vowels in normal speech, especially when the sounds are adjacent but even when they are not. For this reason, there is no such thing as a pure speech sound in running speech. In addition, to ask what a certain phoneme sounds like makes no sense. The answer is that it depends upon the context in which it occurs. Every phoneme has multiple manifestations due to coarticulation. Recall, however, that coarticulation is a learned process, not simply the result of articulatory sloppiness. Coarticulatory patterns differ from language to language (Kingston & Diehl, 1994).

A group of researchers at Haskins Laboratories, home of the spectrogram, have proposed a *gestural* model of phonology that focuses on this aspect of speech production (Browman & Goldstein, 1989; Galantucci, Fowler, & Turvey, 2006; Liberman, Cooper, Shankweiler, & Studdert-Kennedy, 1967; Liberman & Mattingly, 1985). In gestural phonology, each syllable or word is considered as a sequence of articulatory gestures, each of which is a combination of movements of various articulators working together to produce the given output. Thus, in the word "pin," for example, the vocal folds do not suddenly crash together at the beginning of the [ɪ], nor does the velum suddenly fall wide open at the "end" of the [ɪ] or the beginning of the [n]. Rather, the vocal folds gradually come together to vibrate for the vowel and nasal portions of the word, while the velum gradually lowers to allow air to flow into the nasal cavity—well before the listener perceives the nasalized [ɪ] to be over. Like a complicated dance, each articulator moves at its own pace while coordinating with all of the others to create an overall movement pattern that achieves the speech goal. These scientists propose that knowledge of their own articulatory patterns—including these overlaps—makes it possible for listeners to decode each others' messages despite the apparent messiness of real speech. Thus, understanding each others' messages involves not only processing the acoustics of the speech that hits our ears but also taking into account the conditions under which that speech was formed in the speaker's mouth (Lindblom, 1990).

DIVA

How does the infant combine her growing store of perceptual and distributional expectations about the language to which she has been exposed with her developing motor control? One recent model of speech production, termed the "Directions into Velocities of Articulators" (**DIVA**) model (e.g., Guenther, 1995; Guenther, Ghosh, & Tourville, 2006), thoroughly incorporates the role of sensory information, especially auditory, tactile, and proprioceptive information, in supporting speech production. It also associates the speech production process to specific areas of the brain.

Within this theory, the two key aspects of speech production are feedforward and feedback mechanisms that support planning, self-monitoring, and self-correction. The proponents propose that as an adult prepares to speak a familiar word or phrase, **somatosensory** information about the current state of the vocal tract (i.e., sensory information about touch, temperature, and body position from the skin and the internal organs) is retrieved. Then, a pre-established motor program is called up for use, with motor commands adjusted for current conditions into a motor plan sent from the motor planning portion of the cortex—both directly and through the cerebellum—to the actual motor cortex itself and eventually to the muscles. This is the feedforward system. The level of detail in the motor plan depends upon the amount of experience the person has had in producing this particular utterance. *Expertise yields flexibility as well as precision*; the targets are viewed as regions of acceptable production, not as rigidly invariant commands. Thus, they include the potential for adjustments based on the current conditions that have been identified, including both the linguistic context and the physiologic context (e.g., chewing gum while speaking), among other factors.

In addition to this feedforward system for implementing an existing motor program, auditory and somatosensory expectations for how this utterance should sound and feel are aroused in the temporal and parietal cortices of the brain, respectively. These expectations are checked against the actual sensations that are experienced as the person speaks. If they don't match, an error has occurred, and a correction is made. This is the feedback system. Again, it is specific but not rigid (Guenther, 1995; Guenther et al., 2006). For example, adults and children who are given inaccurate feedback about their own vocalizations (i.e., they "hear" themselves producing a different vowel than they are in fact producing) quickly adjust their vocalizations accordingly (Villacorta, Perkell, & Guenther, 2007). If something interferes with a person's articulation (e.g., a device is put in his mouth), he is much more likely to adjust his speech if he can hear the effects (Perrier, 2005).

Thus, the system as modeled by Guenther (1995) and Guenther and colleagues (2006) relies on (1) an auditory target—what the word should sound like; (2) general motor programs that have been stored and are ready to be adapted to the current context; (3) subconscious expectations about what it should feel like to produce the word; and (4) connections from auditory and somatosensory error detection centers to motor adjustment centers for rapid correction. This model is depicted in Figure 3-15, which shows how the target maps (speech goals as auditory and somatosensory targets) are compared to the state maps (perceived actual somatosensory and auditory results of action) to derive the error maps, which determine what needs to be changed and send that information to the motor cortex for correction.

According to the DIVA theory, these components are built up during the prelinguistic period as the child experiences others' vocalizations auditorily (and presumably also visually) and her own vocalizations both auditorily and somatosensorily. Because the expectations are flexible, the infant recognizes matches between her own vocalizations and those of the older people around her (parents, siblings, etc.) despite the large acoustic differences among them. This flexibility and the availability of auditory expectations as well as somatosensory ones allow the baby to recognize which of her utterances remain within the target range even as her vocal tract changes significantly over time (Callan, Kent, Guenther, & Vorperian, 2000; Guenther, 1995). However, toddlers may not be able to use these feedback systems as efficiently as older children and adults; in a recent study, 2-year-olds failed to modify their vowels when they were given misleading feedback about which vowels they were producing (MacDonald, Johnson, Forsythe, Plante, & Munhall, 2012). Thus, the learning process is a protracted one.

Implications of DIVA for Speech Perception Deficits as a Cause of SSDs

Speech perception skills have been hypothesized to be one factor contributing to the difficulties of some children with speech production disorders. Thyer and Dodd (1996) compared the auditory processing skills of children with delayed, nondevelopmental, or variable speech production deficits to those of peers without phonological disorders of any sort and found no differences. However, their results are in contrast to those of several other studies that have demonstrated impaired speech perception in children with SSDs (Broen, Strange, Doyle, & Heller, 1983; Hoffman, Daniloff, Bengoa, & Schuckers, 1985; Johnson, Pennington, Lowenstein, & Nittrouer, 2011; Rvachew & Jamieson, 1989; Shuster, 1998). These deficits often persist into adulthood (Kenney, Barac-Cikoja, Finnegan, Jeffries, & Ludlow, 2006). For example, Bird and Bishop (1992) demonstrated that some children with phonological difficulties were worse at phoneme discrimination than their peers, though they could

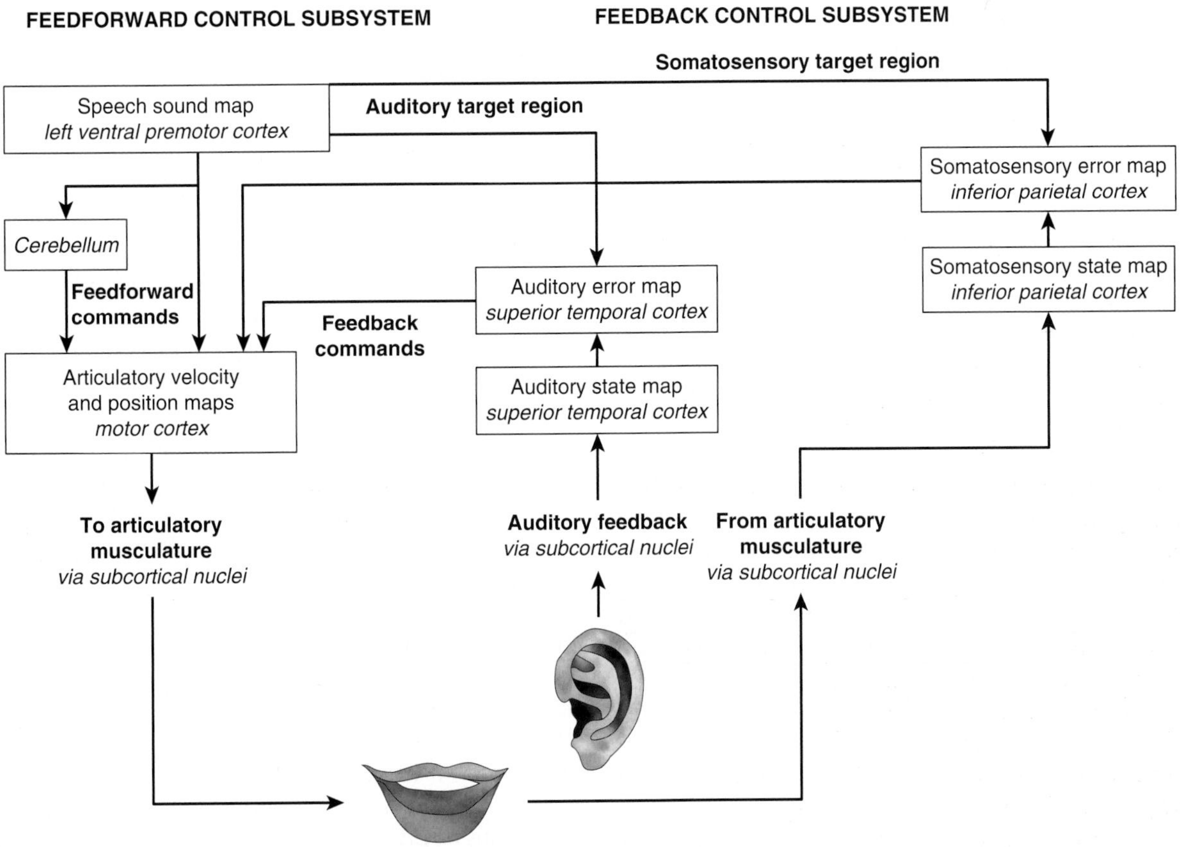

FIGURE 3-15. DIVA model.

discriminate some sounds that they could not produce. Similarly, Edwards, Fox, and Rogers (2002) found children with phonological disorders to be worse at discriminating consonant–vowel–consonant words that differed in the final consonant than age-matched peers who were typically developing. Vocabulary size was also a factor. Rvachew, Rafaat, and Martin (1999a) reported that children with SSDs were more likely to benefit from therapy for sounds for which they were **stimulable** (i.e., that they could produce with modeling and cueing) if they also demonstrated good speech discrimination of those sounds. Furthermore, a combination of stimulability and speech perception treatment facilitated the development of sounds that were previously unstimulable, poorly perceived, or both. Nijland (2009) found that both children classified as having phonological disorders and children with a diagnosis of CAS demonstrated speech perception deficits. Interestingly, the children with phonological disorders only demonstrated "higher-order" perception difficulties (e.g., deficits in phonological awareness, such as rhyming), while those with CAS had difficulty with lower-order tasks (e.g., discrimination between two nonwords) as well as higher-order perception tasks. Children with SSDs are hypothesized to have incomplete or less robust phonological representations as a result of these speech perception challenges (Anthony et al., 2011; Edwards, Fourakis, Beckman, & Fox, 1999; Sutherland & Gillon, 2005); this may contribute to their risk of literacy difficulties.

Despite these findings of poorer speech discrimination among children with speech sound disorders, however, impaired lower-level discrimination does not appear to be a primary cause of SSDs. **Auditory processing disorder** (APD) is a deficit in the ability to analyze and interpret auditory signals received by the ear and passed on to the brain. Specifically, this diagnosis is appropriate for someone who has deficits in some or all of the following areas:

- Sound localization and lateralization
- Auditory discrimination
- Auditory pattern recognition
- Temporal aspects of audition, including temporal integration, temporal discrimination, temporal ordering, and temporal masking
- Auditory performance in competing acoustic signals
- Auditory performance with degraded acoustic signals (ASHA, 2005, p. 2; Richard, 2012)

As a result, children with APD have decreased ability to discriminate speech sounds as well as difficulty following directions, especially under noisy or otherwise adverse conditions. Importantly, APD does not reflect impaired hearing acuity, nor does it suggest that the person is intellectually below age expectations. However, about half of children with APD also have both language impairments and reading disorders (Sharma, Purdy, & Kelly, 2009). Conversely, 70% to 80% of children with specific language impairment also demonstrate deficits in auditory processing (Corriveau, Pasquini, & Goswami, 2007). Surprisingly, children with SSDs are not more likely to demonstrate signs of APD than are children without speech disorders (Thyer & Dodd, 1996).

APD may be the wrong aspect of speech perception in which to seek deficits in children with SSDs, however. If the DIVA model is correct, it may be that auditory self-monitoring, not auditory processing of others' speech, is the source of the problem.

Dynamic Systems Theory

Dynamic systems theory (Thelen & Smith, 1994; Van Lieshout, 2004) provides an even broader scope than DIVA. In this view, development is seen as a dynamic, evolving, self-organizing process. It is reliant on continuous interactions among motor, perceptual, and cognitive functions and the external factors that facilitate or impede them. The emphasis is not on achieving a particular goal (e.g., learning to produce a particular word) but on the emergence of collaborative systems that can be used to achieve various goals. In this process, *periods of instability—as well as periods of stability—are not only expected, but necessary.*

The implications of dynamic systems theory for speech development and speech-language pathology are that a myriad of factors—including language skills, cognitive skills, motivation, and environmental factors (such as parental input and encouragement)—must be taken into account when planning intervention. Furthermore, it reminds us that stability is not always a good thing; sometimes, a child may be "stuck" in a given articulatory pattern. Instability can be a sign of poor perception of the targets, poor storage or underlying representations of the targets, or poor motor programming/planning, but it may also be a sign of a system undergoing much needed change. Subcomponent skills, such as the ability to produce the features of which a given phoneme is composed or the substructures of a word shape, must be at least emerging in the child for it to be possible for her to organize those features into a new whole, the target phoneme or word shape. For example, a child whose production of stops is stable and whose production of fricatives is becoming stabilized as a result of therapy may begin to produce affricates without this class of consonants even being addressed in therapy (Rvachew & Bernhardt, 2010). During the process, a period of confusion or **apparent regression** may be exhibited.

DIVA and Dynamic Systems Concepts as a Framework for a Model of Childhood Apraxia of Speech

CAS is a neuromotor speech disorder that impacts planning and/or programming for speech production. To date, its etiologies are much less well identified than those of dysarthria. As defined in ASHA's (2007) Technical Report on CAS, this disorder is

> *a neurologic childhood (pediatric) SSD in which the precision and consistency of movements underlying speech are impaired in the absence of neuromuscular deficits (e.g., abnormal reflexes, abnormal tone). CAS may occur as a result of known neurologic impairment, in association with complex neurobehavioral disorders of known or unknown origin, or as an idiopathic neurogenic SSD. The core impairment in planning and/or programming spatiotemporal parameters of movement sequences results in errors in speech sound production and prosody. (pp. 3–4)*

Although the vast majority of cases of CAS have no known etiology, a few genetic differences associated specifically with CAS have been identified within the past decades. The first (chronologically) of these is **FOXP2**, a **chromosomal translocation** (movement of some genetic material from its typical location to another location) in the region 7q31 (gene locus 31 on the long arm—q—of chromosome 7). The combination of this translocation and symptoms of apraxia of speech were first identified in a British family known as the "KE" family (Fisher, Vargha-Khadem, Watkins, Monaco, & Pembrey, 1998). Since that time, several additional people with FOXP2 mutations have been located and found to have symptoms of CAS (MacDermot, Bonora, Sykes, Coupe, Lai, et al., 2005; Tomblin, O'Brien, Shriberg, Williams, Murray, et al., 2009). However, this genetic abnormality is associated with a variety of cognitive, language, motor, psychosocial, and possible craniofacial involvements that are not typically seen in people with CAS.

Another genetic source of some cases of CAS is a chromosomal duplication at 7q11.23, the same site at which deletion results in Williams syndrome (Somerville, Mervis, Young, Seo, del Campo, et al., 2005). The facial characteristics associated with this **Dup7** syndrome are much more subtle than those associated with FOXP2 (or with Williams syndrome). They include prominent forehead; high, broad nose; posteriorly rotated ears; long **columella**; short **philtrum**; thin lips; small jaw; dental malocclusion; high-arched palate; hypotonia; and slight facial asymmetries. The vast majority of the 30 or more children and adults with this syndrome studied as of 2011 either have or had histories of oral–motor, motor speech, and/or speech sound disorders. Typically, these SSDs are moderate to severe and include at least some symptoms of CAS (Velleman & Mervis, 2011; Velleman, O'Connor, McGloin, Cormier, Mervis, et al., 2009b). Ongoing research has confirmed these findings.

Shriberg (2006) has also reported on three siblings with CAS apparently resulting from a translocation affecting chromosomes 4 and 16. Only relatively small numbers of cases of these genetic differences have been studied thus far. In short, the incidence and prevalence of heritable chromosomal sources of CAS and the extent to which the symptoms of these types of CAS match those of others with CAS remain to be determined.

As indicated in the ad hoc committee's report (ASHA, 2007), CAS also tends to occur as a secondary diagnosis with certain other genetic neurobehavioral disorders. These include autism spectrum disorders (ASD), epilepsy, **fragile X syndrome**, **galactosemia**, **Rett syndrome**, and VCF. Some authors have also reported co-occurrence of CAS symptoms with Down syndrome (Kumin, 1996; Rupela & Manjula, 2007, 2010; Rupela, Manjula & Velleman, 2010). The frequencies of occurrence of CAS symptoms with each of those disorders have not been definitively established. Additionally, the extent to which the apraxia symptoms associated with these disorders match those of children with apraxia of unknown etiology remains to be explored.

Definitive research to identify the key characteristics of CAS has not been completed. Research to date has been complicated by circularity (i.e., participants selected based upon their CAS symptoms are then studied to determine the symptoms of CAS) and by ambiguous subject selection (e.g., participants selected based upon clinical referral, despite the documented confusion among SLPs about differential diagnosis). However, the ASHA ad hoc committee came to the conclusion that there is a consensus among those who specialize in researching this disorder that three particular speech features are critical to the diagnosis and treatment of CAS: (1) transitions between sounds or between syllables are interrupted or lengthened yielding a choppy quality; (2) repeating the same syllable, word, or phrase in a series (e.g., "baby baby baby baby baby" or [pʌtʌkʌ pʌtʌkʌ pʌtʌkʌ pʌtʌkʌ pʌtʌkʌ]) is likely to result in inconsistent productions of the target, often called **token-to-token variability**; and (3) prosody, especially word stress, is atypical with reduced differentiation of stressed versus unstressed syllables in the word. The latter is described using the cover term **excess equal stress**.

It is important to note, however, that CAS is a syndrome (i.e., a **symptom complex**), not a **unitary disorder**. That is, not all children will demonstrate the same symptoms and symptoms will change over time in a given individual. Thus, a checklist approach to diagnosis is not possible; rather, a pattern of symptoms is key to identification (ASHA, 2007).

With respect to speech production, phonotactic problems are especially common in CAS: delayed or deviant syllable and word shapes; difficulties with multisyllabic words; worse performance with increasing length and complexity of the utterance; and sequencing issues at the phoneme, syllable, morpheme, and word levels (Velleman, 2003). Furthermore, Jacks, Marquardt, and Davis (2006) reported that phonetic accuracy in CAS is determined by phonotactic accuracy, frequency, and complexity. In other words, the structure of the word has a significant impact on the likelihood that the child will produce the consonants and vowels in that word correctly. For example, a child may produce [s] much more accurately in contexts that reflect individually well-established motor patterns (e.g., the child's own name), are frequent in the language he is learning (e.g., [sɪC]—as in "sick, Sid, sill, sin, sip, sis, sit, six"—versus [sʊC]—as in "soot"), and are simple (e.g., a CV word).

The difficulty that children with CAS demonstrate in maintaining the stability and fluidity of articulatory movement has been documented physiologically by Grigos and Kolenda (2010) using a kinematic movement tracking system. Their 3-year-old participant with CAS exhibited slower, less stable, less accurate jaw movements than age-matched children who were typically developing. With focused therapy, his movement control increased. Preston, Molfese, Gumkowski, Sorcinelli, and Harwood (2014) studied neurologic **event-related potentials** just prior to producing speech in children with CAS versus peers who were TD. They found slower response times indicating longer motor planning times in the CAS group. The same participants also exhibited less right hemisphere activity during speech planning for complex words.

As suggested by the DIVA and dynamic systems models, in addition to intact motor and sensory systems, a successful speaker must be able to coordinate these two systems in order to:

1. Determine the current state of the articulators (via feed-forward mechanisms)
2. Create motor programs for the production of words, phrases, and sentences
3. Store those programs that are likely to be needed again at some future time
4. Retrieve pre-existing programs
5. Adjust pre-existing programs both to create motor plans and to adjust plans that are in process to the current targets and to the physiologic, linguistic (e.g., grammatical), and **paralinguistic** (e.g., social) contexts
6. Determine the success of their efforts (via auditory and somatosensory feedback mechanisms) and make ongoing adjustments to the motor plan as appropriate

The types of difficulties shown by children with CAS have led some researchers to propose that in the terms of the DIVA model, CAS is a disorder resulting from an overreliance on feedback rather than feedforward mechanisms. The deficits in speech production may result from an increase in "neural noise" that interferes with motor programming and planning. Alternatively, a decreased ability to collect and use somatosensory information to adapt motor programs to current articulatory conditions before beginning to speak may result in a less reliable feedforward system—inadequate programs that are insufficiently or inappropriately adjusted to the context yielding inadequate or inappropriate plans

(Terband, Maassen, Guenther, & Brumberg, 2009). This proposal is strengthened by findings that children at risk for CAS also demonstrate weaknesses in fine motor skills (Bradford & Dodd, 1996; Highman, Hennessey, Leitao & Piek, 2013). They are impaired on non-speech sensory–motor tasks and also non-speech sequential memory tasks. Furthermore, their scores on non-speech sequential tasks correlate with the severity of their speech disorder (Nijland, Terband, & Maassen, in press). Terband and colleagues (2009) propose that as a result of the faulty feedforward system, the child's motor plans are imprecise or incomplete and she has to rely more heavily—or perhaps even instead—on the auditory and somatosensory feedback systems. Under these conditions, errors are identified after they occur, not prevented in advance. The identification and remediation of errors is a comparatively slow process, yielding inappropriate increases in coarticulation (within the syllable), searching behaviors, variability, and distortions. Similar deficits might account for stuttering behaviors as well. A recent study by Iuzzini-Seigel, Hogan, Guarino, and Green (2015) confirmed this hypothesis. Children with CAS were compared to peers with speech sound disorders or no speech difficulties on a task that required them to speak during auditory masking that made it difficult for them to self-monitor acoustically. With the masking, those with CAS made more errors involving voicing and vowels, which tend to be persistent areas of difficulty in CAS. The other participants were not affected. The authors suggest that the slow, choppy speech of children with CAS may result, at least in part, from an over-reliance on auditory feedback to help them correct for incomplete, imprecise, or irretrievable motor programs. Auditory feedback not only occurs after the articulatory action has already begun but also arrives even later than somatosensory feedback, so speakers with CAS must pause and wait to self-monitor, resulting in decreased rate and a jerky syllable-by-syllable or word-by-word rhythm. Thus, this model shows promise for providing insights into the neuromotor bases of CAS (Terband et al., 2009).

It is a mistake to assume that CAS has only motor consequences, however. According to the ad hoc committee (ASHA, 2007), children with CAS are at increased risk for expressive language and phonological awareness difficulties (which may result in literacy difficulties) as well as for speech production errors. As noted by Highman and team (2013), "a deficit in one domain can, over time, constrain development in other domains" (p. 198). They found that as a group, children at familial risk for CAS demonstrated early weaknesses in expressive language as well as motor speech skills. Even more concerning was an increasing difference between expressive vocabulary scores for those at risk for CAS versus young children without risk factors. Speech production abilities at 9 and 18 months of age (as measured using the Communication and Symbolic Behavior Scales [Wetherby & Prizant, 2002]) were predictive of vocabulary scores at 24 months. Furthermore, Nijland (2009) found that the speech perception difficulties of children with CAS included deficits in both lower-level tasks, such as nonword discrimination, and higher-level tasks, such as rhyming. When event-related potentials are measured during speech perception tasks, children with CAS demonstrate less response to phonemic minimal pairs (e.g., /pɑ/-/bɑ/), which are crucial to phonological contrast and therefore meaning. In contrast, they exhibit more response to allophonic pairs (e.g., [pɑ]-[pʰɑ]), which do not result in meaning differences and are therefore typically ignored by native speaker listeners (Froud & Khamis-Dakwar, 2012). Thus, they are not tuning in to the aspects of the speech signal that are most important for efficient communication. It is not surprising, then, that many studies have demonstrated increased risk for phonological awareness and literacy difficulties in children with CAS (ASHA, 2007). Phonemic awareness deficits in CAS include reduced perception and production of vowels (Maassen, Groenen, & Crul 2003), syllables (Marquardt, Sussman, Snow, & Jacks, 2002), rhymes (Marion, Sussman, & Marquardt, 1993), and phoneme sequences—especially in nonwords (Bridgeman & Snowling, 1988). The nature of these deficits observed in children with CAS suggests impoverished phonemic representations (Marquardt et al., 2004). Reading and spelling difficulties typically ensue (Lewis, Freebairn, Hansen, Iyengar, & Taylor, 2004).

Thus, although CAS is fundamentally a motor speech disorder, there are significant linguistic symptoms as well. It is likely that these reflect the difficulty of generating abstract concepts about phonology based upon impaired motor speech control and insufficient somatosensory information, with the resulting insufficient phonological representations.

Summary

Sensory information about the current state of the articulators (and the rest of the body) makes it possible for the feedforward motor system to adjust motor programs to the context, creating tailor-made motor plans before speech even begins. Sensory feedback through the auditory and somatosensory systems alerts motor planning centers to errors or miscalculations, and repairs are made. Deficits in these sensory–motor programming, planning, and correction systems may result in SSDs, especially CAS.

EXERCISE 3-3

Models of Speech Production and Perception

COGNITIVE(–LINGUISTIC) PRECURSORS TO SPEECH

Neonates' brains are at about 25% of their adult weight. Myelination of neurons within the brain begins at about 6 months' gestation and achieves its peak within the first year of life. Cell density reaches adult levels in the Wernicke area during the same time period. However, neuronal development lags behind in the Broca area, not reaching mature levels there until early childhood. In fact, cell connections in the prefrontal lobes are not adult-like until after adolescence (McLeod & Bleile, 2003). Thus, cerebral maturation is a protracted process.

There is much we still do not know about brain–language connections, let alone cognition–language connections. For example, most studies that have examined the influence of sex on the likelihood of speech-language impairments have found that males are more susceptible to such deficits than are females (Harrison & McLeod, 2010). This relates, no doubt, to the many differences that are found between the brains of members of the two sexes (Good, Johnsrude, Ashburner, Henson, Friston, et al., 2001), but many questions remain about relationships between anatomy and function, let alone anatomy and dysfunction (Herbert, Ziegler, Makris, Bakardjiev, Hodgson, et al., 2003). Furthermore, in infants with focal brain injury, it is difficult to predict which lesion sites will be associated with which (if any) speech or language symptoms; neurologic plasticity provides significant advantages at this age. Yet, according to Dall'Oglio, Bates, Volterra, Di Capua, and Pezzini (1994), just as a child with focal brain injury resulting in significant left-hemisphere damage may appear to develop early language milestones age-appropriately, a child with an injury that has apparently not affected the left hemisphere at all may nonetheless demonstrate significant linguistic delays. Furthermore, some children in their study who had significant nonverbal deficits showed no delays in early communication and language skills and vice versa. Yet, no child developed expressive language before presymbolic gesture use (e.g., using a comb on themselves, holding a telephone up to their ear).

As reviewed above, even neonates have already built up expectations (i.e., have learned) about language based upon their experience in utero, resulting in increased attention to their mothers' voices and to the prosody of their own language(s). Recent psycholinguistic studies have demonstrated that human brains are excellent at gathering statistical information about the world, including but not limited to statistics about language (Kirkham, Slemmer, & Johnson, 2002). This information can be very specific and include not only phonetic details but even socio-phonetic details (e.g., associations between particular speech patterns and gender) (Pierrehumbert, 2001, 2003). This tallying of number of occurrences and co-occurrences of various phonetic elements (e.g., particular consonants and vowels) and structures (e.g., various combinations of specific consonants and vowels, also known as phonotactics) occurs automatically when we are exposed to speech. It is even exhibited when the speech is in a made-up language that follows certain non-English phonetic rules and when the listeners are engaged in some other attention-grabbing task with the artificial language as background noise to which their attention is not called (Saffran, Newport, Aslin, Tunick, & Barrueco, 1997). Humans of any age, including infants, demonstrate by their behavior that they have abstracted phonetic and phonotactic patterns from such artificial languages in as little as two minutes for babies and 20 minutes for children and adults (Johnson & Jusczyk, 2001; Saffran, Aslin, & Newport, 1996). **Phonotactic probability**, the likelihood that two sounds will occur together within the words of a given language, plays an important role in many aspects of language processing and production. Interestingly, adults quickly learn consonant patterns that are based upon word position or vowel type but not based upon the individual speaker's voice (Onishi, Chambers, & Fisher, 2002). Even infants can learn such "rules," even when the patterns embedded in the speech are unnatural (i.e., they do not occur in any of the languages of the world, such as labial consonants co-occurring with only non-round vowels) (Seidl & Buckley, 2005). This type of probabilistic tallying of data is called **implicit learning** because it is done automatically and without attention. It is in sharp contrast to **declarative memory**, which refers to the explicit, conscious learning of facts, word meanings, and the like (McClelland, McNaughton, & O'Reilly, 1995; Ullman, 2001).

The research in this field indicates that implicit learning affects not only the perception but also the production of prelinguistic infants. The influence of frequency continues into early word production of toddlers as well. For example, Welsh children both babble more fricatives and produce more of them in their early words than do children learning other languages, no doubt as a result of the extremely high frequency of these sounds in the language they are learning. Furthermore, it is considered to be a "red flag" for phonological disorder if English-speaking children demonstrate frequent, persistent initial consonant deletion. Yet, this process is common in children learning Finnish, French, Hindi, Estonian, and Welsh (Vihman & Croft, 2007; Vihman & Velleman, 2000a, 2000b). There are at least two features of a language that appear to predispose a child to pay less attention to initial consonant maintenance: (a) the accent falls on the final syllable of the word (as in French), thus calling attention to the end rather than the beginning of the word and (b) **geminates**, consonants that are doubled or even tripled in length, are common in medial position (as in Welsh and Japanese), thus calling attention to the middle of the word (Vihman & Croft, 2007).

Non-motoric features of words continue to impact the child as she progresses further into word production. For example, **neighborhood density**, which represents the number of minimal pairs a word has, affects young children's word repetition ability. Basic words that children learn early are easier for them to repeat if they are from sparse neighborhoods (more distinct). Participants who were better able to recognize such words on an experimental task also had better phonological awareness (Garlock, Walley, & Metsala, 2001). Phonotactic probability and neighborhood density continue to impact word recognition and repetition into adulthood (Storkel, Armbruster, & Hogan, 2006).

Neurocognitive research suggests that the **neocortical** (especially **frontal lobe**) portions of the brain, in addition to the **basal ganglia**, are the centers for generalization from specific instances (tokens) to more abstract patterns (types):

> *This system underlies the learning of new, and the computation of already-learned, rule-based procedures that govern the regularities of language—particularly those procedures related to combining items into complex structures that have precedence (sequential) and hierarchical relations ... the sequential and hierarchical combination...of stored forms and abstract representations into complex structures (Ullman, 2004, p. 245).*

These brain structures are shown in Figures 3-16 and 3-17.

This **procedural learning** is slow and implicit; the learner is consciously aware neither of tallying the occurrences and contexts of the examples nor of making a generalization about a pattern from the examples. Once a pattern has been learned, however, it can be retrieved (subconsciously) and applied rapidly and automatically (Ullman, 2004).

Procedural learning contrasts with **declarative memory**, through which we consciously remember specific experiences as whole events (**episodic memory**) and through which we learn facts, the meanings of words, and irregular grammatical forms (McClelland et al., 1995; Ullman, 2001). The **hippocampus**, the **thalamus**, and portions of the **temporal lobes**, all shown in Figures 3-16 and 3-17, are primarily responsible for this type of learning (Ullman, 2004). Using declarative memory, even infants can associate speaker information (such as gender-related voice characteristics) with phonetic details (such as the speaker's accent—Houston & Jusczyk, 2000; cf. also Rovee-Collier, 1997). This information can be combined with generalizations arrived at via implicit learning to draw linguistic and sociolinguistic inferences.

Ambient-language probabilistic learning effects can be found in children with SSDs as well as in children who are TD. For instance, children with Down syndrome who are learning to speak Kannada, a non-Indo-European language spoken in southern India that also has frequent medial geminates, also exhibit frequent initial consonant deletion (Rupela et al., 2010). Similarly, Chinese children with phonological disorders produce the most frequent diphthongs in their language more accurately than those that are less frequent (Stokes, Lau, & Ciocca, 2002).

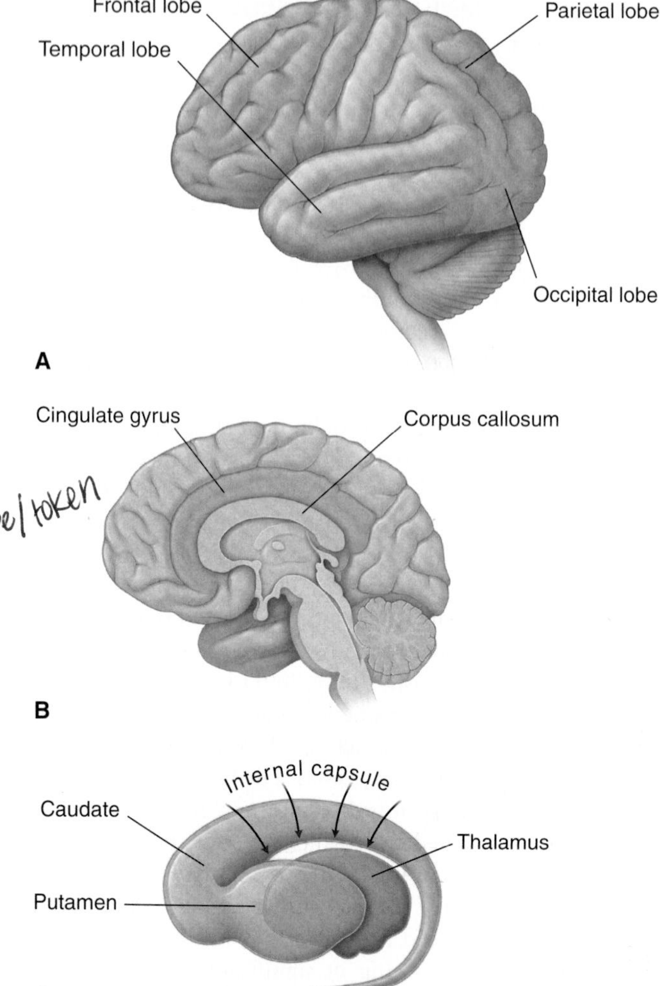

FIGURE 3-16. A. In this lateral view, the cerebral hemispheres are divided into four lobes—frontal, parietal, occipital, and temporal—which are structurally and functionally distinct from each other. **B**. A sagittal view of the cerebral hemispheres shows the corpus callosum and cingulate gyrus. The corpus callosum connects the left and right hemispheres and coordinates their actions. The cingulate gyrus is part of the limbic system; it lies immediately superior to the corpus callosum. **C**. The basal ganglia include the caudate and putamen, which are together known as the striatum, and the globus pallidus (medial to the putamen, not shown). The thalamus lies medial to the basal ganglia. *Arrows* indicate the trajectory of neurons in the internal capsule, a bundle of white matter that carries motor commands from the cortex to the spinal cord.

Storkel, Maekawa, and Hoover (2010) have shown that phonologically delayed children appear to acquire vocabulary words that have both low phonotactic probability (i.e., less common sound sequences) and lower neighborhood density (i.e., fewer similar-sounding words) just as well as children without delays. However, unlike children who are typically developing, those with delays in sound learning find words that have both high phonotactic probability and dense neighborhoods (i.e., frequent sound combinations and many similar-sounding words) to be more challenging to learn well. Storkel and colleagues (2010) hypothesize that weaker/less specific representations make it

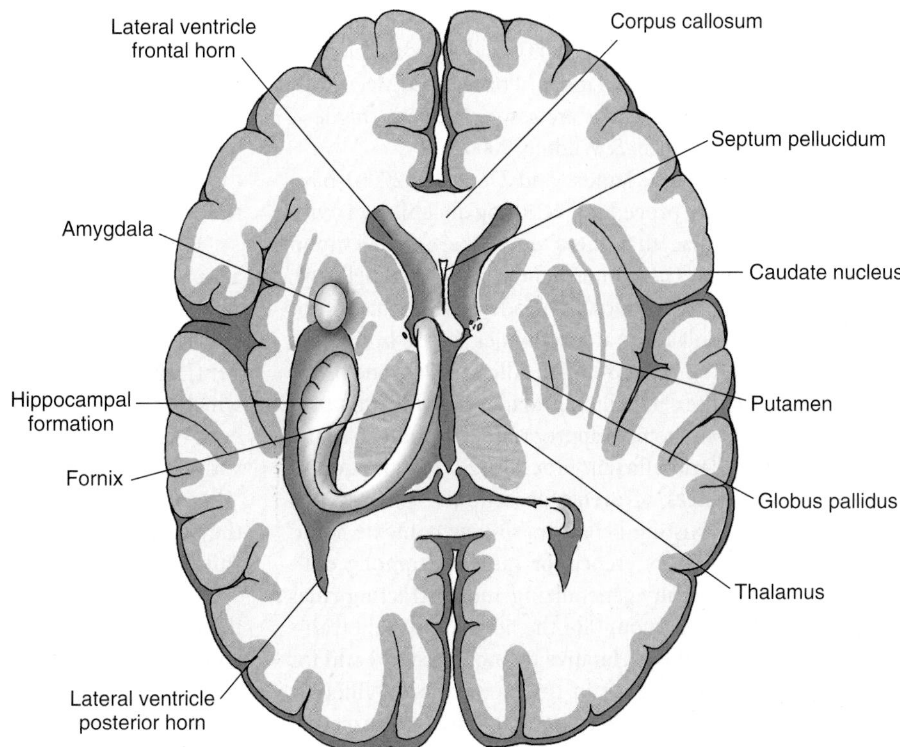

FIGURE 3-17. Hippocampus and thalamus.

more difficult for children with speech sound delays to differentiate between words that they already know and new ones.

Children with specific language impairment are very slow to learn the rules of the languages to which they are exposed. This may result from the fact that they demonstrate deficits on implicit sequential learning tasks, particularly those involving language (Evans, Saffran, & Robe-Torres, 2009). Their learning improves when these patterns are taught through intensive, focused exposure (perhaps facilitating implicit learning) or through explicit training and review of examples of the rules (declarative learning)—just the strategies that are typically used in speech-language intervention. It has been suggested that some of the same underlying neurocognitive mechanisms underlie both language processing and sequential learning (Conway & Pisoni, 2008). Likewise, Conway, Karpicke, and Pisoni (2007) have shown that implicit learning skill is correlated with speech perception skill under degraded listening conditions (such as those experienced by persons with cochlear implants). They hypothesize that individual differences in implicit sequential learning abilities may underlie the wide variety of outcomes associated with cochlear implantation. However, this hypothesis has yet to be explored in depth.

Basic cognitive capacities, such as attention, memory, the ability to make arbitrary associations, and the ability to generalize from specific concrete examples to abstract pattern recognition, are clearly key to the types of learning described above. Children who are cognitively compromised due to head injury, perinatal stroke, anoxia, seizures, prenatal drug or alcohol exposure, high lead levels, or syndromes such as Down syndrome and fragile X syndrome, and children with deficits in attention or organization will clearly be at risk in these respects.

In fact, children with attention deficits—either primary or secondary to some other disorder, such as Tourette, fragile X, and fetal alcohol syndromes—have been shown to be at higher risk of speech-language and learning difficulties. Up to 33% of children with language disorders have comorbid diagnoses of attention disorders; however, the percentage is somewhat lower for those who have speech disorders only (10%) and for those with combined speech-language disorders (23%) (Cantwell & Baker, 1987). Clearly, attention deficits will impact a child's ability to learn from the speech-language models to which they are exposed.

Similarly, memory deficits can have a significant impact upon learning, including speech-language acquisition. Recent models of memory focus on the importance of verbal working memory (VWM) for language and literacy development. Two main subcomponents of VWM that are differentiated by modality have been hypothesized. The first is the **phonological loop** (a.k.a. phonological memory), which is responsible for holding acoustic speech information in short-term memory. The second is the **visual–spatial sketch pad**, which serves a similar function for visual–spatial input (Gathercole & Pickering, 2000). A third component, **working memory** capacity, determines the person's ability to hold items in short-term memory while manipulating them, such as for phonological awareness tasks that require replacement or movement of syllables or phonemes (e.g., Pig Latin). In addition to being a hallmark of reading disability, phonological memory deficits also have been identified in children with Down syndrome

(Laws, 1998, 2004), fetal alcohol syndrome (Pei, Rinaldi, Rasmussen, Massey, & Massey, 2008), and Landau-Kleffner syndrome (Majerus, Van der Linden, Poncelet, & Metz-Lutz, 2004). General memory deficits are associated with fragile X syndrome (Munir, Cornish, & Wilding, 2000).

Mostofsky, Goldberg, Landa, and Denckla (2000) have identified deficits in procedural learning in children with ASD and hypothesize that these deficits are based upon cerebellar differences (i.e., abnormalities in the **cerebellum**). This is in keeping with a proposal by Rodier (2002) that motor deficits in ASD result from abnormalities in the **brainstem** and/or the cerebellum. According to Allen (2006), one of the main functions of the cerebellum is to identify and anticipate temporal patterns and to plan appropriate responses to them, resulting in "rapid and efficient processing or production of coordinated sequences of events or actions" (p. 202). An inability to adjust existing behaviors to new contexts could be one source of the preference for sameness among children with ASD. Difficulty generalizing and abstracting rules from exemplars could account for the need for explicit training (i.e., learning via the declarative memory system) and for extended periods of practice in this population. Williams, Whiten, Suddendorf, and Perrett (2001) hypothesize that differences in the mirror neuron system could account for imitation deficits in children with ASD; however, such differences have yet to be experimentally verified. (See Hamilton, Brindley, & Frith [2007] for an opposing point of view.)

Summary

The interrelationships among cognition, language, and speech are many and complex. Overall, deficits in at least two of the three areas appear to co-occur more often than not, although one may be far more significant than the other(s). Basic cognitive capacities, such as attention, memory, the ability to make arbitrary associations, and the ability to generalize from specific concrete examples to abstract patterns, clearly underlie linguistic learning. Human pattern learning capabilities (e.g., implicit procedural learning) appear to be especially important; deficits in this area often co-occur with speech-language or other communication as well as learning deficits. Attempts to divide speech sound disorders into those that are purely motoric and those that are purely cognitive–linguistic appear to be unenlightening.

EXERCISE 3-4

Cognitive Precursors to Speech

SOCIAL PRECURSORS TO SPEECH

Like the solution to a good mystery novel, communication efficacy depends upon the triad: means, motive, and opportunity (Davis & Velleman, 2008). Means refers to the ability to produce the speech sounds required for one's own language in the proper combinations and sequences. This is the portion of the equation that most speech-language pathologists focus on in their intervention strategies most of the time. However, the ability to produce speech is useless without the other two: the motivation to communicate ideas to someone else and the opportunity to communicate them to a listener who will understand and respond appropriately.

Emotional disorders co-occur with speech disorders about 15% of the time and with speech-language disorders 21% of the time (Cantwell & Baker, 1987). Being a sociable, persistent child reduces one's risk of speech-language disorder (Harrison & McLeod, 2010), but it's difficult to determine which is the cause and which is the effect—or whether there even is a cause–effect relationship present. In any case, motivation is a key factor to successful communication. After all, "It is not sufficient to ensure that children have language; they also must use it to build social and functional relationships" (MacDonald & Carroll, 1992, p. 121).

Of course, before infants can have intent to communicate themselves, they must have the opportunity to learn about communication. This is where caregiver input and responsiveness are vital. In most cultures (though, apparently, not all—see, e.g., Everett, 2008), adults and even young children who interact with babies adjust their prosody, word choices, and grammatical choices according to the infants' age (Tomasello & Mannle, 1985). As previously mentioned, this IDS is also called baby talk and motherese, and it is restricted neither to mothers nor to infants (e.g., many people use "pet talk" as well; Burnham, Kitamura, & Vollmer-Conna, 2002). It is beyond the scope of this book to review all of the vast literature on IDS. We will focus briefly and specifically on the features of this register that relate the most to phonology here. The two main aspects of the register to be emphasized are phonological changes in caregivers' speech and pragmatic changes in the way that they address their babies.

The phonological changes found in IDS include higher pitch, wider pitch ranges, and hyperarticulated vowels. Caregivers' motives in using these features appear to be partly affective (emotional) and partly didactic; for example, the pitch characteristics, but not the carefully articulated vowels, are present in speech to pets as well as to infants (Burnham et al., 2002).

The pragmatic changes in IDS involve caregivers following the child's lead in various ways. Most researchers have focused on **semantic contingency**—the fact that adults tend to talk about the child's focus of interest. Contingency can also be phonetic, however. **Phonetic contingency** involves incorporating phonetic aspects of the child's utterance into one's own. This can start at birth, with the caregiver imitating the infants' pitch patterns, for example. Some parents even copy their babies' **reflexive vocalizations** (burps, grunts, and the like) as well as their **vocal play** (raspberries, etc.). Mothers may be especially likely to be phonetically contingent to their babies' vocalizations during periods when their infants are at the beginning of a new vocal stage (Velleman et al., 1989). When the infant begins to produce canonical babble, it becomes easier for the caregiver to be both semantically and phonetically contingent, incorporating the phonetics of the child's babble into a word that is semantically related to the child's focus. For example, if the infant says [ba] while holding a ball, the parent is likely to say "ball," thus reinforcing both the vocalization and its potential meaning. Many caregivers optimistically interpret their children's babbles as real words, which results in the production of a great deal of phonetically and semantically contingent language. This may facilitate the child's learning of these sound–meaning connections. In fact, research has shown an association between the clarity of a mother's speech when she talks to her infant and that infant's speech perception skills (Liu, Kuhl, & Tsao, 2003).

It would be unethical to deliberately withhold IDS in order to study whether or not it increases the child's rate of language development. However, as reviewed above, it has been shown in a variety of experiments that infants learn better when the verbal stimuli are presented as baby talk than when they are presented using typical adult-to-adult speech patterns (Kaplan, Jung, Ryther, & Zarlengo-Strouse, 1996). In addition, some naturally occurring experiments can be observed and manipulated. For example, Kaplan, Bachorowski, Smoski, and Hudenko (2002) studied infants of depressed mothers. They found that these parents produced less varied prosodic patterns than non-depressed mothers and that all infants were less likely to demonstrate **associative learning** when the verbal stimuli were presented in IDS by depressed mothers rather than being produced in IDS by non-depressed mothers. The infants of depressed mothers learned the typical amount when the stimuli were presented to them by non-depressed strangers. Similarly, Harrison and McLeod (2010) found that mothers' levels of well-being were predictive of the likelihood of children having speech-language problems.

It has been demonstrated that children from lower socioeconomic status homes are exposed to fewer communicative gestures (Rowe & Goldin-Meadow, 2009), fewer words, and shorter utterances than those from more highly educated/more financially stable families and that these differences have a negative impact on the youngsters' vocabularies (Hart & Risley, 1995; Hoff & Tian, 2005; Rowe & Goldin-Meadow, 2009). Children who live in poverty are known to demonstrate language delays relative to those from more advantaged homes (Pungello, Iruka, Dotterer, Mills-Koonce, & Reznick, 2009; Walker, Greenwood, Hart, & Carta, 1994). However, very few studies have addressed the role of SES on children's early speech. Some studies have indicated that vocalization rates are lower in children who live in poverty though the age of onset of babble is not different (Eilers, Oller, Levine, Basinger, Lynch, et al., 1993; Oller, Eilers, Basinger, Steffens, & Urbano, 1995; Oller, Eilers, Steffans, Lynch, & Urbano, 1994). In contrast, Furey, Watkins, and Wardrop (2005) found that there was no difference in **volubility** (number of words spoken by each child per session) between offspring of more versus less well-educated mothers. However, the babble of infants whose mothers have 15 or fewer years of education appears to include fewer different consonants than that of infants whose mothers have higher levels of schooling (Furey, 2003). In contrast, the complexity of babble (e.g., the proportion of syllables that include consonants) does not appear to be impacted by SES (Calvo & Furey, 2007; Eilers et al., 1993; Oller, Eilers, Basinger, et al., 1995; Oller, Eilers, Steffans, et al., 1994). Nor is the complexity of children's early words affected by income levels (Furey & Owen, 2008). Dollaghan, Campbell, Paradise, Feldman, Janosky, and colleagues (1999) found that maternal education impacted some aspects of 3-year-olds' linguistic skills, but not consonant accuracy. Surprisingly, Broomfield and Dodd (2004) actually found a higher incidence of speech disabilities in children from birth through school age from affluent families versus other income levels. Campbell, Dollaghan, Rockette, Paradise, Feldman, and team (2003), on the other hand, identified SES as one predictive factor in the likelihood of a 3-year-old exhibiting a speech delay. Similarly, McDowell, Lonigan, and Goldstein (2007) identified impacts of SES on phonological awareness in children from 2 to 5 years old, especially in the older children. Thus, the effects of SES on speech production and awareness skills are mixed and unclear.

With respect to the child's communication with others, **communicative intents** are the meat of motive—rejecting/avoiding, requesting, giving, showing, greeting, and commenting. Even the most low-functioning child will express aversion—rejecting/avoiding—in some way (e.g., by throwing an object they do not want or turning away from it). But the other intents are often lacking in children with lower intelligence quotients; children in non-stimulating, unsupportive family environments; children with learning disabilities; and children on the autism spectrum.

Furthermore, for a child to make the effort to learn to talk—especially a child who has some type of motor speech disorder for whom this may be a difficult task—she has to know that someone is indeed there not only to hear it but to listen and respond as well. Providing these opportunities may not be as easy as it sounds. In some cases, the child's communicative acts may be so aversive, so subtle, or so atypical that her significant others either do not recognize them as such or are reluctant to reward them with a response. In other cases, the child may not be able to recognize adult responses as communicative.

ASDs are the disorders that most people think of when they consider children whose social/pragmatic skills may interfere with their communicative development. Until recently, up to 50% of children with ASDs did not achieve oral communication (Seal & Bonvillian, 1997). Fortunately, early identification and intervention, as well as improved intervention strategies, have significantly decreased this proportion (Tager-Flusberg, Paul, & Lord, 2005). However, phonetic and phonological deficits are very common in those children with ASDs who do communication orally (see Boucher, 2013 or Velleman, Andrianopoulos, Boucher, Perkins, Averback, et al.,

2009a for reviews). Furthermore, even very intelligent individuals with this syndrome, such as those with high-functioning autism, often retain immaturities in their speech past expected ages or fail to adapt to the speech patterns of their peers (Baron-Cohen & Staunton, 1994; Paul, Bianchi, Augustyn, & Volkmar, 2008). Some ASD researchers, such as Paul and colleagues (2008), attribute these persistent residual speech differences to the pragmatic deficits that are key to this group of disorders. Such scholars hypothesize that these ongoing phonetic immaturities reflect the children's lack of interest in sounding like their peers or perhaps their lack of understanding that their speech errors might pose a problem for listeners. However, many other authors have reported motor deficits in ASDs (e.g., Ming et al., 2007), and some have extended this finding to motor speech deficits (e.g., Boucher, 2013; Prizant, 1996; Szypulski, 2003; Velleman et al., 2009a, 2009b). Thus, the exact roles of pragmatic versus motor speech factors in the phonetic and phonological delays, differences, and disorders exhibited by children with ASDs remain to be delineated.

Summary

Communication requires means, motive, and opportunity. The latter two of these are social factors: the child must have both a reason and a desire to communicate as well as a responsive audience. Children with ASDs appear to have deficits with respect to motive, but they may also demonstrate motor speech difficulties. Furthermore, their attempts at communication may be so atypical that listeners do not recognize them as such. On the other hand, children of depressed mothers and those from lower socioeconomic levels may have reduced opportunities for learning due to exposure to less varied vocabulary and to less responsiveness—or less helpful responses—on the part of their communication partners.

EXERCISE 3-5

Cognitive and Social Deficits

EXERCISE 3-6

Overall Review

CHAPTER SUMMARY

Multiple factors can impact the successful development of oral communication. These include intact anatomy; functional physiology; and neurologic control of sensory–motor integration, motor programming/planning, processing, categorization, generalization, attention, and memory. Furthermore, all of these factors contribute to providing the required means of communication. They are useless without the addition of motive (the desire to communicate) and opportunity (a receptive audience willing and able to interpret the communicative attempts).

Three models of speech production may be useful in conceptualizing the developmental progression of becoming a fluent speaker of a language. Gestural phonology reminds us that we do not produce a series of consonants and vowels; we produce fluid, overlapping articulatory gestures that yield the percept of a series of consonants and vowels. DIVA highlights the importance of feedforward mechanisms for identifying and adjusting for the current state of the system before embarking on action in order to minimize the amount of feedback about miscalculations or inaccuracies that is necessary. Dynamic systems theory integrates the roles of all precursors to speech in a highly complex communication system that is constantly evolving and reorganizing itself for maximum efficiency and effectiveness. It reassures us that flexibility and even instability and errors are key parts of the learning process.

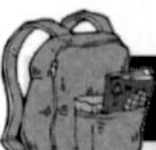

KEY TAKE-HOME MESSAGES

1. Speaking more than one language or dialect or a nonmainstream dialect is a linguistic difference, neither a delay nor a disorder.
2. Prerequisites are necessary antecedents of later development; precursors may contribute but are not crucial.
3. A wide variety of factors can affect speech development. Interactions among these factors and the impacts of these factors may differ from child to child and also over time.
4. Purely motoric or purely cognitive-linguistic speech disorders are not the rule; symptoms overlap in many children with speech sound delays or disorders.
5. Theoretical speech production models, such as DIVA, gestural phonology, and dynamic systems theory, can help us understand disorders such as Childhood Apraxia of Speech.

CHAPTER 3

Precursors to Speech Review

Exercise 3-1: **Anatomy/Physiology and Motor Functions/ Differences**

A. State whether the following statements are true or false:

1. ______Speech motor development is derived from non-speech motor functions (sucking, swallowing, etc.).
2. ______Motor plans are specific to a particular situation or context.
3. ______Children with Down syndrome always have large tongues (macroglossia).
4. ______Ankyloglossia results from intubation of premature infants.

B. Match the following reflexes to the definitions:

1. ______Jaw stretch reflex	a. Sucking movements stimulated by touch on the palate
2. ______Biting reflex	b. Orientation of the head in the direction of a light touch stimulus in the peri-oral area, typically followed/accompanied by mouth opening and sucking or swallowing movements
3. ______Rooting reflex	c. Jaw closing when the area below the lower lip is tapped
4. ______Sucking reflex	d. Mouth closing in response to light touch on the anterior gingiva (gums)

C. Multiple Choice: Choose the correct answer.

1. Motor programs are:
   a. learned through experience.
   b. more contextual than motor plans.
   c. innately determined.
   d. suppressed in infancy.
2. Reflexes:
   a. always decrease after infancy.
   b. do not occur in the oral area.
   c. are exaggerated in children with speech delays.
   d. are automatic.
3. Types of muscle tone do not include:
   a. low.
   b. premature.
   c. high.
   d. fluctuating.

Exercise 3-2: **Sensory and Sensory–Motor Connections**

1. Which of the following are generally believed to play *positive* roles in early speech perception or production?
   a. Phonetic/phonotactic distributional probabilities
   b. Intra-oral tactile sensations
   c. Auditory acuity
   d. Visual information about the speaker's mouth
   e. Otitis media
   f. Infant-directed speech
   g. Mirror neurons
   h. Cochlear implants
   i. Muscle spindles
2. Multiple Choice: Choose the correct answer.
   A. The effects of otitis media on speech development:
      a. are universal.
      b. are primarily sensorineural.
      c. are influenced by socioeconomic status.
      d. rarely impact language skills.
   B. Infants cannot detect:
      a. distributional probabilities.
      b. categorical differences.
      c. prosodic patterns, such as stress.
      d. differences between indeterminate tokens.

Exercise 3-3: **Models of Speech Production and Perception**

A. Multiple Choice: Choose the correct answer.

1. Speech sounds are not produced as individual units according to which model?
   a. Feedback mechanism
   b. DIVA model
   c. Gestural phonology
   d. Dynamic systems theory
2. Key elements of the DIVA model include:
   a. feedforward mechanisms.
   b. feeding functions.
   c. static articulatory targets.
   d. all of the above.
3. In dynamic systems theory, which of the following do not play an important role?
   a. Innate linguistic parameters
   b. Cross-modal interactions
   c. Cognitive functions
   d. Environmental influences

4. Which of the following are not expected to co-occur during the typical process of speech development?
   a. Precision and flexibility
   b. Hypersensitivity and hyposensitivity
   c. Stability and instability
   d. Feedforward and feedback
5. Childhood Apraxia of Speech:
   a. has a consistent genetic basis.
   b. results from feedback, not feedforward, deficits.
   c. may have a neurologic basis.
   d. none of the above.

Exercise 3-4: **Cognitive Precursors to Speech**

Multiple Choice: Choose the correct answer.

1. Human learning:
   a. is slower when teaching is explicit.
   b. is based on patterns in adults but not in infants.
   c. is not possible without focused attention.
   d. includes tallying statistics about linguistic occurrences.
2. Children's speech-language learning is not affected by:
   a. neighborhood density (number of minimal pairs).
   b. phonotactic probability (distinctness).
   c. longitude and latitude.
   d. focal brain injury.
3. Learning differences in children with ASD have been attributed to:
   a. abnormalities in the brainstem and/or the cerebellum.
   b. procedural learning deficits.
   c. differences in the mirror neuron system.
   d. all of the above.

Exercise 3-5: **Cognitive and Social Deficits**

Multiple Choice: Choose the correct answer.

1. Which of the following typically has negative effects on infants' learning?
   a. Maternal depression
   b. Volubility
   c. Infant-directed speech
   d. Maternal educational achievement
2. Children with autism spectrum disorders may exhibit:
   a. decreased procedural learning.
   b. motor speech disorders.
   c. persistent immaturities in their speech.
   d. all of the above.

Exercise 3-6: **Overall Review**

1. For each of the following precursor symptoms, indicate (1) a possible etiology (medical condition, genetic syndrome, etc.) and (2) a possible speech-language implication.
   a. low tone (hypotonia)
   b. high-arched palate
   c. decreased hearing acuity
   d. decreased sensory–motor feedback and/or feedforward
   e. decreased implicit/procedural learning
   f. impaired phonological loop
   g. decreased motivation to communicate
2. Essay question: Using information from this chapter and at least one reference other than this book, learn more about a particular genetic condition or neurodevelopmental syndrome. Choose two of the symptoms from Question 1 that tend to co-occur in children with that diagnosis. Citing your sources, describe:
   a. how these two symptoms manifest in that condition.
   b. their likely impact on speech.
   c. potential interactions between the two. That is, is the impact of the combination of the two symptoms likely to be more significant than the impact of only one of them? Are the two symptoms likely to exacerbate each others' impacts on speech (perception or production)? Why or why not?
   d. how the impacts that these symptoms have on children with this diagnosis would be described within one or more of the models reviewed in this chapter.
3. Essay question: Sheila has Down syndrome. At 18 months, she has successfully survived cardiac surgery, including several weeks of hospitalization. Several deficits remain: low muscle tone, frequent otitis media, an apparently large tongue, and a cognitive impairment. Are these typical of children with Down syndrome? How will these or other features of her syndrome affect her speech development?

References

Allen, G. (2006). Cerebellar contributions to autism spectrum disorders. *Clinical Neuroscience Research*, *6*(3–4), 195–207.

Ambrose, S. E., Berry, L. M. U., Walker, E. A., Harrison, M., Oleson, J., & Moeller, M. P. (2014). Speech sound production in 2-year-olds who are hard of hearing. *American Journal of Speech Language Pathology*, *23*, 91–104.

Anderson, J. L., Morgan, J. L., & White, K. S. (2003). A statistical basis for speech sound discrimination. *Language and Speech*, *46*(2–3), 155–182.

Anthony, J. L., Aghara, R. G., Dunkelberger, M. J., Anthony, T. I., Williams, J. M., & Zhang, Z. (2011). What factors place children with speech sound disorders at risk for reading problems? *American Journal of Speech-Language Pathology*, *20*, 146–160.

Arvedson, J. C. (2000). Evaluation of children with feeding and swallowing problems. *Language, Speech, and Hearing Services in Schools*, *31*, 28–41.

ASHA (2005). (Central) auditory processing disorders: The role of the audiologist. Available at: http://www.asha.org/policy

ASHA (2007). *Childhood Apraxia of Speech [Technical Report]*. Rockville Pike, MD: American Speech-Language-Hearing Association.

Baron-Cohen, H., & Staunton, R. (1994). Do children with autism acquire the phonology of their peers? An examination of group identification through the window of bilingualism. *First Language*, *14*, 241–248.

Bates, E. A. (2004). Explaining and interpreting deficits in language development across clinical groups: Where do we go from here? *Brain and Language*, *88*, 248–253.

Baylis, A. L., Munson, B., & Moller, K. T. (2008). Factors affecting articulation skills in children with velocardiofacial syndrome and children with cleft palate or velopharyngeal dysfunction: A preliminary report. *Cleft Palate-Craniofacial Journal, 45*(2), 193–207.

Bersu, E. T., & Opitz, J. M. (1980). Anatomical analysis of the developmental effects of aneuploidy in man: The down syndrome. *American Journal of Medical Genetics, 5*(4), 399–420.

Bijelac-Babic, R., Bertoncini, J., & Mehler, J. (1993). How do 4-day-old infants categorize multisyllabic utterances? *Developmental Psychology, 29*(4), 711–721.

Bird, J., & Bishop, D. V. M. (1992). Perception and awareness of phonemes in phonologically impaired children. *European Journal of Disorders of Communication, 27*, 289–311.

Bishop, D. V. M. (2002). Motor immaturity and specific speech and language impairment: Evidence for a common genetic basis. *American Journal of Medical Genetics, 114*(1), 56–63.

Blaiser, K. (2011). *Speech sound disorders: Children with hearing loss.* San Diego, CA: American Speech-Language-Hearing Association.

Blamey, P. J., Barry, J. G., & Jacq, P. (2001). Phonetic inventory development in young cochlear implant users 6 years postoperation. *Journal of Speech, Language, and Hearing Research, 44*, 73–79.

Bosma, J. F. (1975). Anatomic and physiologic development of the speech apparatus. In D. B. Tower (Ed.), *The nervous system: Human communication and its disorders, 3.* New York, NY: Raven Press.

Boucher, M. (2013). *Evaluation of motor speech and intervention planning for children with autism.* Doctoral dissertation, University of Massachusetts, Boston, MA (p. 729).

Boysson-Bardies, B. d., Halle, P., Sagart, L., & Durand, C. (1989). A cross-linguistic investigation of vowel formants in babbling. *Journal of Child Language, 16*, 1–17.

Boysson-Bardies, B. d., & Vihman, M. M. (1991). Adaptation to language: Evidence from babbling and first words in four languages. *Language, 67*, 297–319.

Boysson-Bardies, B. d., Vihman, M. M., Roug-Hellichus, L., Durand, C., Landberg, I., & Arao, F. (1992). Material evidence of infant selection from target language: A cross-linguistic phonetic study. In C. Ferguson, L. Menn, C. Stoel-Gammon (Eds.), *Phonological development: Models, research, implications.* Timonium, MD: York Press.

Bradford, A., & Dodd, B. (1996). Do all speech-disordered children have motor deficits? *Clinical Linguistics and Phonetics, 10*(2), 77–101.

Bridgeman, E., & Snowling, M. (1988). The perception of phoneme sequence: A comparison of dyspraxic and normal children. *British Journal of Disorders of Communication, 23*, 245–252.

Broen, P. A., Strange, W., Doyle, S. S., & Heller, J. H. (1983). Perception and production of approximant consonants by normal and articulation-delayed preschool children. *Journal of Speech and Hearing Research, 26*, 601–608.

Broomfield, J., & Dodd, B. (2004). Children with speech and language disability: Caseload characteristics. *International Journal of Language and Communication Disorders, 39*(3), 303–324.

Browman, C. P., & Goldstein, L. (1989). *Articulatory gestures as phonological units. Haskins status report on speech research* (pp. 69–101). New Haven, CT: Haskins Laboratories.

Buccino, G., Binkofskib, F., & Riggioa, L. (2004). The mirror neuron system and action recognition. *Brain and Language, 89*(2), 370–376.

Burnham, D., Kitamura, C., & Vollmer-Conna, U. (2002). What's new, Pussycat? On talking to babies and animals. *Science, 296*, 1435.

Callan, D. E., Kent, R. D., Guenther, F. H., & Vorperian, H. K. (2000). An auditory-feedback-based neural network model of speech production that is robust to developmental changes in the size and shape of the articulatory system. *Journal of Speech, Language, and Hearing Research, 43*, 721–736.

Calvo, J., & Furey, J. E. (2007). *Phonetic complexity in words targeted by children from 12 to 18 months of age.* Paper presented at the American Speech-Language-Hearing Association, Boston, MA.

Cameron, T. H., & Kelly, D. P. (1988). Normal language skills and normal intelligence in a child with de Lange syndrome. *The Journal of Speech and Hearing Disorders, 53*(2), 219–222.

Campbell, T. F., Dollaghan, C. A., Rockette, H. E., Paradise, J. L., Feldman, H. M., Shriberg, L. D., …, Kurs-Lasky, M. (2003). Risk factors for speech delay of unknown origin in 3-year-old children. *Child Development, 74*(2), 346–357.

Cantwell, D. P., & Baker, L. (1987). Prevalence and type of psychiatric disorder and developmental disorders in three speech and language groups. *Journal of Communication Disorders, 20*, 151–160.

Carnoel, S. O., Marks, S. M., & Weik, L. (1999). The speech-language pathologist: Key role in the diagnosis of velocardiofacial syndrome. *American Journal of Speech-Language Pathology, 8*(1), 23–32.

Chen, C.-L., Lin, K.-C., Chen, C.-H., Chen, C.-C., Liu, W. Y., Chung, C.-Y., …, Wu, C.-Y. (2010). Factors associated with motor speech control in children with spastic cerebral palsy. *Chang Gung Medical Journal, 33*(4), 415–423.

Chen, H., & Stevens, K. N. (2001). An acoustical study of the fricative /s/ in the speech of individuals with dysarthria. *Journal of Speech, Language, and Hearing Research, 44*(6), 1300–1314.

Cheng, H. Y., Murdoch, B. E., Goozée, J. V., & Scott, D. (2007). Electropalatographic assessment of tongue-to-palate contact patterns and variability in children, adolescents, and adults. *Journal of Speech, Language, and Hearing Research, 50*(2), 375–392.

Cleland, J., Wood, S., Hardcastle, W. J., Wishart, J., & Timmins, C. (2010). Relationship between speech, oromotor, language and cognitive abilities in children with Down's [sic] syndrome. *International Journal of Language and Communication Disorders, 45*(1), 83–95.

Conway, C. M., Karpicke, J., & Pisoni, D. B. (2007). Contribution of implicit sequence learning to spoken language processing: Some preliminary findings with hearing adults. *Journal of Deaf Studies and Deaf Education, 12*(3), 317–334.

Conway, C. M., & Pisoni, D. B. (2008). Neurocognitive basis of implicit learning of sequential structure and its relation to language processing. *Annals of the New York Academy of Sciences, 1145*, 113–131.

Corriveau, K., Pasquini, E., & Goswami, U. (2007). Basic auditory processing skills and Specific Language Impairment: A new look at an old hypothesis. *Journal of Speech, Language, and Hearing Research, 50*, 647–666.

Crelin, E. S. (1973). *Functional anatomy of the newborn.* New Haven, CT: Yale University Press.

Crelin, E. (1987). *The human vocal tract.* New York, NY: Vantage.

Dall'Oglio, A. M., Bates, E., Volterra, V., Di Capua, M., & Pezzini, G. (1994). Early cognition, communication, and language in children with focal brain injury. *Developmental Medicine and Child Neurology, 36*(12), 1076–1098.

Darley, F., Aronson, A., & Brown, J. (1975). *Motor speech disorders.* Philadelphia, PA: Saunders.

Davis, B., & MacNeilage, P. (1995). The articulatory basis of babbling. *Journal of Speech and Hearing Research, 38*, 1199–1211.

Davis, B. L., & Velleman, S. L. (2008). Establishing a basic speech repertoire without using NSOME: Means, motive, and opportunity. *Seminars in Speech and Language, 29*(4), 312–319.

Dawson, P. W., Blamey, P. J., Dettman, S. J., Barker, E. J., & Clark, G. M. (1995). A clinical report on receptive vocabulary skills in cochlear implant users. *Ear and Hearing, 16*, 287–294.

DeCasper, A. J., & Fifer, W. P. (1980). Of human bonding: Newborns prefer their mothers' voices. *Science, 208*, 1174–1176.

DeCasper, A. J., & Spence, M. J. (1986). Prenatal maternal speech influences newborns' perception of speech sounds. *Infant Behavior and Development, 9*(2), 133–150.

Desjardins, R. N., & Werker, J. F. (1996, 18–21 April). *4-month-old female infants are influenced by visible speech.* Poster presented at the Xth Biennial International Conference of Infant Studies, Providence, RI.

Dollaghan, C. A., Campbell, T. F., Paradise, J. L., Feldman, H. M., Janosky, J. E., & Pitcairn, D. L. (1999). Maternal education and measures of early speech and language. *Journal of Speech, Language, and Hearing Research, 42*, 1432–1443.

Edmonston, N. K. (1982). Management of speech and language impairment in a case of Prader-Willi syndrome. *Language, Speech, and Hearing Services in Schools, 13*, 241–245.

Edwards, J., Fourakis, M., Beckman, M. E., & Fox, R. A. (1999). Characterizing knowledge deficits in phonological disorders. *Journal of Speech, Language, and Hearing Research, 42*, 169–186.

Edwards, J., Fox, R. A., & Rogers, C. L. (2002). Final consonant discrimination in children: Effects of phonological disorder, vocabulary size, and articulatory accuracy. *Journal of Speech, Language, and Hearing Research, 45*, 231–242.

Eilers, R. E. (1977). Context-sensitive perception of naturally-produced stop and fricative consonants by infants. *Journal of the Acoustical Society of America, 61*, 1321–1336.

Eilers, R. E., & Minifie, F. D. (1975). Fricative discrimination in early infancy. *Journal of Speech and Hearing Research, 18*, 158–167.

Eilers, R. E., Oller, D. K., Levine, S., Basinger, D., Lynch, M. P., & Urbano, R. (1993). The role of prematurity and socioeconomic status in the onset of canonical babbling in infants. *Infant Behavior and Development, 16*, 297–315.

Evans, J. L., Saffran, J. R., & Robe-Torres, K. (2009). Statistical learning in children with specific language impairment. *Journal of Speech, Language, and Hearing Research, 52*, 321–335.

Everett, D. L. (2008). *Don't sleep, there are snakes*. New York, NY: Pantheon.

Fadiga, L., Craighero, L., Buccino, G., & Rizzolatti, G. (2002). Speech listening specifically modulates the excitability of tongue muscles: A TMS study. *European Journal of Neuroscience, 15*(2), 399–402.

Fisher, S. E., Vargha-Khadem, F., Watkins, K. E., Monaco, A. P., & Pembrey, M. E. (1998). Localisation of a gene implicated in a severe speech and language disorder. *Nature Genetics, 18*(2), 168–170.

Flanagan, J. E., Landa, R., Bhat, A., & Bauman, M. (2012). Head lag in infants at risk for autism: A preliminary study. *The American Journal of Occupational Therapy, 66*(5), 577–585.

Flipsen, P. J., & Parker, R. G. (2008). Phonological patterns in the conversational speech of children with cochlear implants. *Journal of Communication Disorders, 41*, 337–357.

Friederici, A. D., & Wessels, J. M. (1993). Phonotactic knowledge of word boundaries and its use in infant speech perception. *Perception and Psychophysics, 54*, 287–295.

Froud, K., & Khamis-Dakwar, R. (2012). Mismatch negativity responses in children with a diagnosis of Childhood Apraxia of Speech (CAS). *American Journal of Speech Language Pathology, 21*, 302–312.

Furey, J. E. (2003). *The growth of early phonological and lexical development: A longitudinal investigation*. (Doctoral), University of Illinois, Urbana, IL.

Furey, J. E., & Owen, A. (2008). *Phonetic complexity of toddlers' early words*. Chicago, IL: American Speech-Language-Hearing Association. .

Furey, J. E., Watkins, R. V., & Wardrop, J. L. (2005). *Early phonological development and maternal education*. Paper presented International Child Phonology Conference, Fort Worth, TX.

Galantucci, B., Fowler, C. A., & Turvey, M. T. (2006). The motor theory of speech perception reviewed. *Psychonomic Bulletin and Review, 13*(3), 361–377.

Garlock, V. M., Walley, A. C., & Metsala, J. L. (2001). Age-of-acquisition, word frequency, and neighborhood density effects on spoken word recognition by children and adults. *Journal of Memory and Language, 45*, 468–492.

Garstecki, D. C., Borton, T. E., Stark, E. W., & Kennedy, B. T. (1972). Speech, language, and hearing problems in the Laurence-Moon-Biedl syndrome. *The Journal of Speech and Hearing Disorders, 37*(3), 407–413.

Gathercole, S. E., & Pickering, S. J. (2000). Assessment of working memory in six- and seven-year old children. *Journal of Educational Psychology, 92*, 377–390.

Gaultier, C. (1995). Respiratory muscle function in infants. *The European Respiratory Journal, 8*(1), 150–153.

Gerken, L. A., & Zamuner, T. (2004, June 24). *Exploring the basis for generalization in language acquisition*. Paper presented at the 9th Conference on Laboratory Phonology, University of Illinois at Urbana-Champaign, Urbana, IL.

German, R. Z., & Palmer, J. B. (2006). Anatomy and development of oral cavity and pharynx. *GI Motility online*. Available at: http://www.nature.com/gimo/contents/pt1/full/gimo5.html

Gibbon, F. E. (1999). Undifferentiated lingual gestures in children with articulation/phonological disorders. *Journal of Speech, Language, and Hearing Research, 42*, 382–397.

Good, C. D., Johnsrude, I., Ashburner, J., Henson, R. N. A., Friston, K. J., & Frackowiak, R. S. J. (2001). Cerebral asymmetry and the effects of sex and handedness on brain structure: A voxel-based morphometric analysis of 465 normal adult human brains. *NeuroImage, 14*(3), 685–700.

Goodsit, J. V., Morse, P. A., Ver Hoeve, J. N., & Cowan, N. (1984). Infant speech recognition in multisyllabic contexts. *Child Development, 55*, 903–910.

Green, J. R., Moore, C. A., Higashikawa, M., & Steeve, R. W. (2000). The physiologic development of speech motor control: Lip and jaw coordination. *Journal of Speech, Language, and Hearing Research, 43*, 239–256.

Grigos, M. I., & Kolenda, N. (2010). The relationship between articulatory control and improved phonemic accuracy in childhood apraxia of speech: A longitudinal case study. *Clinical Linguistics & Phonetics, 24*(1), 17–40.

Groenen, P., Crul, T., Maassen, B., & van Bon, W. (1996). Perception of voicing cues by children with early otitis media with and without language impairment. *Journal of Speech, Language, and Hearing Research, 39*, 43–54.

Guenther, F. H. (1995). Speech sound acquisition, coarticulation, and rate effects in a neural network model of speech production. *Psychological Review, 102*(3), 594–621.

Guenther, F. H., Ghosh, S. S., & Tourville, J. A. (2006). Neural modeling and imaging of the cortical interactions underlying syllable production. *Brain and Language, 96*, 280–301.

Halle, P., & Boysson-Bardies, B. d. (1994). Emergence of an early receptive lexicon: Infants' recognition of words. *Infant Behavior and Development, 17*, 119–129.

Halle, P., & Boysson-Bardies, B. d. (1996). The format of representation of recognized words in infants' early receptive lexicon. *Infant Behavior and Development, 19*, 435–451.

Halliday, L. F., & Bishop, D. V. M. (2005). Frequency discrimination and literacy skills in children with mild to moderate sensorineural hearing loss. *Journal of Speech, Language, and Hearing Research, 48*, 1187–1203.

Hamilton, A. F., Brindley, R. M., & Frith, U. (2007). Imitation and action understanding in autistic spectrum disorders: How valid is the hypothesis of a deficit in the mirror neuron system? *Neuropsychologia, 45*(8), 1859–1868.

Harrison, L. J., & McLeod, S. (2010). Risk and protective factors associated with speech and language impairment in a nationally representative sample of 4- to 5-year-old children. *Journal of Speech, Language, and Hearing Research, 53*, 508–529.

Hart, B., & Risley, T. R. (1995). *Meaningful differences in the everyday experience of young American children*. Baltimore, MD: Brookes.

Hasegawa-Johnson, M., Pizza, S., Alwan, A., Cha, J. S., & Haker, K. (2003). Vowel category dependence of the relationship between palate height, tongue height, and oral area. *Journal of Speech, Language, and Hearing Research, 46*(3), 738–753.

Hennequin, M., Faulks, D., Veyrune, J.-L., & Bourdiol, P. (1999). Significance of oral health in persons with Down syndrome: A literature review. *Developmental Medicine and Child Neurology, 41*(4), 275—283.

Herbert, M. R., Ziegler, D. A., Makris, N., Bakardjiev, A., Hodgson, J., Adrien, K. T., ..., Caviness, V. S. J. (2003). Larger brain and white matter volumes in children with developmental language disorder. *Developmental Science, 6*(4), F11–F22.

Highman, C., Hennessey, N. W., Leitao, S., & Piek, J. P. (2013). Early development in infants at risk of childhood apraxia of speech: A longitudinal investigation. *Developmental Neuropsychology, 38*(3), 197–210.

Hirsh-Pasek, K., Kemler-Nelson, D. G., Jusczyk, P. W., Wright-Cassidy, K., Druss, B., & Kennedy, L. (1987). Clauses are perceptual units for young infants. *Cognition, 26*, 269–286.

Hockett, C. (1955). *A manual of phonology*. Baltimore, MD: Waverly Press.

Hoff, E., & Tian, C. (2005). Socioeconomic status and cultural influences on language. *Journal of Communication Disorders, 38*, 271–278.

Hoffman, P. R., Daniloff, R. G., Bengoa, D., & Schuckers, G. (1985). Misarticulating and normally articulating children's identification and discrimination of synthetic [r] and [w]. *Journal of Speech and Hearing Disorders, 50*, 46–53.

Hopkins-Acos, P., & Bunker, K. (1979). A child with Noonan syndrome. *The Journal of Speech and Hearing Disorders, 44*(4), 494–503.

Houston, D. M., & Jusczyk, P. W. (2000). The role of talker-specific information in word segmentation by infants. *Journal of Experimental Psychology: Human Perception and Performance, 26*(5), 1570–1582.

Houston, D. M., Jusczyk, P. W., Kuijpers, C., Coolen, R., & Cutler, A. (2000). Cross-language word segmentation by 9-month-olds. *Psychonomic Bulletin and Review, 7*(3), 504–509.

Iuzzini-Seigel, J., Hogan, T. P., Guarino, A. J., & Green, J. R. (2015). Reliance on auditory feedback in children with childhood apraxia of speech. *Journal of Communication Disorders, 54*, 32–42. Available at: http://dx.doi.org/10.1016/j.jcomdis.2015.01.002

Jacks, A., Marquardt, T. P., & Davis, B. L. (2006). Consonant and syllable structure patterns in childhood apraxia of speech: Developmental change in three children. *Journal of Communication Disorders, 39*, 424–441.

James, D., Rajput, K., Brinton, J., & Goswami, U. (2008). Phonological awareness, vocabulary, and word reading in children who use cochlear implants: Does age of implantation explain individual variability in performance outcomes and growth? *Journal of Deaf Studies and Deaf Education, 13*(1), 117–137.

Johnson, E. K., & Jusczyk, P. W. (2001). Word segmentation by 8-month-olds: When speech cues count more than statistics. *Journal of Memory and Language, 44*, 1–20.

Johnson, E. P., Pennington, B. F., Lowenstein, J. H., & Nittrouer, S. (2011). Sensitivity to structure in the speech signal by children with speech sound disorder and reading disability. *Journal of Communication Disorders, 44*, 294–314.

Jusczyk, P. W. (1998). A reply to Littman and to Denenberg. *Science, 280*, 1176–1177.

Jusczyk, P. W., & Aslin, R. N. (1995). Infants' detection of the sound patterns of words in fluent speech. *Cognitive Psychology, 29*(1), 1–23.

Jusczyk, P. W., Cutler, A., & Redanz, L. (1993a). Infants' sensitivity to predominant stress patterns in English. *Child Development, 64*, 675–687.

Jusczyk, P. W., Friederici, A. D., Wessels, J. M., Svenkerud, V. Y., & Jusczyk, A. M. (1993b). Infants' sensitivity to the sound patterns of native language words. *Journal of Memory and Language, 32*, 402–420.

Jusczyk, P. W., Luce, P. A., & Charles-Luce, J. (1994). Infants' sensitivity to phonotactic patterns in the native language. *Journal of Memory and Language, 33*, 630–645.

Jusczyk, P. W., Murray, J., & Bayly, J. (1979). *Perception of place of articulation in fricatives and stops by infants*. Paper presented at the Biennial Meeting of the Society for Research in Child Development, San Francisco, CA.

Kaplan, P. S., Bachorowski, J.-A., Smoski, M. J., & Hudenko, W. J. (2002). Infants of depressed mothers, although competent learners, fail to learn in response to their own mothers' infant-directed speech. *Psychological Science, 13*(3), 268–271.

Kaplan, P. S., Jung, P. C., Ryther, J. S., & Zarlengo-Strouse, P. (1996). Infant- versus adult-directed speech as signals for faces. *Developmental Psychology, 32*, 880–891.

Kemler-Nelson, D. G., Hirsh-Pasek, K., Jusczyk, P. W., & Wright-Cassidy, K. (1989). How the prosodic cues in motherese might assist language learning. *Journal of Child Language, 16*, 55–68.

Kenney, M. K., Barac-Cikoja, D., Finnegan, K., Jeffries, N., & Ludlow, C. L. (2006). Speech perception and short-term memory deficits in persistent developmental speech disorder. *Brain and Language, 96*, 178–190.

Kent, R. D. (2009). *Biological substrates of speech development*. Paper presented at the Leadership Conference, University of Massachusetts-Amherst.

Kent, R. D., & Netsell, R. (1978). Articulatory abnormalities in athetoid cerebral palsy. *Journal of Speech and Hearing Disorders, 43*(3), 353–373.

Kingston, J., & Diehl, R. L. (1994). Phonetic knowledge. *Language, 70*, 419–454.

Kirkham, N. Z., Slemmer, J. A., & Johnson, S. P. (2002). Visual statistical learning in infancy: Evidence for a domain general learning mechanism. *Cognition, 83*, B35–B42.

Kuehn, D. P., Templeton, P. J., & Maynard, J. A. (1990). Muscle spindles in the velopharyngeal musculature of humans. *Journal of Speech and Hearing Research, 33*(3), 488–493.

Kuhl, P. K., & Miller, J. D. (1975). Speech perception in early infancy: Discrimination of speech-sound categories. *Journal of the Acoustical Society of America, 58* (Suppl 1), S56.

Kumar, D. (1990). Moebius syndrome. *Journal of Medical Genetics, 27*, 122–126.

Kumin, L. (1996). Speech and language skills in children with Down syndrome. *Mental Retardation and Developmental Disabilities Research Reviews, 2*, 109–115.

Kummer, A. W., Lee, L., Stutz, L. S., Maroney, A., & Brandt, J. W. (2007). The prevalence of apraxia characteristics in patients with velocardiofacial syndrome as compared with other cleft populations. *Cleft Palate-Craniofacial Journal, 44*(2), 175–181.

Lalakea, M. L., & Messner, A. H. (2003). Ankyloglossia: Does it matter? *Pediatric Clinics of North America, 50*, 381–397.

Lalonde, K., & Holt, R. F. (2015). Preschoolers benefit from visually salient speech cues. *Journal of Speech, Language, and Hearing Research, 58*, 135–150.

Laures, J. S., & Weismer, G. (1999). The effects of a flattened fundamental frequency on intelligibility at the sentence level. *Journal of Speech, Language, and Hearing Research, 42*, 1148–1156.

Law, Z. W. Y., & So, L. K. H. (2006). Phonological abilities of hearing-impaired Cantonese-speaking children with cochlear implants or hearing aids. *Journal of Speech, Language, and Hearing Research, 49*, 1342–1353.

Laws, G. (1998). The use of nonword repetition as a test of phonological memory in children with Down syndrome. *Journal of Child Psychology and Psychiatry, 39*(8), 1119–1130.

Laws, G. (2004). Contributions of phonological memory, language comprehension and hearing to the expressive language of adolescents and young adults with Down syndrome. *Journal of Child Psychology and Psychiatry, 45*(6), 1085–1095.

Levitt, A. G., Jusczyk, P. W., Murray, J., & Carden, G. (1988). Context effects in two-month-old infants' perception of labiodential/interdental fricative contrasts. *Journal of Experimental Psychology. Human Perception and Performance, 14*, 361–368.

Lewis, B. A., Freebairn, L. A., Hansen, A. J., Iyengar, S. K., & Taylor, H. G. (2004). School-age follow-up of children with Childhood Apraxia of Speech. *Language, Speech, and Hearing Services in the Schools, 35*(2), 122–140.

Lewis, B. A., Freebairn, L. A., Heeger, S., & Cassidy, S. B. (2002). Speech and language skills of individuals with Prader-Willi syndrome. *American Journal of Speech-Language Pathology, 11*, 285–294.

Lewis, B. A., Singer, L. T., Fulton, S., Salvator, A., Short, E., Klein, N., & Baley, J. (2002). Speech and language outcomes of children with bronchopulmonary dysplasia. *Journal of Communication Disorders, 35*, 393–406.

Lewkowicz, D. J., & Hansen-Tift, A. M. (2012). Infants deploy selective attention to the mouth of a talking face when learning speech. *Proceedings of the National Academy of Sciences, 109*(5), 1431–1436.

Liberman, A. M., Cooper, F. S., Shankweiler, D. S., & Studdert-Kennedy, M. (1967). Perception of the speech code, *Psychological Review, 74*, 431–461.

Liberman, A. M., & Mattingly, I. G. (1985). The motor theory of speech perception revised. *Cognition, 21*(1), 1–36.

Lindblom, B. (1990). Explaining phonetic variation: A sketch of H and H theory. In W. J. Hardcastle & A. Marchal (Eds.), *Speech production and speech modelling* (pp. 403–439). Dordrecht, The Netherlands: Kluwer.

Liss, J. M. (1990). Muscle spindles in the human levator palatini and palatoglossus muscles. *Journal of Speech and Hearing Research, 33*(4), 736–746.

Liu, H.-M., Kuhl, P. K., & Tsao, F.-M. (2003). An association between mother's speech clarity and infant's speech discrimination skills. *Developmental Science, 6*(3), F1–F10.

Maas, E., Robin, D. A., Austermann Hula, S. N., Wulf, G., Ballard, K. J., & Schmidt, R. A. (2008). Principles of motor learning in treatment of motor speech disorders. *American Journal of Speech-Language Pathology, 17*, 277–298.

Maassen, B., Groenen, P., & Crul, T. (2003). Auditory and phonetic perception of vowels in children with apraxic speech disorders. *Clinical Linguistics and Phonetics, 17*, 447–467.

MacDermot, K. D., Bonora, E., Sykes, N., Coupe, A.-M., Lai, C. S. L., Vernes, S. C., …, Fisher, S. E. (2005). Identification of FOXP2 truncation as a novel cause of developmental speech and language deficits. *American Journal of Human Genetics, 76*, 1074–1080.

MacDonald, J. D., & Carroll, J. Y. (1992). A social partnership model for assessing early communication development: An intervention model for preconversational children. *Language, Speech, and Hearing Services in Schools, 23*, 113–124.

MacDonald, E. N., Johnson, E. K., Forsythe, J., Plante, P., & Munhall, K. G. (2012). Children's development of self-regulation in speech production. *Current Biology, 22*(2), 113–117.

Majerus, S., Van der Linden, M., Poncelet, M., & Metz-Lutz, M.-N. (2004). Can phonological and semantic short-term memory be dissociated? Further evidence from landau-kleffner syndrome. *Cognitive Neuropsychology, 21*(5), 491–512.

Mandel, D. R., Jusczyk, P. W., & Pisoni, D. B. (1995). Infants' recognition of the sound patterns of their own names. *Psychological Science, 6*(5), 314–317.

Marion, M. J., Sussman, H. M., & Marquardt, T. P. (1993). The perception and production of rhyme in normal and developmentally apraxic children. *Journal of Communication Disorders, 26*, 129–160.

Marquardt, T., Jacks, A., & Davis, B. L. (2004). Token-to-token variability in developmental apraxia of speech: Three longitudinal case studies. *Clinical Linguistics and Phonetics, 18*(2), 127–144.

Marquardt, T. P., Sussman, H. M., Snow, T., & Jacks, A. (2002). The integrity of the syllable in developmental apraxia of speech. *Journal of Communication Disorders, 35*, 31–49.

Masataka, N. (1992). Pitch characteristic of Japanese maternal speech to infants. *Journal of Child Language, 19*(2), 213–223.

Mattys, S. L., Jusczyk, P. W., Luce, P. A., & Morgan, J. L. (1999). Phonotactic and prosodic effects on word segmentation in infants. *Cognitive Psychology, 38*(4), 465–494.

Maye, J., & Weiss, D. (2003). Statistical cues facilitate infants' discrimination of difficult phonetic contrasts. In B. Beachley, A. Brown, & F. Conlin (Eds.), *BUCLD 27: Proceedings of the 27th Annual Boston University Conference on Language Development, 2* (pp. 508–518). Boston, MA: Cascadilla Press.

Maye, J., Werker, J. F., & Gerken, L. A. (2002). Infant sensitivity to distributional information can affect phonetic discrimination. *Cognition, 82*, B101–B111.

McClelland, J. L., McNaughton, B. L., & O'Reilly, R. C. (1995). Why there are complementary learning systems in the hippocampus and neocortex: Insights from the successes and failures of connectionists models of learning and memory. *Psychological Review, 102*(3), 419–457.

McDonald, E. T., & Aungst, L. F. (1970). Apparent independence of oral sensory functions and articulation proficiency. In J. F. Bosma (Ed.), *2nd symposium on oral sensation and perception* (pp. 391–395). Springfield, IL: Charles Thomas.

McDowell, K. D., Lonigan, C., & Goldstein, H. (2007). Relations among socioeconomic status, age, and predictors of phonological awareness. *Journal of Speech, Language, and Hearing Research, 50*, 1079–1092.

McLeod, S., & Bleile, K. (2003). *Neurological and developmental foundations of speech acquisition.* Paper presented at American Speech-Language-Hearing Association, Chicago, IL.

Mehler, J., Jusczyk, P. W., Lambertz, G., Halsted, N., Bertoncini, J., & Amiel-Tison, C. (1988). A precursor of language acquisition in young infants. *Cognition, 29*, 143–178.

Messner, A. H., & Lalakea, M. L. (2000). Ankyloglossia: Controversies in management. *International Journal of Pediatric Otorhinolaryngology, 54*, 123–131.

Miller, J. F., & Leddy, M. (1998). Down syndrome: The impact of speech production on language production. In R. Paul (Ed.), *Exploring the speech-language connection* (pp. 139–162). Baltimore, MD: Brookes.

Ming, X., Brimacombe, M., & Wagner, G. C. (2007). Prevalence of motor impairment in autism spectrum disorders. *Brain and Development, 29*, 565–570.

Miyamoto, R. T., Svirsky, M. A., & Robbins, A. M. (1997). Enhancement of expressive language in prelingually deaf children with cochlear implants. *Acta Otolaryngologica, 117*, 154–157.

Mody, M., Schwartz, R. G., Gravel, J. S., & Ruben, R. J. (1999). Speech perception and verbal memory in children with and without histories of otitis media. *Journal of Speech, Language, and Hearing Research, 42*, 1069–1079.

Moeller, M. P., Hoover, B., Putman, C., Arbataitis, K., Bohnenkamp, G., Peterson, B., …, Stelmachowicz, P. G. (2007). Vocalizations of infants with hearing loss compared to infants with normal hearing, Part II: Transition to words. *Ear and Hearing, 28*, 628–642.

Moon, C., Lagercrantz, H., & Kuhl, P. K. (2013). Language experienced in utero affects vowel perception after birth: A two-country study. *Acta Paediatrica, 102*, 156–160.

Moore, C. A., & Ruark, J. L. (1996). Does speech emerge from earlier appearing oral motor behaviors? *Journal of Speech and Hearing Research, 39*(5), 1034–1047.

Morgan, J. L. (1996). A rhythmic bias in preverbal speech segmentation. *Journal of Memory and Language, 35*, 666–688.

Morgan, J. L., & Saffran, J. R. (1995). Emerging integration of sequential and suprasegmental information in preverbal speech segmentation. *Child Development, 66*, 911–936.

Mostofsky, S. H., Goldberg, M. C., Landa, R. J., & Denckla, M. B. (2000). Evidence for a deficit in procedural learning in children and adolescents with autism: Implications for a cerebellar contribution. *Journal of the International Neuropsychological Society, 6*, 752–759.

Munir, F., Cornish, K. M., & Wilding, J. (2000). Nature of the working memory deficit in Fragile-X syndrome. *Brain and Cognition, 44*(3), 387–401.

Myers, J., Jusczyk, P. W., Kemler-Nelson, D. G., Charles-Luce, J., Woodward, A. L., & Hirsh-Pasek, K. (1996). Infants' sensitivity to word boundaries in fluent speech. *Journal of Child Language, 23*(1), 1–30.

National Institutes of Health (N.D.). Moebius syndrome. *Genetics Home Reference.* Retrieved 3/31/15, from http://www.ghr.nlm.nih.gov/condition/moebius-syndrome

Nijland, L. (2009). Speech perception in children with speech output disorders. *Clinical Linguistics and Phonetics, 23*(3), 222–239.

Nijland, L., Terband, H., & Maassen, B. (2015). Cognitive functions in Childhood Apraxia of Speech. *Journal of Speech, Language, and Hearing Research, 58*, 550–565.

Nittrouer, S., & Burton, L. T. (2005). The role of early language experience in the development of speech perception and phonological processing abilities: Evidence from 5-year-olds with histories of otitis media with effusion and low socioeconomic status. *Journal of Communication Disorders, 38*, 29–63.

Oller, D. K., Eilers, R. E., Basinger, D., Steffens, M., & Urbano, R. (1995). Extreme poverty and the development of precursors to the speech capacity. *First Language, 15*(4), 167–187.

Oller, D. K., Eilers, R. E., Steffens, M., Lynch, M. P., & Urbano, R. (1994). Speech-like vocalizations in infancy: An evaluation of potential risk factors. *Journal of Child Language, 21*, 33–58.

Onishi, K. H., Chambers, K. E., & Fisher, C. (2002). Learning phonotactic constraints from brief auditory experience. *Cognition, 83*, B13–B23.

Paradise, J. L., Dollaghan, C. A., Campbell, T. F., Feldman, H. M., Bernard, B. S., Colborn, K., …, Smith, C. G. (2000). Language, speech sound production, and cognition in three-year-old children in relation to otitis media in their first three years of life. *Pediatrics, 105*(5), 1119–1130.

Paul, R., Bianchi, N., Augustyn, A., Klin, A., & Volkmar, F. R. (2008). Production of syllable stress in speakers with autism spectrum disorders. *Research in Autism Spectrum Disorders, 2*(1), 110–124.

Pei, J. R., Rinaldi, C. M., Rasmussen, C., Massey, V., & Massey, D. (2008). Memory patterns of acquisition and retention of verbal and nonverbal information in children with fetal alcohol spectrum disorders. *Canadian Journal of Clinical Pharmacology, 15*(1), e44–e56.

Pennington, L., Miller, N., & Robson, S. (2010). Speech therapy for children with dysarthria acquired before three years of age (Review). *The Cochrane Library*. doi: 10.1002/14651858.CD006937.pub2

Perrier, P. (2005). Control and representations in speech production. *ZAS Papers in Linguistics, 40*, 109–132.

Pierrehumbert, J. (2001). Stochastic phonology. *GLOT, 5*(6), 1–13.

Pierrehumbert, J. (2003). Probabilistic phonology: Discrimination and robustness. In R. Bod, J. Hay, & S. Jannedy (Eds.), *Probability theory in linguistics* (pp. 177–228). Cambridge, MA: MIT Press.

Polka, L., & Sundara, M. (2003). Word segmentation in monolingual and bilingual infant learners of English and French. In Sole M. J., Recasens D., & Romero, J. (Eds.), *Proceedings of the 15th International Congress of Phonetic Sciences* (pp. 1021–1024). Barcelona, Spain: Causal Productions.

Preston, J. L., Molfese, P. J., Gumkowski, N., Sorcinelli, A., & Harwood, V. (2014). Neurophysiology of speech differences in Childhood Apraxia of Speech. *Developmental Neuropsychology, 39*(5), 385–403.

Prizant, B. M. (1996). Brief report: Communication, language, social and emotional development. *Journal of Autism and Developmental Disorders, 26*(2), 173–178.

Pungello, E. P., Iruka, I. U., Dotterer, A. M., Mills-Koonce, R., & Reznick, J. S. (2009). The effects of socioeconomic status, race, and parenting on language development in early childhood. *Developmental Psychology, 45*(2), 544–557.

Ramus, F. (2002). Language discrimination by newborns: Teasing apart phonotactic, rhythmic, and intonational cues. *Annual Review of Language Acquisition, 2*, 85–115.

Richard, G. J. (2012). Primary issues for the speech-language pathologist to consider in regard to the diagnosis of auditory processing disorder. *Perspectives on Language Learning and Education, 19*, 78–86.

Ringel, R., House, A., Burk, K., Dolinsky, J., & Scott, C. (1970). Some relations between orosensory discrimination and articulatory aspects of speech production. *Journal of Speech and Hearing Disorders, 35*, 1–11.

Roberts, J. (1997). Acquisition of variable rules: A study of (–t, d) deletion in preschool children. *Journal of Child Language, 24*(2), 351–372.

Robin, N. H. (2008). *Medical genetics: Its application to speech, hearing, and craniofacial disorders*. San Diego, CA: Plural.

Rodier, P. M. (2002). Converging evidence for brain stem injury in autism. *Development and Psychopathology, 14*(3), 537–557.

Rovee-Collier, C. (1997). Dissociations in infant memory. *Psychological Review, 104*, 467–498.

Rowe, M. L., & Goldin-Meadow, S. (2009). Differences in early gesture explain SES disparities in child vocabulary size at school entry. *Science, 323*(February 13), 951–953.

Ruark, J. L., & Moore, C. A. (1997). Coordination of lip muscle activity by 2-year-old children during speech and nonspeech tasks. *Journal of Speech, Language, and Hearing Research, 40*, 1373–1385.

Rupela, V., & Manjula, R. (2007). Phonotactic patterns in the speech of children with Down syndrome. *Clinical Linguistics and Phonetics, 21*(8), 605–622.

Rupela, V., & Manjula, R. (2010). Diadochokinetic assessment in persons with Down syndrome. *Asia Pacific Journal of Speech, Language, and Hearing, 13*(2), 109–120.

Rupela, V., Manjula, R., & Velleman, S. L. (2010). Phonological processes in Kannada-speaking adolescents with Down syndrome. *Clinical Linguistics and Phonetics, 24*(6), 431–450.

Rvachew, S., & Bernhardt, B. M. (2010). Clinical implications of dynamic systems theory for phonological development. *American Journal of Speech-Language Pathology, 19*(1), 34–50.

Rvachew, S., & Jamieson, D. G. (1989). Perception of voiceless fricatives by children with a functional articulation disorder. *Journal of Speech and Hearing Disorders, 54*, 193–208.

Rvachew, S., Rafaat, S., & Martin, M. (1999a). Stimulability, speech perception skills, and the treatment of phonological disorders. *American Journal of Speech-Language Pathology, 8*, 33–43.

Rvachew, S., Slawinski, E. B., Williams, M., & Green, C. (1999b). The impact of early onset otitis media on babbling and early language development. *Journal of the Acoustical Society of America, 105*, 467–475.

Sadagopan, N., & Smith, A. (2008). Developmental changes in the effects of utterance length and complexity on speech movement variability. *Journal of Speech, Language, and Hearing Research, 51*(5), 1138–1151.

Saffran, J. R., Aslin, R. N., & Newport, E. L. (1996). Statistical learning by 8-month-old infants. *Science, 274*, 1926–1928.

Saffran, J. R., Newport, E. L., Aslin, R. N., Tunick, R. A., & Barrueco, S. (1997). Incidental language learning: Listening (and learning) out of the corner of your ear. *Psychological Science, 8*, 101–105.

Schmidt, L., & Lee, T. (2005). *Motor control and learning: A behavioral emphasis*. Champaign, IL: Human Kinetics.

Schwauwers, K., Taelman, H., Gillis, S., & Govaerts, P. (2006). *The phonological development in young hearing-impaired children with a cochlear implant*. Paper presented at the Conference on the Emergence of Language Abilities, Lyon, France.

Seal, B. C., & Bonvillian, J. D. (1997). Sign language and motor functioning in students with autistic disorder. *Journal of Autism and Developmental Disorders, 27*(4), 437–466.

Seidl, A., & Buckley, E. (2005). On the learning of arbitrary phonological rules. *Language Learning and Development, 1*(3&4), 289–316.

Sharma, M., Purdy, S. C., & Kelly, A. S. (2009). Comorbidity of auditory processing, language, and reading disorders. *Journal of Speech, Language, and Hearing Research, 52*, 706–722.

Sheppard, J. J., & Mysak, E. D. (1984). Ontogeny of infantile oral reflexes and emerging chewing. *Child Development, 55*(3), 831–843.

Shi, R., Werker, J. F., & Morgan, J. L. (1999). Newborn infants' sensitivity to perceptual cues to lexical and grammatical words. *Cognition, 72*, B11–B21.

Shprintzen, R. J. (2000). *Syndrome identification for speech-language pathology: An illustrated pocketguide*. San Diego, CA: Singular.

Shriberg, L. D. (2006). *Research in idiopathic and symptomatic childhood apraxia of speech*. Paper presented at the 5th International Conference on Speech Motor Control, Nijmegen, The Netherlands.

Shriberg, L. D., Flipsen, P. J., Thielke, H., Kwiatkowski, J., Kertoy, M. K., Katcher, M. L., …, Block, M. G. (2000a). Risk for speech disorder associated with early recurrent otitis media with effusion: Two retrospective studies. *Journal of Speech, Language, and Hearing Research, 43*, 79–99.

Shriberg, L. D., Friel-Patti, S., Flipsen, P. J., & Brown, R. L. (2000b). Otitis media, fluctuant hearing loss, and speech-language outcomes: A preliminary structural equation model. *Journal of Speech, Language, and Hearing Research, 43*, 100–120.

Shuey, E. M., & Jamison, K. (1996). Sotos syndrome. *Language, Speech, and Hearing Services in Schools, 27*(1), 91–93.

Shuster, L. I. (1998). The perception of correctly and incorrectly produced /r/. *Journal of Speech, Language, and Hearing Research, 41*, 941–950.

Smith, A. (2010). Development of neural control of orofacial movements for speech. In W. J. Hardcastle, J. Laver, & F. E. Gibbon (Eds.), *The handbook of phonetic sciences* (pp. 251–296). Malden, MA: Blackwell.

Smith, A., & Zelaznik, H. N (2004). Development of functional synergies for speech motor coordination in childhood and adolescence. *Developmental Psychobiology, 45*(1), 22–33.

Solomon, N. P., & Charron, S. (1998). Speech breathing in able-bodied children and children with cerebral palsy: A review of the literature and implications for clinical intervention. *American Journal of Speech-Language Pathology, 7*(2), 61–78.

Somerville, M. J., Mervis, C. B., Young, E. J., Seo, E.-J., del Campo, M., Bamforth, S., …, Osborne, L. R. (2005). Severe expressive-language delay related to duplication of the Williams-Beuren locus. *New England Journal of Medicine, 353*(16), 1694–1701.

Spencer, L. J., & Tomblin, J. B. (2009). Evaluating phonological processing skills in children with prelingual deafness who use cochlear implants. *Journal of Deaf Studies and Deaf Education, 14*(1), 1–21.

Stager, C. L., & Werker, J. F. (1997). Infants listen for more phonetic detail in speech perception than in word-learning tasks. *Nature, 388*(July), 381–382.

Steeve, R. W., Moore, C. A., Green, J. R., Reilly, K. J., & McMurtrey, J. R. (2008). Babbling, chewing and sucking: Oromandibular coordination at 9 months. *Journal of Speech, Language, and Hearing Research, 51*(6), 1390–1404.

Stokes, S., Lau, J. T.-K., & Ciocca, V. (2002). The interaction of ambient frequency and feature complexity in the diphthong errors of children with phonological disorders. *Journal of Speech, Language, and Hearing Research, 45*, 1188–1201.

Storkel, H. L., Armbruster, J., & Hogan, T. P. (2006). Differentiating phonotactic probability and neighborhood density in adult word learning. *Journal of Speech, Language, and Hearing Research, 49*, 1175–1192.

Storkel, H. L., Maekawa, J., & Hoover, J. R. (2010). Differentiating the effects of phonotactic probability and neighborhood density on vocabulary comprehension and production: A comparison of preschool children with versus without phonological delays. *Journal of Speech, Language, and Hearing Research, 53*, 933–949.

Sundara, M., Namasivayam, A. K., & Chen, R. (2001). Observation-execution matching system for speech: A magnetic stimulation study. *NeuroReport, 12*(7), 1341–1344.

Sutherland, D., & Gillon, G. T. (2005). Assessment of phonological representations in children with speech impairment. *Language, Speech, and Hearing Services in Schools, 36*, 294–307.

Swift, E., & Rosin, P. (1990). A remediation sequence to improve speech intelligibility for students with Down syndrome. *Language, Speech, and Hearing Services in Schools, 21*(3), 140–146.

Szypulski, T. A. (2003). Interactive oral sensorimotor therapy: One more weapon in the arsenal fight to combat the primary deficits of autism. *Advance for Speech & Hearing, 13*(1), 9.

Tager-Flusberg, H., Paul, R., & Lord, C. E. (2005). Language and communication in autism. In F. R. Volkmar, R. Paul, A. Klin, & D. Cohen (Eds.), *Handbook of autism and pervasive developmental disorder, Vol. 1* (3rd ed., pp. 335–364). New York, NY: Wiley.

Teitelbaum, P., Teitelbaum, O. B., Fryman, J., & Maurer, R. (2002). Reflexes gone astray in autism in infancy. *The Journal of Developmental and Learning Disorders, 6*, 15–22.

Terband, H., Maassen, B., Guenther, F. H., & Brumberg, J. (2009). Computational neural modeling of speech motor control in childhood apraxia of speech (CAS). *Journal of Speech, Language, and Hearing Research, 52*, 1595–1609.

Thelen, E., & Smith, L. B. (1994). *A dynamic systems approach to the development of cognition and action.* Cambridge, MA: MIT Press.

Thyer, N., & Dodd, B. (1996). Auditory processing and phonologic disorder. *International Journal of Audiology, 35*(1), 37–44.

Tjaden, K., Rivera, D., Wilding, G., & Turner, G. S. (2005). Characteristics of the lax vowel space in dysarthria. *Journal of Speech, Language, and Hearing Research, 48*(3), 554–566.

Tomasello, M., & Mannle, S. (1985). Pragmatics of sibling speech to one-year-olds. *Child Development, 56*(4), 911–917.

Tomblin, J. B., O'Brien, M., Shriberg, L. D., Williams, C., Murray, J., Patil, S., …, Ballard, K. J. (2009). Language features in a mother and daughter of a chromosome 7;13 translocation involving FOXP2. *Journal of Speech, Language, and Hearing Research, 52*, 1157–1174.

Tomik, B., Krupinski, J., Glodzik-Sobanska, L., Bala-Slodowska, M., Wszolek, W., Kusiak M., & Lechwacka, A. (1999). Acoustic analysis of dysarthria profile in ALS patients. *Journal of the Neurological Sciences, 169*(1–2), 35–42.

Ullman, M. T. (2001). The Declarative/Procedural Model of lexicon and grammar. *Journal of Psycholinguistic Research, 30*(1), 37–69.

Ullman, M. T. (2004). Contributions of memory circuits to language: The Declarative/Procedural Model. *Cognition, 92*, 231–270.

Van Lieshout, P. H. H. M. (2004). Dynamical systems theory and its application in speech. In B. Maassen, R. D. Kent, H. F. M. Peters, P. H. H. M. van Lieshout, & W. Hulstijn (Eds.), *Speech motor control in normal and disordered speech* (pp. 51–81). Oxford, UK: Oxford University Press.

Velleman, S. L. (2003). *Resource guide for childhood apraxia of speech.* Florence, KY: Cengage.

Velleman, S. L., Andrianopoulos, M. V., Boucher, M., Perkins, J., Averback, K. E., Currier, A., …, Van Emmerik, R. (2009a). Motor speech disorders in children with autism. In R. Paul & P. Flipsen (Eds.), *Speech sound disorders in children: In honor of Lawrence D. Shriberg* (pp. 141–180). San Diego, CA: Plural.

Velleman, S. L., Mangipudi, L., & Locke, J. L. (1989). Prelinguistic phonetic contingency: Data from Down syndrome. *First Language, 9*, 159–174.

Velleman, S. L., & Mervis, C. B. (2011). Children with 7q11.23 Duplication syndrome: Speech, language, cognitive, and behavioral characteristics and their implications for intervention. *Perspectives on Language Learning and Education, 18*(3), 108–116.

Velleman, S. L., O'Connor, K., McGloin, S., Cormier, C., Mervis, C. B., & Morris, C. A. (2009b, May 21). *Speech characteristics of children with DUP7 syndrome versus Williams syndrome.* New Haven, CT: Haskins Laboratories.

Velleman, S. L., & Vihman, M. M. (2007). Phonological development in infancy and early childhood: Implications for theories of language learning. In M. C. Pennington (Ed.), *Phonology in context* (pp. 25–50). UK: MacMillan.

Vihman, M. M. (2002). The role of mirror neurons in the ontogeny of speech. In M. I. Stamenov & V. Gallese (Eds.), *Mirror neurons and the evolution of brain and language.* Amsterdam, The Netherlands: John Benjamins. (Advances in Consciousness Research).

Vihman, M. M., & Croft, W. (2007). Phonological development: Towards a "radical" templatic phonology. *Linguistics, 45*(4), 683–725.

Vihman, M. M., & Nakai, S. (2003). Experimental evidence for an effect of vocal experience on infant speech perception. In M. J. Solé, D. Recasens, & J. Romero (Eds.), *Proceedings of the 15th International Congress of Phonetic Sciences*, Barcelona, Spain (pp. 1017–1020).

Vihman, M. M., Nakai, S., DePaolis, R. A., & Halle, P. (2004). The role of accentual pattern in early lexical representation. *Journal of Memory and Language, 50*, 336–353.

Vihman, M. M., & Velleman, S. L. (2000a). Phonetics and the origins of phonology. In N. Burton-Roberts, P. Carr, & G. Docherty (Eds.), *Conceptual and empirical foundations of phonology* (pp. 305–339). Oxford, UK: Oxford University Press.

Vihman, M. M., & Velleman, S. L. (2000b). The construction of a first phonology. *Phonetica, 57*, 255–266.

Villacorta, V. M., Perkell, J. S., & Guenther, F. H. (2007). Sensorimotor adaptation to feedback perturbation of vowel acoustics and its relation to perception. *Journal of the Acoustical Society of America, 122*(4), 2306–2319.

von Hapsburg, D., & Davis, B. L. (2006). Auditory sensitivity and the prelinguistic vocalizations of early-amplified infants. *Journal of Speech, Language, and Hearing Research, 49*, 809–822.

Vorperian, H. K., Kent, R. D., Lindstrom, M. J., Kalina, C. M., Gentry, L. R., & Yandell, B. S. (2005). Development of vocal tract length during early childhood: A magnetic resonance imaging study. *Journal of the Acoustical Society of America, 117*(1), 338–350.

Wake, M., Tobin, S., Cone-Wesson, B., Dahl, H.-H., Gillam, L., McCormick, L., …, Williams, J. (2006). Slight/mild sensorineural hearing loss in children. *Pediatrics, 118*(5), 1842–1851.

Walker, D., Greenwood, C., Hart, B., & Carta, J. (1994). Prediction of school outcomes based on early language production and socioeconomic factors. *Child Development*, *65*, 606–621.

Wallace, A. F. (1963). Tongue-tie. *Lancet*, *2*, 377–378.

Warner-Czyz, A. D., Davis, B. L., & Morrison, H. M. (2005). Production accuracy in a young cochlear implant recipient. *Volta Review*, *105*(2), 151–173.

Webster, R., Erdos, C., Evans, K., Majnemer, A., Kehayia, E., Thordardottir, E., …, Shevell, M. (2006). The clinical spectrum of developmental language impairment in school-age children: Language, cognitive and motor findings. *Pediatrics*, *118* (5), 1541–1549.

Weissenborn, J., Hohle, B., Bartels, S., Herold, B., & Hofmann, M. (2002). *The development of prosodic competence in German infants.* Paper presented at the International Conference on Infant Studies, Toronto.

Werker, J. F., & Stager, C. L. (2000). Developmental changes in infant speech perception and early word learning: Is there a link? In M. Broe & J. Pierrehumbert (Eds.), *LabPhon V: Acquisition and the lexicon* (pp. 181–193). Cambridge, UK: Cambridge University Press.

Werker, J. F., & Tees, R. C. (1984). Cross-language speech perception: Evidence for perceptual reorganization during the first year of life. *Infant Behavior and Development*, *7*, 49–64.

Wetherby, A. M., & Prizant, B. (2002). *Communication and Symbolic Behavior Scales Developmental Profile.* Baltimore, MD: Brookes.

Whalen, D. H., Levitt, A. G., & Wang, Q. (1991). Intonational differences between the reduplicative babbling of French- and English-learning infants. *Journal of Child Language*, *18*, 501–516.

Williams, J. H., Whiten, A., Suddendorf, T., & Perrett, D. I. (2001). Imitation, mirror neurons and autism. *Neuroscience and Biobehavioral Reviews*, *25*(4), 287–295.

Wilson, E. M., Green, J. R., Yunusova, Y., & Moore, C. A. (2008). Task specificity in early oral motor development. *Seminars in Speech and Language*, *29*(4), 257–266.

Wilson, E. M., & Nip, I. S. B (2010). Physiologic studies provide new perspectives on early speech development. *Perspectives on Speech Science and Orofacial Disorders*, *20*, 29–36.

Wood, J. L., & Smith, A. (1992). Cutaneous oral-motor reflexes of children with normal and disordered speech. *Developmental Medicine and Child Neurology*, *34*(9), 797–812. Available at: http://www.ncbi.nlm.nih.gov/pubmed/1526350

Woolridge, M. W. (1986). The 'anatomy' of infant sucking. *Midwifery*, *2*(4), 164–171. Available at: http://www.health-e-learning.com/articles/anatomy_of_latch.pdf

Zelaznik, H. N., & Goffman, L. (2010). Generalized motor abilities and timing behavior in children with specific language impairment. *Journal of Speech, Language, and Hearing Research*, *53*, 383–393.

CHAPTER 4

Basic Principles for Speech Sound Evaluation

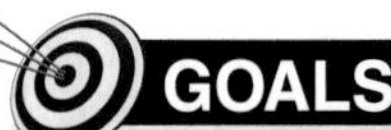

GOALS of This Chapter

1. Review difference versus delay versus disorder.
2. Review the main purposes of evaluation: screening, assessment, diagnosis.
3. Describe the process of carrying out an oral mechanism examination.
4. Review other factors that should be ruled in or out as impacting the child's speech profile.
5. Review assessment types, including standardized tests, non-normed assessment tools, and static versus dynamic assessment.
6. Discuss how a variety of tools can complement each other, yielding a more comprehensive speech profile.

INTRODUCTION: WHAT ARE WE LOOKING FOR?

It is not the purpose of this chapter to provide step-by-step instructions for particular evaluation procedures; those will be provided in great breadth and depth in later chapters, as they relate to specific components of children's phonological systems (phonetics, phonemes, phonotactics, prosody). Here, we provide an overview of the primary purposes, components, and approaches to the evaluation of childhood speech sound disorders (SSDs). Instructions for carrying out a thorough oral motor/motor speech evaluation are also provided here.

Before discussing evaluation principles, however, it is important first to identify what types of problems we may be evaluating. These include delays versus disorders, and physiologic versus more cognitive speech sound problems.

Difference Versus Delay Versus Disorder

A key distinction in speech-language pathology is that among the concepts of **difference**, delay, and **disorder**. A difference is the result of exposure to alternative speech-language models. For example, a child who is raised in a bilingual household or in a home where a non-mainstream dialect is spoken will speak differently than a child who has only been exposed to General American English. Although a difference is not a "pathology," speech-language pathologists (SLPs) are often involved in distinguishing between linguistic differences and problems (delays or disorders). One important role that we play is preventing those with speech or language differences from being inappropriately labeled as having disorders or delays. For example, children who speak African American English (AAE) tend to exhibit phonological characteristics of this dialect even in Mainstream American English (MAE) contexts such as school longer than grammatical characteristics (Craig, Thompson, Washington, & Potter, 2003). Furthermore, many of the characteristics of AAE overlap with features of speech-language delay or disorder. Thus, child AAE speakers are at increased risk of being misdiagnosed with speech-language deficits (Stockman, Boult, & Robinson, 2008; Velleman & Pearson, 2010).

On the other hand, children who speak different languages or dialects (or more than one language or dialect) should have equal access to speech-language services if they would benefit from them. Yet Stow and Dodd (2005) report that primarily Pakistani bilingual children in an 11% minority community in England were far less often referred for evaluation of possible SSDs than were monolingual children (25.74% versus 58.43%), although the prevalence of SSDs should have been expected to be the same. Based on SLPs' self-reports, bilinguals also appear to be less likely to be referred for therapy than are children who are monolingual or who speak the mainstream dialect or language (Kritikos, 2003).

A delay is identified when a child's behavior (in this case, pronunciation) is similar to what one would expect from a younger, typically developing child. Thus, a 10-year-old whose speech production is the same as that of a typical 4-year-old would be described as having a speech delay. A contrasting situation is identified when the client produces words in a way that would not be typical of a younger child at any age, for example demonstrating atypical or "deviant" phonological patterns (such as initial consonant deletion in English). This person's problem would be classified as a disorder.

Another, more subtle, type of disorder is characterized by "**chronological mismatch**," which occurs when some aspects of the child's speech and/or language are significantly (more) delayed in comparison to others. Thus, although some aspects of her phonology may be appropriate to some younger typically developing children, the child's overall profile is not typical for any age group because of one or more mismatches between various components of her phonology. For example, the client might have an age-appropriate consonant repertoire but be unable to combine these sounds into the structures expected for English at that age (e.g., closed syllables, clusters, multisyllabic words).

The distinction between delay and disorder is an important one. For example, most children who are identified as late talkers (i.e., delayed) when they are toddlers are within the normal range with respect to vocabulary by the time they are 3 years old, even if they haven't received speech-language intervention. Although they typically continue to score lower as a group on standardized tests of speech, language, and literacy than do children who were never considered to have delays, these children also typically continue to score within normal limits on these tests (Paul & Roth, 2011). Thus, the prognoses of children with delays are fairly good, though they should continue to be monitored periodically.

On the other hand, in two recent studies, children whose speech sound error patterns had been more than 10% atypical in preschool were more likely to demonstrate deficits in phonological awareness and reading skills at age 8 (Leitao & Fletcher, 2004; Preston, Hull, & Edwards, 2013). Similarly, children who produced more distortions in preschool were more likely to demonstrate more severe persistent speech sound difficulties at school age (Preston, Hull, & Edwards, 2013). Thus, two different signs of disorder (atypical patterns and distortions) early on have been shown to be predictive of more significant related problems later. This indicates that the prognoses of children with SSDs—atypical profiles—are more guarded than are those of children who are only delayed.

Currently, the cover term "SSD" is being used by many SLPs to describe any type of speech production difficulty, whether it be a delay or a disorder (but not differences). It is important not to allow our terminology to blur this distinction.

Sources of Speech Sound Problems

As discussed in Chapter 3, speech sound difficulties can be roughly divided into two primary sources, though these are far from mutually exclusive: anatomic/physiologic and cognitive/linguistic. Anatomic/physiologic causes of SSDs include structural, motor, and sensory differences, such as cleft palate, low muscle tone, hearing impairment, dysarthria, and apraxia. Cognitive/linguistic causes relate to deficits in more abstract neurologically based processes, such as implicit learning, phonological memory, and central auditory processing. All of these aspects should be considered in all evaluations, regardless of the assumptions that may be tempting to make based upon the intake information. Therefore, every comprehensive speech sound assessment should include a thorough oral mechanism examination (as discussed at length later in this chapter), a hearing screening or evaluation, and a language screening or evaluation, as well as any other testing suggested by the presenting profile of strengths and concerns. A potential speech sound delay or disorder cannot be properly diagnosed in a vacuum without proper consideration of prerequisites (such as hearing), precursors (such as use of meaningful gestures), and associated abilities (such as cognition, language, and social skills). In medical contexts, co-occurring deficits or symptoms of disorder are referred to as **co-morbidities**. These may be causal (such as a genetic difference), share a common etiology (such as multiple symptoms of a single neurodevelopmental disorder), or be coincidental. It is not always possible to determine which, but it is important to ask this question.

EVALUATION CONSIDERATIONS

Before preparing for an evaluation, one must first consider the purpose of the process: **identification** of a problem or ruling out a problem; diagnosis; or a thorough assessment of the nature of the difficulties that the child is exhibiting. Several types of assessment tools, analyses, and strategies are available to choose among; typically, a combination of these will be used. These evaluation choices are described further.

Purposes of Evaluations

Evaluation of speech sound delays and disorders occurs at many levels, depending largely on the purpose of the evaluation, as well as upon the setting, the evaluator, and the time available. A **speech screening** is carried out in order

TABLE 4-1 **Key Considerations and Processes for Speech Sound Assessment**

Co-Morbidities, Precursors, and Strengths (History, Observation, and Screenings)	Environmental Factors (History and Observation)	Identify Problem (Screening)	Analyze Speech Sound Strengths and Weaknesses (Assessment)	Identify Speech Sound Delay, Difference, and/or Disorder(s) (Diagnosis)
Genetic or other neurodevelopmental or acquired condition (e.g., Down syndrome, post-natal stroke)	Ambient language(s) or dialect(s)	Intelligibility/ communicative effectiveness	Oral–motor and motor speech abilities (oral mechanism examination)	Profile based on all factors in all other columns
Anatomic differences (e.g., cleft palate)	Cultural/societal patterns and expectations	Social impacts (e.g., frustration levels)	Consonant and vowel repertoires (independent analysis)	
Physiologic differences (e.g., low tone)	Linguistic stimulation	Screening test results	Accuracy of speech production (relational analysis)	
Hearing impairment	Cognitive stimulation	Percent consonants correct (revised)	Phonotactic repertoire (independent analysis)	
Other sensory differences (e.g., vision impairment)	Socioeconomic status	Academic impacts	Accuracy of phonotactic structures (relational analysis)	
Language delay, disorder, strengths			Error patterns (relational analysis)	
Communicative strengths			Prosodic repertoire (independent analysis)	
Cognitive delay, disorder, strengths			Appropriateness of prosody (relational analysis)	
Social–pragmatic delay, disorder (e.g., ASD), strengths			Phonological awareness/ (pre)literacy skills	
Attention disorder, strengths				
Emotional–behavioral disorder, strengths				

to identify whether or not a problem is present. Assessment is far more in-depth and results when possible in a comprehensive profile of the youngster's speech strengths and weaknesses. Diagnosis consists of deciding whether or not the child's speech profile—in the context of his other strengths, weaknesses, and symptoms—warrants a particular label referring to a speech, language, or other condition (such as Childhood Apraxia of Speech [CAS], specific language impairment [SLI], autism spectrum disorder [ASD], etc.). Each of these is discussed in depth below and also delineated in Table 4-1.

Identification

The purpose of identification of a speech problem is to determine whether or not further evaluation is warranted. The recognition of a moderate to severe phonological delay or disorder can be relatively simple; often an experienced SLP can identify the existence of a problem based on a few minutes of observation. For young children, for instance, frustration—on the part of either the child or the caretakers and other stakeholders—is often a salient indicator of lack of communicative success.

Quantitative documentation of a significant condition through speech screening may be much more challenging and time-consuming, however. Intelligibility seems like the most practical way to conceive of typical speech versus a delay or disorder, yet there is no single widely accepted way to measure this. A wide variety of strategies have been used with varying populations.

The primary approach to intelligibility is to measure how much of a person's speech is understood by a naïve listener who tries to write down what the speaker said. The speech to be transcribed may be elicited or imitated words (Gordon-Brannan & Hodson, 2000), elicited or imitated sentences (Chin, Tsai, & Gao, 2003; Gordon-Brannan & Hodson, 2000; Maassen, 1986), or spontaneous connected speech (Barnes, Roberts, Long, Martin, Berni, et al., 2009). A few criterion-referenced tests are available for these purposes, such as the *Children's Speech Intelligibility Measure* (Wilcox & Morris, 1999), which is based on production of similar-sounding words that the listener must try to distinguish, and the *Beginner's Intelligibility Test* (Osberger, Robbins, Todd, & Riley, 1994), which is based on sentence production.

Another way to measure intelligibility is by parent report. When parents are asked to estimate how well strangers would understand their children, they typically estimate that their children are about 50% intelligible by 2;0 to 2;6 (2 years, 0 months to 2 years, 6 months), 75% intelligible by age 3, and 90% to 100% intelligible by age 4 (Coplan & Gleason, 1988). One standardized parent rating scale that is available is the *Intelligibility in Context Scale* (McLeod, Harrison, & McCormack, 2012), which shows good reliability and validity as well as good correlations with the percent of consonants that the child produces correctly (Shriberg, Austin, Lewis, McSweeny, & Wilson, 1997a). However, there is some concern that parents may tend to overestimate their children's intelligibility (Flipsen, 1995), so the comprehension levels of actual strangers may be better measures. Gordon-Brannan and Hodson (2000) suggest that it is cause for significant concern if a child who is 4 years old or older is not at least 66% intelligible in connected speech to unfamiliar listeners who know the topic.

Another strategy is to have listeners use a rating scale (e.g., a 1–5 scale where "1" means "completely unintelligible" and "5" means "completely intelligible") to judge a speaker's spontaneous speech. However, these scales tend not to be used reliably or systematically. In particular, the distance from a "1" to a "2" versus the distance from "3" to "4" may vary from listener to listener, from client to client, or even from time to time (Schiavetti, 1992).

A popular screening measure that is correlated with severity is **percent consonants correct–revised** (PCC-R). It is carried out by transcribing a child's speech, then counting how many of the consonants that she attempted were produced correctly. This metric is correlated with severity. As such, it can be used to differentiate children with typical speech from those with speech deficits (Shriberg & Kwiatkowski, 1982; Shriberg et al., 1997a, 1997b). The calculation and uses of this measure are described in more detail in Chapter 7. As discussed there, limitations of PCC-R include the fact that it is based on spontaneous speech but only intelligible words can be taken into account in the calculation. Thus, a child with a few clear, intelligible words and many indecipherable words may receive an inappropriately high score.

A further complication of using spontaneous connected speech samples is that a wide variety of factors can impact intelligibility, including the phonological and grammatical complexity and the length of the utterance, the position of the word within the utterance, the intelligibility of the other words in the utterance (Weston & Shriberg, 1992), the communication context including whether or not visual or auditory cues are clear, and the listener's familiarity with the content and with the speaker (Chin, Tsai, & Gao, 2003; Kent, Miolo, & Bloedel, 1994).

Nonetheless, Gordon-Brannan and Hodson (2000) found strong correlations among intelligibility measures based on percent intelligibility of imitated sentences, percent intelligibility of imitated words, listener ratings of spontaneous conversational speech, and percentage of occurrence of phonological errors. Similarly, Hustad, Schueler, Schultz, and DuHadway (2012) did not find differences when they compared parent ratings, unfamiliar listener ratings, and transcription percentage correct scores of the speech of children with cerebral palsy. Thus, if one uses a consistent methodology for measuring intelligibility, controlling for the listed factors as well as possible, the results should be reliable and valid within one's own practice.

Assessment

The challenge of most speech-language evaluations is to analyze the phonological system of the individual in order to determine that child's phonological/speech sound profile, including his strengths as well as his weaknesses, thoroughly enough within available time limits that goals can be set efficiently and effectively. This part of the process is the **assessment.** This level of detail is often not available from any one standardized instrument, but can be obtained from such instruments and/or from speech samples if one has a good understanding of the nature of the necessary information and how to extract it. The types of tools that are used for this purpose are described in detail below ("Popular Assessment Tools").

Diagnosis

Having determined the presence (via identification) and nature of a delay or disorder (via a thorough assessment), **diagnosis** is sometimes the next step. The primary diagnosis may be clear-cut, especially when the speech problem is secondary to some syndrome, such as Down syndrome or Williams syndrome, or some other condition, such as ASD. In these cases, the diagnosis has often already been made by someone else, such as a pediatrician, psychologist, or neurologist. In other cases, the primary or secondary diagnosis may be unclear or mixed; for example, many children with SSD—including those with a neurodevelopmental primary diagnosis—display some symptoms of CAS or some symptoms of childhood dysarthria but not enough to warrant such a diagnostic label.

In some cases, there are specific tools available that could be used for assistance in arriving at a diagnosis. For example, the *Screening Test for Developmental Apraxia of Speech* (Blakely, 1980) or *The Apraxia Profile* (Hickman, 1997) could be used when ruling out versus making a diagnosis of CAS, though they are both lacking in many psychometric properties (McCauley & Strand, 2008). However, with respect to the majority of speech-language/communication diagnoses, that is, those that are within the scope of practice of SLPs without extra specialized training, (for example, for making a diagnosis of ASD), the appropriate diagnostic procedures are most often the same as those required for carrying out a thorough assessment, as described below. The determination of a diagnosis is then an extra step in the evaluation analysis procedure. For example, a thorough oral mechanism/motor speech evaluation should be an inherent part of any speech sound disorder evaluation. The child's responses and scores (if normed) on such an evaluation will both provide insight into the nature of the youngster's speech sound delay or disorder (assessment) and be useful when deciding whether or not diagnoses of CAS, dysarthria, speech delay, and/or phonological disorder are warranted. *A diagnosis should never be made without a comprehensive assessment.*

In many cases, the actual diagnostic label is not terribly important in the sense that *the diagnosis does not determine the appropriate goals*. Even the knowledge that a child has a particular syndrome or condition is grossly insufficient for determining that youngster's communicative strengths, weaknesses, and intervention needs.

Types of Assessment

Assessment approaches can be roughly divided into those that are static versus those that are dynamic, and those that are relational versus those that are independent. These distinctions are explained below.

Static Assessment

Static assessment is typically provided through the use of a standardized test that requires the child to produce certain words (usually in a picture-naming task) spontaneously, at a particular moment in time, without cues or suggestions as to how to improve her pronunciation. Some such tests do include phrases or sentences.

Dynamic Assessment

Dynamic assessment, in contrast, is the process of eliciting the child's very best performance while at the same time identifying those strategies—visual, gestural, or tactile cueing; phonetic placement descriptions (e.g., "Put your tongue between your teeth"); imitation; minimal pairs, etc.—that are most facilitatory for that particular client. Although dynamic assessment can be carried out and documented in a systematic way (Glaspey & Stoel-Gammon, 2005, discussed in further detail in Chapter 5), it is by its very nature **criterion referenced** (i.e., intended to compare an individual's performance at one time to the performance of the same individual at another time). It is challenging (though not completely impossible if one is very systematic) to compare one child's performance to that of another because the procedures used vary widely depending upon the child's needs and responses.

Through both the initial static assessment and ongoing dynamic assessment, appropriate intervention strategies should be selected based on the nature of the deficits, their functional impacts, the targeted communicative contexts, and the learning style of the child as well as many other personal factors (age, gender, cognitive status, hearing status, linguistic background and maturity, cultural expectations, family perspectives, etc.). Over time, as in the response to intervention process that is used in special education, the child's learning process and his progress on the goals addressed will determine the levels and types of intervention that he will receive on a long-term basis.

Relational Analysis

The tests that most SLPs use are examples of relational (i.e., contrastive) analysis; that is, they focus on how the child's phonology compares to the adult system. In other words, they identify the child's errors from an adult point of view. In a relational analysis, the child's accuracy at producing specific consonants or specific adult word and syllable shapes (e.g., clusters, multisyllabic words) may be calculated. A relational analysis compares the child's output to the adult output to identify what must be changed in order for the child's phonology to sound adult-like. Substitutions, omissions, and distortions—predictable patterns in which a certain presumed target phoneme or class of phonemes is produced in some other way or omitted completely by the child—are documented.

Both **articulation tests** and phonological process tests are relational. Articulation tests are measures of the client's ability to produce individual consonants (and sometimes clusters and/or vowels) in initial, final, and sometimes medial word positions. Scoring is based on the accuracy of these individual productions. Although clusters are included in some of these tests, usually only the accuracy of the target cluster (e.g., "Was st- produced as st-?") is scored.

In some cases, **stimulability** is also assessed in a standardized form of dynamic assessment. This procedure asks the question, "Can the child produce the sound under any circumstances?" For example, a youngster who mispronounces a word when asked to label a picture might nonetheless produce the word correctly when it is modeled. This is especially likely to happen if the child watches the SLP producing the word or if she is given some information about how to pronounce a difficult sound (such as "Put your tongue between your teeth"). Other tests (such as the *Secord Contextual Articulation Tests [S-CAT]* by Secord & Shine, 1997) focus on contextual factors: Can the child produce the sound in specific phonetic contexts? For example, /ʃ/ may be more accurate before a palatal vowel such as /i/; /ɹ/ may be more accurate before or after a velar, and so on. Phonetic tests of these types are covered in depth in Chapter 7, which focuses on phones and phonemes.

In many cases, the SLP will classify the substitution, omission, or distortion errors that have been identified in terms of phonological patterns that impact classes of sounds (e.g., all fricatives are substituted with stops; thus the child is stopping). Phonological process tests are designed to identify such patterns in the child's speech errors. They are discussed in detail in Chapter 9 as error patterns are the focus of that chapter.

There are several advantages of standardized relational tests. The targets are known, so poor intelligibility is not a factor unless the child's problem is very severe. The targets are selected to represent the majority of the consonants (and sometimes clusters and/or vowels) of the language. Furthermore, these tests are normed, and they yield standardized scores so that the severity of the child's delay or disorder can be estimated and eligibility for special services can be determined and documented. For many SLPs, a primary reason for using such tests is that the educational and healthcare bureaucracies mandate that they do so in order to justify the need for services.

But such relational analyses only tell us what is going wrong—not what is functioning well—in the child's system. For example, a particular child might be producing a consonant that sounds like [s], but only when she is attempting to say /ʃ/. When she attempts /s/, she produces [t] instead. A relational analysis will indicate that neither /s/ nor /ʃ/ are produced correctly and that the child is both fronting (producing the palatal /ʃ/ as an alveolar [s]) and stopping (producing the continuant /s/ as the stop [t]). These conclusions are appropriate, but they miss the fact that the phone [s] is actually being produced by the client, albeit in the wrong words. Independent analysis can reveal such key insights. Using relational analysis tools alone takes the focus off of the child's phonological system as a system that is more or less functional in and of itself. The various components of the system are not analyzed to determine which may be contributing the most (or the least) to the child's current level of communicative effectiveness. Such an approach might be compared to evaluating a malfunctioning car by watching it drive down the road beside an intact vehicle. The mechanic may get some hints as to the general location of the problem—muffler versus windshield washer, etc.—and seeing the well-functioning car will also remind her of her eventual goal for the other one. But she can't determine the actual source of the malfunction until she opens the hood and examines the muffler, carburetor, and so on. Of course, an experienced mechanic may be able to identify which component is malfunctioning just by watching the car drive by. An experienced child phonologist can also often differentiate malfunctioning phonological components simply by listening to the child speak. But to become an experienced mechanic, one first has to learn what the components of the car are, how they work individually, and how they work together. Furthermore, even the expert mechanic verifies her hunches before beginning her repairs.

In short, relational patterns are descriptions of the differences between the child's productions and the adult (presumed target) productions. In many cases, the adult pattern may actually *be* the child's internal phonological target (in other words, the child knows what the correct phoneme or structure [e.g., cluster] is and is trying to produce it, but cannot do so). Under those circumstances, the description of the difference between the child's pronunciation and the adult's pronunciation is also a description of what is going wrong in the child's system. In other cases, the child may think that the target is something else (e.g., may believe that the word "truck" begins with [tʃ] rather than with tr-), and this misconception about what he is supposed to be doing—*not* an inability to say the correct target—may be the actual source of the incorrect production. The standardized test doesn't show whether the speech of a child with a SSD is atypical or simply immature in comparison to that of his typically developing peers. It simply indicates that this child makes more errors than do others his age. It is more difficult to know whether the child's speech is only quantitatively or also qualitatively different from age expectations (i.e., whether his speech is delayed or disordered) without a careful analysis of the child's own system first.

Independent Analysis

An independent analysis is an analysis of the child's system as a system, regardless of the adult target system. Independent analyses consider the child's system as a phonological system in its own right, which may or may not be functioning well. In an independent analysis, the word and syllable shapes, the consonants and vowels, and the stress patterns that the child actually *does* produce are determined. Any phonological system must be sufficiently rich (that is, sufficiently complex) for the level of communication of its user. A child who only attempts 10 words might easily get away with one or two consonant phonemes and one or two vowel phonemes. But as she attempts to acquire more words, her system must add complexity.

There are a variety of options available for expanding a phonological system, and all of them must be assessed. Complexity can be phonotactic (word and syllable shapes available), phonetic (sounds available), phonemic (contrasts), pattern-based (interactions of phones, phonemes, and word structures), or prosodic (suprasegmental patterns available). The child may choose to add complexity to his system in ways that have not been chosen by the adult phonology that surrounds him. This is not the primary focus of an independent analysis. In this type of analysis, the interest lies primarily in whether the phonological system is appropriately rich and which subsystems are contributing to this complexity. If one subsystem is grossly underdeveloped in comparison to others (e.g., the child has many phonemes but all of his words are monosyllabic), that subsystem (e.g., phonotactics) will likely be the target of our intervention.

Thus, an independent analysis gives us a clearer picture of the child's actual phonological capabilities and limitations. One additional major advantage of an independent analysis is that it can be carried out without respect to the presumed target words. Thus, if a child is unintelligible or produces only babble or **jargon**, it is still possible to assess the components of her speech production in order to determine whether they are age-appropriate or severely limited. For instance, one prelinguistic child may produce reduplicated canonical syllables only (e.g., [bɑbɑbɑ]), while another may produce widely varied syllables, even including some primitive stop + glide clusters (e.g., [djudigwɑtʃu]), in varied prosodic contexts (e.g., apparent questions versus statements versus commands). The second child has a far better foundation for word production.

Both independent and relational analyses are important for assessing child phonological disorders. Although the ultimate long-term goal is to make the child's phonology adult-like, it is important to identify the non-functional aspects of the child's current system *as a system* before attempting to fix it. Children who have SSDs may exhibit extreme deficits in one particular subcomponent or in the interactions among subcomponents, and then this subcomponent or this type of phonological interaction must be an important focus of therapy. On the other hand, the purpose of having an intact phonology is to communicate. For this reason, the child should ideally not only have a functional phonology but also have a phonology that is as similar as possible to that of his environment, so that people will understand him. Relational analysis will help to determine which aspects of his phonology are most deviant in this sense and will be another major influence in the goal selection process. Many more examples of both types of analysis and their implications for intervention will be given throughout this book.

Summary

Identification, diagnosis, and assessment are important discrete aspects of the assessment process. Static assessment focuses on the child's ability to function in one context with minimal support (usually labeling pictures without any cues given about errors that she may make). Dynamic assessment focuses on the child's ability to improve her production when various types of cues are given. Independent analysis allows the SLP to look at the child's system as an entity and to identify non-functional components or poor interactions among components. Relational analysis reveals how the child's output differs from the adults'. All of these procedures contribute to the identification of which of the child's speech sound differences has the most important impact on intelligibility.

EXERCISE 4-1

Types of SSDs and Evaluation Processes

ORAL MECHANISM/MOTOR SPEECH EVALUATION

The evaluation of the structures and functions of oral motor and oral sensory systems is typically referred to as an "oral mechanism examination." It includes careful documentation and analysis of the child's oral and other speech-related anatomy and physiology (e.g., respiratory and laryngeal function) and the manner in which he is able to use his oral structures for the purpose of producing speech sounds. There are many standardized oral mechanism protocols available, but few norm-referenced tests; many of these protocols are based upon the most famous among them, the Mayo Clinic protocol.

Comprehensive "oral mechanism" protocols and tests provide instructions for examining the structure and the speech and non-speech functioning of each component structure: lips, tongue, hard palate, soft palate, larynx, and lungs, and each component function: respiration, phonation, resonance, and articulation. Overarching features (i.e., characteristics that are examined globally as well as with respect to the individual structures) include overall muscle tone, symmetry, range of motion, variability, fluidity, and rate.

The Verbal Motor Production Assessment for Children (VMPAC) (Hayden & Square, 1999) is currently the only norm-referenced, standardized oral motor/motor speech test designed specifically for children. It provides systematic instructions and tasks for the anatomic and physiologic assessment of a child's oral mechanism and motor speech skills with basic norms provided. Although it does not demonstrate all types of validity and reliability, the VMPAC is more psychometrically adequate than are other currently available instruments for assessing oral motor and motor speech functioning in children (McCauley & Strand, 2008). However, other instruments are in development (Strand, McCauley, Weigand, Stoeckel, & Baas, 2013).

Many SLPs perform non-standardized, informal oral mechanism examinations. Whether one uses a standardized measure or not, the following components should be included.

Overall Muscle Tone

First, observe the client's overall muscle tone and strength, both while moving (e.g., walking) and while sitting still. Does the child's body appear limp? Does she sit or stand in a rounded posture, W-sit, or lean upon objects for support? Are her joints more flexible than expected? Does her face, or any part of it, appear to droop? Are reflexes slow or absent? Do movements appear slow, weak, or imprecise? Is drooling excessive for the child's age? If the answers to some of these questions are "yes," consider the possibility of hypotonia and refer the child for a neurologic, occupational therapy, and/or physical therapy evaluation if these have not yet been done.

In contrast, hypertonia is characterized by overactive reflexes and muscle rigidity. The joints are less flexible than is typically expected and facial expressions appear stiff or tight as if the child has had a face lift. A child with noticeable hypertonia also should be referred for further evaluation by a neurologist and/or an occupational or physical therapist if these assessments have not already occurred.

Symmetry

Although the two sides of the human body are never identical, the structures, functions, and ranges of motion of the two sides should be very similar. Noticeable differences may be due to asymmetries of neural control. For example, it is quite common for people who have had cardiovascular accidents (CVAs, or strokes) to demonstrate some droop on the side of the face that is controlled by the affected brain hemisphere. A smile that extends farther to one side of the face than the other, a tongue that protrudes laterally instead of directly forward, and similar phenomena can be signs of neurologic abnormalities of various sorts.

Of course, no one's face is perfectly symmetrical. In fact, totally symmetrical faces look odd. Slight asymmetries may be exacerbated in stressful situations, including medical conditions. Furthermore, it is normal for the mouth to open a

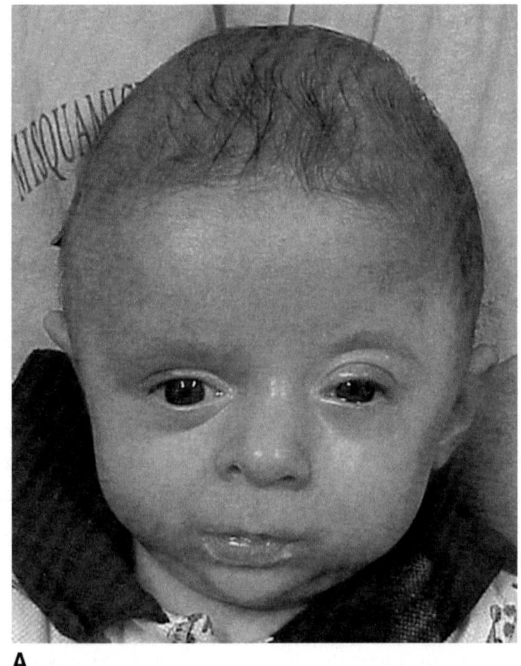
A

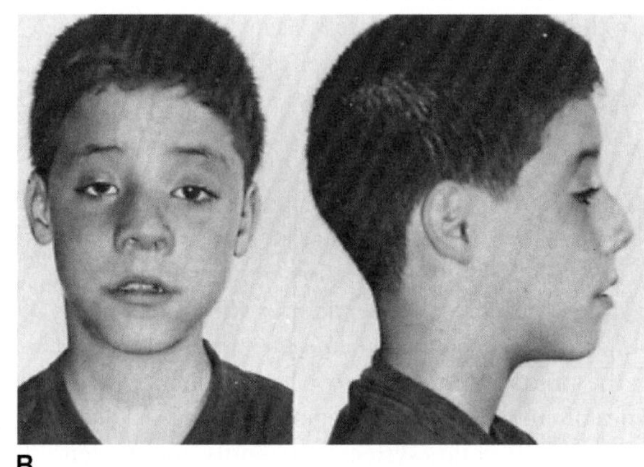
B

FIGURE 4-1. A, B. Facial asymmetry

bit wider on the right during verbal tasks (but not for smiling) (Graves & Landis, 1990). However, noticeable asymmetries can be signs of neurologic differences or genetic syndromes (such as 7q11.23 Duplication syndrome; Velleman & Mervis, 2011). Neither side of the face should appear either droopier or stiffer than the other, and ranges of motion should be roughly the same for both sides. For example, when the child smiles, his mouth should extend the same amount on both sides. When he sticks out his tongue, it should protrude straight out, not deviate to one side or the other. Chewing should occur on both sides in a rotary motion, with the tongue moving the bolus from one side to the other. Some examples of atypically asymmetrical child faces are given in Figure 4-1.

Range of Motion

For all of the moving parts of the oral mechanism (lips, tongue, soft palate), we consider range of motion: How far can the lips and tongue protrude or retract, rise or lower? How far do the tongue and the soft palate rise or lower from their resting states?

Variability

Movements that are performed repeatedly should be fairly consistent across repetitions. **Inconsistency** from one repetition or one trial to the next may be indicative of poor motor planning, programming, or self-monitoring. Inconsistency in multiple repetitions of the same syllable or word in a series (token-to-token variability) is a hallmark of CAS (ASHA, 2007). Rupela and Manjula (2010) also have demonstrated reduced consistency on such tasks among children with Down syndrome.

One common approach to assessing variability is through syllable or word repetitions. Two main types of repetitions are elicited: alternating motion rates (AMRs), which are repetitions of the same syllable (e.g., [pʌpʌpʌpʌ], [tʌtʌtʌtʌ]), and sequential motion rates (SMRs), which are repetitions of alternating syllables (e.g., [pʌtʌkʌ pʌtʌkʌ pʌtʌkʌ]). (These two tasks, collectively, were previously referred to as "diadochokinesis" or "diadochokinetic rates.")

Fluidity

Oral movements or stretches of speech should be smooth and continuous, not rough or choppy. Starts and stops or sudden increases or decreases in loudness, pitch, or rate are not typical and should be carefully documented. Again, AMRs and SMRs can be useful for identifying these patterns.

In very young children who are just beginning to talk, two- to three-word phrases or simple sentences may initially be produced as a series of words. That is, they may lack the prosodic contour that is expected for sentences in the language, thus sounding segregated or choppy. This may occur even if the child previously produced appropriate intonation contours while producing prelinguistic vocalizations (e.g., during the jargon stage). However, this should only last for a few weeks.

Rate

The traditional purpose for administering AMRs and SMRs is to determine rates of production of repeated (AMR) or varied (SMR) syllables. Slowed rate is a well-established finding among children with dysarthria and CAS and has also been reported for children with Down syndrome

(Rupela & Manjula, 2010) and those with ASD (Velleman, Andrianopoulos, Boucher, Perkins, Averback, et al., 2009). Simple AMR and SMR tasks can be carried out even for children between 4 and 6 years old (Rvachew, Ohberg, & Savage, 2006); norms for children are available. However, Williams and Stackhouse (1998, 2000) have demonstrated that rate may be a less useful measure of motor speech disorder than consistency and accuracy for children between the ages of 3 and 5.

Assessment of Individual Structures

Specific aspects of individual structures also receive careful attention, as described further.

Jaw

As noted, it is normal for the jaw to open a bit wider to the right during some oral tasks (but not for smiling) (Graves & Landis, 1990). The jaw should open smoothly, without jerking or sliding to either side, only as far as appropriate for the speech or non-speech task being performed. See also the section on "Teeth."

Lips

Observe the symmetry of the child's lips, both at rest and during movement. Ask the child to smile and pucker and produce [i] and [u], both in isolation and in sequence. Watch for independence of the lips and the jaw (i.e., they don't necessarily move at the same time or to the same extent). Note whether the lips move smoothly from retraction (smile, [i]) to protrusion (pucker, [u]). Observe the child while eating: Do the lips seal enough to keep liquids or solids inside? Does the child effectively use the lips to clear soft food (e.g., pudding) off of a spoon?

Teeth

The alignment of the upper and lower jaws is observed with the person's upper (**maxillary**) and lower (**mandibular**) teeth in contact. It is normal for the upper teeth to protrude slightly (about a quarter of an inch) beyond the lowers and to hide the tops of those lower teeth. If the maxillaries protrude more than that, this is classified as an **overbite** or **open bite**. This can be a feature of cleft palate among other conditions. The reverse state of affairs is called **underbite**. Missing, misaligned, or poorly spaced teeth should also be noted. Ask the child to bite a cookie or cracker and observe for symmetry and function during biting and during chewing.

Tongue

Observe the tongue at rest and while the child produces a prolonged [a]. It should appear to fit comfortably and symmetrically within the oral cavity. If a clear tongue tip is not visible (i.e., if the tongue looks heart-shaped) and/or the child is not able to produce alveolar consonants, assess carefully for tongue tie. Recall that interincisal distance—the distance between the upper and lower teeth when the child opens her mouth as far as possible with the tongue tip on the upper teeth—is the most prognostic measure for determining whether ankyloglossia is likely to impact speech (Messner & Lalakea, 2002).

Ask the child to touch the alveolar ridge with the tongue tip ("Put your tongue on the bump behind your teeth") and also to move the tongue from side to side (from one corner of the mouth to the other). Movements should be smooth and precise, without struggle, tremor, staccato-like motion, or groping (although some children will not have done these things before, so you may need to illustrate). Does the child move the head or the jaw back and forth instead of the tongue? Notice what it takes for the child to perform these movements: oral directions (repeated how many times?), a visual model, tactile cues?

Palate and Oro–Pharyngeal Area

Ask the child to open the mouth with the head slightly back so that you can easily view the hard and soft palate. Look for symmetry and smooth tissue (e.g., no scars or other abnormalities). Using a small flashlight, observe the color of the hard and soft palate. They should be pink and white. If there is a bluish tint at the midline, there could be a submucous cleft. If so, if possible gently rub your gloved finger along the back of the hard palate to see if you can feel a depression in the bone.

Observe the soft palate as the child prolongs [ɑ] and then during [ɑʔɑʔɑʔ]. You should see the soft palate rise smoothly and symmetrically. Note abnormalities of the **uvula**, such as a bifid (split) uvula. Look for redness or swelling of the tonsils or of the faucial pillars at the threshold of the pharynx, which can indicate infection.

Hold a mirror under the child's nose as she produces [papa]. Compare the lack of fogging that occurs with these non-nasal sounds to the fogging on the mirror when the child produces [mama].

Resonance and Voice Quality

Listen for nasality, hoarseness, harshness, or sounds of strain as the client vocalizes. Measure the length of prolongations of [ɑ], [i], and [u]. Note whether these prolongations are smooth and fully voiced or whether there are breaks in the pitch or the voicing. Note swollen tonsils or adenoids that may impact on resonance.

Articulatory Control and Flexibility; Rate and Rhythmicity

Observe the child producing single sounds as well as sequences that challenge the range of motion. These include protrusion–retraction of the lips (e.g., [i—u—i—u]), jaw opening and closing (e.g., [papapa]), tongue lifting and lowering (e.g., [tatata]), and tongue fronting and backing

TABLE 4-2 Differential Symptoms of Dysarthria Versus Childhood Apraxia of Speech

Childhood Apraxia of Speech	Dysarthria
No or mild muscle tone issues	Significant muscle tone issues
More difficulty in volitional contexts	Automatic ~ volitional
Difficulties significantly worse in more complex, sequential contexts	Less increase in difficulty in complex sequential contexts
Sequencing, substitution, complication as well as simplification errors	Distortions, simplifications
Linguistic deficits (e.g., grammar) worse than cognitive expectations	Language abilities parallel cognitive abilities

(e.g., [kʌtʌkʌtʌ]). Are these motions smooth, symmetrical, and rapid? Does the child raise and lower the tongue tip/dorsum rather than raising and lowering the jaw, with the tongue riding along? Are the repeated productions rhythmic?

Dysarthria Versus Apraxia Versus Phonological Disorder

One of the key questions that many SLPs keep in mind as they do an oral mechanism/motor speech evaluation is whether the client shows symptoms of dysarthria, CAS, both, or neither. Table 4-2 summarizes some of the key differentially diagnostic characteristics of CAS versus dysarthria, as discussed in depth in Chapter 3. Table 4-3 contrasts the symptoms of CAS and the symptoms of a cognitive–linguistic speech sound disorder. Many of these characteristics are elucidated in Chapters 5 to 9 of this book.

Summary

The oral mechanism examination is a crucial component of any speech-language assessment. It should include both evaluation of individual structures and more global observations of the entire respiratory/resonatory/articulatory system. The clinician should carefully note signs of atypical muscle tone, range of motion, variability, fluidity, or rate as well as of structural or functional asymmetry.

POPULAR ASSESSMENT TOOL TYPES

It is not a primary purpose of this book to review specific popular assessment tools nor to recommend any one over another. However, different types of evaluation materials will be discussed. It is assumed that all clinicians systematically collect phonological data of some sort before attempting to set therapy goals. The majority of SLPs use marketed tools, often in conjunction with other analyses, for this purpose. These assessment materials fall into three broad categories: articulation tests, process tests, and more comprehensive **phonological analysis procedures**. Some basic differences among these three types of materials will be described in more detail here.

Articulation Tests

Articulation tests are typically thought of as phonetic, because they focus on the child's ability to articulate particular speech sounds, especially consonants. Word shapes and other aspects of context are usually not taken into account. These tests typically include a set of pictures that the child is to label one by one in order for the clinician to score the child's production of each sound in initial, medial, and/or final position (as appropriate). Each error is categorized as a substitution or an omission; in some cases, distortions are also considered. Each misarticulation is considered to be developmentally appropriate or not depending on the predetermined age of acquisition for the target phoneme.

TABLE 4-3 Differential Symptoms of Childhood Apraxia of Speech Versus Cognitive–Linguistic Speech Sound Disorder

Childhood Apraxia of Speech	Cognitive–Linguistic Speech Sound Disorder
Motor symptoms	No or very mild motor symptoms
Phonotactics relatively more impaired than phonetics	Phonetics impaired as much as phonotactics
Prosodic differences especially choppy, excess equal stress	Prosody within normal limits
Persistent weak syllable deletion	Weak syllable deletion fades
Sequencing errors	Few sequencing errors
Vowel deviations	Few or no vowel errors
Inconsistency in multiple repetitions/other types of inconsistency	Consistency/other types of inconsistency
Volitional worse than automatic	No difference or volitional better

In most cases, the child's score is based on the number of errors made, regardless of the nature of the error (e.g., whether a substitution was a typical one or an atypical one).

The major appeal of these articulation tests is their ease of use. Because single words are elicited, decreased intelligibility is not a major problem; the word the child is attempting is known (unless he speaks a different dialect or makes an inappropriate assumption of what is depicted on the test page). Items are carefully chosen to include all phonemes in the target language, thus minimizing the effects of avoidance of sounds that the child knows he cannot produce. Often, target transcriptions are provided on the answer form, so the examiner does not have to transcribe extensively. Only the target sounds need to be considered, not the other sounds within the words. Another major advantage is that articulation tests are generally normed so that standard scores and percentiles can be determined, allowing the clinician to compare the child's speech sound skills for producing elicited single words to those of other children of similar ages. This is often required in school systems and other settings where accountability is vital.

A few articulation tests include vowels; many include at least a few consonant clusters in different word positions; many include at least some multisyllabic as well as monosyllabic words. However, the child's overall ability to produce clusters or multisyllabic words is not the focus of the scoring procedures of tests such as these. Only the accuracy of individual consonants (and sometimes clusters and/or vowels) within monosyllabic or multisyllabic words is scored. Sound classes (e.g., fricatives) are typically not considered as such. Although the use of these articulation tests may be sufficient for identifying a speech sound problem (by comparing the child's score to norms), they often do not make it possible to differentiate a delay from a disorder. Most phonologists now believe that the data that articulation tests yield are too superficial for the level of assessment that is required for determining remediation targets.

The drawbacks of using articulation tests include the small sets of words assessed, which tend to be restricted to nouns. Most phonemes are only sampled once in each word position, and some (or all) vowel phonemes or uncommon phonemes (such as /ʒ/) may not be sampled at all. Furthermore, word complexity is rarely appropriately controlled. As mentioned above, these tests were designed to identify segmental errors only, based on the traditional assumption that all articulation disorders result from a motoric deficit in the ability to form the articulatory positions required for certain sounds. The identification of whole-syllable and whole-word patterns is difficult. If a test that does not include phrase or sentence-level productions is used, the production of single words only may be a disadvantage as well as an advantage: the lack of phrase- or sentence-level effects enhances intelligibility and transcribability. But if these effects are not observed, they cannot be analyzed and treated. How can we tell that the child needs to work on producing [s] in sentences if we don't test [s] in sentences? Finally, the articulation test speech production context is not natural; younger, lower class, and non-white children may be particularly unfamiliar with picture-naming tasks and may not demonstrate their true phonological capabilities. According to Morrison and Shriberg (1992):

> *In comparison to the validity of conversational speech samples for integrated speech, language, and prosodic analyses, articulation tests appear to yield neither typical nor optimal measures of speech performance (p. 259).*

Eisenberg and Hitchcock (2010) concur:

> *Use of the data from a single standardized test of articulation or phonology would not be sufficient for inventorying a child's consonant and vowel production and selecting targets for therapy (p. 488).*

(See also Shriberg and Kwiatkowski [1980] for further discussion of these ideas.)

Although the limitations of assessing children's speech sounds one by one without considering more general phonological patterns have been clear for three decades or more, many sound-based articulation tests remain popular nonetheless for the reasons described previously. They clearly have a place within a comprehensive speech sound evaluation as long as they are supplemented with speech sample analysis.

Some SLPs use articulation test word targets to facilitate more in-depth phonological analysis. In this procedure, each of the child's word productions is transcribed as a whole rather than only the child's production of the target sound for each stimulus item (e.g., "house" is transcribed as [aʊt] instead of simply marking that the [h] was omitted). Using such transcriptions, especially if they can be supplemented by samples of spontaneous speech, the SLP can carry out further analyses to facilitate the investigation of particular classes of sounds (including vowels) that occur (or not) in initial, medial, or final positions or within clusters. Influences of certain sounds or sound classes on others can also be investigated, as can the influence of structural contexts (e.g., accuracy in singletons versus clusters). In addition, some useful information may be gleaned from the child's productions of multisyllabic words, which are also included (rather unsystematically) in most articulation tests despite the fact that no syllable production data are explicitly collected during standardized test administration.

There are some real advantages and some important limitations to this idea of using transcriptions of articulation test items for broader analysis. The advantages are that the picture stimuli are already gathered with the intent of representing a variety of English sounds. The pictures have been designed to be attractive and recognizable to young children. Furthermore, when a child labels a picture, the clinician usually knows what the child's target word is (though, of course, it is always possible that he is calling a lobster a crab, etc.). This can be very important with some unintelligible children. Phrase-level phonological effects (i.e., connected speech processes, such as pronouncing "did you" as [dʒu]), which may complicate identification of target words as well as their analyses, are also absent in single-word productions. Finally, comparisons among children are facilitated by the fact that all of the children tested produce the same stimuli. The limitations are those described previously.

Process Tests

Other tests have as their aim the identification of error **patterns**, most commonly called phonological processes (see Chapter 9, "Patterns"). These tests, like articulation tests, typically include specific stimulus words that the child is to produce. Most often the words are to be produced singly and spontaneously, although some tests elicit entire sentences containing target sounds and in some cases imitative productions are expected or at least considered to be acceptable. Once these word productions have been elicited, they are analyzed with respect to the presence or absence of specific patterns. These typically include substitution processes in which the child produces the incorrect place (e.g., velar as in velar fronting), manner (e.g., continuant as in stopping of fricatives), or voicing features (as in voicing or devoicing) of a class of sounds (e.g., velars, continuants, or voiced/voiceless consonants). They also identify phonotactic processes, such as final consonant deletion, weak syllable deletion, consonant cluster reduction, etc.

COMMON *Confusion*

IS IT ARTICULATION OR IS IT PHONOLOGY?

A great deal of heat and much less light has been shed on the issue of the (sensory–)motor versus cognitive bases of SSDs, with many efforts to distinguish articulatory or phonetic (i.e., motoric) errors from phonological (cognitive–linguistic) errors. As discussed in Chapter 3, speech production always has a sensory–motor basis. Developmentally, speech perception (the identification and categorization of speech sounds that are relevant for communication) and articulation (the production of phones) precede the expressive use of sounds for meaning (phonemes). In this sense, sensory–motor functioning is a foundation for phonology. On the other hand, communication is not possible without a certain amount of cognitive activity, including implicit/procedural learning of the rules of the ambient language.

Distortions of /ɹ/ or /s/ (lisps) and the like appear to be good candidates for pure articulation disorders. Yet, many SLPs believe that if a pattern can be identified, the problem must be "phonological." But a frontal lisp can affect a whole class of sounds (all sibilant fricatives) and can be described as "fronting:" Does the fact that there's a process name for the phenomenon prove that it's not motoric? Clearly not. Does the fact that an error pattern has a motoric basis (e.g., backing from labial to velar as a result of Moebius syndrome) mean that we should ignore the fact that an entire class of sounds is affected? In other words, should we refrain from labeling a pattern as such just because it has a motor basis? Clearly not.

What would a purely "phonological" disorder look like? A person who is learning a second language and tries to apply the rules of her first language to the second language is a good example of someone whose primary difficulty is phonological (though this would of course be a phonological *difference*, not a disorder). However, the phonological rules of languages do reflect articulatory factors (such as production of places and manners of articulation) and perceptual factors (such as identification of places and manners of articulation) as well as cognitive–linguistic factors. The abstract processing of phonemes and phonological processes is built upon physiologic experiences of phones. The premise that SSDs often have some linguistic basis is supported by the fact that SSDs and language impairments (LI) often co-occur (Shriberg, Tomblin, & McSweeny, 1999). The premise that there is a motoric element even in SSDs accompanied by LI (which are more likely to be cognitive–linguistic [i.e., phonological] disorders) is supported by the fact that adults with a history of SSD and LI (whose children also have SSDs) perform worse on oral motor skills than do adults with histories of SSDs but not of language impairments (whose children also have SSDs) (Lewis, Freebairn, Hansen, Miscimarra, Iyengar, et al., 2007). Furthermore, children with specific language impairment (SLI) have significantly worse gross and fine motor skills than do those without SLI (Zelaznik & Goffman, 2010). In addition, 5% to 8% of children with persistent SLI also demonstrate SSDs (Shriberg, Tomblin, & McSweeny, 1999). Thus, even clearly linguistic disorders such as language impairment are often accompanied by motor deficits.

Another challenge in making the distinction between articulatory and phonological disorders is that even trained SLPs are often not able to distinguish these by ear. In a study by Gibbon (1999), errors were judged by SLPs to be phonological or phonetic. When electropalatography was used to visualize the children's articulation patterns, all of the errors were found to result from undifferentiated control of the blade of the tongue.

In short, it is likely that most—though not all—SSDs include both sensory–motor and cognitive components, although one or the other may be predominant in a given child. Tables 4-2 and 4-3 are intended to facilitate the determination of whether the characteristics of dysarthria, CAS, or cognitive–linguistic speech-sound disorder are primary. However, any of these types of problem may yield a pattern of errors, so *the presence of a pattern does not tell us which causative factors are primary.* Of course, intervention should focus on the dominant symptoms using those strategies that yield the best outcomes for a given child, as discussed in depth in the next chapter and beyond.

Like articulation tests, process tests generate a useful set of word productions that can be analyzed in other ways as well as in the ways recommended in the manual. These tests also are typically standardized and yield norms that allow a comparison to age expectations and severity levels. Furthermore, they can point us in the direction of the types of further analyses that might be appropriate.

Of course, many tests that are currently available combine these two functions. Typically, the child produces a set of words, often in response to picture stimuli. Then the SLP can score those productions individually (segment by segment, as for an articulation test) or as patterns (as for a process test), or both. In fact, some process tests, such as the Khan-Lewis Phonological Analysis (Khan & Lewis, 2002), are designed to use children's responses to an articulation test (e.g., the Goldman-Fristoe Test of Articulation; Goldman & Fristoe, 2000) as the data on which process scoring is based. The difference is in the nature of the analysis, not in the elicitation procedure.

Comprehensive Phonological Analysis Procedures

Several manuals are available for carrying out a more detailed phonological analysis based upon a longer transcribed free speech sample. Each describes the process of thoroughly sampling and assessing various aspects of the child's speech production patterns based upon theoretical principles that reflect the individual authors' views of child phonology. These procedures typically provide a fairly comprehensive view of the child's phonology. However, a lengthy sample of (preferably) spontaneous speech must be elicited from the child and carefully transcribed and then analyzed by the clinician. The time involved in obtaining and transcribing such a sample when added to the time required for carrying out such detailed analyses is seen as prohibitive by many practicing clinicians.

In the best of all possible worlds, there would always be enough time for all SLPs to carry out an in-depth quantitative phonological analysis on every child evaluated or seen for treatment. Unfortunately, reality is far from that ideal. Most of us have a minimum of time available for phonological analysis. Yet, addressing inappropriate, inefficient, or unachievable goals is a true waste of valuable therapy time (and as a result, money). Thus, the time taken to choose remediation targets carefully is a worthwhile investment.

If quantitative data (percentages) and/or age norms are not needed, many aspects of the child's phonological system can be assessed much more simply and quickly using a spontaneous speech sample, a sample from the administration of a standard articulation or process test, or preferably both. The combination provides a set of elicited single-word utterances with known targets plus a set of spontaneous utterances from a more naturalistic context, some of which may be partially or totally unintelligible. Interesting differences may emerge from the comparison of conversational versus elicited speech samples. Most clinicians record a language sample, obtained either in conversation with the child or through observation of even more naturalistic interactions (e.g., in a familiar classroom context or at play with another child). The language sample can be transcribed in the international phonetic alphabet (IPA) later. Then the transcribed words from the articulation test plus the language sample can be analyzed, with the results checked off, estimated, or calculated on a worksheet to identify the phonological system used by the child. Any immature or deviant patterns identified can be more thoroughly quantified later to set baselines in therapy.

Many child phonologists have their own worksheets or even phonological analysis software that they have developed over years of phonological analyses, but the typical SLP lacks the time required for developing such protocols. Therefore, worksheets for speech sample analyses of children's word productions will be provided in Chapters 5 through 9 of this book. These provide the clinician with quick ways to analyze different aspects of a child's speech in more detail without having to carry out an entire phonological analysis. The worksheets can be used either with spontaneous speech samples or with elicited word productions such as those that would be obtained through the administration of a traditional articulation test. Ideally, the clinician would administer such a test and *also* transcribe the child's language sample (or at least a portion of it) in IPA in order to take advantage of the benefits of each data-gathering procedure. In this way, comparisons can be made between elicited single-word and spontaneous conversational speech.

Although these worksheets are not standardized and they provide an overview at best of the child's phonological system, they do provide a means of sketching each aspect of phonology within a feasible time frame. Furthermore, they are more user-friendly than are many of the in-depth analysis procedures on the market. Finally, the worksheets provided here can be used at three different levels of accuracy, allowing the clinician to select the depth of analysis that is appropriate to the client, the time available, and the clinician's own experience level.

The use of speech sample worksheets cannot replace in-depth phonological analysis in cases that require careful quantitative documentation, nor can it provide age equivalencies or scores. However, such worksheets can serve as efficient, flexible assessment tools that will facilitate goal-setting and, later, reassessment.

Summary: Pros and Cons of Various Assessment Tools and Strategies

A child's phonology can be assessed in a variety of different ways: using an articulation test to score correct or incorrect productions of one target phoneme per word, using a process test to identify patterns of errors with elicited words, or using an in-depth analysis of spontaneous speech. Each of these procedures has its pros and cons. The real advantage of articulation tests is their simple format and scoring system as well as their norms. Many young or very active children cannot be induced to name more than a small set of large colorful pictures and would therefore not be appropriate candidates for longer elicitation procedures. However, the amount of information that can be gleaned from one production of each phoneme in each position may be quite limited. More in-depth analyses require spontaneous connected speech, which is certainly more natural but is also far more challenging and time-consuming to elicit and transcribe. Furthermore, data from unintelligible children may often be very difficult to use because the target words are unknown.

In making the final selection of assessment tools for a particular client at a particular time, many factors must be taken into account. The first is the purpose of the assessment. If the goal is to document the presence or the extent of a delay or disorder, or to differentiate delay from disorder, norms are likely to be needed. In these cases, a standardized test (articulation or process) is most appropriate.

The complexity of the problem is also an important factor, of course. For a child with just a few errors or one with simple speech errors that are clearly motoric in nature (e.g., a lisp), a single-word articulation test may provide the needed documentation. A client with a more complex disorder (whether it is primarily motor-based or cognitive–linguistic) will be better served by a pattern-based test, a speech sample-based analysis, or both. The clinician's experience, knowledge, and skills should also influence the selection of an assessment tool; there is no sense in using a tool that one cannot administer, score, or interpret properly. The reality of the time and level of effort available for assessment also unfortunately cannot be ignored.

To identify appropriate goals, independent as well as relational analysis is strongly recommended; as described above, independent analysis leads to the identification of strengths—existing capabilities—upon which new skills can be built. Appropriate intervention strategies will be determined initially via dynamic assessment, through which the range of the child's abilities is explored by assessing her speech in a variety of contexts and with a variety of supports provided (e.g., multimodal cues). Ongoing adjustments to therapy strategies and to the client's prognosis will be made through criterion-referenced assessments, which would include repeated baseline performance measurements and also independent analysis. As described in further depth in Chapter 5, Glaspey and MacLeod (2010) have documented the usefulness and validity of systematically measuring not only the client's performance but also the client's ability to perform in different contexts and with or without the support of various types of cues.

Each clinician must assess each child's linguistic and behavioral capabilities as well as the clinician's own limitations in time, knowledge, and skills in order to determine the most efficient and effective method for assessing the child's phonology.

EXERCISE 4-2

Popular Assessment Tool Types

SPEECH EVALUATION OF BILINGUAL/ BIDIALECTAL CHILDREN

It is neither feasible nor ethical for SLPs to remain ignorant of basic principles of assessment and treatment of children learning more than one language, including the impact of cultural factors, in the 21st century world (International Expert Panel on Multilingual Children's Speech, 2012). As of 2005, some 5.2 million bilingual children were enrolled in American schools (Goldstein & Fabiano-Smith, 2007), and this number will continue to rise. As noted above, SLPs must be especially cautious about either under-diagnosing or over-diagnosing children with speech differences as having SSDs or delays. This is not necessarily an either–or proposition. Many children who demonstrate errors resulting from the influence of one language on another (a.k.a., **interference** or **transfer** errors) may nonetheless demonstrate difficulty with speech motor control, phonological rule learning, and/or phonological awareness (Preston & Seki, 2011). Teasing apart these possibilities is extremely challenging for the majority of American SLPs. In a 2011 American Speech-Language-Hearing Association survey, SLP respondents were asked to rate their ability to "address cultural and linguistic influences on service delivery and outcomes" on a scale of 1 ("Not at all qualified") to 5 ("Very qualified"). Fewer than 37% rated themselves at the level of 4 to 5; the numbers were even lower (less than 31%) among school SLPs (ASHA, 2011). A few key principles can help to inform the process.

First, one bilingual is not the sum of two monolinguals. Bilinguals' linguistic systems are different from those of monolinguals from infancy. It is not clear whether bilingual children initially attempt to construct a single linguistic system (Ray, 2002) or not (Garcia-Sierra, Rivera-Gaxiola, Percaccio, Conboy, Romo, et al., 2011). It may be that they have two separate linguistic systems but that these influence and support each other (Goldstein & Fabiano-Smith, 2007). In any case, exposure to multiple languages makes them remain more open to later ages to shifting their linguistic systems as a result of implicit learning.

Second, the nature and timing of their exposure to the two (or more) languages, including their age, may impact the learning of multilingual children. **Simultaneous bilingualism** occurs when two languages are learned at once (e.g., from birth or shortly thereafter) whereas **sequential bilinguals** are those who acquire much of one language before beginning to learn another. **Compartmentalization** occurs when the two languages are spoken in distinct contexts (e.g., one at home and one at school); unsurprisingly, exposure to language mixing typically results in a child who also mixes the languages, including **code switching** (incorporating more than one language within one utterance or conversation) (Barlow & Enriquez, 2007).

Third, bilingualism does not cause or even exacerbate disorders; nor does code switching. Code switching is a natural, systematic linguistic process (Kohnert, Yim, Nett, Kan, & Duran, 2005). Although some bilingual children may initially appear to be acquiring language more slowly (Fabiano-Smith & Goldstein, 2010) or may demonstrate slightly less mature phonological skills than do their monolingual peers (Burrows & Goldstein, 2010), most catch up without intervention. Furthermore, encouraging a bilingual family to raise a speech-disordered child as a monolingual will not cure the disorder. In fact, such a child would be at a considerable communication disadvantage in his own cultural context (Kohnert, 2008).

An assessment of the phonology of a bilingual child should ideally take place in both languages. If this is not possible, testing in the dominant language is preferable (Peña & Bedore, 2011). Typically developing bilingual children are likely to score similarly on standardized tests in both languages (Holm & Dodd, 1999). Although there is some evidence that the basic nature of the problem (e.g., delay versus disorder) may be the same in both languages (Holm & Dodd, 1999), the orders of acquisition of specific sounds and structures may vary from language to language (Stokes & Surendran, 2005) and even from dialect to dialect (Pearson, Velleman, Bryant, & Charko, 2009; Velleman & Pearson, 2010). Thus, one cannot assume that if a child has mastered a certain sound or structure in one language or dialect that she has also mastered it in the other.

Goldstein and Fabiano-Smith (2007) recommend doing both independent and relational analyses of the child's production in both languages, using samples of single words and of conversational speech. As for any child, analyses should focus on phonetic and phonotactic repertoires and error patterns. In addition, **contrastive analysis**—a comparison of the sound systems of the two languages—will provide some insight into the errors that the speaker is likely to make in the second language. For example, if the first language lacks velar consonants (such as /k, g, ŋ/) and the second has them, the learner may have more difficulty learning velars in the second language than do children who are learning that second language as their only communication system. Similarly, if [ʃ] is an allophone of /s/ in the first language but the two are separate phonemes in the second language, the learner is likely to confuse the two second-language phonemes because she is not used to having to differentiate them for comprehension or production. If two sounds are essentially interchangeable in one's first language, one learns to ignore the differences between them. Having learned to ignore something (such as the voiced [ɦ] versus voiceless [h] allophones for an English speaker) can be harder to overcome than not ever having heard it before (as might be the case, for example, for an English speaker trying to learn to produce clicks in Xhosa or uvular fricatives in French).

This interference, however, is less of a factor in the phonological development of children learning multiple languages than some had expected. Similarly, bilingual children do tend to master shared sounds (sounds that occur in both languages) before unshared sounds, but this has proven to be a less strong effect than had previously been assumed (Fabiano-Smith & Goldstein, 2010). Of course, phonological structures (e.g., consonant clusters) as well as individual sounds may be impacted by transfer (Burrows & Goldstein, 2010).

Other errors may be identified as resulting from the child's learning strategies as she has applied them to the second language. These include analogy (as in assuming that because the plural of "mouse" is "mice," the plural of "house" will be "hice") and spelling pronunciation (as in producing the name of the Massachusetts city of "Worcester" with three syllables—[ˈwɑɚsɛstɚ] instead of two [ˈwʊstɚ]).

While standardized assessment tools are available for some languages other than English, especially Spanish, this is not true of many others. In these cases, it is even more important to carry out a careful analysis based on a speech sample. Often, there is at least some research available regarding phonological development among monolingual speakers of the language, if not regarding bilingual development. While it is not appropriate to judge bilinguals based upon norms developed from monolinguals, such literature can at least help one to determine whether or not the child is demonstrating error patterns that are unusual in both languages—a greater cause for concern than patterns that do occur in one or both of the languages (Yavas & Goldstein, 1998). Dynamic assessment will further help the SLP determine whether there are conditions under which the child can produce sounds or structures that may be in error in one language or the other and how the child learns best.

Summary

Evaluating children who are learning two linguistic codes—languages or dialects—is a complex process, ideally carried out by an SLP who is fluent in the same codes as the child. Assumptions about speech development cannot be made based upon norms developed by testing monolingual children in either language. For a small number of languages, standardized bilingual assessment tools are available. However, in most cases, the SLP will have to carry out independent and relational analyses based upon speech samples in both or all languages and dialects. Norms will typically not be available.

This section provides only a brief overview of the issues associated with the speech evaluation of children who speak more than one language or dialect. Many of these concepts will be revisited in later chapters of this book. For further information, readers also are encouraged to consult sources such as Kohnert (2013).

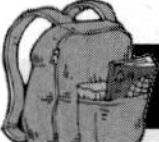

KEY TAKE-HOME MESSAGES

1. The evaluation tools you choose should depend on the purpose(s) of the evaluation (e.g., identification, assessment, diagnosis).
2. A wide variety of tools, from informal and non-normed to standardized normative tests, is available.
3. Bilingual children's phonologies are qualitatively different and require appropriate assessment tools and strategies.
4. Use of a comprehensive, complementary set of evaluation tools yields a broader, deeper understanding of the child's speech profile, and facilitates decisions about intervention goals, tools, and strategies.

EXERCISE 4-3

Assessing Bilingual Children

SUMMARY OF EVALUATION

Evaluation procedures range from screenings intended to identify whether or not there is a problem to comprehensive assessments that yield a full communication profile of the child and have direct implications for intervention. Evaluation processes may include intelligibility estimates, articulation testing, process testing, or comprehensive independent and relational analyses. Assessment may be static—based on the child's performance when no cues or other supports are provided—or dynamic. The evaluation of children who are exposed to more than one language or dialect is even more complex and challenging.

CHAPTER 4

Basic Principles for Speech Sound Evaluation Review

Exercise 4-1: **Types of SSDs and Evaluation Processes**

A. *Essay question.*

Identify a situation in which each of the following assessment procedures would be most appropriate if you were only able to do one:

- Intelligibility testing
- Independent analysis
- Standardized articulation test
- Dynamic assessment

Cite information from this chapter or other sources to support your choices.

B. *Choose the best answer for each question.*

1. Which of the following would be considered consistent with a speech *disorder*?
   a. Chronological mismatch
   b. Non-mainstream dialect
   c. Immature speech patterns
   d. Bilingualism
2. Independent analysis:
   a. focuses on the child's phonological system per se.
   b. yields standardized norm-referenced scores.
   c. highlights the client's phonetic errors.
   d. identifies substitutions, omissions, and distortions.

Exercise 4-2: **Popular Assessment Tool Types**

A. *Essay questions.*

1. Choose three activities from an oral mechanism/motor speech examination (as described in this chapter), and describe how you could make them more child-friendly by using toys, incorporating them into a game, etc. For example, you could elicit a prolonged [ɑ] sound by playing a game in which you pretend to take a nap, saying "ahhhhh" as you put your head down on the pillow.
2. Based on the information in this chapter, if you were to design a speech sound test, which of the test feature choices listed below would you prioritize? Cite information from this chapter or other sources to justify your choices.
   - Singletons versus clusters
   - Consonants versus vowels
   - Initial versus medial versus final position
   - Monosyllabic versus multisyllabic words
   - Single words versus phrases versus sentences
   - Sound-by-sound errors versus error patterns

B. *Choose the best answer for each question.*

1. *Advantages* of most articulation tests include which of the following?
   a. Word targets are known.
   b. Vowels are often not tested.
   c. Word complexity is not controlled.
   d. Only single words are produced.
2. Unlike articulation tests, process tests focus on:
   a. consonant production.
   b. vowel production.
   c. independent analysis.
   d. error patterns.
3. The purpose of independent analysis is:
   a. to determine whether or not the child is delayed.
   b. to analyze the child's system as such.
   c. to compare the child's system to the adult system.
   d. to generate standardized norms.
4. Dynamic assessment differs from static assessment in the sense that:
   a. pictures are not used as stimuli.
   b. cues and feedback are given.
   c. norms are provided.
   d. it does not facilitate goal-writing.

Exercise 4-3: **Assessing Bilingual Children**

A. *Essay questions.*

1. A child learning both English and French pronounces "beau" (handsome) /bo/ and "bon" (good) /bõ/

inconsistently, sometimes as [bo] and sometimes as [bõ]. Provide two possible explanations for this error: (1) one based on linguistic transfer and (2) one based on a physiologic deficit.

2. What are the challenges of carrying out a speech sound evaluation of a child who is bilingual? Describe a hypothetical child's background information (e.g., Is the child a simultaneous or sequential bilingual? How old? Are the parents fluent in English or not? What languages are spoken in the home, and with what frequency?) and describe what strategies you would use to evaluate the child's speech sound development, assuming that you are monolingual in English. Cite information from this chapter or other sources to support your choices.

B. *State whether the following statements are true or false.*

1. _____ If a child who has been being exposed to two languages is diagnosed with a communication disorder, the parents should be counseled to choose one language and use that one at all times.
2. _____ If it's not possible to test a child in both languages to which he has been exposed, it's best to test in the dominant language.
3. _____ Bilingual children may learn the same sounds in different orders in her two (or more) languages.
4. _____ Contrastive analysis is a process of comparing a child's productions to adult productions in order to identify his errors.
5. _____ Bilingual children generally have less mature linguistic skills than do those who are monolingual.

References

ASHA. (2007). *Childhood Apraxia of Speech* [Technical Report]. Rockville Pike, MD: American Speech-Language-Hearing Association.

ASHA. (2011). *2011 Membership survey. CCC-SLP survey summary report: Number and type of responses.* Rockville, MD: American Speech-Language-Hearing Association.

Barlow, J. A., & Enriquez, M. (2007). Theoretical perspectives on speech sound disorders in bilingual children. *Perspectives on Communication Disorders and Sciences in Culturally and Linguistically Diverse Populations, 14*(2), 3–10.

Barnes, E., Roberts, J., Long, S. H., Martin, G. E., Berni, M. C., Mandulak, K. C., & Sideris, J. (2009). Phonological accuracy and intelligibility in connected speech of boys with Fragile X syndrome or Down syndrome. *Journal of Speech, Language, and Hearing Research, 52*, 1048–1061.

Blakely, R. (1980). *Screening Test for Developmental Apraxia of Speech.* Tigard, OR: CC Publications.

Burrows, L., & Goldstein, B. (2010). Whole word measures in bilingual children with speech sound disorders. *Clinical Linguistics & Phonetics, 24*(4–5), 357–368.

Chin, S. B., Tsai, P. L., & Gao, S. (2003). Connected speech intelligibility of children with cochlear implants and children with normal hearing. *American Journal of Speech-Language Pathology, 12*(4), 440–451.

Coplan, J., & Gleason, J. R. (1988). Unclear speech: Recognition and significance of unintelligible speech in preschool children. *Pediatrics, 82*, 447–452.

Craig, H. K., Thompson, C. A., Washington, J. A., & Potter, S. L. (2003). Phonological features of child African American English. *Journal of Speech, Language, and Hearing Research, 46*(3), 623–635.

Eisenberg, S. L., & Hitchcock, E. R. (2010). Using standardized tests to inventory consonant and vowel production: A comparison of 11 tests of articulation and phonology. *Language, Speech and Hearing Services in Schools, 41*, 488–503.

Fabiano-Smith, L., & Goldstein, B. (2010). Phonological acquisition in bilingual Spanish-English speaking children. *Journal of Speech, Language, and Hearing Research, 53*(1), 160–178.

Flipsen, P. Jr. (1995). Speaker–listener familiarity: Parents as judges of delayed speech intelligibility. *Journal of Communication Disorders, 28*(1), 3–19.

Garcia-Sierra, A., Rivera-Gaxiola, M., Percaccio, C., Conboy, B. T., Romo, H., Klarman, L., … Kuhl, P. K. (2011). Bilingual language learning: An ERP study relating early brain responses to speech, language input, and later word production. *Journal of Phonetics, 39*, 546–557.

Gibbon, F. E. (1999). Undifferentiated lingual gestures in children with articulation/phonological disorders. *Journal of Speech, Language, and Hearing Research, 42*, 382–397.

Glaspey, A. M., & MacLeod, A. A. N. (2010). A multi-dimensional approach to gradient change in phonological acquisition: A case study of disordered speech development. *Clinical Linguistics & Phonetics, 24*(4–5), 283–299.

Glaspey, A., & Stoel-Gammon, C. (2005). Dynamic assessment in phonological disorders: The Scaffolding Scale of Stimulability. *Topics in Language Disorders, 25*(3), 220–230.

Goldman, R., & Fristoe, M. (2000). *Goldman-Fristoe Test of Articulation* (2nd ed., GFTA-2). Bloomington, MN: Pearson Assessments.

Goldstein, B. A., & Fabiano-Smith, L. (2007). Assessment and intervention for bilingual children with phonological disorders. *The ASHA Leader Online* (February).

Gordon-Brannan, M., & Hodson, B. W. (2000). Intelligibility/severity measurements of prekindergarten children's speech. *American Journal of Speech-Language Pathology, 9*, 141–150.

Graves, R., & Landis, T. (1990). Asymmetry in mouth opening during different speech tasks. *International Journal of Psychology, 25*, 179–189.

Hayden, D., & Square, P. (1999). *Verbal Motor Production Assessment for Children (VMPAC).* San Antonio, TX: Psychological Corporation.

Hickman, L. A. (1997). *The Apraxia Profile: A Descriptive Assessment Tool for Children.* San Antonio, TX: Communication Skill Builders.

Holm, A., & Dodd, B. (1999). Differential diagnosis of phonological disorder in two bilingual children acquiring Italian and English. *Clinical Linguistics & Phonetics, 13*(2), 113–129.

Hustad, K. C., Schueler, B., Schultz, L., & DuHadway, C. (2012). Intelligibility of 4-year-old children with and without cerebral palsy. *Journal of Speech, Language, and Hearing Research, 55*(4), 1177–1189.

International Expert Panel on Multilingual Children's Speech (2012). *Multilingual children with speech sound disorders: Position paper.* Retrieved August 3, 2014 from http://www.csu.edu.au/research/multilingual-speech/position-paper

Kent, R. D., Miolo, G., & Bloedel, S. (1994). The intelligibility of children's speech: A review of evaluation procedures. *American Journal of Speech-Language Pathology, 3*(2), 81–95.

Khan, L. M., & Lewis, N. P. (2002). *Khan-Lewis Phonological Analysis* (2nd ed.). Circle Pines, MN: American Guidance Service, Inc.

Kohnert, K. (2008). Second language acquisition: Success factors in sequential bilingualism. *The ASHA Leader* (February).

Kohnert, K. (2013). *Language disorders in bilingual children and adults.* San Diego, CA: Plural Publishing.

Kohnert, K., Yim, D., Nett, K., Kan, P. F., & Duran, L. (2005). Intervention with linguistically diverse preschool children: A focus on developing home language(s). *Language, Speech and Hearing Services in Schools, 36*, 251–263.

Kritikos, E. P. (2003). Speech-language pathologists' beliefs about language assessment of bilingual/bicultural individuals. *American Journal of Speech-Language Pathology, 12*(1), 73–91.

Leitao, S., & Fletcher, J. (2004). Literacy outcomes for students with speech impairment: Long-term follow-up. *International Journal of Language and Communication Disorders, 39*(2), 245–256.

Lewis, B. A., Freebairn, L. A., Hansen, A. J., Miscimarra, L., Iyengar, S. K., & Taylor, H. G. (2007). Speech and language skills of parents of children with speech sound disorders. *American Journal of Speech-Language Pathology, 16*, 108–118.

Maassen, B. (1986). Marking word boundaries to improve the intelligibility of the speech of the deaf. *Journal of Speech and Hearing Research, 29*, 227–230.

McCauley, R. J., & Strand, E. A. (2008). A review of standardized tests of nonverbal oral and speech motor performance in children. *American Journal of Speech-Language Pathology, 17*, 81–91.

McLeod, S., Harrison, L. J., & McCormack, J. (2012). The intelligibility in context scale: Validity and reliability of a subjective rating measure. *Journal of Speech Language and Hearing Research, 55*, 648–656.

Messner, A. H., & Lalakea, M. L. (2002). The effect of ankyloglossia on speech in children. *Otolaryngology- Head and Neck Surgery, 127*(6), 539–545.

Morrison, J. A., & Shriberg, L. D. (1992). Articulation testing versus conversational speech sampling. *Journal of Speech and Hearing Research, 35*, 259–273.

Osberger M. J., Robbins A. M., Todd S. L., & Riley A. I. (1994). *The Beginner's Intelligibility Test (BIT)*. Indianapolis, IN: Indiana University School of Medicine.

Paul, R., & Roth, F. P. (2011). Characterizing and predicting outcomes of communication delays in infants and toddlers: Implications for clinical practice. *Language, Speech and Hearing Services in Schools, 42*, 331–340.

Pearson, B. Z., Velleman, S. L., Bryant, T. J., & Charko, T. (2009). Phonological milestones for African American English-speaking children learning Mainstream American English as a second dialect. *Language, Speech, and Hearing Services in the Schools, 40*, 229–244.

Peña, E. D., & Bedore, L. M. (2011). It takes two: Improving assessment accuracy in bilingual children. *The ASHA Leader* (November).

Preston, J. L., Hull, M., & Edwards, M. L. (2013). Preschool speech error patterns predict articulation and phonological awareness outcomes in children with histories of speech sound disorders. *American Journal of Speech Language Pathology, 22*, 173–184.

Preston, J. L., & Seki, A. (2011). Identifying residual speech sound disorders in bilingual children: A Japanese-English case study. *American Journal of Speech-Language Pathology, 20*(2), 73–85.

Ray, J. (2002). Training phonological disorders in a multilingual child: A case study. *American Journal of Speech-Language Pathology, 11*, 305–315.

Rupela, V., & Manjula, R. (2010). Diadochokinetic assessment in persons with Down syndrome. *Asia Pacific Journal of Speech, Language, and Hearing, 13*(2), 109–120.

Rvachew, S., Ohberg, A., & Savage, R. (2006). Young children's responses to maximum performance tasks: Preliminary data and recommendations. *Journal of Speech-Language Pathology and Audiology, 30*(1), 6–13.

Schiavetti, N. (1992). Scaling procedures for the measurement of speech intelligibility. In R. D. Kent (Ed.), *Intelligibility in speech disorders* (pp. 11–34). Philadelphia, PA: John Benjamins.

Secord, W. A., & Shine, R. E. (1997). *Secord contextual articulation tests (S-CAT)*. Sedona, AZ: Red Rock Educational Publications.

Shriberg, L. D., Austin, D., Lewis, B. A., McSweeny, J. L., & Wilson, D. L. (1997a). The Percentage of Consonants Correct (PCC) metric: Extensions and reliability data. *Journal of Speech, Language, and Hearing Research*, 40(4), 708–722.

Shriberg, L. D., Austin, D., Lewis, B. A., McSweeny, J. L., & Wilson, D. L. (1997b). The Speech Disorders Classification System (SDCS): Extensions and lifespan reference data. *Journal of Speech, Language, and Hearing Research, 40*, 723–740.

Shriberg, L. D., & Kwiatkowski, J. (1980). *Natural process analysis: A procedure for phonological analysis of continuous speech samples*. Hoboken, New Jersey: John Wiley & Sons.

Shriberg, L. D., & Kwiatkowski, J. (1982). Phonological disorders I: A diagnostic classification system. *Journal of Speech and Hearing Disorders, 47*, 226–241.

Shriberg, L. D., Tomblin, J. B., & McSweeny, J. L. (1999). Prevalence of speech delay in 6-year-old children and comorbidity with language impairment. *Journal of Speech, Language, and Hearing Research, 41*(6), 1461–1481.

Stockman, I. J., Boult, J., & Robinson, G. C. (2008). Multicultural/multilingual instruction in educational programs: A survey of perceived faculty practices and outcomes. *American Journal of Speech Language Pathology, 17*, 241–264.

Stokes, S. F., & Surendran, D. (2005). Articulatory complexity, ambient frequency and functional load as predictors of consonant development. *Journal of Speech, Language and Hearing Research, 48*(3), 577–591.

Stow, C., and Dodd, B. (2005). A survey of bilingual children referred for investigation of communication disorders: A comparison with monolingual children referred in one area in England. *Journal of Multilingual Communication Disorders, 3*(1), 1–23.

Strand, E. A., McCauley, R. J., Weigand, S. D., Stoeckel, R. E., & Baas, B. S. (2013). A motor speech assessment for children with severe speech disorders: Reliability and validity evidence. *Journal of Speech, Language, and Hearing Research, 56*, 505–520.

Velleman, S. L., Andrianopoulos, M. V., Boucher, M., Perkins, J., Averback, K. E., Currier, A., … Van Emmerik, R. (2009). Motor speech disorders in children with autism. In R. Paul & P. Flipsen (Eds.), *Speech sound disorders in children: In honor of Lawrence D. Shriberg* (pp. 141–180). San Diego: Plural.

Velleman, S. L., & Mervis, C. B. (2011). Children with 7q11.23 Duplication syndrome: Speech, language, cognitive, and behavioral characteristics and their implications for intervention. *Perspectives on Language Learning and Education, 18*(3), 108–116.

Velleman, S. L., & Pearson, B. Z. (2010). Differentiating speech sound disorders from phonological dialect differences: Implications for assessment and intervention. *Topics in Language Disorders, 30*(3), 176–188.

Weston, A. D., & Shriberg, L. D. (1992). Contextual and linguistic correlates of intelligibility in children with developmental phonological disorders. *Journal of Speech and Hearing Research, 35*, 1316–1332.

Wilcox, K., & Morris, S. (1999). *Children's Speech Intelligibility Measure (CSIM)*. San Antonio, TX: Psychological Corporation.

Williams, P., & Stackhouse, J. (1998). Diadochokinetic skills: Normal and atypical performance in children aged 3–5 years. *International Journal of Language and Communication Disorders, 33*(suppl. 1), 481–486.

Williams, P., & Stackhouse, J. (2000). Rate, accuracy, and consistency: Diadochokinetic performance of young, normally developing children. *Clinical Linguistics & Phonetics, 14*(4), 267–293.

Yavas, M., & Goldstein, B. (1998). Phonological assessment and treatment of bilingual speakers. *American Journal of Speech-Language Pathology, 7*(2), 49–60.

Zelaznik, H. N., & Goffman, L. (2010). Generalized motor abilities and timing behavior in children with specific language impairment. *Journal of Speech, Language, and Hearing Research, 53*, 383–393.

CHAPTER 5

Basic Treatment Principles

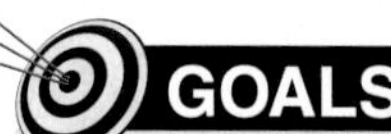

GOALS
of This Chapter

1. Compare/contrast primary features of motor intervention versus cognitive/linguistic intervention.
2. Describe key principles of motor intervention, including:
   a. stimulus and stimulus presentation choices
   b. response choices
   c. feedback choices
   d. achieving generalization
3. Describe key principles of cognitive-linguistic intervention, especially communicative efficacy.
4. Describe intervention strategies for children with sensory processing disorders or social deficits, for bilinguals, and for older children.

INTRODUCTION

The purpose of this chapter is to provide an overview of intervention principles that are applicable across a variety of speech sound deficits, clients, and settings. In the process of reviewing these principles, major perspectives on speech sound intervention will be reviewed. Detailed, step-by-step procedures will not be provided in this chapter; those will follow in the context of in-depth discussion of specific aspects and types of speech sound deficits in later chapters.

Selecting goals and strategies for intervention is a complex process that requires taking many factors into account. Goal development cannot be undertaken without a thorough assessment of all of the aspects of the child's oral motor, motor speech, phonetic, phonotactic, sound pattern, and prosodic strengths and weaknesses discussed in Chapters 3 and 4. Sensory, cognitive, and social variables are also critical, especially for determining age-appropriate, engaging strategies that will simultaneously challenge and be rewarding to the youngster. As treatment progresses, these factors will change due to maturation, intervention (speech-language and possibly other therapies), education, and possibly health differences over time. Both diagnostic therapy and thorough periodic re-evaluations are likely to be warranted depending on the severity and the progression of the child's difficulties.

Prior to consideration of any of these factors, however, it is necessary for the SLP to understand some basic facts and principles about speech sound intervention. These are presented below. Following that, we compare motoric versus cognitive–linguistic approaches to speech sound therapy. Along the way, many options for session design, stimulus selection, response requirements, and feedback types are discussed. Finally, considerations for special populations are presented.

DOES TREATMENT WORK?

Speech sound therapy (a.k.a. "articulation therapy") is the most frequent speech-language service provided to preschool children in the United States, representing 70% of such services. 92% of these preschoolers receive individual therapy—63% once a week and another 27% twice a week. About 41% of their sessions are 46 to 60 minutes long; 38% are 21 to 30 minutes (ASHA, 2011a).

The great news is that these services pay off; speech sound production therapy works (Broomfield & Dodd, 2005; Law, Garrett, & Nye, 2004; Nelson, Nygren, Walker, & Panoscha, 2006 as cited by Lancaster, Keusch, Levin, Pring, & Martin, 2010; Baker & McLeod, 2011a, 2011b). As of 2008, data from ASHA's National Outcomes Measurement System (NOMS) indicated that 70% of the preschool children for whom data were recorded benefited from phonological treatment, demonstrating increased intelligibility and enhanced communicative functioning. Half of those who had previously been unintelligible had become intelligible, even to strangers (Gierut, 2008).

A variety of different therapies have been shown to make a positive difference, at least for some children, when they are provided frequently enough. Approaches that have demonstrated benefits have included traditional articulatory therapy (Almost & Rosenbaum, 1998; Hesketh, Adams, Nightingale, & Hall, 2000); **minimal pairs therapy** (Almost & Rosenbaum, 1998); **Metaphon** (Dean, Howell, Waters, & Reid, 1995; Reid, Donaldson, Howell, Dean, & Grieve, 1996 as cited by Lancaster et al., 2010); **multiple oppositions therapy** (Allen, 2013); therapy provided by trained parents (Law et al., 2004); phonemic perception therapy (Rvachew, Nowak, & Cloutier, 2004; Rvachew, Ohberg, Grawburg, & Heyding, 2003); and phonological awareness training (Gillon, 2000, 2002; Hesketh et al., 2000; Major & Bernhardt, 1998). For children with Childhood Apraxia of Speech (CAS), three approaches have been documented to show promise: integral stimulation/**dynamic temporal and tactile cueing** (DTTC), **rapid syllable transition treatment**, and integrated phonological awareness intervention (Murray, McCabe, & Ballard, 2014). All of these approaches will be discussed in greater depth in later chapters.

A meta-analysis by Law and colleagues (2004) indicated that for children with SSDs, interventions focusing on expressive phonology are more effective than no therapy, especially when the treatment lasts more than eight weeks and is performed by a speech-language pathologist (as opposed to a trained parent). The effectiveness of receptive phonological therapy, such as auditory bombardment activities carried out by parents, was not confirmed by these researchers. It is important to note, however, that many of these studies—like most SLPs—actually included components of more than one treatment approach in their interventions. Such eclectic approaches also do work (Lancaster et al., 2010).

Many of these intervention strategies—or combinations of strategies—have been shown to work well with some children, but not with others (see Lancaster et al., 2010 for a review). For example, a morpho-syntactic approach may be more beneficial than a straight phonological approach for children with concomitant language deficits (Tyler, 2002). This is good news, in a sense; many approaches, including eclectic approaches, are successful. As stated by Baker and McLeod (2011a, 2011b), "at the moment, there are few studies that show that one intervention approach is unequivocally superior to another with a particular client group" (p. 115). This state of uncertainty places the burden on the SLP to keep up to date on the literature on evidence-based practice in speech sound disorders as well as to consider each child's profile carefully (including personality as well as other linguistic and cognitive skills) and to monitor progress, adjusting the treatment program as needed along the way.

Frequency of therapy is an important factor in treatment outcomes (Lancaster et al., 2010). Several reports support the truthfulness of the frequently used phrase "more is better:" more therapy results in better outcomes (Allen, 2013; ASHA, 2011a, 2011b; Gierut, 2008; Jacoby, Lee, Kummer, Levin, & Creaghead, 2002; Law et al., 2004). Furthermore, children receiving individual therapy for only phonology make more progress than do those receiving group therapy. The therapy setting (individual versus group) makes less difference for those with multiple areas of speech-language need. Completion of a home program in addition to direct therapy services increases the benefits even more (ASHA, 2011b).

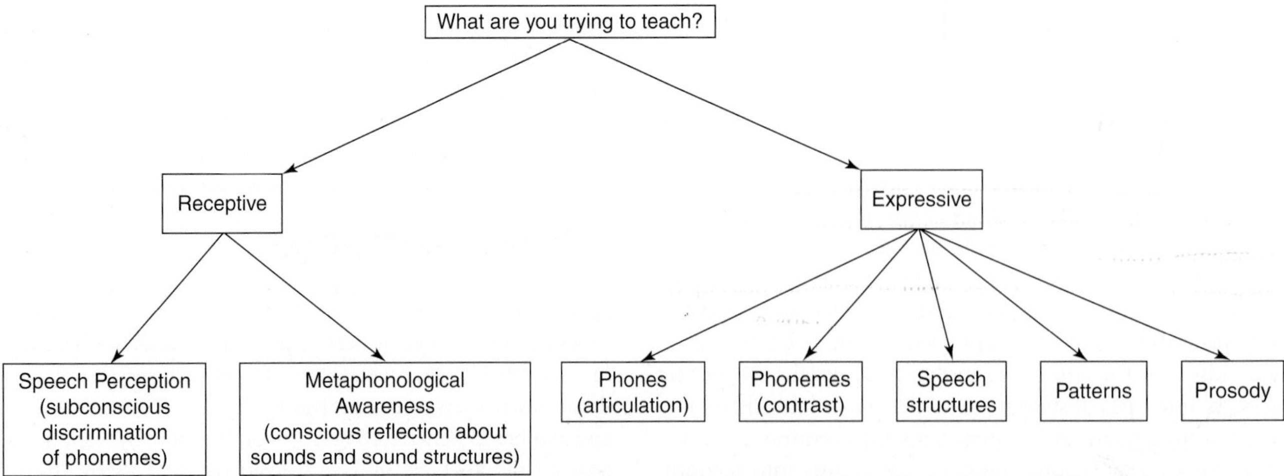

FIGURE 5-1. Primary intervention choices.

CORE TREATMENT CONCEPTS

In planning intervention, the most basic question is "What am I trying to teach?" (Stoel-Gammon, Stone-Goldman, & Glaspey, 2002). This question has many facets, including which aspect of the process is the focus. Is the immediate objective to improve the client's perception of sounds (e.g., the recognition that /p/ and /t/ are two different phonemes in English), the actual production of the sounds or sound patterns, metalinguistic awareness of sounds (e.g., the recognition that /p/ is the first sound in "pat"), some combination of these, or something else entirely? Some of these choices are indicated in Figure 5-1. Once these primary decisions have been made, I consider what phonological level/which phonological components I am targeting: sounds, features, sound classes, syllables, words, phrases, sentences, discourse? Or does the goal focus on articulatory gestures, such as the trajectory for producing a CVCV word that starts with a velar consonant and has a medial bilabial? Furthermore, what is the desired outcome? Is the SLP hoping to stimulate the phonological system, thereby triggering change? Is the goal increased intelligibility or articulatory accuracy—two distinct aims that are not always distinguished by practicing SLPs? These choices are depicted in Figure 5-2. They may reflect the clinician's underlying assumptions about phonological development and processing as well as about the challenges faced by the specific child in question.

Another way to word this most basic question is what does this child need to acquire? The answer to this question relies on abstract conceptual underpinnings, on sensory–motor structures and skills, and on the specific characteristics of the client in question. The resulting goals may include the child's development of such disparate abilities as:

- The motor skills to produce the sounds or structures, alone or in combination with others
- The ability to generate, store, and retrieve motor programs for producing sounds, syllables, and words
- The awareness that two sounds or two classes of sounds are different, that some words end with consonants, etc.
- The awareness of the (morpho-)phonological rules of the language (e.g., that word stress shifts when the morpheme "ity" is added to a word)

These are not necessarily mutually exclusive. For example, Saben and Ingham (1991) suggest that some children need a combination of a linguistic approach (such as therapy that focuses on the communicative value of distinguishing two phonemes from each other) and a more motoric approach focusing on imitation and cues about articulatory placement.

Where to begin? When considering therapy goals for a child with SSD, ease of production and ease of perception factors must be considered. Traditionally, those sounds, sound classes, and sound patterns that are generally easier for children to produce were addressed before targeting those that are articulatorily more difficult. This assumption has been called into question more recently, but research results have been inconsistent. As a result, there is ongoing disagreement in the field on this issue, as will be discussed further in Chapter 7.

> COMMON *Confusion*
>
> ### INTELLIGIBILITY VERSUS ACCURACY
>
> It is often assumed that accuracy is required for intelligibility. Of course, this is true at a basic level: if the listener cannot recognize the speaker's target words, then communication cannot occur. However, there are many ways to improve intelligibility when precision is not possible. For instance, some very young children are so inaccurate and inconsistent that they are not understood. For them, adult-like word pronunciations are not likely to be possible for some time. Therefore, more appropriate immediate goals include producing key words (**core vocabulary**) distinctly and consistently enough that the important people in the child's life will recognize those words as intended. Of course, because of implicit learning, *adults should always pronounce these target words correctly*, but they should also accept the child's best word approximations.
>
> Other examples are provided by older children with low muscle tone, such as those with Down syndrome, who often have been unable to completely eliminate distortions from their conversational speech despite many years of therapy. For them, goals may include the following:
>
> - Listener awareness, triggering repairs when necessary
> - Producing speech sounds distinctly (e.g., /s/ may be distorted but it sounds different from both /ʃ/ and /θ/)
> - Using prosodic patterns—such as pauses between grammatical phrases and emphasis on key words—that facilitate the listener's task
> - Slowing down their production of words that are either semantically important or phonologically challenging to make sure that they are understood
>
> In short, precision is not always required for intelligibility. The SLP must take the client's communication needs and capabilities into account when deciding upon the nature of the goals to write. All of these considerations and strategies will be discussed in more depth in later chapters.

Choosing goals based upon ease of production includes taking both the child's physiologic limitations (e.g., cleft palate, low tone) and his current phonological system (e.g., consonant and vowel repertoires and sound patterns) into account; both of these will impact how likely it is that the child will be able to produce the sound, syllable, or word accurately.

Furthermore, the phrase "ease of perception" has two interpretations, both of which must be considered. First of all, there is the question of which changes in the child's current phonological system are most likely to increase her intelligibility, thereby easing the *listener's* burden and improving the child's communicative effectiveness. However, the child's

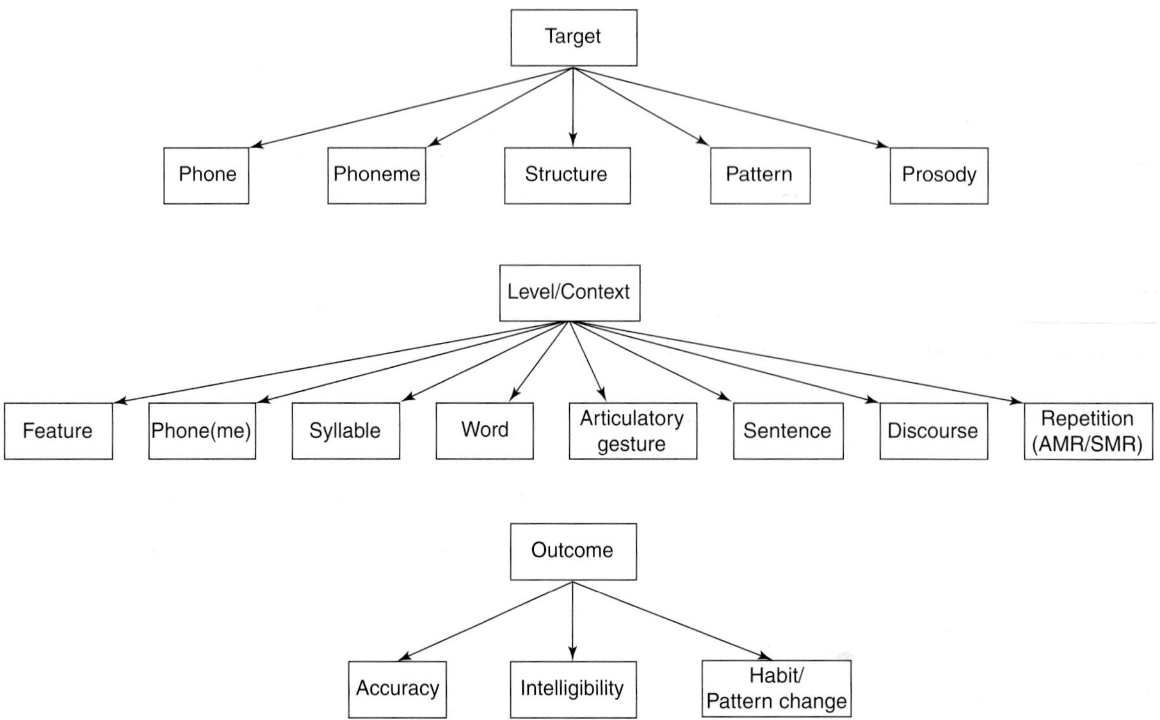

FIGURE 5-2. Production intervention choices.

perceptual system must not be forgotten either. An attempt must be made to determine those sounds and sound patterns that appear to be most perceptually salient to the child. Attempting to facilitate the child's learning of a contrast that the client is not aware of may (or may not, in the perspective of some scholars) be a waste of time. In these cases, one may target a pattern of which the child is aware but which is not yet produced in an adult-like manner instead. Or one may use discrimination training, which is intended to increase the child's awareness of a contrast that is not yet produced. These issues also will be discussed further in Chapter 7.

The first step of any intervention is to use the assessment results to write goals for the client. Those goals are statements about what we believe the child can achieve in a given length of time. But how can we know that our intervention has been successful? It is easy to focus on **performance**—the client's behavior during a given training session. However, performance is not clearly predictive of whether the new skill or information has actually been learned in a lasting way. Two other measures are more indicative of that. The first is **maintenance**, the **retention** of a skill or of some knowledge once the training session is over (e.g., as tested in a probe at the beginning of the next session). The second is **generalization**. Generalization refers to the transfer of learned knowledge or skills (i.e., the ability to use the learned skill in a new way or in a new context). Note that in terms from the Directions into Velocities of Articulators (DIVA) model (e.g., Guenther, 1995; Guenther, Ghosh, & Tourville, 2006; see Chapter 3), retention means the child has an appropriate motor program and can use it reliably to generate (or perhaps retrieve) the same successful motor plan, even after a delay. Generalization means that the motor program is general, abstract, and flexible enough to be applied to new sounds, structures, and/or contexts. This is the ultimate goal so that we don't have to teach the child to pronounce every word in the language in every communicative context. Traditionally, a symptom that was described as a hallmark of CAS was "lack of progress in therapy." This resulted from intervention strategies that only focused on developing motor programs or plans for individual words; children with CAS did not generalize, and therefore, their improvement was limited to the specific words or phrases that had been trained. We know better now.

As summarized by Miccio and Powell (2010), a learner may generalize in various ways:

- **Stimulus generalization** is the transfer of knowledge or skills from one set of stimulating conditions (e.g., labeling an object) to another (e.g., using the same word to label a picture or to request something outside of the therapy context).
- **Response generalization** is the transfer of knowledge or skills to a different output (e.g., from producing /s/ correctly in the word "bus" to producing it correctly in the word "glass").
- **Within-class generalization** is the transfer of learning from one item (e.g., /s/) to another item in the same category (e.g., another fricative, such as /ʃ/).
- **Across-class generalization** is the transfer of learning from an item in one class (e.g., a fricative) to an item in another class (e.g., an affricate).

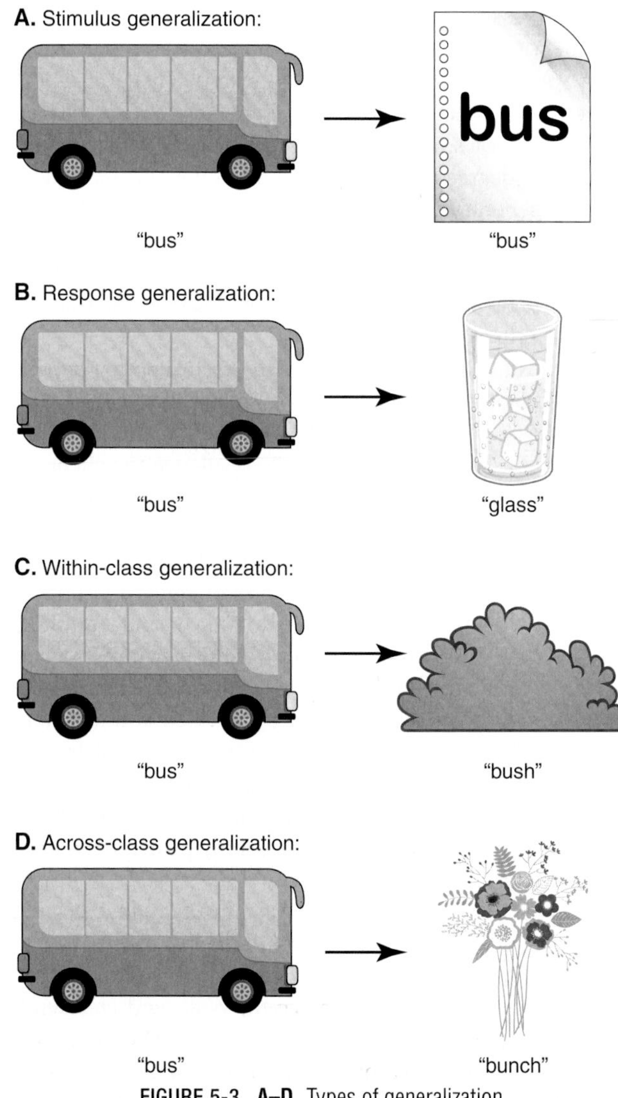

FIGURE 5-3. A–D. Types of generalization.

Note that within-class generalization and across-class generalization are types of response generalization. These are illustrated in Figure 5-3.

Of course, many factors will impact performance, maintenance, and generalization. These include many of the factors discussed in Chapter 3: physiologic, linguistic, cognitive, sensory, and social characteristics that enhance or interfere with the client's ability to benefit from intervention. Attention, motivation, and effort as well as stimulability and ability to self-monitor are key (Kwiatkowski & Shriberg, 1998). Choosing intervention targets and strategies that match the child's state of readiness and learning profile is one of the most crucial and difficult tasks facing the SLP (Guadagnoli & Lee, 2004). The primary choices one can make are between motoric intervention approaches and cognitive–linguistic approaches; of course, various combinations of these two are always options as well.

EXERCISE 5-1

Basic Treatment Principles

Motoric Intervention Approaches

don't help speech use w/ caution

Non-Speech Oral–Motor Exercises

A current controversy in our field relates to the use of non-speech oral–motor exercises (NSOME), such as activities used to train blowing, tongue clicking, chewing, and other articulatory movements that are not used for speech or not practiced in a speech context. However, studies of the motor and sensory demands of speech in comparison to other oral–motor activities have demonstrated that the coordinative organization, task demands, and sensory influences are different for tasks in these two categories (Wilson, Green, Yunusova & Moore, 2008). For example, the strength needed for these non-speech tasks is typically greater than that required for speech; in contrast, speech requires far more coordination and flexibility. Feeding patterns (sucking, chewing) are much more rhythmic than speech; in fact, the infant has to overcome the tendency for strict rhythmicity in order to produce more varied speech-like rhythms. Steeve, Moore, Green, Reilly, and McMurtrey (2008) have demonstrated that the muscle activation patterns for sucking, chewing, and speech are distinct from each other by 9 months of age, as most children are just entering the canonical babble stage. Specifically, speech relies upon co-contraction of **antagonist** (opposing) **muscle** groups; although they have opposite effects, they work together for this function. In contrast, the same antagonist muscle groups are activated in a reciprocal manner (i.e., one muscle is inhibited while the other is activated) for chewing. Other differences in muscle coordination patterns have been reported for the lips, tongue, facial muscles, and the levator veli palatini for speech versus non-speech tasks performed by children and/or adults. Furthermore, jaw motions for speech actually mature earlier than those for the adult-like rotary chew (Wilson et al., 2008). Additionally, neuroimaging studies show that different portions of the brain are activated for speech versus non-speech movements (Bunton, 2008). At this time, there is no appropriate research evidence to suggest that non-speech oral–motor activities will have any impact on speech production (McCauley, Strand, Lof, Schooling, & Frymark, 2009). Thus, *the current state of the literature indicates that non-speech oral–motor therapy will not improve speech production skills.* 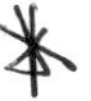

Some people have assumed that those who caution against reliance on non-speech motor treatment claim that motor speech deficits should not be directly addressed in intervention (Marshalla, 2008). This is not the case. As discussed shortly, principles of motor learning are relevant and appropriate to incorporate in therapy for motor speech disorders. The key difference is that motor speech therapy targets speech or movements that are directly related to speech.

For chronologically young or developmentally young children, as with other children with speech sound delay or disorders, to improve speech, you have to work on speech (Forrest, 2002; Forrest & Iuzzini, 2008).

For these reasons, the use of non-speech oral–motor activities should be extremely limited. Their use should be the exception, not the norm. If used at all, non-speech oral–motor activities should be used only for the following and *only if clearly appropriate to the individual client*:

- Increasing general imitation skills
- Increasing general sequencing skills
- Improving muscle tone
- Increasing awareness of oral structures
- Decreasing tactile defensiveness
- Improving non-speech functions (e.g., feeding skills)

It is not clear whether increasing imitation or sequencing skills in non-speech contexts will carry over to speech contexts or whether increasing awareness of oral structures or decreasing tactile defensiveness will have any impact on the success of speech therapy. Therefore, any such activities should be brief—a very small portion of the overall intervention session, if any—and should be carefully selected to specifically address one or more of the goals listed above.

Principles of Motor Learning

The fact that non-speech oral–motor exercises are not appropriate for remediating speech does not mean that motor speech therapy is not appropriate. If the child's speech sound disorder has a motoric component, then principles of motor learning are relevant as long as they are applied to speech tasks. Children's speech motor control is significantly associated with their intelligibility; thus, it is vital that it be addressed promptly and thoroughly (Namasivayam, Pukonen, Goshulak, Yu, Kadis, et al., 2013). In particular, many motor factors may impact the extent of generalization. Some motoric factors relate to the client; children who are stimulable for a sound (i.e., can produce it in some contexts with some degree of support such as tactile cues) are more likely to generalize. Others relate to the clinician: SLPs who use active learning techniques in which the child is more involved in the intervention activities achieve better results (Ertmer & Ertmer, 1998). Many others relate to the training task as discussed shortly.

The result of all of the choices the clinician has to make in designing a therapy activity is ensuring that that activity falls at the client's **challenge point** for that skill—that point at which the task is difficult enough to challenge the client for maximal learning but not difficult enough to be impossible or too discouraging to maintain motivation. At the right level of difficulty, the client understands the task and knows how to approach it given certain cues or other appropriate supports. Careful planning (feedforward) and monitoring (internal feedback) are required, thus providing a good learning opportunity. External feedback—of an appropriate type for that client at that time—is provided at a level and a rate at which the client can process it and benefit from it (Guadagnoli & Lee, 2004). This balance between too hard to achieve and too easy to benefit is difficult to reach, but it should always be our goal. Motor learning principles help us to think through how to get there.

Principles of motor learning have been studied at great length as they apply to non-speech tasks but only to a limited extent with respect to speech. As summarized by Maas, Robin, Austermann Hula, Freedman, Wulf, and colleagues (2008), there are three main considerations: (1) **prepractice**, (2) **practice conditions**, and (3) **feedback conditions**.

Prepractice refers to preparing the child for the speech-learning task. This includes explaining the task clearly (what will happen, and what is the child expected to do?), directing the child's attention to the process and materials to be used, and motivating the client to do it. The latter includes selecting goals and **exemplars** (word or phrase targets) about which the client cares.

Practice conditions include practice amount, distribution, variability, and schedule. Studies indicate that more practice is better than less: 100 trials are not too much for one 15-minute therapy block, and the results are better with that many (Edeal & Gildersleeve-Neumann, 2011). However, there are some indications that the benefits of such intensive practice depend also on the number of different targets that are practiced within the session. If the same target is practiced too many times in a row in exactly the same context, the long-term benefits are significantly reduced. This most likely results from the fact that the same motor plan is being used over and over rather than retrieving a variety of motor programs and generating a variety of motor plans, learning from the results

> **Common MISCONCEPTION**
>
> The fact that non-speech oral–motor exercises do not improve speech does *not* imply that oral mechanism examinations should be eliminated. *A thorough oral mechanism examination is vital for any child with a suspected speech delay or disorder* for the following reasons:
>
> 1. An oral mechanism exam may reveal the cause of a speech delay or disorder.
> 2. Both physiologically based and non-physiologically based speech delays or disorders should be treated with *speech* therapy (not NSOMEs). However, the nature of the speech therapy may differ if there is a physiologic basis for the problem.
> 3. An oral mechanism examination may reveal a physiologic symptom that requires medical assessment or intervention, such as a tremor that may suggest a neurologic condition.

to refine both the motor programs and the motor plan generation processes (Maas et al., 2008). This massed practice of only one or very few exemplars was the traditional—far less successful—approach to treating children with CAS.

Thus, amount of practice interacts with distribution—the amount of practice of a given target within a given amount of time. One distribution option is **massed practice**—many training sessions or many trials of the same target many times in a short amount of time. With respect to sessions, this could mean that therapy would be provided intensively for a short length of time (e.g., three 1-hour sessions per week for four weeks). With respect to trials, this could mean that each therapy session is devoted to only one target (e.g., an entire hour devoted to producing /s/ in final position). The other distribution option is **distributed practice**—training sessions or trials of a particular target spread out over a longer time period. This could be achieved either by having training sessions more spread out (e.g., one session a week for 16 weeks) or by focusing on more than one target per session (so that the child receives, for example, an hour of work on target A per week by working on it for 20 minutes three times a week instead of for a full hour once a week) (Maas et al., 2008).

The level of variability is another choice that must be made. Will the same target be practiced in the same context (e.g., /s/ in final position of one-syllable words) throughout the entire session in a **constant practice** format? Or will the target or the context be varied (e.g., a variety of fricatives in final position or /s/ in a variety of positions) in a **variable practice** format? Further choices include the presentation of targets within the session: either all trials of a given target are practiced together before moving on to the next target in **blocked practice** or trials of various targets are intermixed in **random practice** (Maas et al., 2008). These two sets of distinctions are exemplified in Table 5-1.

Although research applying these concepts to speech has been limited, studies of non-speech motor learning suggest that the benefits of these options depend in part on the learner's ability level. The client's challenge point will vary depending on her familiarity and experience with the task. More intensive practice—massed, blocked practice—generally appears to be useful for beginning to learn a new skill. However, distributed, randomized practice actually facilitates retention and transfer of new motor skills in the long run (Maas et al., 2008; Schmidt & Lee, 2005). Studies of speech therapy for adults with Apraxia of Speech have confirmed that although randomized practice may yield less impressive immediate results, learning is better overall under this condition (Kim, LaPointe, & Stierwalt, 2012), perhaps because it encourages the learner to create more general, flexible motor programs and to practice using them to generate and evaluate the success of a greater variety of motor plans. However, one study comparing random versus blocked practice in children with CAS yielded mixed inconclusive results (Maas & Farinella, 2012). Many treatment approaches incorporate a variety of practice conditions, depending upon the client's profile (Dale & Hayden, 2013).

Another aspect of variability in practice relates to how many exemplars (target words within a given pattern) are targeted at once. There are three primary choices: **training broad** (the horizontal approach), in which many varied exemplars within a broad category (e.g., many different words with various fricatives in final position) are trained to criterion; **training narrow** (the deep or vertical approach), in which massed practice is provided on a few exemplars (e.g., a few similar words with word-final /s/) that are trained to criterion (Elbert & Gierut, 1986; Williams, 2000); and **cycles**, in which a small set of exemplars is trained for a certain period of time (e.g., two to three months), then the goal is shifted regardless of the amount of progress the child has achieved. Training broad is a type of distributed variable practice, which some say is more advantageous; a larger, more varied set of exemplars leads to better generalization in the long run (Strand, 2004; Strand & Skinder, 1999). Other authors say that there is no evidence as of yet as to which of these is more facilitatory of speech motor learning (Maas et al., 2008).

The rationale for the cycles approach is that it could stimulate the entire phonological system and that gradual change on shifting goals is more like the speech sound development of typically developing children. Cycling goals results

TABLE 5-1 Types of Practice

Type of Practice		Session Portion		
Constant vs. Variable Stimuli	**Blocked vs. Random Trials**	**1**	**2**	**3**
Constant	Blocked	*A* × 100	*B* × 100	*C* × 100
Constant	Random		ABACCBCAABBCACBBBABC...	
Variable	Blocked	a1,a2,a3...	b1,b2,b3...	c1,c2,c3...
Variable	Random		b1,c3,a2,a1,b2,c2,c1,a3,b3,b2,a1,c1...	

Key: *A* = /k/ in "cow;" *B* = /st/ in "stick;" *C* = /ɹ/ in "Mary."
a1, a2, a3, etc. = /k/ in a variety of positions, word shapes, words (e.g., "cow, back, buckle, Christmas...")
b1, b2, b3, etc. = /st/ in a variety of positions, word shapes, words (e.g., "stick, misty, best, gesticulate...")
c1, c2, c3, etc. = /ɹ/ in a variety of positions, word shapes, words (e.g., "Mary, rope, butter, careen, crime...")

in work on each goal being spread out over a longer period of time, which is another type of distributed practice. Thus, in a sense, this is a combination of short periods of massed practice on just a few exemplars in the larger context of distributed practice of varied goals (Hodson, 2006; Hodson, Scherz, & Strattman, 2002). This model has not yet been subjected to controlled experimental scrutiny.

As noted above, there is some debate in the field as to whether more generalization results from targeting more complex goals or simpler goals. Those studies that have shown advantages to addressing more complex targets (e.g., Gierut, 2001; Morrisette & Gierut, 2002) have typically been single-subject studies, but there have been several of them. Studies showing that it is better to address simpler goals have been more rigorous and have had larger sample sizes (e.g., Rvachew & Bernhardt, 2010; Rvachew & Nowak, 2001). In a compromise approach, Skelton (2004) and Skelton and Funk (2004) have demonstrated that therapy that mixes easier with more challenging tasks (e.g., production of the target sound in a single syllable versus in a word versus in a short phrase) yields good generalization to untaught exemplars.

In summary, a great deal of research remains to be done on practice conditions for speech learning. However, preliminary findings suggest that from a motor point of view, the ideal therapy session provides a well-prepared motivated client with a great deal of practice on several exemplars, focusing on more than one goal.

Feedback conditions are the final major piece of the puzzle, according to Maas and team (2008). **Reinforcement** can be provided either on a **continuous** schedule (100%) or a **variable** schedule (less frequently, less predictably). There is some reason to believe that systematic blocked feedback is most helpful for a brand new task (Guadagnoli & Lee, 2004), while less frequent more variable reinforcement leads to better generalization in the later stages of learning because it encourages the client to self-evaluate when external feedback is not provided (Strand, 2004). Self-monitoring is important (Koegel, Koegel, & Ingham, 1986 as cited by Ertmer & Ertmer, 1998; Miccio & Powell, 2010; Shriberg & Kwiatkowski, 1990) because this involves training the internal feedback system to monitor output and respond efficiently and effectively. The successes and failures of various motor plans lead to further refinement of general, abstract motor programs and of the process of generating future motor plans to fit the relevant physiologic, linguistic, and social contexts.

In addition to frequencies of feedback, there are also different types of feedback to choose among. These range from motoric, to linguistic, to social. The child's attention may be drawn either to internal factors (such as the articulators) or external factors (such as the sounds produced or whether or not the listener understood the speech). Thus, one may provide **knowledge of performance**, the most internal, motoric type of feedback; did the client perform the articulatory gesture correctly (e.g., was the tongue tip raised to the alveolar ridge?). Studies of non-speech motor learning suggest that this is helpful but that retention of the skills is better if performance feedback is not provided 100% of the time; 33% feedback on performance may yield better long-term outcomes (Kordus & Weeks, 1998). Alternatively, one may provide **knowledge of results**, which is a more linguistic, external form of feedback: Was the production right? In other words, was the attempt successful? This type of feedback may focus on articulatory accuracy (did it sound like [tʃ]?) or communicative effectiveness (did the listener recognize the target word, understand the message, etc.?). Here, too, more is not necessarily better; the client may retain the skills longer if this type of feedback is given randomly and less often (Guadagnoli & Lee, 2004). Of these two types, knowledge of results appears to yield better retention of new skills than knowledge of performance (Young & Schmidt, 1992 as cited by Kim et al., 2012). Alternatively, one may reinforce the effort only, providing social affirmation, as most SLPs do during standardized testing (e.g., "You're working so hard").

Finally, feedback can be immediate or delayed (typically five seconds or so); **delayed feedback** may be more beneficial (Maas et al., 2008), especially once the person has developed some level of skill. The delay provides time for self-evaluation (which, as noted above, is more likely to yield positive changes in motor programming and motor planning skills).

These motor learning principles and the preliminary information we have about when they are best applied are summarized in Table 5-2.

A further variable is whether or not an **error-free learning** approach is used, in which only goals for which the child is stimulable (can sometimes produce the sound or structure accurately) are selected for maximal success and minimal challenge. The cycles approach emphasizes error-free learning so that the child does not practice mistakes (Hodson, 2006; Hodson et al., 2002). On the other hand, one may learn from one's errors; they provide as much information to the motor programming/planning system as the successes do (Maas et al., 2008). Clearly, a balance must be struck between the frustration and the learning that may result from errors.

Additional Considerations

In addition to the above principles of motor learning, there are several other conditions that need to be taken into account when planning any motor intervention activities. The first of these is the child's pre-existing motor programs, including reflexes and any habitual speech or non-speech patterns that may interfere with the target pattern. The rapidity, duration, and modalities of both the stimuli and the expected response can also have significant effects on performance, especially from a trade-off point of view; a rapid response may be far less accurate and vice versa.

A hierarchy of cueing is available for the clinician's selection. For example, the stimulus may be modeled—for immediate imitation, for delayed imitation, or for those who

TABLE 5-2 **Applicability of Motor Learning Principles**

Parameter	Initial Learning Stages	Later Learning Stages
Amount of practice	High	High
Distribution of practice	More concentrated	More distributed
Variability, scheduling	Massed, blocked practice	Varied, random practice
Number of exemplars	Training narrow (fewer)	Training broad (more)
Feedback schedule	More frequent	Less frequent
Feedback type	Knowledge of performance (e.g., articulatory accuracy)	Knowledge of results (e.g., communicative success)
Level of challenge	Low (decrease frustration)	Higher (learn from errors)
Amount of cueing	More	Less

cannot imitate, simultaneously (concurrent with the child's production) (Strand & Debertine, 2000; Strand & Skinder, 1999; Strand, Stoeckel, & Baas, 2006). Cues may be auditory (a question or some other form of elicitation, or a model), visual (a sign, a gesture, an object, a picture, or a written word), tactile, or some combination of these. These options are depicted in Figure 5-4.

Over time, the more supportive cues are gradually withdrawn, giving the child increasing responsibility for retrieving, planning, and producing the target. These cueing strategies have been systematized within Strand's integral stimulation and DTTC approaches (Strand & Debertine, 2000; Strand & Skinder, 1999; Strand et al., 2006), as shown in Figure 5-5.

Similar choices are available with respect to the nature of the desired response: the expected rapidity of the response (e.g., immediate versus delayed imitation) and the duration of the response (for how long or how many times should the child produce the target?) should be made clear to the client in advance. In addition, there are many modalities that the child could use to respond. The two primary choices are oral (imitation or elicited) and gestural. Potential gestural responses include pointing to the correct picture or object, signing or using a meaningful gesture, writing or drawing a picture, and performing a tactile cue on herself, on the SLP, or in the air near her own or the SLP's face.

For some children, the use of multiple modalities (e.g., signing or gesturing while speaking) may facilitate production of the target; for others, the need to activate several systems in order to produce more than one type of cue may exacerbate motor planning or execution problems. From an input perspective, the same is true: multi-modal input

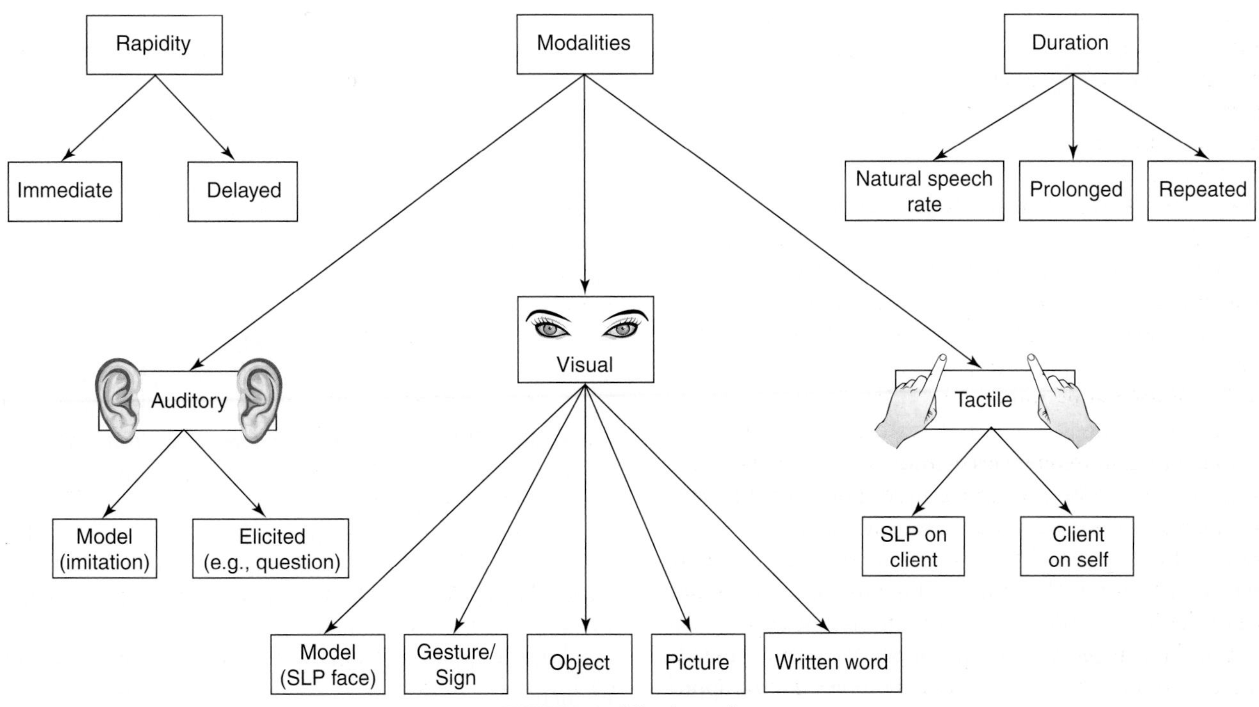

FIGURE 5-4. Stimulus options.

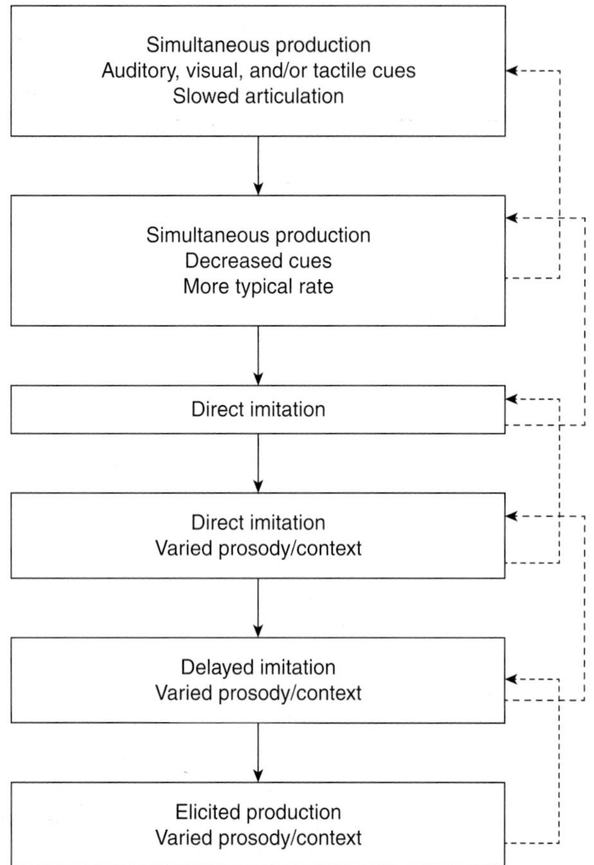

FIGURE 5-5. Dynamic tactile and temporal cueing. Based upon Strand and Skinder (1999); Strand and Debertine (2000); Strand, Stoeckel, and Baas (2006).

COMMON *Confusion*

It is the clinician who *models* the target production as an example for the client to imitate. Similarly, the SLP *elicits* the production from the child, using whatever means are appropriate or necessary to cause him or her to produce the desired target.

The client neither models nor elicits the target; she or he produces it.

is often but not always helpful; children may respond quite differently to auditory, visual, tactile, or multi-modal inputs. A comprehensive system of dynamic tactile cues, known as the **PROMPT** approach (Hayden, 2006; Hayden & Square, 1994), appears to be helpful for children with CAS in particular (Dale & Hayden, 2013). Recall that the amount and the intensity of the stimulus also matter; a balance must be struck between the level of input that stimulates the appropriate response and the level that may overload the system (Guadagnoli & Lee, 2004).

Summary

In short, many varied factors will determine the challenge point (i.e., the conditions under which the client can learn a maximal amount without being so challenged that his system is overwhelmed). These include internal factors, such as stimulability, attention, and motivation; task factors, such as practice amount, distribution, variability, and schedule, as well as supports provided (e.g., auditory, visual, or tactile cues); and feedback factors, such as the frequency and nature of the feedback.

EXERCISE 5-2

Motor-Based Approaches

Cognitive–Linguistic Approaches

The goal of a cognitive–linguistic approach is to change the child's phonological system, typically by adding or expanding classes of phonemes or by making the child aware of language-appropriate phonological patterns. The assumption of these approaches is that the problem is not motoric—relating neither to motor programming/planning deficits (as in CAS) nor to motor execution difficulty (as in dysarthria). Rather, the client's knowledge of the sound system of the language to which she has been exposed is assumed to be incomplete or incorrect. This may be due to faulty phonological acquisition (from the ***nativist*** point of view, in which linguistic knowledge is presumed to be innately given with the learner's task being to select which of many linguistic options a given language represents) or to faulty learning (from a *social-cognitivist* point of view). From either perspective, the child may not have the proper underlying representations for words. In this case, minimal pairs therapy and variations on this approach are likely to be used, as described in Chapter 7 (Phones and Phonemes). Alternatively, she may be using incorrect patterns for realizing (i.e., producing) those words, in which case, process therapy is typically used, as described in Chapter 9 (Patterns).

Regardless of one's theory of phonological development, generalization from one task, one stimulus, one target, one listener to others is a primary goal in all types of intervention for clients of any age. The likelihood of transfer occurring is not limited to only motoric factors. Children who demonstrate that they have some **phonological knowledge** of a sound, a structure, or a pattern are more likely to learn quickly than those who do not. For example, a child who omits final nasals but nasalizes the vowel before the target nasal is thus indicating some awareness that there should be a nasal consonant there or at least that there is nasality in the word, and so he is more likely to learn to produce the nasal consonant correctly (Elbert & Gierut, 1986; Gierut, Elbert, & Dinnsen, 1987). A child who consistently substitutes [f] for /θ/ may not be aware that these two phonemes are different, while one who produces /θ/ in a variety of ways is showing that he is aware that this is a separate phoneme, even though he has not yet figured out how to pronounce it (Velleman, 1988). Phonological knowledge on the part of the clinician is also important; according to Bernhardt

(2004), SLPs with undergraduate degrees in linguistics achieve better results (specifically, their clients make faster progress in word structure development). It is not possible to go into extensive detail about these issues without further discussion about typical and atypical child phonological systems, which will be discussed in far greater depth in Chapters 7 (Phones and Phonemes) and 9 (Patterns).

The cognitive aspects of generalization represent a critical issue for children with global learning deficits. Therefore, it is even more important with this population to diversify therapy stimuli, conditions, and targets with a focus on functionality—responding within the classroom, at home, and on the playground to teachers, family members, and peers alike for a variety of communicative functions. A naturalistic therapy context will encourage generalization to "real life" (Camarata, 1993; Skelton, 2004; Tyler & Lewis, 2005). On the other hand, too many variables may dilute the learning to an inappropriate extent: it must be clear to the client what is expected and when and where those expectations apply.

Attention and memory are additional important considerations (Kwiatkowski & Shriberg, 1998). Implicit/procedural learning is responsible for much of language acquisition in typically developing children. Those with deficits in these areas, such as children with SLI or ASDs, may need more targeted stimulation. This can be provided by modeling phonological elements or structures in an intense, focused manner such that the child is bombarded with many exemplars of the same principle and/or by providing more explicit teaching than usually occurs in the natural course of communication. These are exactly the types of strategies that are typically used in speech-language intervention.

Additional Intervention Considerations

Regardless of whether a more motoric approach or a more cognitive–linguistic approach is used, the SLP must ask how learning works for the individual child in question. First, will learning take place in a bottom–up or a top–down manner? Bottom–up learning involves focusing on the details (e.g., the production of a particular sound) in order to generalize to broader categories (e.g., other sounds within the same category such as other fricatives or other palatals) (Miccio & Ingrisano, 2000). Top–down learning is the reverse: one begins with broader categories (e.g., a whole sound class) or a broader goal (e.g., differentiating two classes of sounds—such as fricatives versus stops—so that they are recognizable to a listener, regardless of whether they are articulatorily accurate). Research suggests that the latter is better; one can learn more efficiently if the focus is on broader patterns (Miccio & Powell, 2010). As we have seen, a more recent debate concerns the appropriateness of building upon that which is already known (e.g., Rvachew & Bernhardt, 2010; Rvachew & Nowak, 2001) versus challenging the system by focusing therapy on unknown elements or categories (Gierut, 2001, 2007). This issue will be discussed in greater depth in Chapter 7.

Another factor that will have to be decided is word position: Will the phoneme be targeted in initial, medial, or final position? If it is a consonant, will the initial focus be on singleton productions or clusters? Do more specific factors related to adjacent segments need to be considered, like the other consonants in the cluster? Adjacent vowels? (Bates, Watson, & Scobbie, 2002). For instance, production of [s] may be facilitated by an adjacent alveolar within a cluster (e.g., st- or -ns) (Swisher, 1973 cited by Kent, 1982). Children may be more likely to produce a final consonant if the preceding vowel is lax (Demuth, Culbertson, & Alter, 2006; Kehoe & Stoel-Gammon, 2001) or if the onset + vowel sequence that precedes it is a more common combination in the ambient language (Zamuner, Gerken, & Hammond, 2004).

The selection of target level is also important: Will it be a syllable, a word, a phrase, a sentence, a conversation? The elicitation of single consonants (e.g., "Say [p]") is not recommended as it provides neither a functional outcome (unless it's a consonant that has meaning in and of itself, such as "shhh" or "mmmm") nor production practice within a speech-like context. Speaking requires the production of series of consonants and vowels, with the proper formant transitions and other coarticulatory gestures between them. Even baby birds learning to sing have to practice the transitions between elements, not the single elements themselves (Marcus, 2013). Furthermore, most SLPs who try to elicit single consonants actually model syllables anyway (e.g., "Say [pʌ]").

Another consideration is how phonetically and semantically complex the target will be. For example, will it be a real word or a nonsense word? Real words are typically viewed as being preferable for children with limited vocabularies; it seems a waste to devote their time to producing a nonfunctional utterance. However, older children with well-ingrained habits may benefit from practicing new sounds and structures in nonsense words (Gierut, Morrisette, & Ziemer, 2010). If the target is a phrase, sentence, or conversation, what is the appropriate level of phonetic, semantic, grammatical, and discourse complexity? The answer to this question depends upon many factors relating to the client's physiologic, linguistic, and social strengths and weaknesses as well as the purpose of the task. It may not always be obvious. Whether it is easy to answer or not, it is vital that this question always be asked—in other words, that the complexity levels be consciously considered, selected, and evaluated.

The format of speech sound therapy depends largely upon the child's chronologic or mental age and level of motivation. For young children, especially those with concurrent language deficits, **play therapy**, in which the activity is flexible and child-centered and the SLP maximizes opportunities to model, elicit, and reinforce speech and language production together, is often most appropriate (Tyler, 2002). For older children, **drill play**, in which some game—typically a board game—is modified such that the child must demonstrate a particular behavior (e.g., produce a certain word) in order to be allowed to take another turn, is one option. **Drill**, in

Common MISCONCEPTION

Goals of the form, "The client will produce /x/ with 90% accuracy" are popular, but they are often inappropriate. There are many other choices, as illustrated by the following examples:

- The client will produce /s/ as distinct from [ʃ] 90% of the time.
- The client will produce liquids in appropriate words five times per session.
- The client will identify the phoneme in the word the SLP produced (/p/ versus /b/) 90% of the time.
- The client will produce high vowels as such regardless of front-back accuracy 90% of the time.
- The client will produce consonant voicing (voiced or voiceless) appropriately 90% of the time regardless of accuracy of place or manner of articulation.
- The client will produce a final consonant when appropriate (i.e., when the target word ends with a final consonant) 90% of the time regardless of articulatory accuracy.
- The client will produce two consonants in a row when target-appropriate 90% of the time regardless of articulatory accuracy.

Of course, many other details would be included in such goals, such as word position, the nature of the stimulus (e.g., "in response to a picture prompt"), the nature of the task (e.g., "by pointing," "in a carrier phrase"), and the type of support that will be provided (e.g., "with tactile and gestural cues").

which the child is explicitly asked to repeatedly perform the target behavior out of context and explicit reinforcement is typically provided verbally ("Good job!") and/or in the form of some tangible reward (sticker, token, etc.), is another.

Therapy scheduling is the source of ethical dilemmas for many SLPs; they want to provide as much therapy as the child needs but their schedules are full. Three aspects of scheduling must be considered: **frequency**—number of sessions per week; **duration**—number of minutes per session; and **intensity**—individual versus group sessions and number of repetitions of the target per session (which is clearly related to the issue of session format). As noted above, the amount of therapy that is provided directly relates to the amount of progress that is made in children with SSDs—generally, more is better (ASHA, 2011a, 2011b; Gierut, 2008; Jacoby et al., 2002; Law et al., 2004). Frequency also matters; children who receive 24 sessions of multiple opposition therapy over eight weeks (i.e., three times a week) make more progress than those who receive 24 sessions of the same therapy over 24 weeks (i.e., once a week) (Allen, 2013).

Many other client-specific questions also arise. Kwiatkowski and Shriberg (1998) stress the importance of maintaining the child's attention, motivation, and effort. They also emphasize that cognitive–linguistic constraints (such as intellectual functioning level and language level) and psychosocial constraints (such as social anxiety) cannot be ignored if the client is to be an active, engaged learner. Linguistic considerations include the language or languages to which the child has been and is being exposed; intervention for bilingual children is discussed in more depth below.

Strategies for Children with Sensory Processing Disorders

Children with hyposensitivity or hypersensitivity present special challenges for the SLP; the sensory environment can have significant impacts on their ability to attend and to learn. Neither a child who is falling asleep nor one who is in a hypervigilant state of anxiety will be able to benefit from intervention. Whenever possible, the wisest course is to collaborate with an occupational therapist who specializes in this area—either via co-therapy or consultation. Sensory integration therapy may improve attention in children with these types of disorders (Miller, Coll, & Schoen, 2007). If an OT is not available to provide guidance, some general rules of thumb are to provide less stimulating, calming, predictable input to the hypersensitive—for example, constant deep pressure, cool colors, low lights, and rhythmic sounds (Hayden-Sloane, *personal communication*, 1999). Introduce new stimuli gradually, having forewarned the child in advance of what is about to happen (http://www.sensory-processing-disorder.com/treatment-guidelines.html). In contrast, more stimulating input will "wake up" the sensory systems of those who are hyposensitive: quick, light touch; bright, shiny colors; and varied sounds (Hayden-Sloane, *personal communication*, 1999). These recommendations are summarized in Table 5-3.

Strategies for Children with Social Deficits

For children with social deficits, communicative motivation is critical for progress to occur and is also extremely challenging. However, every child has something that he wants to communicate, even if it is simply rejection of certain stimuli. Opportunity is another vital component; such children may

TABLE 5-3 Stimuli for Children with Sensory Modulation Disorders

Sense	Hypersensitive	Hyposensitive
Tactile	Constant touch (e.g., wrap, hug) Slow, even, rhythmic touch or rub	Quick, short, irregular, light touch
Gustatory (taste)	Sweet	Bitter, sour, salty; cold
Visual	Cool colors, low lights, large objects	Bright shiny colors for objects of interest
Auditory	Rhythmic; even tone, loudness, pitch; predictable/predictive	Intermittent, changing, varied

Adapted from Hayden-Sloane, *personal communication*, 1999.

initially communicate in unconventional ways (e.g., via idiosyncratic gestures or vocalizations or via echolalia) that may not be recognized as communicative at first. Responsiveness to these communications can lay the foundation for teaching more conventional communication strategies (Zubow & Hurtig, 2014). Basic non-speech skills, such as attention and imitation, may need to be addressed before speech can be usefully targeted.

Facilitating communicative connections is critical; interventions designed to increase communication during the prelinguistic stage result in better linguistic outcomes (Brady, Steeples & Fleming, 2005; Girolametto, Pearce, & Weitzman, 1997; Girolametto, Weitzman & Clements-Baartman, 1998; Norris & Hoffman, 1990). This includes the use of non-vocal communicative means. Many people fear that making sign language, picture exchange communication symbols (PECS), or other alternative systems available to a delayed child will decrease his oral output. In fact, the reverse has been the case in the vast majority of studies. In a recent meta-analysis of the literature on this topic, for example, Millar, Light, and Schlosser (2006) reported that "None of the 27 cases [that met the standards for evidence-based practice] demonstrated decreases in speech production as a result of AAC intervention, 11% showed no change, and the majority (89%) demonstrated gains in speech" (p. 248). With the advent of the iPad and similar devices, it has become even cheaper and easier to design electronic systems. Thus, it is neither necessary nor appropriate to choose between oral and non-oral communication as goals, although in many cases, one will serve only as a supplement to the other.

The fact that increases in communicative intent in other modalities result in increases in vocal communication underscores the importance of assessing and treating motive and opportunity as well as means; they are highly interactive and interdependent. (See Chapter 6 and also materials provided by the Hanen Center at hanen.org as well as Davis and Velleman [2008] for further intervention suggestions for children who lack communicative intent.)

Intervention for Children Learning More Than One Language

Intervention for children who are learning two languages (or more) should ideally take place in both languages—though not necessarily simultaneously—and be provided by a bilingual SLP. How evident the child's phonological deficits are in each language, the relative impact of the SSD on communication function in each, how frequently the child uses each, how long he has been speaking each of them, how proficient he is in other aspects (e.g., grammar) of each one, where and with whom he uses each language, and the family's goals for the child are all factors that should be taken into account when deciding whether one language will be the focus of intervention before the other and if so, which one (Goldstein & Fabiano-Smith, 2007).

Selecting the most efficacious goals for bilingual children depends, as always, upon having completed thorough, appropriate assessments—again, ideally in both languages. Naturally, error patterns that represent a delay or disorder in the given languages should be the targets; age-appropriate language-appropriate immaturities are not useful foci of intervention. There is some evidence that phonological therapy provided in one of a child's languages will result in some generalization to the other language(s) (Fabiano-Smith & Goldstein, 2010; Goldstein & Fabiano-Smith, 2007; Ray, 2002). If this is the case, then treating error patterns that impact both languages may result in the greatest levels of generalization and the most improvement in the child's overall communication function. However, the likelihood of this type of generalization may depend on the nature of the deficit (i.e., motoric/articulatory generalization may be more likely than linguistic generalization). In some cases, the benefits may be broad (e.g., an overall improvement in intelligibility in both languages) rather than specific (e.g., an improvement in the production of a particular sound in both languages) (Barlow & Enriquez, 2007). In addition, a child's strengths in one language may carry over to remediate weaknesses in the other. For example, English-Mandarin children's ability to produce the Mandarin (non-round) /r/ can help them to master the production of the English (round) /ɹ/ (Lin & Johnson, 2010).

Yavas and Goldstein (1998) suggest that one should first "treat phonological patterns that are exhibited with similar error rates" (p. 57) in both languages. These are typically the patterns with the most impact on intelligibility, such as unstressed syllable deletion. In identifying such deficits, one must ensure that the error pattern chosen has similar implications in the two languages. For example, final consonant deletion has a considerable impact on communicative efficacy in English because most words end with consonants. However, in languages such as Vietnamese, there are so few final consonants that this goal is not appropriate. Similarly, weak syllable deletion is important in languages with many multisyllabic words. Some languages (such as Kannada, per Rupela & Manjula, 2006) are highly multisyllabic and actually have almost no one-syllable words; some others (such as Khmer, per Cheng, 1993) have very few polysyllabic words; English falls in between. These language-specific tendencies must be taken into account (Yavas & Goldstein, 1998).

The second priority for goal selection for bilingual children, per Yavas and Goldstein (1998), is error patterns that impact both languages but with different frequency levels and different implications for intelligibility in the two (or more) languages. The lowest priority goals are those error patterns that impact only one language.

Finally, it is important to remember the communication functions of speech. Kohnert, Yim, Nett, Kan, and Duran (2005) emphasize the utility of using a social–cognitive functional approach with children learning multiple languages, ensuring carryover to all of the child's contexts, including not just therapy and the classroom but also other school settings, the home, and the community.

The same principles discussed above apply to children learning more than one dialect. As noted in Chapter 4, in some cases (e.g., a child learning both AAE and Mainstream American English), dialect features may appear to be symptoms of a speech sound or language disorder. Thus, the issues are not trivial.

Diagnostic Therapy/Dynamic Assessment

Dynamic assessment straddles evaluation and treatment. In truth, all evaluation procedures should be dynamic; that is, one should always be taking note of which types of tasks, stimuli, prompts, and reinforcement are the most effective for the child. Similarly, all intervention should be diagnostic; that is, one should always be assessing the child's progress both on the target goals and contexts and in other domains. However, few SLPs carry out these procedures in a systematic manner. Glaspey and colleagues (Glaspey, 2012; Glaspey & MacLeod, 2010; Glaspey & Stoel-Gammon, 2005) have recently developed the Glaspey Dynamic Assessment of Phonology (GDAP; Glaspey, 2006), which can be used for both purposes. Using this tool, the SLP assesses the child's ability to produce the target in various contexts: repetition, label (i.e., in response to "What's this?"), carrier phrase (e.g., "Tell me about this. Start with 'It's a...'"), novel phrase or sentence, or story. Cue levels include the following:

- Maximum support: prolongation, segmentation, simultaneous production, tactile cues, etc.
- Medium support: verbal instruction or model only
- Mild support: articulatory placement cue (e.g., circle gesture formed with the fingers to cue lip rounding)
- Minimum support: spontaneous or delayed imitation

The results are used to determine a starting point for therapy. Throughout therapy, the scaffolding scale can be used to document progress in detail yet with minimum effort for the clinician.

Considerations for Older Children: Listener Awareness and Repair Strategies

As children get older, intensive focus on the accuracy of production of particular consonants and vowels may provide diminishing returns. For many clients with low muscle tone or other physiologic differences (e.g., some children with Down syndrome), 100% accuracy may not be a feasible goal. For these children, the emphasis needs to shift to communicative effectiveness and intelligibility. This requires a gradual increase, from early school age through young adulthood, of responsibility for successful communication. The SLP should help the client develop an increasing awareness of listeners, their needs, and appropriate repair strategies for various contexts. Often, a few carefully selected clear content words (particularly nouns and verbs) can successfully convey the intended message despite an otherwise unintelligible sentence. This is especially true if the speaker has made sure to establish the topic. Redundancy—such as using a quantitative word (a number, "some" or "many," etc.) as well as a plural marker or an adverb of time as well as the past tense marker (e.g., "*Yesterday*, I walk*ed* up *three* hill*s*")—also helps to express meaning. Prosodic cues, such as stressing key words and pausing in between the subject and the verb of the sentence, can also make communication far more effective. These prosodic strategies will be revisited in Chapter 10.

EXERCISE 5-3

Cognitive–Linguistic–Social and Other Approaches

SUMMARY

The choices a speech-language pathologist must make when treating a child with a speech sound production disorder are many and varied. A plethora of factors must be considered. Furthermore, there are many aspects of intervention that cannot be discussed here or cannot be discussed in depth because critical concepts have not yet been introduced; they will be the focus of intervention sections of later chapters. It is often difficult to make these decisions about treatment. The key is to know what questions to ask as one is deciding and to continue to ask them as the assessment or treatment progresses, adjusting as appropriate.

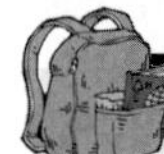

KEY TAKE-HOME MESSAGES

1. The ultimate goal of intervention is generalization.
2. A wide variety of choices must be made when planning intervention, based upon the whole child and his or her context.
3. Different motor intervention strategies are appropriate for initial learning of new skills versus maintenance and generalization of skills.
4. Production accuracy is not the only possible intervention goal. Others include awareness of communication contrast, ability to produce sounds or words distinctly, and changing speech production habits or patterns.

CHAPTER 5

Basic Treatment Principles Review

Exercise 5-1: **Basic Treatment Principles**

A. *Essay question.*

Write a letter to a doctor or an insurance company explaining why a school-aged child with Down syndrome can still benefit from speech therapy even though her low muscle tone does not permit her to produce every consonant within a sentence accurately.

B. *Choose the best answer for each question.*

1. Speech sound therapy:
   a. is a small part of school SLPs' caseloads.
   b. is only effective if it includes phonological awareness training.
   c. is effective if the focus is on expressive phonology.
   d. is only effective if it is eclectic.
2. With respect to therapy for SSD:
   a. more is better.
   b. a motoric approach is better.
   c. a linguistic approach is better.
   d. group therapy is better.
3. The ultimate goal of therapy is:
   a. retention.
   b. generalization.
   c. performance.
   d. feedback.
4. Which of the following would be an example of stimulus generalization?
   a. Using a newly learned target sound or structure (e.g., a cluster) in a new word
   b. Using a newly learned target word in a new context (e.g., in class versus in therapy)
   c. Using a new sound from the same sound class as the target
   d. Using a new sound from a different sound class as the target

Exercise 5-2: **Motor-Based Approaches**

A. *Essay questions.*

1. Why are non-speech oral–motor exercises unlikely to improve speech production? Given that non-speech oral–motor exercises are unlikely to improve speech production, why do SLPs carry out oral mechanism examinations?
2. Explain Table 5-2 with reference to the DIVA model described in Chapter 2.

B. *Choose the best answer for each question.*

1. The evidence against non-speech oral–motor exercises includes the following:
   a. Speech requires more strength than NSOMEs do.
   b. Speech is more rhythmic than chewing.
   c. Different portions of the brain are used for speech than for other oral functions.
   d. Lung capacity is often lower in children with speech sound disorders.
2. Research shows that for better long-term learning in the later stages of acquiring new motor skills:
   a. blocked practice yields better skill retention.
   b. rapidity and accuracy increase simultaneously.
   c. both goals and levels of difficulty should be mixed.
   d. intense multi-modal input is superior for all children.
3. Training broad would include:
   a. practicing a few exemplars many times.
   b. practicing certain exemplars for a pre-specified amount of time.
   c. practicing fewer times with a higher level of focus.
   d. practicing many exemplars within a certain category.
4. Client-internal feedforward and feedback processes are LEAST improved by:
   a. massed practice of a single exemplar.
   b. delayed reinforcement.
   c. variable reinforcement.
   d. allowing the client to make errors.

C. *Fill in the grid.*

Applicability of Motor Learning Principles

Parameter	Initial Learning Stages	Later Learning Stages
Amount of practice		
Distribution of practice		
Variability, scheduling		
Number of exemplars		
Feedback schedule		
Feedback type		
Level of challenge		
Amount of cueing		

Exercise 5-3: Cognitive–Linguistic–Social and Other Approaches

A. Essay question.

Motor learning theorists contrast two kinds of feedback: knowledge of performance and knowledge of results. Which of those two would be more appropriate within a cognitive–linguistic intervention approach? Why?

B. Choose the best answer for each question.

1. Cognitive–linguistic approaches to speech sound therapy are based on the assumption that:
   a. the child doesn't understand how to move his articulators.
   b. the child's phonological system is intact.
   c. phonological awareness is innate.
   d. the child's phonological representations or rules are not adult-like.
2. Research supports the benefits of which of the following intervention strategies?
   a. Focusing on broader patterns
   b. Focusing on bottom–up learning
   c. Focusing on final consonants that follow a tense vowel
   d. Focusing on single consonants rather than syllables
3. Research supports the benefits of which of the following intervention strategies?
   a. Bright colors for children who are hypersensitive
   b. Multiple communication modalities for children with social deficits
   c. Focusing on one language at a time for bilingual children
   d. Maximum cue levels throughout therapy
4. For older children with persistently decreased intelligibility, which of the following are recommended?
   a. Intensive focus on accuracy
   b. Reduction of redundancy
   c. Prosodic highlighting of key words
   d. Listeners taking increased responsibility

References

Allen, M. M. (2013). Intervention efficacy and intensity for children with speech sound disorder. *Journal of Speech, Language, and Hearing Research, 56*(3), 865–877.

Almost, D., & Rosenbaum, P. (1998). Effectiveness of speech intervention for phonological disorders: A randomized controlled trial. *Developmental Medicine & Child Neurology, 40*(5), 319–325. doi: 10.1111/j.1469-8749.1998.tb15383.x

ASHA. (2011a). *National Outcomes Measurement System: Pre-kindergarten national data report 2011*. Rockville, MD: National Center for Evidence-Based Practice in Communication Disorders.

ASHA. (2011b). *National Outcomes Measurement System: Pre-Kindergarten National Data Report 2006-2010*. Rockville, MD: American Speech-Language-Hearing Association.

Baker, E., & McLeod, S. (2011a). Evidence-based practice for children with speech sound disorders: Part 1 narrative review. *Language, Speech, and Hearing Services in Schools, 42*(2), 102–139.

Baker, E., & McLeod, S. (2011b). Evidence-based practice for children with speech sound disorders: Part 2 application to clinical practice. *Language, Speech, and Hearing Services in Schools, 42*(2), 140–151.

Barlow, J. A., & Enriquez, M. (2007). Theoretical perspectives on speech sound disorders in bilingual children. *Perspectives on Communication Disorders and Sciences in Culturally and Linguistically Diverse Populations, 14*(2), 3–10.

Bates, S. A. R., Watson, J. M. M., & Scobbie, J. M. (2002). Context-conditioned error patterns in disordered systems. In M. J. Ball & F. E. Gibbon (Eds.), *Vowel disorders* (pp. 145–185). London, UK: Butterworth-Heinemann. Reprinted as Bates, S., Watson, J. & Scobbie, J. M. (2013). Context-conditioned error patterns in disordered systems. In F. Gibbon & M. Ball (Eds.), *Handbook of vowels and vowel disorders* (pp. 288–325). New York, NY: Psychology Press.

Bernhardt, B. (2004). Maximizing success in phonological intervention. *Child Language Teaching & Therapy, 20*(3), 195–198.

Brady, N. C., Steeples, T., & Fleming, K. (2005). Effects of prelinguistic communication levels on initiation and repair of communication in children with disabilities. *Journal of Speech, Language, and Hearing Research, 48*(5), 1098–1113.

Broomfield, J., & Dodd, B. (2005). Clinical effectiveness. In B. Dodd (Ed.), *Differential diagnosis and treatment of children with speech disorder* (2nd ed., pp. 211–229). London, UK: Whurr.

Bunton, K. (2008). Speech versus non-speech: Different tasks, different neural organization. *Seminars in Speech and Language, 29*(4), 267–275.

Camarata, S. (1993). The application of naturalistic conversation training to speech production in children with speech disabilities. *Journal of Applied Behaviour Analysis, 26*(2), 173–182.

Cheng, L. R. L. (1993). Asian-American cultures. In D. Battle (Ed.), *Communication disorders in multicultural populations* (pp. 38–77). Boston, MA: Andover Medical Publishers.

Dale, P. S., & Hayden, D. A. (2013). Treating speech subsystems in Childhood Apraxia of Speech with tactual input: The PROMPT approach. *American Journal of Speech Language Pathology Papers in Press, 22*, 644–661. doi: 10.1044/1058-0360

Davis, B. L., & Velleman, S. L. (2008). Establishing a basic speech repertoire without using NSOME: Means, motive, and opportunity. *Seminars in Speech and Language, 29*(4), 312–319.

Dean, E. C., Howell, J., Waters, D., & Reid, J. (1995). Metaphon: A metalinguistic approach to the treatment of phonological disorder in children. *Clinical Linguistics and Phonetics, 9*(1), 1–19.

Demuth, K., Culbertson, J., & Alter, J. (2006). Word-minimality, epenthesis, and coda licensing in the early acquisition of English. *Language and Speech, 49*(2), 137–174.

Edeal, D. M., & Gildersleeve-Neumann, C. E. (2011). The importance of production frequency in therapy for Childhood Apraxia of Speech. *American Journal of Speech-Language Pathology, 20*(2), 95–110.

Elbert, M., & Gierut, J. (1986). *Handbook of clinical phonology: Approaches to assessment and treatment.* San Diego, CA: College-Hill Press.

Ertmer, D. J., & Ertmer, P. A. (1998). Constructivist strategies in phonological intervention: Facilitating self-regulation for carryover. *Language, Speech, and Hearing Services in Schools, 29*(2), 67–75. doi: 10.1044/0161-1461.2902.67

Fabiano-Smith, L., & Goldstein, B. (2010). Phonological acquisition in bilingual Spanish-English speaking children. *Journal of Speech, Language, and Hearing Research, 53*(1), 160–178.

Forrest, K. (2002). Are oral-motor exercises useful in the treatment of phonological/articulatory disorders? *Seminars in Speech and Language, 23*(1), 15–26.

Forrest, K., & Iuzzini, J. (2008). A comparison of oral motor and production training for children with speech sound disorders. *Seminars in Speech and Language, 29*(4), 304–311.

Gierut, J. A. (2001). Complexity in phonological treatment: Clinical factors. *Language, Speech, and Hearing Services in the Schools, 32*(4), 229–241.

Gierut, J. A. (2007). Phonological complexity and language learnability. *American Journal of Speech-Language Pathology, 16*(1), 6–17.

Gierut, J. (2008). Treatment efficacy summary: Phonological disorders in children. In ASHA (Ed.), *Treatment efficacy studies* (pp. 7216). Rockville, MD: ASHA.

Gierut, J. A., Elbert, M., & Dinnsen, D. A. (1987). A functional analysis of phonological knowledge and generalization learning in misarticulating children. *Journal of Speech and Hearing Research, 30*(4), 462–479.

Gierut, J. A., Morrisette, M. L., & Ziemer, S. M. (2010). Nonwords and generalization in children with phonological disorders. *American Journal of Speech-Language Pathology, 19*(2), 167–177.

Gillon, G. T. (2000). The efficacy of phonological awareness intervention for children with spoken language impairment. *Language, Speech, and Hearing Services in Schools, 31*(2), 126–141.

Gillon, G. T. (2002). Follow-up study investigating benefits of phonological awareness intervention for children with spoken language impairment. *International Journal of Language and Communication Disorders, 37*(4), 381–400.

Girolametto, L., Pearce, P. S., & Weitzman, E. (1997). Effects of lexical intervention on the phonology of late talkers. *Journal of Speech, Language, and Hearing Research, 40*(2), 338–348.

Girolametto, L., Weitzman, E., & Clements-Baartman, J. (1998). Vocabulary intervention for children Down syndrome: Parent training using focused stimulation. *Infant-Toddler Intervention: A Transdisciplinary Journal, 8*(2), 109–125.

Glaspey, A. (2012). Stimulability measures and dynamic assessment of speech adaptability. *Perspectives on Language Learning and Education, 19*(1), 12–18.

Glaspey, A. M., & MacLeod, A. A. N. (2010). A multi-dimensional approach to gradient change in phonological acquisition: A case study of disordered speech development. *Clinical Linguistics and Phonetics, 24*(4–5), 283–299.

Glaspey, A., & Stoel-Gammon, C. (2005). Dynamic assessment in phonological disorders: The Scaffolding Scale of Stimulability. *Topics in Language Disorders, 25*(3), 220–230.

Goldstein, B. A., & Fabiano-Smith, L. (2007). Assessment and intervention for bilingual children with phonological disorders. *The ASHA Leader* (online) (February).

Guadagnoli, M. A., & Lee, T. D. (2004). Challenge point: A framework for conceptualizing the effects of various practice conditions in motor learning. *Journal of Motor Behaviour, 36*(2), 212–224.

Guenther, F. H. (1995). Speech sound acquisition, coarticulation, and rate effects in a neural network model of speech production. *Psychology Review, 102*(3), 594–621.

Guenther, F. H., Ghosh, S. S., & Tourville, J. A. (2006). Neural modeling and imaging of the cortical interactions underlying syllable production. *Brain Language, 96*, 280–301.

Hayden, D. (2006). The PROMPT model: Use and application for children with mixed phonological-motor impairment. *International Journal of Speech-Language Pathology, 8*(3), 265–281.

Hayden, D. A., & Square, P. A. (1994). Motor speech treatment hierarchy: A systems approach. *Clinics in Communication Disorders, 4*, 162–174.

Hesketh, A., Adams, C., Nightingale, C., & Hall, R. (2000). Phonological awareness therapy and articulatory training approaches for children with phonological disorders: A comparative outcome study. *International Journal of Language and Communication Disorders, 35*(3), 337–354.

Hodson, B. W. (2006). Identifying phonological patterns and projecting remediation cycles: Expediting intelligibility gains of a 7 year old Australian child. *Advances in Speech-Language Pathology, 8*(3), 257–264.

Hodson, B. W., Scherz, J. A., & Strattman, K. H. (2002). Evaluating communicative abilities of a highly unintelligible preschooler. *American Journal of Speech-Language Pathology, 11*(3), 236–242.

Jacoby, G. P., Lee, L., Kummer, A. W., Levin, L., & Creaghead, N. A. (2002). The number of individual treatment units necessary to facilitate functional communication improvements in the speech and language of young children. *American Journal of Speech-Language Pathology, 11*(4), 370–380.

Kehoe, M. M., & Stoel-Gammon, C. (2001). Development of syllable structure in English-speaking children with particular reference to rhymes. *Journal of Child Language, 28*(2), 393–432.

Kent, R. D. (1982). Contextual facilitation of correct sound production. *Language, Speech, and Hearing in Schools, 13*(2), 66–76.

Kim, I.-S., LaPointe, L. L., & Stierwalt, J. A. G. (2012). The effect of feedback and practice on the acquisition of novel speech behaviors. *American Journal of Speech Language Pathology, 21*, 89–100.

Koegel, L. K., Koegel, R. L., & Ingham, J. C. (1986). Programming rapid generalization of correct articulation through self-monitoring procedures. *Journal of Speech and Hearing Disorders, 51*(1), 24–32.

Kohnert, K., Yim, D., Nett, K., Kan, P. F., & Duran, L. (2005). Intervention with linguistically diverse preschool children: A focus on developing home language(s). *Language, Speech, and Hearing in Schools, 36*(3), 251–263.

Kordus, R. N., & Weeks, D. L. (1998). Relative frequency of knowledge of performance and motor skill learning. *Research Quarterly for Exercise and Sport, 69*(3), 224.

Kwiatkowski, J., & Shriberg, L. D. (1998). The capability-focus treatment framework for child speech disorders. *American Journal of Speech Language Pathology, 7*(3), 27–38.

Lancaster, G., Keusch, S., Levin, A., Pring, T., & Martin, S. (2010). Treating children with phonological problems: Does an eclectic approach to therapy work? *International Journal of Language and Communication Disorders, 45*(2), 174–181.

Law, J., Garrett, Z., & Nye, C. (2004). The efficacy of treatment for children with developmental speech and language disorder: A meta-analysis. *Journal of Speech Lang Hear Res, 47*(4), 924–943.

Lin, L.-C., & Johnson, C. J. (2010). Phonological patterns in Mandarin-English bilingual children. *Clinical Linguistics and Phonetics, 24*(4–5), 369–386.

Maas, E., & Farinella, K. A. (2012). Random versus blocked practice in treatment for Childhood Apraxia of Speech. *Journal of Speech, Language, and Hearing Research, 55*, 561–578.

Maas, E., Robin, D. A., Austermann Hula, S. N., Freedman, S. E., Wulf, G., Ballard, K. J., & Schmidt, R. A. (2008). Principles of motor learning in treatment of motor speech disorders. *American Journal of Speech-Language Pathology, 17*, 277–298.

Major, E. M., & Bernhardt, B. H. (1998). Metaphonological skills of children with phonological disorders before and after phonological and metaphonological intervention. *International Journal of Language and Communication Disorders, 33*(4), 413–444.

Marcus, G. (2013). How birds and babies learn to talk. *The New Yorker* (May). http://www.newyorker.com/online/blogs/elements/2013/05/how-birds-and-babies-learn-to-talk.html

Marshalla, P. (2008). Oral motor treatment vs. non-speech oral motor exercises. *Oral Motor Institute, 2*(2). http://www.oralmotorinstitute.org

McCauley, R. J., Strand, E. A., Lof, G. L., Schooling, T., & Frymark, T. (2009). Evidence-based systematic review: Effects of nonspeech oral motor exercises on speech. *American Journal of Speech-Language Pathology, 18*, 343–360.

Miccio, A. W., & Ingrisano, D. R. (2000). The acquisition of fricatives and affricates: Evidence from a disordered phonological system. *American Journal of Speech-Language Pathology, 9*(3), 214–229.

Miccio, A. W., & Powell, T. W. (2010). Triangulating speech sound generalization. *Clinical Linguistics and Phonetics, 24*(4–5), 311–322.

Millar, D. C., Light, J. C., & Schlosser, R. W. (2006). The impact of augmentative and alternative communication intervention on the speech production of individuals with developmental disabilities: A research review. *Journal of Speech, Language, and Hearing Research, 49*(2), 248–264.

Miller, L. J., Coll, J. R., & Schoen, S. A. (2007). A randomized controlled pilot study of the effectiveness of occupational therapy for children with sensory modulation disorder. *American Journal of Occupational Therapy, 61*(2), 228–238.

Morrisette, M. L., & Gierut, J. A. (2002). Lexical organization and phonological change in treatment. *Journal of Speech, Language, and Hearing Research, 45*(1), 143–159.

Murray, E., McCabe, P., & Ballard, K. J. (2014). A systematic review of treatment outcomes for children with Childhood Apraxia of Speech. *American Journal of Speech Language Pathology, 23*, 486–504.

Namasivayam, A. K., Pukonen, M., Goshulak, D., Yu, V. Y., Kadis, D. S., Kroll, R., …, De Nil, L. F. (2013). Relationship between speech motor control and speech intelligibility in children with speech sound disorders. *Journal of Communication Disorders, 46*, 264–280.

Nelson, H. D., Nygren, P., Walker, M., & Panoscha, R. (2006). Screening for speech and language delay in preschool children: Systematic evidence review for the US preventive services task force. *Pediatrics, 117*(2), e298–e319.

Norris, J. A., & Hoffman, P. R. (1990). Language intervention within naturalistic environments. *Language, Speech, and Hearing Services in Schools, 21*(2), 72–84.

Ray, J. (2002). Training phonological disorders in a multilingual child: A case study. *American Journal of Speech-Language Pathology, 11*(3), 305–315.

Reid, J., Donaldson, M. L., Howell, J., Dean, E. C., & Grieve, R. (1996). The effectiveness of therapy for child phonological disorder: The Metaphon approach. In M. Aldridge (Ed.), *Child language* (pp. 165–175). Clevedon, Avon: Multilingual Matters.

Rupela, V., & Manjula, R. (2006). Phonotactic development in Kannada: Some aspects and future directions. *Language Forum: A Journal of Language and Literature, 32*(1–2), 83–93.

Rvachew, S., & Bernhardt, B. M. (2010). Clinical implications of dynamic systems theory for phonological development. *American Journal of Speech-Language Pathology, 19*(1), 34–50.

Rvachew, S., & Nowak, M. (2001). The effect of target-selection strategy on phonological learning. *Journal of Speech, Language, and Hearing Research, 44*(3), 610–623.

Rvachew, S., Nowak, M., & Cloutier, G. (2004). Effect of phonemic perception training on the speech production and phonological awareness skills of children with expressive phonological delay. *American Journal of Speech-Language Pathology, 13*(3), 250–263.

Rvachew, S., Ohberg, A., Grawburg, M., & Heyding, J. (2003). Phonological awareness and phonemic perception in 4-year-old children with delayed expressive phonology skills. *American Journal of Speech-Language Pathology, 12*(4), 463–471.

Saben, C. B., & Ingham, R. J. (1991). The effects of minimal pairs treatment on the speech sound production of two children with phonological disorders. *Journal of Speech and Hearing Research, 34*(5), 1023–1040.

Schmidt, L., & Lee, T. (2005). *Motor control and learning: A behavioral emphasis*. Champaign, IL: Human Kinetics.

Shriberg, L. D., & Kwiatkowski, J. (1990). Self-monitoring and generalization in preschool speech-delayed children. *Language, Speech, and Hearing Services in Schools, 21*(3), 157–170.

Skelton, S. L. (2004). Concurrent task sequencing in single-phoneme phonologic treatment and generalization. *Journal of Communication Disorders, 37*(2), 131–155.

Skelton, S. L., & Funk, T. E. (2004). Teaching speech sounds to young children using randomly ordered, variably complex task sequences. *Perceptual and Motor Skills, 99*(2), 602–604.

Steeve, R. W., Moore, C. A., Green, J. R., Reilly, K. J., & McMurtrey, J. R. (2008). Babbling, chewing and sucking: Oromandibular coordination at 9 months. *Journal of Speech, Language, and Hearing Research, 51*(6), 1390–1404.

Stoel-Gammon, C., Stone-Goldman, J., & Glaspey, A. (2002). Pattern-based approaches to phonological therapy. *Seminars in Speech and Language, 23*(1), 3–14.

Strand, E. A. (2004). *Dynamic Temporal and Tactile Cueing (DTTC): A treatment approach for severe Childhood Apraxia of Speech*. Paper presented at the American Speech-Language Hearing Association, Philadelphia.

Strand, E. A. & Debertine, P. (2000). The efficacy of integral stimulation intervention with developmental apraxia of speech. *Journal of Medical Speech-Language Pathology, 8*, 295–300.

Strand, E. A., & Skinder, A. (1999). Treatment of developmental apraxia of speech: Integral stimulation methods. In A. J. Caruso & E. A. Strand (Eds.), *Clinical management of motor speech disorders in children* (pp. 109–148). New York, NY: Thieme.

Strand, E. A., Stoeckel, R., & Baas, B. (2006). Treatment of severe Childhood Apraxia of Speech: A treatment efficacy study. *Journal of Medical Speech-Language Pathology, 14*(4), 297–307.

Swisher, W. E. (1973). *An investigation of physiologically and acoustically facilitating phonetic environment on the production and perception of defective speech sounds*. Madison, WI: University of Wisconsin.

Tyler, A. A. (2002). Language-based intervention for phonological disorders. *Seminars in Speech and Language, 23*(1), 69–82.

Tyler, A. A., & Lewis, K. E. (2005). Relationships among consistency/variability and other phonological measures over time. *Topics in Language Disorders, 25*(3), 243–253.

Velleman, S. L. (1988). The role of linguistic perception in later phonological development. *Journal of Applied Psycholinguistics, 9*, 221–236.

Williams, A. L. (2000). Multiple oppositions: Theoretical foundations for an alternative contrastive intervention approach. *American Journal of Speech-Language Pathology, 9*(4), 282–288.

Wilson, E. M., Green, J. R., Yunusova, Y., & Moore, C. A. (2008). Task specificity in early oral motor development. *Seminars in Speech and Language, 29*(4), 257–266.

Yavas, M., & Goldstein, B. (1998). Phonological assessment and treatment of bilingual speakers. *American Journal of Speech-Language Pathology, 7*(2), 49–60.

Young, D. E., & Schmidt, R. A. (1992). Augmented kinetic feedback for motor learning. *Journal of Motor Behaviour, 24*(3), 261–273.

Zamuner, T. S., Gerken, L. A., & Hammond, M. (2004). Phonotactic probabilities in young children's speech production. *Journal of Child Language, 31*(3), 515–536.

Zubow, L., & Hurtig, R. (2014). Supporting the use of rudimentary vocalizations. *Perspectives on Augmentative and Alternative Communication, 23*(3), 132–139.

CHAPTER 6

Beginnings: Pre-Speech and First Words

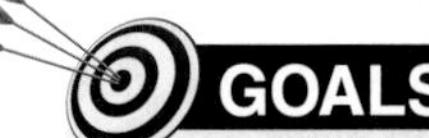

GOALS *of This Chapter*

1. Describe major prelinguistic and early linguistic stages of speech development, including the manners in which prelinguistic vocalizations lay the foundation for early speech.
2. Describe the relative impacts of universals (human physiology including learning capacities), exposure to the ambient language, and individual learning styles and preferences on early speech development.
3. Describe interactions among early linguistic, cognitive, and social-pragmatic development that can be used to facilitate intervention.
4. Describe strategies for leading the child into meaningful communication.

Chuckie, a 2-year-old, vocalizes frequently. However, he relies almost exclusively on his "favorite babble" [əwawawa] in almost all situations. His very few other vocalizations are also reduplicated—the same syllable repeated multiple times. Only one of these appears to have meaning: he typically says [dadada] when he sees his father coming home from work. However, he has invented a set of gestures and signs to express other meanings. For example, he "knocks" on his head with his knuckles when someone comes to the front door, holds his hand up to his ear when the phone rings, and shakes his hand as if in pain to comment that something is hot. Should his parents be concerned about his speech development?

INTRODUCTION

As seen in Chapter 3, many factors that arise long before the first words have important impacts on the child's eventual production of meaningful speech. The importance of including speech-language services within early intervention is no longer debated. Infancy and toddlerhood communication experiences can make a critical difference to a child's eventual communication outcome.

In this chapter, stages of infant vocal development are presented followed by an overview of some theories about the sources of these developments. Finally, prelinguistic and early linguistics assessment and treatment are delineated.

FROM BURPS TO BABBLE: HOW DO SPEECH-LIKE VOCALIZATIONS DEVELOP?

Why Do We Care About Prelinguistic Vocalizations?

Jakobson (1968) claimed that there was a "silent period" between children's production of babbling and their early words and that there was no important connection between these two stages. We now know very differently: prelinguistic vocalizations set the stage for meaningful speech in a variety of ways. Several of the phonetic and phonotactic characteristics of infants' and toddlers' utterances are predictive of their later linguistic profiles (McCathren, Yoder, & Warren, 1999; Paul, 1991; Paul & Jennings, 1992; Stoel-Gammon, 1989; Whitehurst, Smith, Fischel, Arnold, & Lonigan, 1991). We consider several of these in this section.

One basic quantitative fact about babies' productions is simply how often they occur; this is referred to as volubility. In a review of the research, Stoel-Gammon (1992) reported that the number of vocalizations a 3- to 6-month-old produces per minute is correlated not only with her volubility at 13 months but also with her attention to reading at 8 months, her Gesell Developmental Quotient (cognitive level) at 9 months, her Bayley Verbal Scale score at 11 to 15 months, and even her vocabulary size at 27 months. These relationships may reflect the child's fundamental linguistic capacity, the fact that parents are more verbally responsive to a child who vocalizes more, both, or other unknown factors. Based on data from their own and other studies, Iyer and Oller (2008) conclude that hearing loss (Clement, 2004; van den Dikkenberg-Pot, Koopmans-van Beinum & Clement, 1998; Moeller, Hoover, Putman, Arbataitis, Bohnenkamp, et al., 2007; Nathani, Oller, & Neal, 2007; Petinou, Schwartz, Mody, & Gravel, 1999) and cleft palate (Chapman, Hardin-Jones, Schulte, & Halter, 2001) do not affect volubility, although Fagan (2014) reports that vocalization frequency rises from below expectations to typical levels when children with profound hearing loss are provided with cochlear implants. In any case, socioeconomic status does impact volubility (Oller, Eilers, Steffens, Lynch, & Urbano, 1994). Combined with the fact that socioeconomic status has a significant impact on how often parents talk to their children (Hart & Risley, 1995), this finding suggests that volubility may be "contagious;" that is, the more a baby is talked to, the more likely she is to vocalize back. If so, infants' cultural contexts should also be taken into account when judging the relevance of volubility levels to a potential delay or disorder.

With respect to vocalization quality, the distinction between speech-like and non-speech-like vocalizations appears to be differentially diagnostic for autism spectrum disorders (ASD). Children with ASD produce a higher proportion of atypical (non-speech-like) vocalizations (Paul, Fuerst, Ramsay, Chawarska, & Klin, 2011), especially distress vocailzations (Plumb & Wetherby, 2013).

The most important measure of the quality of an infant's vocalizations appears to be the frequency with which he produces what are called **true consonants**. In this context, true consonants are considered to be those that are **supraglottal** (e.g., not [h] and [ʔ], which are produced at the glottis) and those that are not glides (e.g., not [j] and [w]). The percentage of an infant's vocalizations that contain at least one true consonant is correlated with the age at which that child reaches a productive vocabulary of 50 words, the maturity of the child's vocalizations at 29 and 36 months (Vihman, Ferguson, & Elbert, 1986; Vihman & Greenlee, 1987), and even the child's preschool language scale score at 6 years of age (Stoel-Gammon, 1992)! The proportion of infants' babble that includes true consonants may account for up to 40% of the variance in their language skills at 30 months (Whitehurst et al., 1991). Furthermore, the consonant variety of children with ASD or at risk for ASD is predictive of their later developmental levels (Paul et al., 2011; Plumb & Wetherby, 2013). More generally, children's sound production skills at 9 and 18 months predict their vocabulary scores at 24 months (Highman, Hennessey, Leitao, & Piek, 2013).

Of course, these predictive data are not proof that prelinguistic vocalizations are either necessary or sufficient for normal speech-language development. Correlations do not prove causation: For example, there could be some other factor(s), such as the children's individual inborn linguistic capacity, that are responsible for all of these measures. We do not know whether increasing a child's volubility or her percentage of vocalizations with true consonants would actually impact later speech-language measures. But these correlations suggest that best practices should include intervening as well as we know how and as early as possible to improve the quality and the quantity of vocalizations produced by infants who are at risk for speech-language difficulties.

Milestones: Infant Vocalization Stages

Infants are certainly not born non-vocal, but they do have very few vocal options at birth. As shown in Table 6-1, during the first stage of development, their primary vocalizations are reflexive cries, coughs, burps, and other **vegetative sounds** associated with feeding and movement (e.g., sighs and grunts). By 2 to 4 months of age, they are producing some sounds that appear to be more voluntary, especially coos and laughter, and taking vocal turns with their caregivers. Infants imitate caregivers' vowel vocalizations by 12 weeks of age (Kuhl & Meltzoff, 1996) as well as their pitch patterns if those vowels or pitch patterns are already in their own repertoires.

At 4 to 6 months, vocal play emerges as the child produces more varied, more prolonged **closants** (incompletely closed consonant-like sounds) and vocants (non-fully resonant

TABLE 6-1 Vocalization Stages

Age Range	Stage Name	Predominant Vocalization Types
0–2 mo	Vegetative	Cry, burp, cough, sigh, grunt
2–4 mo	Phonation	Coo, laugh
4–6 mo	Vocal play, expansion	Prolonged closants, vocants Squeal, growl, trill, click, friction Marginal babble
6–12 mo	Canonical babble	Reduplicated babble Variegated babble
10–15 mo	Jargon	Jargon
12+ mo	Transition to words	Protowords, grunts First true words

vowel-like sounds) at wider ranges of pitch and loudness, as well as growls, squeals, clicks, trills, and friction noises.

Marginal babble may also emerge during this time. This type of babble is similar to true canonical babbling in that it is rhythmic and it does consist of syllable-like combinations of closants and vocants or even fully resonant vowels, but the timing of these elements is not yet speech-like.

Speech-like syllable timing, including the production of true consonants, arises between 6 and 12 months during the next phase, canonical babbling, which includes both **reduplicated babbling** (e.g., [bɑbɑbɑ], [dididi]) and **variegated babbling** (in which consonants and/or vowels change within the syllable strings, e.g., [bɑdidɑbu]) (Holmgren, Lindblom, Aurelius, Jalling, & Zetterstrom, 1986; Mitchell & Kent, 1990; Smith, Brown-Sweeney, & Stoel-Gammon, 1989).

Finally, at 10 months or later, native language-like prosody is applied to sentence-like strings of variegated syllables, referred to as jargon. This is the stage at which parents tend to report that the child is "telling stories" or "speaking Chinese" (sometimes referred to as "speaking English" by Russians!). It sounds like adult conversational speech, but the words don't match words of the language. Now the infant has broken free of stereotyped rhythmic babble and is using the more complex rhythms of his own language.

Note that the age ranges in Table 6-1 overlap; the earlier types of vocalizations do not cease just because the later types emerge. These different types of babble may co-occur for several weeks.

Common MISCONCEPTION

SOUNDS IN BABBLE

There is a popular myth that babies produce all of the sounds from all languages of the world in their babble. This is no doubt an overgeneralization based upon the "exotic" fricative and trill sounds that many infants produce during the vocal play period. However, these closants do not yet display the timing characteristics of true consonants. This is the reason that many phoneticians advise against transcribing infant speech using the International Phonetic Alphabet (IPA) before the canonical babble stage. Furthermore, although these pre-canonical babble sounds are widely varied, few infants produce more than a few exotic sounds.

As the child's vocalizations mature, certain gestures or vocalizations may become associated with certain context-specific meanings. One of the earliest types of sound–meaning correspondence may be provided by some children's use of **communicative grunts**. These appear to arise through the child's noticing that she tends to grunt reflexively during effort. Grunts then begin to be used for mental effort, when the toddler is paying close attention to something. They gradually take on communicative intent, as when the child makes eye contact and grunts just before or just after doing something that was hard physical work or while trying to attract an adult's attention to an action or object (McCune, Vihman, Roug-Hellichius, Delery & Gogate, 1996). Similarly, **deictic gestures**, such as pointing and reaching, may emerge as early as 10 months (Caselli, 1990). **Referential** (labeling) **gestures**, such as sniffing at the sight of a flower, typically appear a couple of months later.

Similar early meaningful vocal expressions also are limited to restricted contexts and often don't appear to be intended to communicate with others. For example, a quiet high-pitched squeal may be uttered each time the child sees the family cat—but not in response to a cat on television, a picture of a cat in a book, etc. Such context-limited vocalizations that lack an adult true word model are called **phonetically consistent forms** (PCFs) or **protowords**. In some cases, they may emerge from a gestural or vocal routine, such as clapping and saying "yay" at the end of a song. Gradually, they begin to be used in more generalized, explicit ways, acquiring the functions of a true communicative word (Dore, Franklin, Miller, & Ramer, 1976; Menn, 1978).

Somewhere between 10 and 18 months, the first true words emerge. Parents' claims about the timing of such occurrences are notoriously variable, as some caretakers will label the infant's first [dɑdɑ] as a word, whereas others don't credit the child with meaningful language until she is speaking in clear adult-like words or even phrases. These reporting differences may reflect cultural expectations, socioeconomic status, or a variety of other factors. Vihman and McCune (1994) have proposed that the criteria for identifying a word include the context as well as the form of the vocalization, plus the consistency with which the child produces that vocalization in an appropriate context. That is, if the child says [dɑdɑ] when there is no Daddy present nor any items or activities that the child associates with Daddy, then that production is not considered to be a production of the word "Daddy" unless it has already been established that the child does consistently use [dɑdɑ] to refer to "Daddy" when the latter or reminders of him are present.

EXERCISE 6-1

Early Vocal Development

Theories of Early Vocal Development

Where does babbling come from? One source of insight into this question exists in the work of Thelen (1981). She documented the many **rhythmic stereotypies** that infants demonstrate, listed in Table 6-2.

These stereotypic patterns are hypothesized to be instigated by a neural central pattern generator that triggers automatic bilateral rhythmic motions that "tune up" various

TABLE 6-2 Rhythmic Stereotypies

Age	Type of Stereotypy
Birth	Sucking
2–3 mo	Kicking
5 mo	Lip sucking
6 mo	Body rocking
6–7 mo	Toe sucking
6–9 mo	Hand banging
6–12 mo	Canonical babble

parts of the body for later, more voluntary movement. The existence of such a system has been documented in other animals, although only indirect evidence is available for its presence in humans (Wilson, Green, Yunusova, & Moore, 2008). Through repeated rhythmic motion, sensory–motor associations are made among muscles, joints, and tendons so that the infant learns how to plan and program movements and adjust them based upon proprioceptive and kinesthetic feedback. Canonical babble is proposed to be one such rhythmic stereotypy. In theory, it begins as involuntary "jaw wagging," which may initially occur without voicing. It gradually becomes more and more voluntary as the infant accidentally moves the jaw in this way while vocalizing, then makes the sensory–motor associations necessary for voluntary control and learns that he receives positive social feedback when he babbles. This theory is bolstered in a report by Meier, McGarvin, Zakia, and Willerman (1997) of silent babbling in both hearing and deaf children between the ages of 8 and 13 months.

It has often been assumed that such jaw movements for speech arise from the rhythmic sucking and masticatory (chewing) jaw movements that are presumed to be more basic both phylogenetically and ontogenetically. However, differences in muscle coordination patterns have been reported for the lips, tongue, facial muscles, and the levator veli palatini for speech versus non-speech tasks performed by children and/or adults. Furthermore, jaw motions for speech actually mature earlier than do those for the adult-like rotary chew (Wilson et al., 2008). This research suggests that silent babbling is a precursor to speech, not a continuation of sucking motions or practice for the movements needed for chewing.

In the view of Davis and colleagues, (Davis & MacNeilage, 1990; Davis & MacNeilage, 1995; MacNeilage & Davis, 2000; MacNeilage, Davis, Kinney, & Matyear, 2000), these voiced rhythmic jaw wags provide the frame for three primary types of "**ballistic**" **babble syllables**: (1) labial consonant + central vowel (e.g., [bʌ]), for both of which the tongue is not involved at all; (2) alveolar consonant + high front vowel (e.g., [di]), for both of which the tongue tip is raised to or toward the alveolar ridge; and (3) velar consonant + high back vowel (e.g., [gu]), for both of which the tongue dorsum is raised to or toward the velum. These types of babble require no intra-syllabic tongue motion; the infant can virtually create the vocant after the closant just by lowering his jaw. Very little motor planning is required. Davis and colleagues have demonstrated a predominance of such patterns in the early words of children from a variety of languages. They have also shown that many languages demonstrate a statistical preference for these types of syllables even in the adult lexicon. Gildersleeve-Neumann, Davis, and MacNeilage (2000) even extended this result with slightly less robust results to the later-developing consonants that are relatively rare in babbling.

However, Tyler and Langsdale (1996) found little evidence of such "**CV associations**" with the exception of velar + back vowel in their study of nine children between the ages of 18 and 24 months. Furthermore, Vihman (1992) showed that there is an effect of the ambient language on young children's CV combinations, with English toddlers producing more C+i syllables (reflecting English baby-talk words such as "daddy, mommy, piggie, baby, icky," etc.) and Japanese toddlers producing more [ko] syllables, reflecting their input. Similarly, while Chen and Kent (2005) did identify patterns similar to those described by Davis and MacNeilage in 24 infants learning Mandarin Chinese, they also identified language-specific CV co-occurrence patterns as well. Thus, both physiology and the ambient language appear to affect even such apparently motoric aspects of canonical babble as which consonants and vowels tend to be combined into syllables.

This raises the question of the **universality** versus **language specificity** of babble and very early words. Locke (1983) demonstrated that overall, the sounds most common in children's babble and early words are also those that are most common in the languages of the world, as illustrated in Table 6-3.

The astute reader will note some exceptions to this trend: liquids and sibilants are far less frequent in babble and early words than language universals would lead one to expect, no

TABLE 6-3 Correspondences Between Sound Use in Babble and Languages

Sound Class	% of Languages	% of Babble	% Use in Early Words
Stops	100	43	100
Nasals	99.6	9.2	100
Liquids	95.9	1.22	0
Sibilants	90.6	1.6	50
Glides	86	17	60
Other fricatives	73	1.8	30
[h]	63	23.7	50

From Maddieson, I. (1984). *Patterns of sounds.* Cambridge, UK: Cambridge University Press; Locke, J. L. (1983). *Phonological acquisition and change.* New York, NY: Academic Press.

doubt due to production difficulty. Glides and especially [h] are more frequent, no doubt due to ease of production. In any case, Locke (1983) proposed that there is a common core of consonants physiologically "available" to the prelingual child and that this approximates a core of consonants that are frequent universally. The Davis and MacNeilage model of speech arising from basic ballistic syllable types and Thelen's theories about the physiologic basis for babbling also highlight the child's biologic givens.

Yet, it would be highly inappropriate to model the vocal system as automatically unfolding on a biologically established timetable with no outside influences. The infant's exposure to an ambient language (or more than one, in many contexts) affects her perception of speech from the very beginning of life and her own vocal production from not terribly long thereafter. For example, 3-month-olds use more speech-like vocalizations in response to adults who take vocal turns using speech-like vocalizations with them. This is a form of "vocal contagion" (Bloom, Russell, & Wassenberg, 1987; Bloom, 1988; Masataka, 1993) that may be attributable to mirror neurons (Velleman & Vihman, 2002a), motor neurons in the Broca area that fire when a person observes someone else perform an action that is within his own motor repertoire (see Chapter 3). Furthermore, the infant's emerging familiarity with the structures of her language begins to be evident in her vocalizations between 6 and 12 months of age. During this time, babies produce pitch contours that match those of their language, for example, mostly falling for English versus approximately equal proportions of falling and rising for French (Whalen, Levitt, & Wang, 1991). By 10 months, the formants of their vowels also differ according to their linguistic exposure (Boysson-Bardies, Halle, Sagart & Durand, 1989). Boysson-Bardies and Vihman (1991) showed that frequencies of occurrence of consonant manner and place of babies between 9 ½ and 17 months match those of their languages (French, English, Japanese, Swedish); however, both babble and words were included in their counts. Lee, Davis, and MacNeilage (2010) carried out a similar study but included only babble; they reported that between 7 to 8 and 12 months, the frequencies of occurrence of English and Korean infants' vowels in their babble reflect their ambient languages; consonant frequencies also tend to match those of the language but not statistically significantly so. Focusing on early words, Vihman and de Boysson-Bardies (1994) found that fricatives and liquids are used far more frequently by toddlers learning French, in which these sounds each make up about 21% of consonant usage, than in English, in which the proportion of each is only about 16%. Thus, frequency of exposure does appear to have an impact on infant babble.

How about infants who are exposed to more than one language? Oller, Eilers, Urbano, and Cobo-Lewis (1997) showed that babies exposed to two languages were neither delayed nor advanced in their babbling development with respect to age of onset of canonical babbling and proportion of CV syllables. Furthermore, Poulin-DuBois and Goodz (2001) found that babies exposed to both French and English but predominantly to French produce babbles that are more similar to those of French monolinguals, with little or no mixing in of features associated with English monolingual babble only. Thus, there is reason to believe in both a physiologic and a cognitive basis for late babble and early words.

A third influence that emerges is that of the child's individual experiences (e.g., her own name, labels of salient objects, frequently used verbs) and preferences. During the canonical babble and the jargon stages, many children exhibit "favorite babbles," certain sequences of consonants (a.k.a. "vocal motor schemes") or syllables that recur frequently in their speech. These children tend to select words with these same articulatory patterns when they begin producing their first meaningful words (McCune & Vihman, 1987). This makes sense with respect to the DIVA model described in Chapter 3; the baby has developed motor programs for these sequences of consonants and vowels that are therefore ready and waiting to be used for words.

Although there is a common core of consonants produced by most babies the world over, some babies also produce unusual consonants in their babble. For instance, French infants sometimes babble [h] even though this phone is not used in that language, most likely because it is so easy to produce. "Hard" consonants that are babbled nonetheless by specific toddlers tend to show up in those infants' early words. One example of this is Laurent (not his real name, which did begin with "L"), a French baby who, very unusually, included [l] in his babble by the age of 10 months. His early words included [l] as well, sometimes in words that did not even require it (e.g., [bolo] for "chapeau") (Vihman, 1993). It is possible that this child's unusual preference for [l] was inspired, at least in part, by the frequency with which he heard the [l] at the beginning of his own name.

These three influences on babble and early words—human physiology, the ambient language(s), and individual experiences and preferences—are summarized in Table 6-4.

Jakobson (1968) proposed that babble and first words were independent with no influence of prelinguistic vocalizations on spoken language. Yet, as we have seen, features of the language being learned are already present during the prelinguistic period. It would violate all notions of biologic efficiency to propose that these gains are lost and that the child starts again from scratch as word learning begins. The carryover that is evident from babble to words also belies such a theory.

The strong foundation for speech that is laid during the prelinguistic experience also helps explain the mystery that Chomsky (1975), Pinker (1994), and others proposed to account for with their theories of innate knowledge of phonological universals (and grammar). They have argued that **positive evidence**—that is, direct evidence of what is

TABLE 6-4 **Evidence of Influences on Babble and Early Words**

Age Range	Physiologic Influences		Ambient Language Influences		Child-Specific Influences	
	Perception	Production	Perception	Production	Perception	Production
Birth	Words by number of syllables Languages by rhythm Function vs. content words by prosody		Prosody of own language		Own mother's voice Passages read aloud by mother late in pregnancy	
1–2 months	Place, manner, voicing of consonants in syllables; from any language Vowels [i], [ɑ], [u]					
2 months	Pitch, duration		Infant-directed speech (IDS) vs. adult-directed speech (ADS) Syllables in trisyllables if in IDS			Copy pitch patterns, vowels from own repertoire
4 months			Pauses that do/don't interrupt grammatical clauses	Imitate mother's pitch contour if exaggerated	Own name	
6 months			Words, conversational speech in own vs. other language	Proportion of inspiratory/ expiratory phonation		Imitate vocalizations from own repertoire
6–12 months				Falling vs. rising pitch proportions match own language		
7.5 months			Words trained in a list when presented in a passage if in own or similar language and if trochaic			
9 months			Words trained in a list when presented in a passage if in own or similar language, even if iambic			
10 months		Frequent use of [h] in babble	Stress patterns in own vs. other language Consonants, consonant–vowel sequences in own vs. other language Medial consonant sequences in own vs. other language	Vowel formants Utterance length in syllables (monosyllabic vs. disyllabic) Consonant place of articulation (proportion of labials)		

TABLE 6-4 **Evidence of Influences on Babble and Early Words (*Continued*)**

Age Range	Physiologic Influences		Ambient Language Influences		Child-Specific Influences	
	Perception	Production	Perception	Production	Perception	Production
10–12 months			Discrimination of non-native contrasts *decreases*			
11 months			Recognize specific words from own language Words that are/are not interrupted by pauses			
12 months: Babble					Consonants that they do/don't yet produce themselves	
12+ months: First words				Use of [h], labials language specific		First words match "vocal motor schemes" for infants with favorite babbles

Based upon Vihman, M. M. (2014). *Phonological development: The first two years* (2nd ed.). Somerset, NJ: Blackwell-Wiley.

allowed (which infants get through observation)—is not sufficient for language learning without additional **negative evidence**—that is, direct evidence of what is not allowed (which is available only extremely rarely, considering the amount of input the child receives in parent corrections). The speech and language evidence that children receive, they argue, is not enough, because the brain cannot store enough data about what has occurred to use probabilities as evidence for the rules that govern elements or structures that occur only rarely or as evidence that elements or structures that have not occurred must be ruled out. Thus, Chomsky and others conclude that neonates must have inborn knowledge of the grammatical (including phonological) linguistic possibilities—the linguistic universals. Listening to their own languages allows them to select which of those possibilities are the appropriate ambient choices. Certain pieces of information (e.g., hearing a particular grammatical structure) trigger the selection process.

However, the implicit learning research reviewed in Chapter 3 "Precursors" is "very bad news for yesterday's nativists [believers in the innateness of language knowledge, such as Chomsky], because they underscore the extraordinarily plastic and activity-dependent nature of cortical specialization, and buttress the case for an **emergentist** approach to the development of higher cognitive functions" (Bates, Thal, Aram, Nass, & Trauner, 1997, p. 3). These findings make it clear that, in fact, our brains are capable of acquiring, retaining, sorting, associating, and analyzing a great deal of information about probabilities of occurrence and co-occurrence of linguistic elements and structures throughout our lifetimes. Several authors (e.g., Pierrehumbert 2001; Lotto, Kluender, & Holt 2000) have proposed that probabilistic procedural learning leads to pattern detection and abstraction to the cognitive equivalent of subconscious linguistic rules. Thus, in Pierrehumbert's (2001) words, "statistical underrepresentation must do the job of negative evidence" (p. 13); the fact that the infant has not heard certain sounds or combinations that would have been expected based upon probabilities shapes his knowledge of the linguistic system to which he has been exposed.

This model is not only possible, it is preferable. Innate linguistic "switches" flipped on by easily available data, as proposed by Chomsky and others, should lead to the prediction that every person learning a given language would end up with the exact same linguistic system as every other (Macken, 1995). Yet, this is clearly not true; individual speakers have flexible individual **idiolects** (personal ways of speaking), depending upon the socio-cultural, geographical, and ethnic dialects to which they've been exposed and when and how this exposure occurred, not to mention whether or not the speaker has a speech-language disorder. Even 2-year-olds have been shown to use or adjust different aspects of their personal phonetic and phonotactic repertoires as appropriate to the sociolinguistic situation (Docherty, Foulkes, Tillotson, & Watt, 2006). For example, 3- to 5-year-old children are already beginning to use features of infant-directed speech to their baby siblings (Tomasello & Mannle, 1985). A model of phonological learning that predicts such flexibility and variability is much appropriate than one that does not.

EXERCISE 6-2

Theories of Early Vocal Development

IMPORTANT CONCEPTS FROM CHILD PHONOLOGY

The functionality of a child's phonology needs to be considered in the light of all of the subcomponents and elements that are used in adult phonologies (reviewed in Chapter 2). However, there are some special issues that arise in the discussion of immature phonologies. The source of most of these issues is the fact that while even adult phonologies may adjust slightly to the linguistic environment over time, a child's phonology is in a state of rapid change, as are the child's body and mind. Although an immature phonology may be functional for the child at one point in time, new cognitive, physical, or environmental factors may make additional communicative demands on the child at any moment. Similarly, new cognitive, physical, or environmental developments may increase the child's potential for phonological development. In this section, some of the consequences of this state of affairs will be addressed.

Presystematic Versus Systematic Phonology

Children's very early phonology differs in some important ways from their later phonology. Many studies have shown that the first words are learned with very little phonological regularity. For example, the presumed target /f/ in initial position in one word may be stopped ([p]), whereas another target initial /f/ may be produced quite accurately, and a third is omitted altogether. It doesn't seem as though the child has any particular way to produce /f/; he is simply attempting to produce *words*. If one word is short and simple, he may be able to get all the details right. If another is longer or more complex, he may get the gist of it without worrying about the individual phones or their exact order. Or, he may produce one word in a surprisingly adult-like manner, as Hildegard Leopold initially did for the word "pretty:" [pɹ̥ti] (Leopold, 1939). Like a new reader may do with sight words, the child at this age is learning words and short phrases in toto, without recognizing many relationships among the sounds in different words. If a phonological analysis of a child's system is attempted at this stage, consistency or patterns may be unidentifiable, both between the target and the production as well as among the productions, as in the data from Molly given in Table 6-5 (Vihman & Velleman, 1989).

TABLE 6-5 Molly's Unsystematic Early Words

Target	Child's Production
baby	[bæpæ]
cracker	[pɑkæ], [kwɑ], [wæʰk], [pækwɑ], [kʌk]
moo	[meʔje]
night-night	[hʌn:ʌ], [noʊnæ]

Note that Molly appears to have recognized that there is at least one velar stop in "cracker" but she may not be quite sure how many; her knowledge of vowels or her ability to produce them or both are quite limited. She is not very careful—or very aware—of how many syllables occur in each word.

Typically when the child's vocabulary reaches 25 to 100 words, often at the same time as she begins to combine words (around 18 months), the child appears to begin to systematize. The toddler identifies those word shapes that he is comfortable producing and "decides" to focus on those. Thus, the typical sign of such systematization may be that the child will begin to selectively learn words that fit her preferred production patterns (i.e., that fit her system) and will avoid attempting words that she does understand but that cannot be adapted to her preferred word shape. Vihman's (1976) daughter, "V," for example, avoided saying the words for "mommy" and "daddy" in her native Estonian for months because she only knew how to handle words with a low vowel followed by a high vowel (as in the English words "mommy" and "daddy"). The Estonian words (/ema/ and /isa/) have the opposite pattern of a higher vowel followed by a lower one, which she could not (or would not) produce. Velleman and Vihman (2002b) provided similar data from a Finnish-learning child, Atte, who was typically developing. This child favored the VCV (vowel-consonant-vowel) word form. He selected words for his early vocabulary that matched his preference, as shown in Table 6-6. That is, he only tried to say VCV (and one VCVCV) words. It is important to consider such selection and avoidance patterns when attempting to increase the expressive vocabularies of such children.

The challenge of deciphering a child's early messages may be exacerbated for so-called **expressive** children. Contrary to those toddlers whose data tend to show up in articles and textbooks (the **referential** label learners), these children tend to learn phrases rather than individual words. These phrases are typically "formulaic" or "unanalyzed"—that is, the children don't appear to have parsed them into individual

TABLE 6-6 Atte's Selected VCV Words

Target Word	Meaning
apina	monkey
auto	car
aiti	mother
isi	father
aani	sound
ajaa	drives
Antti	(name)
ankka	duck
ukko	old man

pronouns, verbs, etc. Rather, they learn chunks such as "What do you want," "I love you," and "Open the door" as gestalt wholes. Furthermore, the prosody of these utterances tends to be more accurate than the actual segments. These children should not be assumed to be disordered; most of them will gradually deconstruct their phrases into single words, and their speech will eventually be just as intelligible as that of the referential children (Nelson, 1981; Peters, 1983, 1990).

Regardless of the type of learner a child may be, signs of systematization can be expected to gradually emerge. As the child's vocabulary approaches 50 to 100 words, we begin to identify clear phonological patterns in his speech. These patterns may be phonetic or phonotactic, but they are indicative that the toddler is beginning to systematize his use of particular sounds, syllables, or articulatory gestures. This is the first step in the direction of a phonological system.

Often but not always, the patterns that emerge are then spread to words with different adult forms. In these cases, they are referred to as **templates** (Velleman & Vihman, 2002a) when "roughly similar [target] words are mapped onto much more similar output forms" (Menn, Schmidt, & Nicholas, 2009, p. 295). For example, Molly—whose very early words were provided previously—felt comfortable producing words that ended with a nasal + vowel syllable (such as "fun**ny**," "mom**my**," "Grand**ma**," etc.) so much that she changed other words to fit this pattern (saying, e.g., [ɪnni] for "Nicky;" (Vihman & Velleman 1989). Similarly, V changed the Estonian words for "mommy" and "daddy" around so that she could pronounce them, saying [ami] for "ema" and [asi] for "isa." Atte adapted words to his VCV template, as well, as shown in Table 6-7. He produced CVCV words with the correct vowels and medial consonants, but dropped the initial consonants to fit his preferred VCV format.

Vihman and Croft (2007) and Menn and colleagues (2009) describe the key words at the hearts of these templates, the child's preferred output patterns, as "attractors"—output forms that attract other target words to be produced with the same or similar output patterns. For Atte, for example, his VCV name could have been the attractor that drew him to select the other VCV words in Table 6-6 and then to adapt the "adapted" words in Table 6-7 to fit that pattern. A powerful attractor in one child's phonology or an attractor that is powerful at one point in a child's phonology may be powerless for another child or at another time for the same child. In this sense, the "attractor" or the template is like the most popular student or the most popular lifestyle choices within the culture of a junior high school: it is hard for all but the most recalcitrant to resist, but that high level of popularity rarely lasts for long.

It is important to note that while it may lead to more adult-like productions of some words, the establishment of such patterns often results in apparently worse productions of other words. Words that were previously distinct may become homonyms; words that were previously clear may seem garbled. Parents may become concerned because the child seems to be losing ground phonologically. This apparent regression is not in fact regression at all. We believe that children who begin to overgeneralize the regular past tense, plural, etc., at a certain age (saying "eated" for "ate," "tooths" for "teeth," and so on) do so because they are searching for regularities in the morphology. Similarly, children who begin to demonstrate phonological systematicity are demonstrating that they are rule-learners in this respect as well. They have hit upon a phonological pattern that (in most cases) is a viable pattern for a subgroup of the words of their languages (just like "-ed" is for the past tense), and they try to make all words fit that pattern. Although this may be frustrating to the SLP or to parents, it is a good sign. That child has discovered the basic truth that language in general and phonology in particular are **rule governed**. That child now has a phonological *system*. It is important to note as well that as children begin to combine words into phrases and sentences, phonetic or phonotactic accuracy may decrease. This reflects their limited capacity for dealing with phonological complexity and grammatical complexity at the same time (Nelson & Bauer, 1991).

Not all children go through a clear-cut systematization period. The establishment of patterns such as those described above is not necessary, though there is some evidence that children who use sounds in more systematic ways may tend to be earlier talkers (McCune & Vihman, 1987). The hypothesis is that having a set of well-practiced motor programs provides a phonetic foundation for producing words that fit those pre-existing plans.

TABLE 6-7 Atte's Adapted VCV Words

Target Word	Meaning	Child's Production
kala	fish	ala
pallo	ball	allo
sammui	extinguished	ammu
loppu	all done	oppu
heppa	horse	eppa
kello	clock	ello
nalle	teddybear	alle

Phonological Idioms

Children's early words that do not fit with other aspects of their phonological patterns are referred to as **phonological idioms**. Phonological idioms may be advanced in comparison to the rest of the child's system, or they may be simpler. One child may say "pretty" accurately very early in her word learning, even though this is expected to be a relatively difficult word (Leopold 1947). Another may hang onto a very early gross simplification of some word even when she is phonologically capable of producing similar words more accurately; this early version of the word becomes a **frozen form**.

For example, one child named "Mickey" studied by this author called herself [didi]. This was one of her very first words, so it was not a surprise that she simplified it. However, her persistent mispronunciation was not a result of a perceptual confusion; she didn't respond if she was called "Deedee" by others. Even when she was able to produce more difficult similar words (such as "monkey"), she persisted in saying her own name as [didi]. Just as the most common nouns and verbs hang onto their old-fashioned conjugations (e.g., "women, men, children;" "ate, sat, went") even when the rest of the language changes, the child's most frequently used words are likely to be most resistant to modification (Menn, 1983; Menn et al., 2009). For this reason, it is sometimes recommended that new or less familiar words or even nonsense words be used in speech sound therapy, although functionality (ensuring that the child can say the words that matter the most to him in an intelligible manner) may take priority over this consideration.

These characteristics of early phonology must be kept in mind when analyzing the phonologies of children with small vocabularies. Lack of a system or persistence in using words that are not consistent with a system at an early stage may be perfectly normal (Stoel-Gammon & Stone 1991). However, this lack of system does not mean that it is impossible to carry out any type of phonological analysis. This is where the ability to assess other aspects of the child's phonology, especially the phonotactic and phonetic repertoires, can play a vital role. Phonetic, phonotactic, and suprasegmental characteristics can be assessed, even in children who are still in the babbling or jargoning stages. A very young child at the onset of word learning should still produce a variety of phones (typically four to six), usually in a few different word shapes (e.g., CV, VC, CVCV, CVC) with pitch patterns that are appropriate to the context (question, request, demand, etc.). And as the child's vocabulary grows, there should be signs of emerging systematicity.

Vihman (1996) summarizes these phases of early development as follows:

1. Presystematic: No single word production pattern is apparent; few inter-word relationships are revealed either in the child's forms or in the words attempted.
2. First signs of organization:
   A. Crystallization (the less common type)
      - Selective targeting of adult forms with particular phonetic characteristics
      - Increase in variability in the production of certain word shapes, suggesting "experimentation"

   OR

   B. Controlled expansion
      - Gradual relaxation of production constraints
      - Expansion in the range of adult targets attempted
3. Emergence of system: One or more of the child's word shapes assume the status of "canonical forms" or production templates (especially noticeable in the case of "crystallization"). These forms begin to dominate production; adult models are restructured to fit the template. At the same time, systematic treatment of problematic aspects of adult forms may result in the first regular adult-model–child-form relationships, expressible as "phonological rules" or "processes." (p. 151)

In other words, the first few words typically have no discernable common production pattern. They may be quite accurate (Vihman, Keren-Portnoy, & DePaolis, 2013) or quite different from the target. As the child develops, she may demonstrate a preference for certain sounds and structures (crystallization, templates) or she may simply gradually begin to produce a wider variety of forms. At the third stage—typically the point at which the child has about 25 to 50 words in her expressive vocabulary, by parent report—specific, consistent patterns (such as reduplication, final consonant deletion, and particular substitutions) can often be identified.

It has been suggested (Leonard, Devescovi, & Ossella, 1987; Leonard & McGregor, 1991; Leonard, 1992) that children with phonological disorders may be even more likely than children whose phonologies are developing normally to demonstrate idiosyncratic phonological patterns as their systems develop. Leonard (1992) proposes that this tendency may be due in part to the children's efforts to acquire larger lexicons using less sophisticated phonological systems.

Summary

At the beginnings of word learning, children's phonologies may be unsystematic with no detectable regularities. As they begin to systematize, selection, avoidance, and preferred production patterns (**word recipes**) may be identified. Phonological idioms may occur as either surprisingly sophisticated early productions or as a few simplified forms that do not improve even as the child's phonology changes to accommodate more phones and word shapes. Similar patterns may be seen and may be even more pervasive in the phonologies of children with phonological disorders.

EVALUATION

Speech sound evaluation at any age should include thorough consideration of physiologic (including motor and sensory), cognitive, and social precursors of phonology. These have been discussed in depth in Chapter 3. Here, we focus on assessing the child's prelinguistic and very early linguistic vocalizations per se.

It may seem daunting to evaluate the prelinguistic vocalizations of an infant or young toddler who, by definition, produces no meaningful utterances. Clearly, one cannot identify "errors" in the speech of such a child because he has no particular speech targets. There are very few valid, reliable, multiculturally appropriate, standardized, published evaluation tools available to administer to such young children (Crais, 2011) and those that do exist don't focus on speech development per se. Many infant/toddler developmental tests (such as the *Bayley Scales of Infant and Toddler Development: Bayley-III*; Bayley, 2006) include a few questions about vocalization types and functions, but they are quite general and do not focus on the specific nature of the child's vocalizations. The Communication and Symbolic Behavior Scales (CSBS; Wetherby & Prizant, 1993) does include a "vocal communicative means" subscale based upon a spontaneous speech sample that allows one to determine whether the child's vocal production is age-appropriate overall. The subscale includes both phonetic measures (e.g., variety of consonants produced) and phonotactic measures (syllable shapes). This subscale (like most of the other subscales of the CSBS) is predictive of a child's later expressive vocabulary (McCathren, Yoder, & Warren, 2000) as is the "speech composite score" of the briefer CSBS-Developmental Profile (CSBS-DP; Wetherby & Prizant, 2002) (Wetherby, Allen, Cleary, Kublin, & Goldstein, 2002). However, even these tests do not include specific analyses of which aspects of the child's vocalizations are appropriate or inappropriate. Thus, they are excellent for identification of a problem but may not provide the information we need to diagnose or treat the speech deficits per se.

Therefore, under most circumstances, our evaluations of very young or other prelinguistic children's speech will be based upon analyses of the children's spontaneous speech samples, ideally from interactions both with the SLP and with familiar caregivers, sampling both the child's typical behavior and her performance when prompted or cued by the SLP (Crais, 2011). Such samples may be composed of various types of babble perhaps as well as vocal play or even less mature vocalizations. Such an evaluation can be broken down into two major areas—quantity and quality.

With respect to quantity, recall that the frequency of an infant's vocalizations is predictive of several later speech and language milestones. Thus, a basic measure of how many times per minute a baby vocalizes is the first step in assessing his prelinguistic skills. Vihman and McCune (1994) reported averages of 130 to 240 vocalizations produced by 12- to 13-month-olds per half-hour home recording session, or approximately five vocalizations per minute. These children's American parents had volunteered them for a research study and were making efforts to encourage the children to talk during the recording sessions, so means may be lower for children of less-motivated parents, for children from different cultural backgrounds in which parents are less pushy, or for children in different social contexts. Iyer and Oller (2008) reported that hearing children produced about eight vocalizations per minute during the pre-canonical babbling period and four per minute during canonical and post-canonical babbling. However, they noted that there is considerable variability not only across children but also for the same child in different sessions. For example, one child produced 3.27 vocalizations per minute in one session and 15.66 in another. Thus, it is important to measure more than one session per child.

The two major approaches to measuring the quality of infants' vocalizations consist of either comparing the sounds the baby produces to those that are typical at that age or calculating frequencies of occurrence of various categories of sounds. The first rough division of vocalizations into categories should include the following:

- No vocalizations
- Coos, screeches, grunts, clicks, raspberries, or other non-speech sounds with pitch or loudness changes (vocal play)
- Vocants or vowels
- Closants or consonants (e.g., prolonged nasals, trills, fricative-like sounds, etc.)
- Semi-rhythmic/non–speech-like CV combinations (marginal babble)
  - Closant + vocant
  - Consonant + vowel
- Rhythmic CV combinations (canonical babble)
  - Repetitive (reduplicated babble)
  - Varied (variegated babble)
- Non-meaningful speech-like vocalizations with speech-like prosody (jargon)
- Words

(Davis & Velleman, 2008)

With respect to determining whether a child's repertoire is age appropriate, there are a variety of published studies that have yielded the stages listed in the milestones section above. For more detail and clinical utility, Proctor (1989) developed a protocol for developmental vocal assessment. A modified, expanded version of her chart, which indicates what types of vocalizations, consonants, vowels, and vocal behaviors (e.g., vocal imitation) are considered typical at different ages between birth and 1 year, is included as Table 6-8.

As noted above, the proportion of babble that includes consonants is a key index of later language outcomes. One clinically useful measure of prelinguistic vocalizations that captures this factor is **Mean Babble Level** (Stoel-Gammon, 1989; Smith et al., 1989). For this metric, each vocalization that the child produces is ranked according to the number of different true consonants it contains:

Level 1: No true consonants: only vowels, glottals ([h, ʔ]), and/or glides

Examples: [ʔʌʔʌ], [wɑ], [ɛː]

Level 2: Only one true consonant, one or more times. Consonants that differ by voicing only (e.g., [p], [b]) count as the same consonant

Examples: [bɑ], [tiditu], [gugugugk]

Level 3: More than one true consonant, with consonants differing by more than voicing

Examples: [dɪp], [bɑki], [dʌdʌdʌdʌnʌ]

TABLE 6-8 **Vocal Development Checklist**

Child's Name:______________________ DOB:__________ Examiner:__________

Diagnosis:______________________

Medical Factors:______________________

Social Factors:______________________

Assessment Dates:

Date	Age (CA or GA)	Vocal Level	Comments

O: Observed R: Reported E: Emerging (use with O or R) C: Consonant V: Vowel

Stage 1: Birth to 2 Months

Rating	Behavior	Frequency/Transcription/Comments
O R E	Crying with sudden pitch shifts, extremely high pitch	
O R E	Fussing/discomfort	
O R E	Vegetative sounds (burps, feeding sounds)	
O R E	Neutral sounds (sighs, grunts)	
O R E	Ingressive vocalizations (vocalizing during inspiration)	
O R E	V-like sounds:	
	front V-like [i, ɪ, e, ɛ, æ]	
	mid V-like [ʌ, ə]	
	back V-like [u, ʊ, o, ɔ, a]	
O R E	C-like sounds [k, h, ʔ, g, x, j, l, r]	
O R E	Clicks, friction noises	
O R E	Trills (front, mid, back, uvular)	

Stage 2: 2 to 4 Months

Rating	Behavior	Frequency/Transcription/Comments
O R E	Marked decrease in crying after 12 weeks	
O R E	Transition from primarily reflexive sounds	
O R E	Differential vocalizations related to state and context	
O R E	Vocalizes responsively+	
O R E	Mainly V-like sounds: [i, ɪ, e, ɛ, æ, ʌ, ə, u, ʊ, ɔ, a]	
O R E	Occasional diphthongs	
O R E	Unrounded, often nasalized, central vowels	
O R E	Back V-like sounds frequent	
O R E	More C-like sounds emerge: [b, d, g, n, t, k, w, l, j, v, z, θ, h]	
O R E	Back/glottal C-like sounds [g, h, x, k, ʔ]	
O R E	More distinct friction sounds, trills	
O R E	Liquids (mainly trills)	
O R E	Voiced fricatives	
O R E	Nasals (syllabic nasals, nasalized vowels)	
O R E	Combinations of "C" with "V": coo/goo; [ʔʌ] or [gʊ]	
	single units (early stage 2)	
	in series/combination [əɣʊɣʊ] (mid-late stage 2)	

+: Not listed in original DVAP

TABLE 6-8 **Vocal Development Checklist (*Continued*)**

Stage 3: 4 to 6/7 Months

Rating	Behavior	Frequency/Transcription/Comments
O R E	Laughter emerges; voiced/voiceless alternations (haha)	
O R E	Vocal imitation (within own repertoire)+	
O R E	Pitch variations: rise, fall, fall-rise, rise-fall, rise-fall-rise	
O R E	Vocal play:	
	extreme pitch patterns	
	yell, squeal	
	low-pitched growl	
	variations in vocal quality	
	friction sounds: "raspberries," trills, smacks, snorts	
O R E	More varied V-like sounds [i, ɪ, e, ɛ, æ, ʌ, ə, u, ʊ, o, ɔ, a]	
O R E	# of C-like sounds increases:	
	English-like: [m, n, b, d, g, p, t, k, w, l, j, v, z, θ, h]	
	other: [ɣ, x, ʔ, ɸ, ɲ, ʀ, ɰ, ç, ɕ]	
O R E	Marginal babble:	
	phonation interrupted by one C-like sound	
	series of C-like interruptions to phonation	

+: Not listed in original DVAP

Stage 4: 6/7 to 10 Months

Rating	Behavior	Frequency/Transcription/Comments
O R E	Marked change: vocalizations far more speech-like overall	
O R E	Consistent variation of intonation contours	
O R E	Varied, distinct Vs [i, ɪ, e, ɛ, æ, ʌ, ə, u, ʊ, o, ɔ, a]	
O R E	Diphthongs increase [aɪ, oʊ, aʊ, eɪ]	
O R E	Cs increase with fully stopped stops	
	English-like: [m, n, b, d, g, p, t, k, w, l, j, v, z, θ, h]	
	other: [ɣ, x, ʔ, ɸ, ɲ, ʀ, ɰ, ç, ɕ, β, ʃ, ʒ, ð]	
O R E	Series of canonical babble syllables	
	reduplicated, rhythmic (babababa)	
	smooth transitions between C and V; between syllables	
	produced in turn-taking routines with caregiver+	
	syllabic imitation (within own repertoire)+	
	variegated: change in V or C within sequence*	
	jargon: speech-like intonation contour*	
O R E	Parents identify "first word" (e.g., mama) (10 mos.)*	

+: Not listed in original DVAP
*: May not emerge until next stage.

TABLE 6-8 Vocal Development Checklist (*Continued*)

Stage 5*: 10 to 12 *Months

Rating	Behavior	Frequency/Transcription/Comments
O R E	Sentence-like prosodic contours:	
	falling (as in declaratives)	
	steadily rising (as in Y/N questions)	
	sharp rise (as in imperatives)	
O R E	Increasingly varied more speech-like vocalizations:	
	variegated babble : change in V or C within sequence	
	speech-like intonation contour (jargon)	
	syllables not restricted to CV*	
	more fricatives and "other" C's in jargon+	
O R E	Meaningful vocal communication:	
	phonetically consistent forms (e.g., squeal at cat)+	
	approximations of single words	
	approximations of phrases (e.g., "I love you")+*	
	"fills in the blanks" in verbal routines (e.g., book)+*	

+: Not listed in original DVAP

*: May not emerge until next stage.

Voicing is not used to differentiate consonants for Mean Babble Level (MBL) for a couple of reasons. First of all, infants and toddlers are inconsistent in their productions of voice onset time without the clear-cut voiced and voiceless categories that they will eventually learn as appropriate to their language of exposure. Most likely as a result of this, transcribers are quite unreliable in their transcription of voicing in infant vocalizations. The infants' productions often fall on or near category boundaries, making it difficult for a transcriber to decide whether a voiced or voiceless consonant is being heard (Stoel-Gammon, 1989; Smith et al., 1989).

The child's MBL is the sum of the individual babble levels (1+1+2+3+2...) divided by the total number of babbles. Thus, the MBL will always add up to somewhere between 1.0 and 3.0. Table 6-9 gives approximate age expectations for MBL for children who are typically developing and for late talkers, based on several different studies.

In a meta-analysis of several studies, Morris (2010) concluded that lower-than-expected MBL levels indicate that the child is at risk of not developing meaningful speech by 24 months of age. For example, Fasolo, Majorano, and D'odorico (2008) demonstrated a significant relationship between MBL at 18 to 20 months and vocabulary at 24 months in Italian-learning children. Importantly, however, MBL values differ by language (Fasolo et al., 2008; Morris, 2010).

MBL is a useful tool for clinical settings as well as in research due to its simplicity and reliability. It is easy to learn to rank vocalizations in this way, even "online" (i.e., to keep a tally of a client's babble levels throughout a therapy session):

Level 1	Level 2	Level 3
𝍸 𝍸 𝍸	𝍸 III	II

$$(1 \times 15) + (2 \times 8) + (3 \times 2) = 37$$

$$37/25 = 1.48 = \text{MBL}$$

Thus, progress can be measured over time to document changes in the types of babbles that the at-risk baby is producing. The primary differences in babble quality that it documents are the number of true consonants in the babble and the distinction between reduplicated babble in which the same syllable is repeated (e.g., [didididi]) and variegated babble in which consonants (and vowels) vary from one syllable in the vocalization to the next ([didɑgumo]). Infants, including those with Down syndrome, are expected to produce approximately equal amounts of canonical and variegated babble throughout the prelinguistic period (Smith & Stoel-Gammon, 1996).

Several other babble measures have been used or suggested in research. These include the **C:V ratio**—the ratio of

TABLE 6-9 **Mean Babble Levels for Typically Developing and Late-Talking Infants and Toddlers Learning English**

Age (months)	MBL: Typically Developing	MBL: Late Talking
9	1.3	1.19
15	1.58	1.48
18	1.65	1.53
23	1.9	1.8

Based on data from Stoel-Gammon, C. (1989). Prespeech and early speech development of two late talkers. *First Language, 9*, 207–224; Thal, D., Oroz, M., & McCaw, V. (1995). Phonological and lexical development in normal and late-talking toddlers. *Applied Psycholinguistics, 16*, 407–424; Fasolo, M., Majorano, M., & D'odorico, L. (2008). Babbling and first words in children with slow expressive language development. *Clinical Linguistics & Phonetics, 22*, 83-94; Morris, S. R. (2010). Clinical application of the mean babbling level and syllable structure level. *Language, Speech, and Hearing in Schools, 41*(2), 223–230.

number of consonants or closants used divided by the number of vowels or vocants used (a.k.a., the "closant curve"). Based on small samples, this ratio tends to increase from approximately 0.8 at 10 to 11 months up to 1.3/1.4 between 20 and 28 months (Robb & Bauer, 1991). A similar measure is the **babbling ratio**—the proportion of the child's syllables that are of consonant + vowel form (i.e., the number of CV syllables divided by the total number of syllables produced). Oller and Eilers (1988) proposed a cutoff of 0.2 as the criterion for the onset of canonical babbling; when 20% of the infant's syllables are CV (i.e., include a true consonant), the infant has entered the canonical babble stage. In Kent and Bauer's (1985) study of five typically developing 13-month-olds, approximately 38% of the participants' speech vocalizations included CV syllables. The vocalizations themselves ranged from V alone (60% of vocalizations), CV alone (19%), and VC alone (2%) to VCVCV (1%). In other words, 80% of the vocalizations were monosyllabic. It is important to note that these results were based on infants exposed to English; results would likely be quite different for children from different language backgrounds.

All three of these measures focus on the frequency at which the baby produces true consonants. MBL also takes variety into account in differentiating Levels 2 and 3: to be a Level 3 babble, the vocalization must include two different consonants. However, a child could have a mean babble level of 3 by producing, for example, [bidi] many times. This is not a hypothetical problem; some toddlers are limited to just a few vocalizations that they produce repeatedly (sometimes even ad nauseum) throughout the day. Thus, it is important to measure the diversity of a child's vocalizations as a group, not just the diversity that occurs within a given vocalization.

One simple measure of diversity is calculated just by counting the number of different consonants (or vowels) the baby produces. Stoel-Gammon (1988) reported that children with normal hearing who were studied from ages 4 to 18 months demonstrated an increase of consonant types from 4.5 to 8.7. In contrast, infants with severe to profound hearing impairment actually decreased from 4.3 to 3.2 consonant types during the same time period. Of course, when using a measure such as this, it is important to control for a child's volubility; otherwise, a child who produces 10 different consonants in 20 utterances will receive a higher score than would a child who produces the same 10 different consonants in 150 utterances.

To address vocal variety with more validity, Bauer (1988) proposed two phonetic diversity measures: **Consonant diversity** is calculated by dividing the number of different consonants (i.e., the number of consonant types) the child produced by the total number of consonants produced (i.e., the number of consonant tokens) in the sample. Similarly, **vowel diversity** is calculated by dividing the number of vowel types the child produced by the number of vowel tokens produced during the sample. Measures such as these have been helpful in demonstrating that, for example, 15-month-olds with cleft palate demonstrate less phonetic diversity than do their typically developing peers (Salas-Provance, Kuehn, & Marsh, 2003).

Finally, given the reports about ballistic syllables by Davis and colleagues (Davis & MacNeilage, 1990; Davis & MacNeilage, 1995; MacNeilage & Davis, 2000; MacNeilage, et al., 2000), it is important to consider syllable diversity—the number of different combinations of consonants and vowels that the child produces. For example, does the infant always use labials with the low back vowel [ɑ], or do labial consonants combine with a variety of different vowels? An infant who only babbles [bɑ] and [di], for example, is less advanced than is one who also babbles [bi] and [dɑ].

Jakielski (2000) and Jakielski, Maytasse, and Doyle (2006) developed a measure of the overall sophistication of a child's early words, the **Index of Phonetic Complexity** (IPC). Rules for calculating this measure are given in Table 6-10. Despite its name (the word "phonetic"), this tool includes syllable and word shapes as well as vowel and consonant types. Points are given for the use of more complex sounds (such as velars and fricatives) and sound combinations (such as clusters and multisyllabic words). Morris (2009) demonstrated that the IPC has good test–retest reliability.

The usefulness of this index has been shown in several research studies. For example, Jakielski and colleagues (2006) demonstrated increases in IPC values by age, especially between 20 and 27 months, when IPC values jumped from a mean of 1.26 at 20 to 23 months to a mean of 2.21 at 24 to 27 months. Calvo and Furey (2007) and Furey and Owen (2008) demonstrated gradual increases in the IPC values of both the target words attempted by 12- to 18-month-olds and also their actual productions of those words. Twenty-three 12-month-olds from lower and middle socioeconomic status (SES) families exhibited IPCs ranging from 0 (no word attempts) to 2.26 with a mean of slightly less than 1.0.

TABLE 6-10 Index of Phonetic Complexity

Points Assigned for:	No Points for:	One Point Each for:
Consonant by place	Labials Coronals	Dorsals (velars)
Consonant by manner	Stops Nasals Glides	Fricatives Affricates Liquids
Vowel by class	Monophthongs Diphthongs	Rhotics
Word shape	Ends with a vowel	Ends with a consonant
Word length in syllables	Monosyllables Disyllables	Three + syllables
Singleton consonants place variation	Reduplication	Variegated by place
Contiguous consonants	No clusters	Consonant clusters
Cluster by type	**Homorganic**	**Heterorganic**

Examples of word complexity ratings:
"Mommy" = 0 points
"Coat" = 1 point
"Horse" = 3 points
"Pizza" = 2 points
"School" = 5 points

From Jakielski, K. J. (2000). *Quantifying phonetic complexity in words: An experimental index.* Paper presented at the International Child Phonology Conference, University of Northern Iowa; Jakielski, K. J., Maytasse, R., & Doyle, E. (2006). *Acquisition of phonetic complexity in children 12-36 months of age.* Paper presented at the American Speech-Language-Hearing Association, Miami, FL.

TABLE 6-11 Word Complexity Measure

Feature	Number of Points Possible	Number of Points Earned
More than two syllables	1 per word	
Unstressed first syllable	1 per word	
Final consonant	1 per word	
Cluster	1 per cluster	
Velar	1 point each	
Liquid (including syllabics)	1 point each	
Rhotic vowel	1 point each	
Fricative	1 point each	
Affricate	1 point each	
Fricative or affricate is voiced	1 extra point each	
Total points	~~~~~~~	

From Stoel-Gammon, C. (2010). The Word Complexity Measure: Description and application to developmental phonology and disorders. *Clinical Linguistics and Phonetics, 24*(4–5), 271–282.

The same children at 18 months of age had IPC values that ranged from 0.40 to 2.62 with a mean of about 1.5. There was a consistent gap between the IPC values of the targets (the words the children were trying to produce as pronounced by an adult) and the productions (the forms they actually produced). Differences were not noted in these studies between children from low SES families versus those from middle-income families.

Furey and Harrold (2009) demonstrated that a great deal (20%) of the phonetic complexity in both children's targets and their productions, as measured by IPC, is attributable to challenging manner classes (e.g., fricatives). Word shapes (e.g., presence of clusters, number of syllables per word) accounted for another 20% of the complexity in the children's targets. One specific aspect of word shape, the use of non-homorganic consonant clusters (i.e., clusters in which the two consonants are from different places of articulation), accounted for another 20% of the complexity in the children's actual productions.

Stoel-Gammon's (2010) **Word Complexity Measure** also takes into account not only the complexity of the consonants that the child produces but also the syllable and word structures produced. For example, extra points are given for clusters, final consonants, and iambic stress patterns (i.e., a produced unstressed first syllable) as well as for affricates and liquids. The rules for this measure are given in Table 6-11. The vocalizations of three 17-month-olds had WCM values ranging from 0.60 to 1.02. Those of two toddlers who were 21 and 22 months old were 0.93 and 1.49, respectively.

Although MBL, IPC, and WCM can all be used for children who are not yet producing words, both IPC and WCM have been used to study early word productions as well. Some other tools can be used only for children who are speaking in words. For instance, Ingram (1992) developed the **Phonological Mean Length of Utterance** (PMLU) as a comprehensive tool to compare to the traditional mean length of utterance that is measured in morphemes. However, unlike IPC and WCM, this measure is based only on segments, not syllable or word shapes. It consists of counting one point for every consonant or vowel that the child produces in the word (but not more than the total number of segments in the target word) plus one additional point for every consonant that is correct (but not for vowels). Because it does not consider phonotactics, it does not "reward" children who rise to the language's structural challenges by producing final consonants, clusters, and multisyllabic words. Therefore, the correct production of a word like "banana" receives the same number of points (3 consonants + 3 vowels + 3 consonants correct = 9) as a word like "splash" (4 consonants + 1 vowel + 4 consonants correct = 9). This is a serious limitation of this PMLU measure.

Paul and Jennings (1992) extended MBL to real words and word-like utterances as well as babbles. They added consonant clusters to Level 3 and named this modified measure **Syllable Structure Level** (SSL). Morris (2009) then demonstrated that "syllable structure level" has good test–retest reliability. When this measure was applied to the intelligible speech of late talkers versus language age-matched children who were typically developing (TD) (and therefore younger) by Paul and Jennings (1992), the late talkers (LT) actually had higher SSLs. However, the later talkers' mean babble levels (which did not include word attempts) were lower. Pharr, Ratner, and Rescorla (2000), on the other hand, identified differences between LTs and age-matched peers who were TD. In this case, the TD children performed better (e.g., mean SSL of 2.18 for TD children versus 1.43 for LT children at 24 months; 2.39 for TD versus 2.19 for LT at 36 months). The differences between these two studies no doubt result from matching the groups by language age (in which case the older LTs did better) versus chronologic age (in which case the more linguistically advanced TDs did better).

O'Connor, Velleman, McGloin, Connelly, and Mervis (2010) used a variety of babble measures to compare five pairs of children between 1;9 and 3;1 who were matched for age and roughly for developmental level (as measured by the Mullen Scales of Early Learning; Mullen 1995). In each pair, one child had Williams syndrome (WS) and the other had 7q11.23 Duplication syndrome (Dup7). Two of the pairs of children were compared at two different ages (1;9 versus 3;0 in one case; 2;0 versus. 3;0 in the other). Overall, the children with WS outperformed the children with Dup7 on all measures. With just a few exceptions, they were more voluble (i.e., they produced more words and more syllables per half-hour session) and their MBL, IPC, WCM, and PMLU scores were higher. The two children with Dup7 whose speech was analyzed twice were responsible for several of the exceptions at age 1;9 to 2;0, but they both lost significant ground in comparison to their WS matches at age 3. The authors drew two conclusions. First, children with Dup7 are at significant risk of speech delay, which does not dissipate over time even if intervention is provided (as is typically the case for children with WS). Secondly, none of the measures of phonological complexity proved to be more enlightening than the others overall when applied to this limited sample of five pairs of children.

EXERCISE 6-3

Prespeech and Early Speech Assessment

TREATMENT

We focus here on treatment for vocal means (i.e., strategies for increasing the quantity and quality of vocalizations that an infant or toddler or a severely impaired older child produces). However, this emphasis should not be taken to imply that other aspects of communication—especially communicative intent (a.k.a. communication motivation; see Chapter 3)—are not important.

As ironic as it may seem, providing non-vocal communication modalities for children who cannot or do not yet communicate orally is often the most useful first step toward speech. Parents often fear that if their children are taught alternatives to oral communication, they will choose never to communicate orally. Of course, family's preferences must always be respected. However, the use of sign language, picture exchange (PECS), or simple electronic devices does not decrease the likelihood that a child will establish oral communication. On the contrary, it is likely to not only enhance the child's overall communicative effectiveness, thus markedly decreasing frustration and increasing learning opportunities, but also to increase oral communication capacities (Millar, Light, & Schlosser, 2006; DeThorne, Johnson, Walder, & Mahurin-Smith, 2009; Oommen & McCarthy, 2014).

At the same time, speech should also be a primary focus at these young ages—even for children who are likely to remain partially reliant upon non-oral communication systems. For some children, this may mean shaping vocalizations that don't appear to be meaningful, don't sound like words, or both so that they become more speech-like and associated with meanings. This starts with identifying the potential meanings of any vocalizations that the child produces and reinforcing them, even if they are quite rudimentary and atypical (Zubow & Hurtig, 2014). Building upon whatever vocalizations the child may have, even if they are not speech-like, is the first step. These productions should be brought under the child's voluntary control and each associated with a particular meaning in order to reinforce the concept that speech is an effective means of interaction and achieving one's ends. Modeling and reinforcing such sound–meaning associations as a grunt when moving a heavy object (McCune et al., 1996), a hissing sound while pretending to spray a hose, or snoring while pretending to sleep will stimulate the child to use available non-speech vocalization capacities to communicate. These stimulations are used in a meaningful context and incorporate means, motive, and opportunity for the purpose of encouraging meaningful oral communication.

DeThorne and colleagues (2009) also recommend minimizing communication pressure. For children with Childhood Apraxia of Speech, especially, "automatic" (non-conscious) speech is easier than that which is elicited (Velleman & Strand, 1994; Velleman, 2003). The more the focus is on the child's speech, the less likely she is to speak. Imitating the child's vocalizations—also known as phonetic contingency (Velleman, Mangipudi, & Locke, 1989)—reinforces her productions and keeps the interaction going in a positive way. Speaking with somewhat exaggerated intonation and a slightly slowed rate—although speech should be neither over-intoned nor slowed to such an extent that sounds are distorted—and providing multisensory input and feedback are also very helpful (DeThorne et al., 2009).

Voluntary differentiated control of specific speech motor programs (so that various vocalizations can be identified as distinct from each other; see Chapter 5) is augmented by maximizing the number of specific uses of the targeted forms per session in a meaningful, playful way (such as saying "cup, cup, cup" while setting the table or "moo, moo, moo" while playing with toy cows). Once the child is able and willing to produce a certain vocalization in a certain context, it can be shaped using adapted principles of motor learning (see Chapter 5 and Davis & Velleman, 2008) into a more refined, word-like utterance.

If the child's vocalizations do not incorporate speech-like rhythm (e.g., are marginal babble), modeling canonical vocalizations paired with rhythmic movement (e.g., banging or bouncing) can be helpful. To encourage the transition from canonical babble-like vocalizations to jargon-like babble, songs can be sung using simple syllables (e.g., ba, ba, ba) instead of words. Repetitions of real words with CV shapes (e.g., "go, go, go") can also be paired with appealing activities (Davis & Velleman, 2008). At this level, it is important to model speech-like rhythms and prosody rather than stereotyped, robotic patterns.

For children who do not produce any consonants, meaningful consonant-alone vocalizations may be an appropriate first goal. These could include, for example, "shhh" and "mmmm." In addition, many emotional words are composed of glottals and glides combined with vowels: "uh-oh," "yeah," "wow," "whee," and "haha." Once the clients can approximate these, then the goal becomes other meaningful CV and VC syllables with early occurring consonants ([b], [p], [m], [n], [w]) (Davis & Velleman, 2008).

GOAL-WRITING

Recall that goals do not have to be "with 90% accuracy." The concept of accuracy is often nonsensical at this level; how can babble be accurate? Alternative goals include the following:

- Will produce __# of different consonants/vowels/syllables per session/vocalization/word-like unit
- Will produce __# different identifiable words per session
- Will produce syllables with true consonants __% of the time
- Will produce vocalizations with communicative intent __% of the time
- Will produce core vocabulary words with target consistent forms __% of the time

Homonymy, the same production corresponding to a variety of meanings, and variability, the same word pronounced inconsistently from time to time, often contribute to the unintelligibility of very young children and children with severe SSDs (as discussed at much greater length in Chapter 7). In the case of homonymy (e.g., [bɑ] used to mean "ball," "bottle," "baby," and "bath"), the goal is to split the overused production into one different form per meaning. Often, the homonymy is the result of a template, a pattern such as reduplication or harmony, that the child imposes on all or most words. In this case, different patterns need to be introduced through modeling and selective responding. For example, if the child uses [bɑ] and [bɑbɑ] interchangeably for both "ball" and "bottle," the adults in her environment should respond as if she always means "ball" when she says [bɑ] and "bottle" when she says [bɑbɑ] to help her learn that the number of syllables in a word matters. Of course, both words should always be modeled correctly even though these approximations are accepted when the child produces them.

COMMON *Confusion*

VARIABILITY VERSUS VARIETY

Variability refers to a type of inconsistency: one sound or word produced in many different ways. As such, variability interferes with intelligibility because the form of the word is unpredictable. Parents of children whose words are significantly misproduced but consistent are far more able to learn to understand their offspring than are those whose children's productions are inconsistent.

If it is present on a long-term basis, variability is a negative feature of a child's phonological system and is an appropriate target for remediation. On a short-term basis, variability may indicate that the child's system is undergoing change—for the better, it is hoped. For example, a child who produces "thumb" variably as [fʌm], [sʌm], and [tʌm] is likely aware that /f/ and /θ/ are different phonemes, but hasn't figured out how to pronounce [θ] yet. In such a situation, variability may be viewed as a positive sign of ongoing change.

Variety refers to the size of the child's repertoire of sounds or words. The more elements the child has at her disposal, the more different meanings she will be able to express (assuming that the sounds are used distinctly and appropriately). For example, one can form far more different words with 12 consonants and four vowels than with only two consonants and two vowels. Variety also refers to the number of different consonants and vowels or of different syllable shapes that children can incorporate into the same word (thus avoiding reduplication, or consonant or vowel harmony). Thus, variety is a desirable aspect of a child's phonological system.

The more variety within the repertoire, the more communication opportunities are available. The more variability the child exhibits, the harder it will be for the listener to determine her intended message. Thus, in general:

VARIABILITY INTERFERES WITH COMMUNICATION.
VARIETY ENHANCES COMMUNICATION.

Selective responding can also be used when excessive variability is the problem: for example, only [bɑ]—not [bʌ], [dɑ], [ɑ]—etc., is taken to mean "ball." Again, maximizing production opportunities can help the child develop more stable motor patterns for producing individual words.

EXERCISE 6-4

Prespeech and Early Speech Intervention

SUMMARY

In summary, an infant at the threshold of word learning is by no means a "tabula rasa" (blank slate), as once assumed. An extensive foundation for meaningful speech already has been laid by his perceptual and production experience in the languages to which he has been exposed. For children who are not able to benefit sufficiently from "incidental" exposure to language, many strategies are available for stabilizing motor patterns, maximizing implicit learning, and encouraging vocal communication.

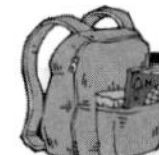

KEY TAKE-HOME MESSAGES

1. Prelinguistic vocalizations lay the foundation for early speech development.
2. Early linguistic, cognitive, and social development are interrelated.
3. Frequency of use of "true consonants" in early vocalizations is especially predictive of later speech skills.
4. A variety of measures of early speech have been developed to quantify a child's progress during this developmental time period.
5. Variability interferes with communication; variety enhances communication.
6. It is not necessary to choose between stimulating oral and non-oral forms of communication; enhancing communication in either modality facilitates the development of both.
7. Early speech sound intervention goals focus on communication and developing a phonological system.

CHAPTER 6

Beginnings: Pre-Speech and First Words Review

Exercise 6-1

A. Essay question: Why is it important to begin speech-language intervention before the child begins producing words? Use sources from this chapter and/or other evidence-based literature to support your answer.

B. Multiple choice: Choose the best answer.

1. Infants' volubility levels are correlated with:
   a. hearing loss.
   b. socioeconomic status.
   c. cleft palate.
   d. number of true consonants.
2. Which is an expected order of emergence of vocalization types?
   a. Phonation, vocal play, canonical babble
   b. Canonical babble, jargon, phonation
   c. Vegetative, jargon, phonation
   d. Phonation, vocal play, vegetative

Exercise 6-2

A. Essay question: Linguist Werner Jakobson believed that babble and word production were unrelated and that the nature of babble was universal (i.e., all infants' babble repertoires are the same). Argue otherwise, using sources from this chapter and/or other evidence-based literature.

B. Multiple choice: Choose the best answer.

1. Which of the following is not an important influence on infant speech perception and production?
   a. Mastication
   b. Human physiology
   c. The ambient language
   d. Personal experiences and preferences
2. Babies babble:
   a. all of the sounds of the languages of the world.
   b. only in response to infant-directed speech.
   c. based in part on words to which they have been exposed.
   d. the same regardless of the language they hear.

C. 1. Consider the following data from the babble and early words of Emma (Studdert-Kennedy & Goodell, 1992).

Favorite babbles: [ɑbinəbinə] [bedəbedə] (and similar combinations)

Early words:

- "berry, bird, booster" [bu:di:]
- "pillow, playdough" [be:də]
- "airplane" [ɑpi:n]
- "tomato" [me:nə]
- "raisin" [we:di:]
- "Happy birthday, cranberry, raspberry" [ɑbu:di:]

Questions:

a. What is the articulatory pattern underlying Emma's favorite babbles and early words?

b. What implications do these data have for theories about the impact of prelinguistic vocalizations on speech (i.e., word production) development?

2. Consider the following data from Marina, aged 3;11 (Velleman, 1994)

Fish	[dɪs]
Mom	[mɑm] (not stimulable for 'mommy'
Paula	[bɑwɑ]
Baby	[bɑbɑ, didi] (not stimulable for [bɑbi] or [bebi]

Questions:

a. What are the syllable types that Marina does/does not produce?

b. Do these data support the Davis and MacNeilage theory of ballistic syllables? Why or why not?

Exercise 6-3

A. *Case study questions.*

1. Chuckie, a 2-year-old, vocalizes frequently. However, he relies almost exclusively on his "favorite babble" [əwɑwɑwɑ] in almost all situations. His very few other vocalizations are also reduplicated—the same syllable repeated multiple times. Only one of these appears to have meaning: he typically says [dɑdɑdɑ] when he sees his father coming home from work. However, he has invented a set of gestures and signs to express other meanings. For example, he "knocks" on his head with his knuckles when someone comes to the front door, holds his hand up to his ear when the phone rings, and shakes his hand as if in pain to comment that something is hot. Should his parents be concerned about his speech development? Use information from this and other chapters and/or other sources to justify your answer.
2. Keesha, a 36-month-old who had a perinatal stroke, is sent to you for an evaluation of her speech. She vocalizes using true consonants and full vowels, but has no meaningful speech. The diagnostic question is whether speech production limitations are a factor in her communication delay. You can use one of the assessment tools described in this chapter to address this question. Which would you use, and why? What other factors would you assess for and why? Justify your answer using sources cited in this chapter, Chapter 3, and/or other evidence-based literature.
3. Kelly is 24 months old and vocalizes rarely. Her utterances do not appear to have specific meanings. Consider her total vocalizations from a 30-minute play session:

[bʊtʊ]	[beme]
[dæ]	[tæʔ]
[ʌbɛbi]	[ʌmæməm]
[ʌbɛbʊ]	[dɑtɑtɑ]
[heɪ]	[ʌbʊbʊ]
[ʌjɛjɛ]	[ʌbɑpi]

Questions:

a. Is Kelly's volubility typical for her age? Explain.

b. Calculate Kelly's mean babble level. Is it age appropriate (as far as you can tell from this limited sample)?

c. How many different consonant types did she produce?

d. What is her index of phonetic complexity score? Is it age appropriate (as far as you can tell from this limited sample)?

Multiple choice: Choose the best answer.

1. Kelly's MBL is:
   a. 1.0.
   b. 1.5.
   c. 2.5.
   d. 2.0.
2. Kelly's babble is predominantly:
   a. canonical.
   b. linguistic.
   c. marginal.
   d. jargon.

B. *Multiple choice: Choose the best answer.*

1. Which measure is not appropriate for tracking prelinguistic vocal development (i.e., babble)?
   a. Word complexity measure
   b. Phonological mean length of utterance
   c. Mean babble level
   d. Index of Phonetic Complexity
2. Which measure does take phonotactic variety into account?
   a. Phonological mean length of utterance
   b. Mean babble level
   c. Index of Phonetic Complexity
   d. Consonant variety
3. Evidence that a given child has rule-governed phonology does not include:
   a. variability from word to word.
   b. apparent regression.
   c. templates.
   d. avoidance of certain patterns.
4. Signs of atypical phonological development in the prelinguistic period may include:
   a. frozen forms.
   b. phonological idioms.
   c. decreased volubility.
   d. apparent regression.

Exercise 6-4

A. Case study questions.

1. By completing the evaluation described in Exercise 6-3, you discover that Keesha has (a) a small consonant repertoire, (b) a small vowel repertoire, (c) primarily vowel-only syllables, and (d) a favorite babble pattern ([ʔuʔoʔuʔo]) that she produces constantly. In addition, she lacks the "naming insight:" the realization that speech sounds can communicate meaning. Write three goals for the child, each with two objectives, including strategies that you would use to address them and rationales for both the goals and the strategies.
2. Use the below transcript from Bobby to answer the questions. Assume that Bobby's multisyllabic vocalizations are rhythmic in a speech-like way.
   1. What is Bobby's approximate vocal age (based upon the DVAP in Table 6-8)?
   2. What prelinguistic vocal stage is Bobby at?
   3. What is Bobby's mean babble level?
   4. What are Bobby's relative strengths? His relative weaknesses?
   5. Write two goals for Bobby. Describe your first intervention session with him.

1. [bʊbʊ]
2. [no]
3. [tʌʔ]
4. [ʊpʊ]
5. [ɑnɑ]
6. [jæ]
7. [bɛdɛ]
8. [heɪ]
9. [ɣi]
10. [βeβe]
11. [dʌ]
12. [əbɛbʊ]
13. [wæwæ]
14. [dʊ]
15. [tɑ]
16. [bɪ]
17. [tʌɣʌ]
18. [bʊdi]
19. [bɛ]
20. [dit]
21. [ɑɪ]
22. [mʌ]
23. [əbebi]
24. [əmʌm]
25. [bʊɣʊ]
26. [bɔ]
27. [ðɑʊ]
28. [mi]
29. [ðo]
30. [mipi]
31. [hæhæ]
32. [dʊ]
33. [bɑ]
34. [bɑβɑ]
35. [tɛnɛ]
36. [dik]
37. [əjɛjɛ]
38. [et]
39. [əpæpi]
40. [əbɑbɑ]
41. [wɛdɛ]
42. [pʊ]
43. [nʊ]
44. [bɑpɑ]
45. [bɑbɑ]
46. [əbubu]
47. [dɑnɑ]
48. [əðɛðɑɪ]
49. [tætæ]
50. [ju]

Note: The voiced fricatives [β, ð, ɣ] should be considered closants, not consonants, in this context.

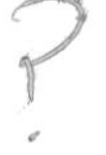

B. Multiple choice: Choose the best answer.

1. Which of the following would be an appropriate therapy goal for a child with no meaningful vocalizations?
   a. Increase non-vocal communication.
   b. Increase homonymy.
   c. Increase variability.
   d. Increase monotony.
2. Therapy for a child with no meaningful vocalizations might include:
   a. modeling communicative grunts.
   b. modeling sound effects.
   c. modeling emotion words.
   d. All of the above.
3. Variability:
   a. may interfere with communication.
   b. is an indicator of motor control.
   c. is the same as variety.
   d. rarely occurs in typically developing children.

References

Bates, E., Thal, D., Aram, D., Nass, R., & Trauner, D. (1997). From first words to grammar in children with focal brain injury. *Developmental Neuropsychology, 13*, 239–274. Special Issue on Origins of Language Disorders.

Bauer, H. R. (1988). The ethological model of phonetic development: I. Phonetic contrast estimators. *Clinical Linguistics & Phonetics, 2*(4), 347–380.

Bayley, N. (2006). *Bayley scales of infant and toddler development: Bayley-III.* Harcourt Assessment, Psych. Corporation.

Bloom, K. (1988). Quality of adult vocalizations affects the quality of infant vocalizations. *Journal of Child Language, 15*(3), 469–480.

Bloom, K., Russell, A., & Wassenberg, K. (1987).Turn taking affects the quality of infant vocalizations. *Journal of Child Language, 14*(2), 211–227.

Boysson-Bardies, B. D., & Vihman, M. M. (1991). Adaptation to language: Evidence from babbling and first words in four languages. *Language, 67*, 297–319.

Boysson-Bardies, B. D., Halle, P., Sagart, L., & Durand, C. (1989). A cross-linguistic investigation of vowel formants in babbling. *Journal of Child Language, 16*, 1–17.

Calvo, J., & Furey, J. E. (2007). *Phonetic complexity in words targeted by children from 12 to 18 months of age.* Paper presented at the American Speech-Language-Hearing Association, Boston, MA.

Caselli, M. C. (1990). Communicative gestures and first words. In V. Volterra & C. J. Erting (Eds.), *From gesture to language in hearing and deaf children* (pp. 56–67). New York, NY: Springer-Verlag.

Chapman, K. L., Hardin-Jones, M., Schulte, J., & Halter, K. A. (2001). Vocal development of 9-month-old babies with cleft palate. *Journal of Speech, Language, and Hearing Research, 44*, 1268–1283.

Chen, L.-M., & Kent, R. D. (2005). Consonant-vowel co-occurrence patterns in Mandarin-learning infants. *Journal of Child Language, 32*, 507–534.

Chomsky, N. (1975). *Reflections on language.* New York, NY: Pantheon.

Clement, C. J. (2004). *Development of vocalizations in deaf and normally hearing infants.* (Doctoral Dissertation), Netherlands Graduate School of Linguistics, Amsterdam.

Crais, E. R. (2011). Testing and beyond: Strategies and tools for evaluating and assessing infants and toddlers. *Language, Speech, and Hearing Services in the Schools, 42*, 341–364.

Davis, B. L., & MacNeilage, P. F. (1990). Acquisition of correct vowel production: A quantitative case study. *Journal of Speech and Hearing Research, 33*(1), 16–27.

Davis, B., & MacNeilage, P. (1995). The articulatory basis of babbling. *Journal of Speech and Hearing Research, 38*, 1199–1211.

Davis, B. L., & Velleman, S. L. (2008). Establishing a basic speech repertoire without using NSOME: Means, motive, and opportunity. *Seminars in Speech and Language, 29*(4), 312–319.

DeThorne, L. S., Johnson, C. J., Walder, L., & Mahurin-Smith, J. (2009). When "Simon Says" doesn't work: Alternatives to imitation for facilitating early speech development. *American Journal of Speech-Language Pathology, 18*, 133–145.

Docherty, G. J., Foulkes, P., Tillotson, J., & Watt, D. J. L. (2006). On the scope of phonological learning: Issues arising from socially structured variation. In L. Goldstein, D. Whalen, & C. Best (Eds.), *Laboratory Phonology, 8* (pp. 393-421). Berlin, Germany: Mouton de Gruyter.

Dore, J., Franklin, M. B., Miller, R. T., & Ramer, A. L. H. (1976). Transitional phenomena in early language acquisition. *Journal of Child Language, 3*(1), 13–28.

Fagan, M. K. (2014). Frequency of vocalization before and after cochlear implantation: Dynamic effect of auditory feedback on infant behavior. *Journal of Experimental Child Psychology, 126*, 328-338.

Fasolo, M., Majorano, M., & D'odorico, L. (2008). Babbling and first words in children with slow expressive language development. *Clinical Linguistics & Phonetics, 22*, 83-94.

Furey, J. E., & Harrold, K. (2009). *Early words: What factors add complexity?* Paper presented at the International Child Phonology Conference, Austin, TX.

Furey, J. E., & Owen, A. (2008). *Phonetic complexity of toddlers' early words.* Paper presented at the American Speech-Language-Hearing Association, Chicago, IL.

Gildersleeve-Neumann, C., Davis, B. L., & MacNeilage, P. F. (2000). Contingencies governing the acquisition of fricatives, affricates, and liquids. *Applied Psycholinguistics, 21*, 341–363.

Hart, B., & Risley, T. R. (1995). *Meaningful differences in the everyday experience of young American children.* Baltimore, MD: Brookes.

Highman, C., Hennessey, N. W., Leitao, S., & Piek, J. P. (2013). Early development in infants at risk of childhood apraxia of speech: A longitudinal investigation. *Developmental Neuropsychology, 38*(3), 197–210.

Holmgren, K., Lindblom, B., Aurelius, G., Jalling, B., & Zetterstrom, R. (1986). On the phonetics of infant vocalization. In B. Lindblom & R. Zetterstrom (Eds.), *Precursors of early speech* (pp. 51–63). New York, NY: Stockton Press.

Ingram, D. (1992). Early phonological acquisition: A cross-linguistic perspective. In C. A. Ferguson, L. Menn & C. Stoel-Gammon (Eds.), *Phonological development: Models, research, implications* (pp. 423–435). Timonium, MD: York Press.

Iyer, S. N., & Oller, D. K. (2008). Prelinguistic vocal development in infants with typical hearing and infants with severe-to-profound hearing loss. *The Volta Review, 108*(2), 115–138.

Jakielski, K. J. (2000). *Quantifying phonetic complexity in words: An experimental index.* Paper presented at the International Child Phonology Conference, University of Northern Iowa.

Jakielski, K. J., Maytasse, R., & Doyle, E. (2006). *Acquisition of phonetic complexity in children 12-36 months of age.* Paper presented at the American Speech-Language-Hearing Association, Miami, FL.

Jakobson, R. (1968). *Child language, aphasia, and phonological universals* (A. R. Keiler, Trans.). The Hague, Netherlands: Mouton.

Kent, R. D., & Bauer, H. R. (1985). Vocalizations of one-year-olds. *Journal of Child Language, 12*, 491–526.

Kuhl, P. K., & Meltzoff, A. N. (1996). Infant vocalizations in response to speech: Vocal imitation and developmental change. *Journal of the Acoustical Society of America, 100*(4, Part 1), 2425–2438.

Lee, S. A., Davis, B., & MacNeilage, P. (2010). Universal production patterns and ambient language influences in babbling: A cross-linguistic study of Korean- and English-learning infants. *Journal of Child Language, 37*, 293–318.

Leonard, L. B. (1992). Models of phonological development and children with phonological disorders. In C. A. Ferguson, L. Menn, & C. Stoel-Gammon (Eds.), *Phonological development: Models, research, implications* (pp. 495–508). Timonium, MD: York Press.

Leonard, L. B., & McGregor, K. K. (1991). Unusual phonological patterns and their underlying representations: A case study. *Journal of Child Language, 18*(2), 261–272.

Leonard, L., Devescovi, A., & Ossella, T. (1987). Context-sensitive phonological patterns in children with poor intelligibility. *Child Language Teaching and Therapy, 3*(2), 125–132.

Leopold, W. (1939). *Speech development of a bilingual child: A linguist's record* (Volume I: Vocabulary growth in the first two years). Evanston, IL: Northwestern University Press.

Leopold, W. (1947). *Speech development of a bilingual child: A linguist's record* (Volume II: Sound learning in the first two years). Evanston, IL: Northwestern University Press.

Locke, J. L. (1983). *Phonological acquisition and change.* New York, NY: Academic Press.

Lotto, A. J., Kluender, K. R., & Holt, L. L. (2000). Effects of language experience on organization of vowel sounds. In M. Broe & J. Pierrehumbert (Eds.), *Laboratory phonology V: Language acquisition and the lexicon* (pp. 219–228). Cambridge, UK: Cambridge University Press.

Macken, M. A. (1995). Phonological acquisition. In J. A. Goldsmith (Ed.), *The handbook of phonological theory* (pp. 671–698). Oxford, UK: Blackwell.

MacNeilage, P. F., & Davis, B. L. (2000). On the origin of internal structure of word forms. *Science, 288*, 527–531.

MacNeilage, P. F., Davis, B. L., Kinney, A., & Matyear, C. L. (2000). The motor core of speech: A comparison of serial organization patterns in infants and languages. *Child Development, 71*(1), 153–163.

Maddieson, I. (1984). *Patterns of sounds.* Cambridge, UK: Cambridge University Press.

Masataka, N. (1993). Effects of contingent and noncontingent maternal stimulation on the vocal behavior of three-to-four month-old Japanese infants. *Journal of Child Language, 20*(2), 303–312.

McCathren, R. B., Yoder, P. J., & Warren, S. F. (1999). The relationship between prelinguistic vocalization and later expressive vocabulary in young children with developmental delay. *Journal of Speech, Language, and Hearing Research, 42*, 915–924.

McCathren, R. B., Yoder, P. J., & Warren, S. F. (2000). Testing predictive validity of the communication composite of the communication and symbolic behavior scales. *Journal of Early Intervention, 23*(1), 36–46.

McCune, L., & Vihman, M. M. (1987). Vocal motor schemes. *Papers and Reports on Child Language Development, 26*, 72–79.

McCune, L., Vihman, M. M., Roug-Hellichius, L., Delery, D. B., & Gogate, L. (1996). Grunt communication in human infants (Homo sapiens). *Journal of Comparative Psychology, 110*(1), 27–37.

Meier, R. P., McGarvin, L., Zakia, R. A., & Willerman, R. (1997). Silent mandibular oscillations in vocal babbling. *Phonetica, 54*(3–4), 153–171.

Menn, L. (1978). Phonological units in beginning speech. In A. Bell & J. B. Hooper (Eds.), *Syllables and segments* (pp. 157–171). Amsterdam, Netherlands: North-Holland Publishing Co.

Menn, L. (1983). Development of articulatory, phonetic, and phonological capabilities. In B. Butterworth (Ed.), *Language production, 2* (pp. 3–50). London, United Kingdom: Academic Press.

Menn, L., Schmidt, E., & Nicholas, B. (2009). Conspiracy and sabotage in the acquisition of phonology: Dense data undermine existing theories, provide scaffolding for a new one. *Language Science, 31*(2–3), 285–304.

Millar, D. C., Light, J. C., & Schlosser, R. W. (2006). The impact of augmentative and alternative communication intervention on the speech production of individuals with developmental disabilities: A research review. *Journal of Speech, Language, and Hearing Research, 49*, 248–264.

Mitchell, P. R., & Kent, R. D. (1990). Phonetic variation in multisyllable babbling. *Journal of Child Language, 17*(2), 247–265.

Moeller, M. P., Hoover, B., Putman, C., Arbataitis, K., Bohnenkamp, G., Peterson, B., . . . Stelmachowicz, P. G. (2007). Vocalizations of infants with hearing loss compared to infants with normal hearing—Part II: Transition to words. *Ear and Hearing, 28*, 628–642.

Morris, S. R. (2009). Test-retest reliability of independent measures of phonology in the assessment of toddlers' speech. *Language, Speech, and Hearing Services in Schools, 40*, 46–52.

Morris, S. R. (2010). Clinical application of the mean babbling level and syllable structure level. *Language, Speech, and Hearing in Schools, 41*(2), 223–230.

Mullen, E. M. (1995). *Mullen Scales of Early Learning*. Circle Pines, MN: American Guidance Service.

Nathani, S., Oller, D. K., & Neal, A. R. (2007). On the robustness of vocal development: An examination of infants with moderate to severe hearing loss and additional risk factors. *Journal of Speech, Language, and Hearing Research, 50*, 1425–1444.

Nelson, K. (1981). Individual differences in language development: Implications for development and language. *Developmental Psychology, 17*(2), 170–187.

Nelson, L. K., & Bauer, H. R. (1991). Speech and language production at age 2: Evidence for tradeoffs between linguistic and phonetic processing. *Journal of Speech and Hearing Research, 34*, 879–892.

O'Connor, K. M., Velleman, S. L., McGloin, S., Connelly, T., & Mervis, C. B. (2010). *Complexity of speech in Williams and Duplication 7 syndromes*. Paper presented at the International Child Phonology Conference, University of Memphis.

Oller, D. K., & Eilers, R. E. (1988). The role of audition in infant babbling. *Child Development, 59*(2), 441–449.

Oller, D. K., Eilers, R. E., Steffens, M., Lynch, M. P., & Urbano, R. (1994). Speech-like vocalizations in infancy: An evaluation of potential risk factors. *Journal of Child Language, 21*, 33–58.

Oller, D. K., Eilers, R. E., Urbano, R., & Cobo-Lewis, A. B. (1997). Development of precursors to speech in infants exposed to two languages. *Journal of Child Language, 24*, 407–425.

Oommen, E. R., & McCarthy, J. W. (2014). Natural speech and AAC intervention in childhood motor speech disorders: Not an either/or situation. *Perspectives on Augmentative and Alternative Communication, 23*(3), 117–123.

Paul, R. (1991). Profiles of toddlers with slow expressive language development. *Topics in Language Disorders, 11*, 1–13.

Paul, R., & Jennings, P. (1992). Phonological behavior in toddlers with slow expressive language development. *Journal of Speech, Language, and Hearing Research, 35*(1), 99–107.

Paul, R., Fuerst, Y., Ramsay, G., Chawarska, K., & Klin, A. (2011). Out of the mouths of babes: Vocal production in infant siblings of children with ASD. *Journal of Child Psychology and Psychiatry, 52*(5), 588–598.

Peters, A. M. (1983). *The units of language acquisition*. Cambridge, UK: Cambridge University Press.

Peters, A. M. (1990). *The morphosyntactic development of a phrasal child*. Paper presented at the Fifth International Congress for the Study of Child Language, Budapest, Hungary.

Petinou, K., Schwartz, R. G., Mody, M., & Gravel, J. S. (1999). The impact of otitis media with effusion on early phonetic inventories: A longitudinal prospective investigation. *Clinical Linguistics and Phonetics, 13*, 351–367.

Pharr, A. B., Ratner, N. B., & Rescorla, L. (2000). Syllable structure development of toddlers with expressive specific language impairment. *Applied Psycholinguistics, 21*, 429–449.

Pierrehumbert, J. (2001). Stochastic phonology. *GLOT, 5*(6), 1–13.

Pinker, S. (1994). *The language instinct*. New York, NY: William Morrow.

Plumb, A. M., & Wetherby, A. M. (2013). Vocalization development in toddlers with Autism Spectrum Disorder. *Journal of Speech, Language, and Hearing Research, 56*, 721–734.

Poulin-DuBois, D., & Goodz, N. (2001). Language differentiation in bilingual infants: Evidence from babbling. In J. Cenoz & F. Genesee (Eds.), *Trends in bilingual acquisition* (pp. 95–106). Philadelphia, PA: John Benjamins.

Proctor, A. (1989). Stages of normal noncry vocal development in infancy: A protocol for assessment. *Topics in Language Disorders, 10*(1), 26–42.

Robb, M. P., & Bauer, H. R. (1991). The ethologic model of phonetic development II: The closant curve. *Clinical Linguistics & Phonetics, 5*(4), 339–353.

Salas-Provance, M. B., Kuehn, D. P., & Marsh, J. L. (2003). Phonetic repertoire and syllable characteristics of 15-month-old babies with cleft palate. *Journal of Phonetics, 31*, 23–38.

Smith, B. L., & Stoel-Gammon, C. (1996). A quantitative analysis of reduplicated and variegated babbling in vocalizations by Down syndrome infants. *Clinical Linguistics & Phonetics, 10*(2), 119–129.

Smith, B. L., Brown-Sweeney, S., & Stoel-Gammon, C. (1989). A quantitative analysis of reduplicated and variegated babbling. *First Language, 9*, 175–190.

Stoel-Gammon, C. (1988). Prelinguistic vocalizations of hearing-impaired and normally hearing subjects: A comparison of consonantal inventories. *The Journal of Speech and Hearing Disorders, 53*(3), 302–315.

Stoel-Gammon, C. (1989). Prespeech and early speech development of two late talkers. *First Language, 9*, 207–224.

Stoel-Gammon, C. (1992). Prelinguistic vocal development: Measurement and predictions. In C. A. Ferguson, L. Menn & C. Stoel-Gammon (Eds.), *Phonological development: Models, research, and implications* (pp. 439–456). Monkton, MD: York Press.

Stoel-Gammon, C. (2010). The Word Complexity Measure: Description and application to developmental phonology and disorders. *Clinical Linguistics and Phonetics, 24*(4–5), 271–282.

Stoel-Gammon, C., & Stone, J. R. (1991). Assessing phonology in young children. *Clinics in Communication Disorders, 1*(2), 25–39.

Studdert-Kennedy, M., & Goodell, E. W. (1992). Gestures, features, and segments in early child speech. *Haskins Laboratories Status Report on Speech Research, 111*/112, 89–102.

Thal, D., Oroz, M., & McCaw, V. (1995). Phonological and lexical development in normal and late-talking toddlers. *Applied Psycholinguistics, 16*, 407–424.

Thelen, E. (1981). Rhythmical behavior in infancy: An ethological perspective. *Developmental Psychology, 17*, 237–257.

Tomasello, M., & Mannle, S. (1985). Pragmatics of sibling speech to one-year-olds. *Child Development, 56*(4), 911–917.

Tyler, A. A., & Langsdale, T. E. (1996). Consonant-vowel interaction in early phonological development. *First Language, 16*(47), 159–191.

van den Dikkenberg-Pot, I., Koopmans-van Beinum, F. J., & Clement, C. J. (1998). Influence of lack of auditory speech perception on sound productions of deaf infants. *University of Amsterdam Proceedings, 22*, 47–60.

Velleman, S. L. (1994). The interaction of phonetics and phonology in developmental verbal dyspraxia: Two case studies. *Clinics in Communication Disorders, 4*(1), 67–78.

Velleman, S. L. (2003). *Childhood Apraxia of Speech resource guide*. Clifton Park, NY: Delmar/Thomson/Singular.

Velleman, S., & Strand, K. (1994). Developmental verbal dyspraxia. In J. E. Bernthal & N. W. Bankson (Eds.), *Child phonology: Characteristics, assessment, and intervention with special populations* (pp. 110–139). New York, NY: Thieme Medical Publishers, Inc.

Velleman, S. L., & Vihman, M. M. (2002a). Whole-word phonology and templates: Trap, bootstrap, or some of each? *Language, Speech, and Hearing Services in the Schools, 33*, 9–23.

Velleman, S. L., & Vihman, M. M. (2002b). The emergence of the marked unfaithful. In A. Carpenter, A. Coetzee & P. De Lacy (Eds.), *University of Massachusetts Occasional Papers in Linguistics 26: Papers in Optimality Theory II* (pp. 397–419). Amherst, MA: GLSA.

Velleman, S. L., Mangipudi, L., & Locke, J. L. (1989). Prelinguistic phonetic contingency: Data from Down syndrome. *First Language, 9*, 159–174.

Vihman, M. M. (1976). From pre-speech to speech: On early phonology. *Stanford Papers and Reports in Child Language Development, 12*, 230–243.

Vihman, M. M. (1992). Early syllables and the construction of phonology. In C. A. Ferguson, L. Menn., & C. Stoel-Gammon (Eds.), *Phonological development: Models, research, implications*. Timonium, MD: York Press.

Vihman, M. M. (1993). Variable paths to early word production. *Journal of Phonetics, 21*, 61–82.

Vihman, M. M. (1996). *Phonological development: The origins of language in the child*. Cambridge, MA: Blackwell Publishers Inc.

Vihman, M. M. (2014). *Phonological development: The first two years* (2nd ed.). Somerset, NJ: Blackwell-Wiley.

Vihman, M. M., & Croft, W. (2007). Phonological development: Towards a "radical" templatic phonology. *Linguistics, 45*(4), 683–725.

Vihman, M. M., & de Boysson-Bardies, B. (1994). The nature and origins of ambient language influence on infant vocal production. *Phonetica, 51*, 159–169.

Vihman, M. M., & Greenlee, M. (1987). Individual differences in phonological development: Ages one and three years. *Journal of Speech and Hearing Research, 30*, 503–521.

Vihman, M. M., & McCune, L. (1994). When is a word a word? *Journal of Child Language, 21*, 517–542.

Vihman, M. M., & Velleman, S. L. (1989). Phonological reorganization: A case study. *Language and Speech, 32*, 149–170.

Vihman, M., Ferguson, C., & Elbert, M. (1986). Phonological development from babbling to speech: Common tendencies and individual differences. *Applied Psycholinguistics, 7*, 3–40.

Vihman, M. M., Keren-Portnoy, T., & DePaolis, R. (2013). *The role of production in infant word learning*. Paper presented at the International Child Phonology Conference, Nijmegen, The Netherlands.

Wetherby, A. M., & Prizant, B. M. (1993). *Communication and Symbolic Behavior Scales manual: Normed edition*. Chicago, IL: Riverside.

Wetherby, A. M., & Prizant, B. (2002). *Communication and Symbolic Behavior Scales Developmental Profile*. Baltimore, MD: Brookes.

Wetherby, A. M., Allen, L., Cleary, J., Kublin, K., & Goldstein, H. (2002). Validity and reliability of the communication and behavior scales developmental profile with very young children. *Journal of Speech, Language, and Hearing Research, 45*, 1202–1218.

Whalen, D. H., Levitt, A. G., & Wang, Q. (1991). Intonational differences between the reduplicative babbling of French- and English-learning infants. *Journal of Child Language, 18*, 501–516.

Whitehurst, G. J., Smith, M., Fischel, J. E., Arnold, D. S., & Lonigan, C. J. (1991). The continuity of babble and speech in children with specific expressive language delay. *Journal of Speech and Hearing Research, 34*, 1121–1129.

Wilson, E. M., Green, J. R., Yunusova, Y., & Moore, C. A. (2008). Task specificity in early oral motor development. *Seminars in Speech and Language, 29*(4), 257–266.

Zubow, L., & Hurtig, R. (2014). Supporting the use of rudimentary vocalizations. *Perspectives on Augmentative and Alternative Communication, 23*(3), 132–139.

CHAPTER 7

Phones and Phonemes

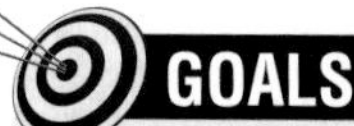

GOALS of This Chapter

1. Review factors impacting the development of speech sounds in monolingual and bilingual children who are typically developing and children who have speech sound disorders due to a variety of etiologies.
2. Describe motoric and linguistic, independent and relational approaches for assessing youngsters' production and perception of speech sounds.
3. Describe motoric and linguistic approaches for remediating speech sound delays and disorders.

Amy, age 5, produces eight different consonants and five vowels. However, her consonant repertoire (1) does not include any stops or glides and (2) is used apparently randomly with two types of inconsistency; the same target consonant is produced in different ways in different words, and *the same target consonant is produced in different ways in the same word on different occasions. The consonants that she can say are not necessarily produced correctly; for example, she produces [f] but not when it is the target consonant.*

May, Amy's twin sister, produces four different consonants and five vowels. When the target word contains a consonant or vowel that she can produce, she produces it accurately. That is, she matches the target whenever possible. Her substitutions are completely predictable, regardless of the word or word position.

Which of the twins has the more severe phonological disorder? Which is likely to be more intelligible? Which is likely to make more rapid progress in therapy?

INTRODUCTION

Speech sounds have traditionally been regarded as the basic building blocks for speech. Most phonologists and speech scientists now recognize that speech is actually most often processed at the syllable level or above. Although we talk about consonants and vowels, the articulatory/acoustic transitions between the brief steady states that we perceive as consonants and vowels are at least as important to the actual processes of perception and production as are the relatively steady-state segments themselves. The portions that we perceive to be between them help to define the segments. Some theories of speech production, such as gestural phonology, have claimed that articulatory gestures (motor movements from one articulatory position to the next) form the basis for phonetic development from infancy onward and that speech sounds (phones or phonemes) and features emerge from gestural regularities (Goodell & Studdert-Kennedy, 1991; Kent, 1997; Lindblom, 1992; Studdert-Kennedy & Goodell, 1992). Expressive children, whose first words are predominantly phrases (e.g., "Iloveyou," "What'sthat?") with even less clear articulation and more variability than the early meaningful utterances of referential children, provide support for these concepts (Nelson, 1981; Peters, 1977). Clearly, part of the articulatory knowledge that every speaker has includes the impact of context on the production of a given segment. A competent speaker is able to adjust her motor plan to the surrounding consonants and vowels, rate of speech, stress placement, etc., as well as to non-linguistic factors (such as eating while speaking, a sore tongue, the impact of Novocaine, etc.). Similarly, a competent listener is able to adjust his expectations to include phonetic variants resulting from such conditions (Munson, Edwards, & Beckman, 2005).

However, listeners' knowledge also includes the categorization of the many speech sounds as they are actually produced into discrete collections associated with more abstract concepts (such as "the 's' sound") (Munson et al., 2005). The fact remains that at a conscious level, it is easier for us to think of speech as a stream of consecutive sounds, like beads on a string. What we perceive as a misproduction of a particular consonant may in fact be a miscoordination of the transition from a preceding vowel into that consonant or from that consonant into the following vowel, but our perception that something was awry at the consonantal level is nonetheless valuable information. A child who has difficulty with oral–motor timing or spatial coordination will be perceived as being unable to produce certain sound segments or classes of sound segments of her native language. Furthermore, children who have difficulty producing a certain consonant (or vowel) in one context often also have difficulty producing the same consonant in another context, despite the fact that the transitions differ. Therefore, it is still appropriate to analyze the sound segments within a child's sound repertoire as if they were discrete entities. However, care must be taken to remember that these sounds are not used in isolation and that contextual factors (word position, syllable shape, stress patterns, and the influence of other sounds within the word as well as rate, semantic and syntactic context, and so on) are extremely important to consider.

The same speech sounds—phones, or segments—may function in different ways in different languages. Recall that those phones that are in contrast with each other (i.e., differentiate words) within a language are referred to as phonemes; others that occur but not contrastively are called allophones. In Chapter 2, the major sets of sounds and phonetic features that tend to occur within languages were reviewed, including phonetic universals and markedness. In this initial section of this chapter, we focus on phonetic development in children learning English and other languages. Phonetic universals, markedness and defaults, sound systems, and distribution requirements will each be discussed with respect to their effects on child phonetic repertoires. Later in the chapter, the focus is on how these phones function within individuals' speech systems to create the contrast that makes communication successful.

PHONETIC DEVELOPMENT

Child Phonetic Inventories

At age 1, infants produce primarily bilabial consonants, although consonant types do vary by word position. Stops are predominant in CV vocalizations (i.e., in initial position), while fricatives and nasals are most common in VC syllables (i.e., in final position) (Kent & Bauer, 1985). In addition, consonant place preferences differ in babble, in which dental and alveolar consonants predominate, versus in words, in which bilabials predominate (Vihman, Macken, Miller, Simmons, & Miller, 1985).

TABLE 7-1 Sound Classes Used by 24-Month-Olds

Sound Class	Initial Position		Final position	
	50%	90%	50%	90%
Stop	b, d, g, t, k	b, d	p, t, k	t
Nasal	m, n		n	
Fricative	f, s		s	
Liquid/glide	w, h		ɹ	

From Stoel-Gammon, C. (1987). Phonological skills of 2-year-olds. *Language, Speech, and Hearing Services in Schools, 18*, 323–329.

Stoel-Gammon (1987) reported that the consonants used by at least 50% of thirty-three 24-month-old American English-speaking children were stops, nasals, fricatives, glides, and liquids. Those phones that were present in 90% of the children's inventories were [b, d] in initial position and [t] in final position. In general, a wider variety of phones occurred in initial position than in final position. Her specific findings are listed in Table 7-1.

Similarly, McIntosh and Dodd (2008) reported that 90% of 32 children between 25 and 29 months of age had nasals, voiced and voiceless stops, and at least one glide and one fricative, typically: [m, n, p, b, t, d, k, g, s, w]. By 30 to 35 months of age, 90% of their 30 participants in this age group had additional members of these classes, typically: [m, n, ŋ, p, b, t, d, k, g, s, h, w, j]. Fasolo, Majorano, and D'odorico (2008) reported that 12 typically developing 20-month-old Italian-learning toddlers had a mean of 10.5 consonants in their inventories, most often including [p, b, t, d, k, m, n, ɲ, l, w, j]. In contrast, 12 late-talking Italian toddlers at the same age had 4.42 consonants on average, typically: [p, b, t, k, m, n, w]. Thus, there are similarities but also differences across languages. Furthermore, inventory size can be an indicator of delay (or possibly disorder).

Overall, however, those sounds that are used most commonly in the languages of the world tend to be those that children babble and use in their first words. Presumably, these are the sounds in which the balance between ease of perception and ease of production is most easily maintained, although ease of production is clearly given more weight by children and ease of perception is relatively more important to adults. These same unmarked sounds also tend to be those that are produced correctly by the majority of 2-year-old children (Locke, 1983).

Dinnsen (1992) identified a hierarchy of phonetic repertoires among the languages of the world that also fits English-speaking children with functional phonological disorders. He hypothesized that such children's phonetic repertoires would fall into one of the following levels and that remediation can be expected to facilitate the child's transition from one level to the next, more phonetically elaborate level. The levels that he proposed are given in Table 7-2.

TABLE 7-2 Phonetic Class Levels

Level A: vowels, glides, voiced stops, nasals, glottals
Level B: Level A sounds + voicing contrast for stops
Level C: Level B sounds + some fricatives and/or affricates
Level D: Level C sounds + one liquid consonant (lateral [l], non-lateral [ɹ])
Level E: Level D sounds + more liquids *or* more obstruents (e.g., fricatives and/or affricates)

From Dinnsen D. A. (1992). Variation in developing and fully developed phonologies. In C. A. Ferguson, L. Menn, & C. Stoel-Gammon (Eds.), *Phonological development: Models, research, implications* (pp. 191–210). Timonium, MD: York Press.

Similarly, Kent (1992) proposed a hierarchy of articulatory complexity with a focus on the aspects of motor control demonstrated at each level. At the lowest level, children have enough laryngeal control to initiate the vibration of the vocal folds for voiced sounds. They also demonstrate the ability to produce rapid versus slower movements as exemplified in contrasts between stops versus glides versus vowels. In addition, they can control the opening/closing of the velopharyngeal port in order to produce nasal versus oral consonants. The tongue can be raised to the alveolar ridge, and the lips can be closed or rounded. These articulatory abilities yield the consonants [p, m, n, w, h]. Note that this set differs from Dinnsen's Level A in that Dinnsen leads us to expect voiced stops first, while Kent posits a voiceless consonant as the first stop to appear.

At the next level, the child develops the ability to grade the amount of force applied to the articulators (tongue, lips, etc.)—more for stops, less for fricatives. Added lingual control contributes palatal and velar places of articulation. Additionally, voicing control improves so that voiced–voiceless consonant pairs emerge. The typical consonants added to the set above are [b, d, g, k, j, f]. Note that this second level of Kent's corresponds to a combination of Dinnsen's Levels B and C.

At Kent's Level 3, tongue control becomes even more precise, and [t, ɹ, l, ŋ] are added as in Dinnsen's Level D. Further refinements in lingual control and in gradations of force at Level 4, as in Level E, yield the interdental place of articulation as well as the production of more challenging palatal consonants and the addition of the affricate manner of articulation. The fricative consonants [s, z, ʃ, ʒ, tʃ, dʒ, v, θ, ð] result.

The levels proposed by both Dinnsen (1992) and Kent (1992) are in keeping with the adult universals described in Chapter 2; all languages have stops and vowels, 97% have nasals, and 86% have glides, and sibilants and liquids are relatively frequent among adult languages but are not as frequent in babble or early words. Similarly, sibilants are most often incorrectly produced by normally developing 2-year-olds. It is not a surprise, then, that stops, vowels, nasals, and glides are present in even the simplest of phonetic repertoires among phonologically delayed children and that liquids and sibilants are not. The early addition of a voicing contrast for stops is also not surprising in light of the fact that many languages use this type of contrast as they expand their stop series.

However, the exact nature and complexity of the voicing (or other laryngeal) contrasts in a particular language may have a significant effect on a child's acquisition of the contrast (Kim & Stoel-Gammon, 2011). This serves as a reminder of the influence of the language of exposure on the child's phonetic development. In another example of this sort, Stokes and Surendran (2005) used Kent's hierarchy to estimate the roles of articulatory complexity versus language-specific functional loads (importance for contrast) and ambient frequencies (frequency of occurrence in the language). They found that about 40% of children's accuracy of consonant production was attributable to articulatory complexity in English. However, articulatory complexity played a lesser role in Cantonese and Dutch.

Stoel-Gammon (1985) reported on phonetic inventories for 34 normally developing English-learning children from 15 to 24 months of age. The initial-consonant inventories that she identified in at least 50% of these children at each age fall into Dinnsen's (1992) categories, as indicated in Table 7-3. Note that, as predicted by Dinnsen but not Kent, their stops tended to be voiced.

Thus, the children in the early phonological period (at 15 months) were pre-Level A, and children at 18 to 21 months produced Level A sounds. Rapid changes apparently occurred between 21 and 24 months, with 2-year-olds producing a far wider range of Level C (Kent's Level 2) sounds. When Stoel-Gammon divided the children further into groups according to their ages of onset of word use, she found that those children who talked relatively early (first words by 15 months) had larger phonetic inventories (i.e., were at higher levels) at each time period than did the children who talked later (at 18 months) or very late (at 21 months). Thus, a large phonetic inventory was predictive

TABLE 7-3 Stoel-Gammon Data/Dinnsen Levels

Age (months)	No. of Subjects	Dinnsen Levels	Phone Classes
15	7	pre-A	voiced stops, h
18	19	A	voiced stops, nasals, glide w, h
21	32	A	voiced stops, nasals, glide w, h
24	33	C	voiced and voiceless stops, nasals, glides, fricatives

From Dinnsen D. A. (1992). Variation in developing and fully developed phonologies. In C. A. Ferguson, L. Menn, & C. Stoel-Gammon (Eds.), *Phonological development: Models, research, implications* (pp. 191–210). Timonium, MD: York Press; Stoel-Gammon, C. (1985). Phonetic inventories, 15–24 months: A longitudinal study. *Journal of Speech and Hearing Research, 28*(4), 505–512.

of earlier lexical acquisition. These differences diminished somewhat with age.

Note that these data are not strictly in keeping with other universals that were discussed in Chapter 2. For instance, languages with only one glide are more likely to have [j], and most languages (71%) that have [w] also have [j]. Yet, the majority of these children produced [w] but not [j]. Bernhardt and Stoel-Gammon (1996) hypothesized several factors that, in addition to universal markedness, may affect whether or not young children produce certain sounds, including misperception, undergeneralization and overgeneralization, articulatory immaturity, and frequency of occurrence in the ambient language. It is not known which of these affect the development of glides.

Dinnsen (1992) reported that all of the phonetic inventories of 40 young children with moderate to severe SSD could be uniquely assigned to one of his proposed five distinct levels of complexity. In addition, whether every element at a given level was addressed in treatment or not, no child progressed beyond that level without acquiring all of the phonetic features within that level. For example, several children acquired a liquid consonant along the way as they progressed from Level C to Level E without treatment on liquid sounds.

Gierut, Simmerman, and Neumann (1994) confirmed that the phonetic repertoires of children with SSD can be uniquely assigned to Dinnsen's four levels. It is important to note that this level schema may be less appropriate for children with extremely small lexicons (e.g., 10 to 20 words), however; they may have more unusual sets of sounds (Dinnsen, 1992).

Summary

Those sounds and sound classes that are universally preferred also tend to occur more frequently in children's babbling and early words and to be produced correctly early on in phonological development, although ambient language effects are also important. Ease of perception has more of an influence on adult phonologies than on children's phonologies. The latter tend to be determined by production factors far more than by listeners' needs.

Children's Markedness and Defaults

Recall that defaults are the least marked (i.e., most common) elements in a repertoire (or in a language). Timmy, a typically developing child whose early phonology was described by Vihman, Velleman, and McCune (1994), is a perfect example of defaults in child phonology. His most frequent babbles were composed primarily of the syllable [bɑ]. Although he produced his first words between 12 and 14 months, it was not until 16 months that any of them contained any vowel other than [ɑ]. Furthermore, even when [i] finally appeared at 16 months and [u] at 16.5 months, their uses were restricted to certain words and certain phonotactic contexts. For Timmy, then, [ɑ] was a default vowel.

Another child, Alice (described by Vihman et al., 1994 and Vihman, 1992) provides an example of a less expected default. Palatals are typically marked in young children's phonologies, just as they are less common than are labials and coronals in adult phonology. However, Alice produced many palatals in her babble and in her early words. Although she quickly began producing a wider variety of consonant and vowel sounds, many of her words continued to be at least occasionally produced with a palatal or palatalized consonant or with a palatal vowel ([ɪ] or [i]). At 14 months, for instance, she produced "daddy" in several different forms, including [jæɪji] and [tɑɪdi]. Thus, Alice's unmarked, preferred place of articulation for both consonants and vowels was palatal. (Note that another possible interpretation of Alice's pattern is given later in the chapter.)

Summary

Sounds may either be universally marked (or unmarked) or marked within a certain linguistic system, including a child's linguistic system. Thus, just as particular languages have default—highly preferred—sounds, so do particular children's phonologies.

Sound Systems

Consonant Inventories

Within Dinnsen's (1992) hierarchy of levels of phonetic development, it is important to note that the first task appears to be that of filling in one systematic gap (i.e., entire sound classes that were missing) at a time (voiced stops, then fricatives/affricates, then liquids, etc.). By the time they reach Level E, however, children (in Dinnsen's view) are dealing primarily with accidental gaps (i.e., sounds for which the child had already mastered the same features in other sounds), adding more liquids, fricatives, or affricates to a system that already includes some members of each of these classes. Grunwell (1985), too, proposed a stage model of phonetic development that demonstrates this concept of a patterned phonetic repertoire in which most (if not all) features available at each stage are used fully. New phones are added that share some of the features of the old phones, and as new features are added, the new combination possibilities are exploited. Although these and other (e.g., Robb & Bleile, 1994) phonologists report slightly different patterns of acquisition for the phonetic repertoire of English, they agree on the notion that children acquire sounds in a patterned manner, not randomly.

Stoel-Gammon (1985) studied the phonetic inventories of children from 9 to 24 months of age and reported on the development of those inventories from the onset of words (which ranged from 15 to 24 months) to 2 years of age. As proposed by Dinnsen (1992), her subjects' inventories generally followed a universal developmental progression. It is

TABLE 7-4 Phonetic Inventories 9–24 Months

	labial	alveolar	velar	glottal
15 MONTHS:				
STOP				
Voiced	b	d		
FRICATIVE				h
18 MONTHS:				
STOP				
Voiced				
NASAL				
GLIDE				
FRICATIVE				h
21 MONTHS:				
STOP				
Voiced	b	d		
Voiceless		t		
NASAL	m	n		
FRICATIVE				h
24 MONTHS:				
STOP				
Voiced	b	d	g	
Voiceless		t	k	
NASAL	m	n		
GLIDE	w			
FRICATIVE	f	s		h

Based on Stoel-Gammon, C. (1985). Phonetic inventories, 15–24 months: A longitudinal study. *Journal of Speech and Hearing Research, 28*(4), 505–512.

interesting to look at the detail of her subjects' consonant development over time; this is given in Table 7-4. This table illustrates that the subjects did not simply acquire individual sounds in a random order; their consonant repertoires appeared to develop in a patterned manner.

Although these children had many systematic gaps to fill in, they appeared to do so in a patterned way that took advantage of accidental gaps whenever possible. Note, for instance, that when nasals first appeared, they occurred at the places of articulation that had already been used for voiced stops, as did fricatives later.[1] Similarly, when the velar place of articulation was introduced, both voiced and voiceless features (which were already in use for [d] and [t]) were applied.

Norms for the development of consonants by children acquiring American English have been provided in various studies. It is important to note, however, that these represent relational analysis—consonants that children produce accurately. The studies cited above were based on independent analysis; they reported the consonants that children produce, regardless of the target (i.e., regardless of accuracy). A child may produce a consonant frequently enough that it would

[1]Technically, [f] is labiodental, but as there is no strictly labial fricative in English, these two places of articulation are considered together.

TABLE 7-5 Norms from the Nebraska Articulation Norms Project

Acquired by Age	Females	Males
<3;0	m, n, h, w, p, b, t, d, k, g, **f**	m, n, h, w, p, b, t, d, k, g
3;0	**s**	
3;6	j	j, f
4;0	**v, ð, ʃ, tʃ**	**dʒ**
4;6	**l**, dʒ	v
5;0	**z**	s, ʃ, tʃ
5;6	**ŋ, θ**	ð, ɹ
6;0	ɹ	ŋ, θ, z, l

Sounds mastered earlier by one sex than the other are in bold and slightly larger font. Adapted from Smit, A. B., Hand, L., Freilinger, J. J., Bernthal, J. E., & Bird, A. (1990). The Iowa articulation norms project and its Nebraska replication. *Journal of Speech and Hearing Disorders, 55*(4), 779–798.

be considered phonetically mastered in an independent analysis, despite the fact that it is never produced accurately. "Ellie" (from Menn, Schmidt, & Nicholas, 2009) is a case in point: She produced [ʃ] in "out" ([aʊʃ]), "this" ([dɪʃ]), "black" ([bæʃ]), and other words, but not in words in which it was a target, such as "fish" ([bis]) or "push" ([bʊs]).

It is useful to know specifically which consonants are usually mastered at which ages. One large study of consonant ages of acquisition based on relational analysis is the Nebraska Articulation Norms Project, described by Smit, Freilinger, Hand, Bernthal, and Bird (1990). For this study, the criterion was 75% correct productions averaged over initial and final positions (for most consonants—some were not tested in both positions). Their results from testing 463 children from urban and rural Nebraska between the ages of 3 and 9 are given in Table 7-5. They investigated differences by gender and found that girls generally acquire several sounds earlier than do boys, with boys only acquiring two sounds before girls.

Perspicacious readers will note with frustration and confusion the large amounts by which the results of various studies vary. These differences result, at least in part, from the use of independent versus relational analysis as well as differences in word stimuli, elicitation techniques, standards for "correct" production/mastery (e.g., Are distortions considered correct? Is the criterion 75% or 90%?), word positions taken into account, and the geographic backgrounds of the participants. Table 7-6 is an attempt by this author to reconcile the differences among various studies by roughly averaging the ages of acquisition reported by several different authors.

With respect to children with SSDs, Bernhardt and Stoel-Gammon (1996) found that 22 children with moderate to severe phonological disorders did follow universal expectations for acquisition order to a large extent. However,

TABLE 7-6 Consonant Ages of Mastery (Initial Position) Averaged over Several Studies

1. Ages are approximate. Results vary widely from study to study.
2. Many of these sounds emerge long before their ages of mastery but may be distorted or inconsistently produced correctly depending upon the phonetic context (e.g., word-initial versus intervocalic versus in a cluster) or utterance complexity.

Age	Consonants Mastered
2;0	[b], [d], [t]
2;6	[p], [b], [m], [n], [w], [h], [f]
3;0	Above + 1–2 more fricatives, [l]
3;6	Above + [t], [k]
4;0	Above + [g]
5;6	[v], [l]
6;0	[ð]
6;6	[ʃ], [tʃ], [dʒ]
7;0	[θ]
8;0	[ɹ]
9;0	[s], [z]

Based upon data provided by Stoel-Gammon (1987), Dyson (1988), Smit and colleagues (1990), McIntosh and Dodd (2008), Pearson and colleagues (2009).

several of them differed in some respects as well, including substitutions of fricatives for stops (perhaps due to an inability to achieve firm closure, resulting, for example, from lower muscle tone), voicing of initial obstruents (probably reflecting difficulty coordinating the timing of the vocal folds with that of the supraglottal articulators), and sibilants (e.g., [s], [ʃ]) produced without proper grooving, perhaps resulting from decreased fine motor control of the tongue tip).

Vowel Inventories

Some studies have shown that the vowel repertoires to which children have been exposed have exerted an influence on the babble vowel space by 10 months of age (de Boysson-Bardies, Sagart, Halle, & Durand, 1986). As they enter the period of word production, children's vowel inventories, like their consonant inventories, tend to grow in a patterned manner, mirroring the shapes of adult vowel systems. Timmy's vowel repertoire, for example, developed into a predictable three-vowel system. His only vowel was [ɑ] in all words from 12 to 15.5 months. Finally, at 16 months, he produced some words with [i], and at 16.5 months, he also added [u]. Thus, just like the majority of languages that have three-vowel systems, Timmy's early three-vowel system at 16 months included the three corner vowels, [ɑ, i, u].

Based upon a review of the literature, Otomo and Stoel-Gammon (1992) state that these three unmarked (i.e., universally preferred) corner vowels are often acquired early in children who are developing normally. Their own study of the acquisition of the English unrounded vowels (/i, ɪ, e, ɛ, æ, ɑ/) of six normally developing children from 22 to 30 months of age confirmed the early development of [i] and [ɑ]. (The rounded vowel /u/ was not studied.) Selby, Robb, and Gilbert (2000) report a great deal of variety in the vowels of four children between 15 and 36 months with respect to height (high, middle, and low vowels), advancement (front, mid, and back vowels), and the tense/lax distinction. However, Menn and Vihman (2011) state that it is not uncommon for English-speaking children's first vowel contrast (i.e., the first pair of vowels to differentiate words in the child's production lexicon) to be between the relatively close neighbors at the bottom of the triangle, [ɑ] and [æ]. The differences among these studies may result, in part, from the fact that some of the studies focused on independent analysis (i.e., the occurrence of various vowels, regardless of whether or not there was a meaningful target or what that target was, as in Selby et al. [2000]) while others were assessing lexical mastery (i.e., the ability to produce a given vowel correctly in a specific word for communicative purposes).

Some others have looked at vowels in both respects: use and accuracy. Stoel-Gammon and Herrington (1990) compared the vowel systems of two children with SSD to those of another group of children who were developing normally. All of these children, like the children discussed above, showed earlier acquisition and higher accuracy rates for corner vowels. However, the authors also reported early acquisition and high accuracy for [o] for both groups of children. Their findings indicated that unstressed vowels (e.g., [ə]) caused difficulty for children with SSD but not for children with normally developing phonologies.

Pollock and Keiser (1990) also studied the vowel errors of 15 children with SSD. Among their subjects, /i, u, ɔ/ were most often produced correctly (more than 95% of the time). The vowels /ɑ/ and /o/ also had high accuracy rates (above 90%). Pollock and Keiser additionally performed analyses of the children's productions of diphthongs and **rhotic vowels** (vowels that are affected by [ɹ], such as the vowels in "bird" [bɝd] and "store" [stoɚ]). These vowel types are less common among the languages of the world (and therefore considered to be universally marked), and they were especially difficult for the children with SSD to produce accurately. Thus, those vowels that are universally marked appear to frequently be marked in individual children's systems as well.

In a follow-up study, Pollock and Hall (1991) studied the vowel productions of five children between the ages of 8 and 11 who had been diagnosed with Childhood Apraxia of Speech (CAS). These children also exhibited particular difficulty with the marked rhotic vowels and diphthongs. Among the less marked vowels, /ɑ/ was most often correctly produced (100%), with accuracy rates also above 90% for /i, o, ɔ, ʌ/.

Velleman, Huntley, and Lasker (1991) did a similar study of younger children (ages 2 to 7 years), comparing a group of phonologically delayed/disordered children with many characteristics of CAS versus a group of children who were also phonologically delayed/disordered but with few such characteristics. In keeping with the Pollock studies, they also reported particularly high error rates on rhotic vowels (except for the simplest rhotic, [ɚ]) and on diphthongs for all of the children. No errors were reported for /i/; few were reported for /ʌ, ɚ, u, ɑ/. Furthermore, [ɑ] was the vowel that most often served as a substitute for incorrect vowels (i.e., it was the most common intrusive vowel). The children with many (more than 14) characteristics of CAS had higher vowel error rates (as measured by vowel deviations on the *Assessment of Phonological Processes—Revised*, Hodson, 1986), but their actual *patterns* of errors did not differ substantially from those of the children with speech sound delay/disorder.

Universal Versus Ambient Language Effects

Feature complexity is a factor that affects mastery. Some consonants and vowels are more difficult (i.e., more marked) than are others in senses that can be measured across languages. For example, in Cantonese, the complexity of diphthongs, as measured by the number of features (height, front/backness, tenseness, roundness) by which the first and second vowel components differ, influences their order of acquisition. Thus, /oʊ/ is mastered before /ɔɪ/, for instance, because the two elements of /oʊ/ are more similar than are those of /ɔɪ/ (Stokes, Lau, & Ciocca, 2002). Similarly, the categories of sounds that are acquired earlier versus later by monolingual and bilingual English and Spanish learners also match general markedness hierarchies. However, there is more variability among bilingual than monolingual children (Fabiano-Smith & Goldstein, 2010a). In addition, bilingual preschoolers may be expected to make more errors than monolingual children, even if they are typically developing (Gildersleeve-Neumann, Kester, Davis & Pena, 2008).

As discussed elsewhere, the language to which the child is exposed will have a significant impact on the child's order of mastery of consonants and vowels. This is true in the most obvious sense; children will tend not to learn sounds to which they have not been exposed (although even this is not an absolute truth since some children do incorporate sounds in their repertoires that do not come from the ambient language). It is also true in a relative sense; the same phones may be among the earliest acquired in one language but later in another. For example, Cataño, Barlow, and Moyna (2009) replicated Dinnsen, Chin, Elbert, and Powell's (1990) study of levels of sound categories using data from 16 predominantly Spanish-speaking children between 18 months and 4.5 years of age. Their findings were similar to those of Dinnsen with a few exceptions, notably that the Spanish participants had mastered /l/ already at Level A (which is at Level D for English speakers).

Furthermore, although stops, nasals, and glides do tend to be acquired early in all languages, the specifics of which members of these feature classes are first may differ widely from language to language. For example, /k/ is mastered before /p/ in Spanish monolinguals, but the reverse is the case in English monolingual children (Fabiano-Smith & Goldstein, 2010a). These authors compared the consonant mastery of eight monolingual English-speaking children between 3 and 4 years of age to a similarly aged group of eight monolingual Spanish speakers. The consonants mastered (produced correctly more than 90% of the time) by the English speakers were /b, d, g, p, n, w, f, z, h/. In contrast, the Spanish speakers had mastered /m, n, ɲ, t/.

Furthermore, the process of learning two languages may affect the two languages differently. Fabiano-Smith and Goldstein (2010b) report that bilingual children may show different relative delays in acquiring sound classes that are shared by their two languages, such as delays in mastering glides in Spanish, stops in English, and fricatives in both. In the Fabiano-Smith and Goldstein (2010a) study, a group of eight bilingual Spanish–English speakers had mastered /b, w, f, h/ only in English and /n, ɲ, β, f/ only in Spanish. Thus, bilingual children do not necessarily learn the sounds of each language in the same order (or at the same rate) as monolinguals; bilinguals had a subset of English sounds as compared to English monolinguals and a different set of sounds as compared to Spanish monolinguals. Furthermore, even shared consonants were not acquired at the same time in both languages: While the bilingual children had mastered /f/ in both languages, for example, they had acquired /n/ in Spanish only.

In a much larger study comparing a group of 10 3- to 4-year-old monolingual English (ME)-speaking children to 20 English–Spanish bilinguals who were primarily English dominant (PE) and to a much smaller group of three bilinguals with equal exposure and ability in both languages (ES), Gildersleeve-Neumann and colleagues (2008) found that the ES group had most difficulty with English sounds that are typically acquired late, such as liquids. Children from this same group and, to a lesser extent, children from the PE group also tended to include some Spanish sounds (such as fricative allophones) in their English words.

These language-based differences also affect children who are learning different dialects of the same language. For example, Pearson, Velleman, Bryant, and Charko's (2009) study showed that consonantal developmental milestones were not the same for 537 children who were learning African American English (AAE) as their first dialect as for 317 children learning General American English (GAE) only. Although AAE speakers were generally later to master final consonants (due to the fact that consonants are often optional in final position in AAE), they mastered some initial consonants (/ɹ, s/) and even certain final consonants (/s, z/) at earlier ages than did GAE-only learners. Consonant mastery (90% correct) data for these two dialects are provided in Table 7-7. Although the dialect influences were less clear, the findings still held up for children from the two dialect groups who also had SSD (Velleman & Pearson, 2010).

Frequency of exposure is responsible for many of the acquisition differences between languages; consonants and vowels that occur more frequently in a given language

TABLE 7-7 Developmental Milestones for Consonants: AAE vs. GAE

Initial Singletons		Initial Clusters		Age of Mastery (by year)	Final Singletons		Final Clusters	
AAE	GAE	AAE	GAE		AAE	GAE	AAE	GAE
(p)*, b, t, d, k, g, w, j, m, n f, h, ʃ, tʃ, dʒ, l		**kl, pl, kɹ**	**tɹ**	4	m, n, p, ŋ, f, ʃ, tʃ, ɹ		mp	
ɹ, s					**s, z**	**b, t, d, k, g v, dʒ, l**		**nt, ŋk, ld, lt ks, ɹl, ɹf**
v, z		**pɹ, gɹ, sp, st** *tɹ*	*kl, pl*	5	*b, dʒ l*		**ɹs** *ŋk, ks, ɹl*	**ɹd**
θ		spl		6	*k, g, v*	*s, z*	*ɹf*	**ft, sk, ɹt** *ɹs*
	ɹ, s	**skɹ**	*pɹ, kɹ, gɹ, sp, st*					
	ð		**stɹ, ʃɹ, θɹ** *skɹ*	8	*t, d*		*nt, ɹd*	**st**
		θɹ		10		**θ, ð**	*ld, ɹt*	**ɹθ**
ð		*ʃɹ, stɹ*		12+	*θ, ð*		*lt, ft, sk, st, ɹθ*	

Bold: 90% criterion reached earlier in that dialect.
Italic: 90% criterion reached later in that dialect.
Neither bold nor italic: 90% criterion reached at the same time in both dialects (non-contrastive).
Initial singleton /p/ was omitted by oversight. It is placed in the 4-year-old box based on the findings of Smit and colleagues (1990). Initial /p/ is included in the initial clusters /pɹ/, /pl/, and /sp/.
Based upon data provided by Pearson and colleagues (2009).

generally emerge and are mastered sooner. For example, Pye, Ingram, and List (1987) demonstrated that children learning Quiche Mayan may acquire [tʃ] and [l] earlier due to the frequencies of these sounds in their language. Frequency in the language is a second variable that accounts for diphthong acquisition in Cantonese (Stokes et al., 2002) as well. Additionally, Welsh and Finnish both incorporate lengthened (geminate) medial consonants, but these are more frequent in Welsh, and Welsh children produce correspondingly more long medial consonants at an earlier age (Menn & Vihman, 2011).

Summary

The order and process of phonetic development, according to Lindblom, Krull, and Stark (1993), is affected by several factors. These include ease of production/markedness, the language to which the child is being exposed, and the system upon which the child has to build at any given time. Important aspects of the child's pre-existing system that may impact further learning include the combinatorial possibilities of the elements (both features and phones) that the child has already learned.

Like those of adult languages, children's sound systems are not random collections of articulatorily or perceptually easy sounds. Each child's system tends to maximize the use of the features that are already available by incorporating sounds with all possible combinations of those features. When a new feature (e.g., [nasal] or [velar]) is learned, the entire class of sounds associated with that feature (in combination with existing features) may then be learned more quickly, even in children with SSDs (Miccio & Ingrisano, 2000). In other words, the child tends to spontaneously fill in all accidental gaps created by the addition of a new feature.

Children's vowel systems tend to mirror the simplest vowel systems of the languages of the world. The corner vowels [i, u, ɑ], which usually occur in languages with simple three-vowel systems, are typically produced earlier and more accurately by young children, children with SSD, and children with CAS. Other back vowels (e.g., [o, ɔ]) also appear to be acquired sooner than front vowels ([e, ɛ]) by all of these groups of English-speaking children.

EXERCISE 7-1

Phonetic Development

CONTRAST IN CHILD PHONOLOGY

Recall that the ultimate goal of a phonological system is the ability to communicate a wide variety of messages. To do that, one must have relatively large sets of consonants and vowels and relatively many options for combining them into contrasting syllable and word shapes. Children have smaller numbers of phones and word shapes than adults do to use in forming words with a resulting decrease in the number of contrasts that are available to them. However, they also have smaller vocabularies, so less contrast is needed.

Do children avoid homonymy, which reduces intelligibility? Do they change their word use to limit its occurrence? In other words, do they give priority to ease of production (minimizing articulatory complexity at the cost of clarity) or ease of perception (maximizing communicative effectiveness)? There has been some discussion of this point in the child phonology literature.

Ingram (1975) hypothesized that some unexpected, atypical phonological patterns in children's early words may be attributable to their attempts to avoid homonymy. Vihman (1981), on the other hand, argued that homonymy is viewed by the child as a small price to pay in order to use the smallest number of word forms possible. Indeed, she claimed that some children actually seek homonymy as a means of maximizing their vocabularies in the face of limited phonological capacities. A young child who reuses the same word form for several word meanings can have a larger vocabulary without greater articulatory effort.

Ingram (1985) proposed a broader perspective that encompasses both of these points of view. His proposal was based upon the give-and-take among three factors in early phonology: vocabulary size, phonetic inventory size, and amount of homonymy. If the vocabulary grows beyond the phonetic capacity, he argued, homonymy will increase. This will be tolerated to a certain point. However, eventually, the increase in homonymy will exert pressure upon the system, encouraging the child to explore new phonetic options. In this view, alternating periods of increasing and decreasing homonymy would be expected in early phonology.

Ingram (1981) provided an analysis of a child with a high degree of homonymy. This child, Joan (initially described by Velten, 1943), produced a large number of homonyms at age 1;10. One cause—or effect—of this was the fact that she already had a vocabulary of 175 words. She also produced a relatively wide variety of speech sounds for a child of her age. However, she had a strong preference for monosyllables, which restricted the number of different word shapes she could produce. Some of her most overused homonymic forms are listed in Table 7-8 with the words that they were used to represent[2] (adapted from Ingram, 1981). Even with contextual cues, such a high level of homonymy must surely have caused confusion for Joan's listeners.

Lleó (1990) took the homonymy issue beyond the very earliest periods of phonological development in her study of a child who was being raised trilingual (German, Spanish, and Catalán), demonstrating that the tolerance of homonymy is a strategy that is available to the child later in phonology as well. She provided examples to show that limitations on the phonetic repertoire and also on the phonotactic repertoire may motivate the child to be more tolerant of higher levels of homonymy in order to expand her vocabulary. The child, Laura, whom Lleó studied, for instance, actually demonstrated increased homonymy during a period when her phonetic repertoire was increasing. This is unexpected; a larger phonetic repertoire should have improved the potential for contrast. Lleó's explanation is that the child was also attempting far more multisyllabic words at this time but was only able to produce monosyllabic and disyllabic word shapes. She could not produce all of the syllables in the words that she wanted to say. Therefore, longer words were reduced to homonymous disyllabic forms. For example, the long words "escombraries" (garbage), "sabatilles" (slippers), and "Tobias" (a name) were merged into a single two-syllable form, [ˈpies], for a time. The lack of available phonotactic contrast (no more than two syllables per word) was a more overwhelming factor than was the increased availability of phonetic contrast (more sounds). When the child's phonotactic repertoire eventually grew to include trisyllabic forms, the amount of homonymy in her lexicon decreased.

TABLE 7-8 Joan's Homonyms

Child Form	Meanings
[bɑt]	bought, buckle, button, pocket, spot, bad, bark, bent, bite, black, pat, block
[bu]	bowl, boy, pea, pear, ball, bare, bear, beer, blow, blue
[bʊt]	bread, break, brick, pig, put, bead, bed, bird, board, boat, boot

From Ingram, D. (1981). *Procedures for the phonological analysis of children's language.* Baltimore, MD: University Park Press.

In short, the multiple factors that operate on a developing phonology—including vocabulary size, phonetic inventory, and phonotactic inventory—will influence the amount of contrast that is available within the system. If the number of possible contrasts is too small for the child's lexicon, homonymy may increase. This state of affairs may be relatively acceptable for the child whose motivation during that period is lexical rather than phonological. That is, if the child is able to communicate despite many homonymous forms, she will be less motivated to vary her phonetic and phonotactic repertoires. This is quite common in early phonology, when children's attempts at communication are fairly context bound and adults are usually able to guess at their meanings despite ambiguous phonological information. As the child's vocabulary and semantic intent continue to grow, however, lack of contrast begins to have a noticeable impact on her communicative effectiveness. At this time, homonymy will be less tolerable. Either the system will have to grow in some respect in order to accommodate an unmanageable vocabulary size or frustration and decreased intelligibility will result. The latter is typical of children with SSDs.

[2]Denise Segal (personal communication) noted that some of these homonyms may also have had semantic sources. "Button" and "buckle," for example, could easily be grouped into one semantic category by a child of this age.

Thus, it is important to consider the possible consequences of prioritizing increased expressive vocabularies in children with significantly delayed or disordered phonological systems. Although of course we do want children to learn new words, it is sometimes essential to improve the child's phonology first or at least simultaneously so that the new vocabulary words can be understandable to listeners.

Clinical Priorities

It is understandably instinctive to prioritize a goal to increase a child's expressive vocabulary if this is an area of deficit. A small lexicon is an obvious source of communication failure. Furthermore, vocabulary is frankly more fun to address in therapy than is speech production. However, one must keep in mind the possible consequences of building up the vocabulary of a child who has an SSD; if the child, the caretakers, or other significant people in the youngster's life are already frustrated due to poor intelligibility, a larger potential set of word targets will only make this worse. Adding a new word that sounds identical to one the child already says will likely add more aggravation than meaning to the child's communication attempts. Therefore, increasing the child's potential for contrast and targeting vocabulary words that are less likely to result in homonymy should be considered seriously.

Summary

Children do not consistently avoid homonymy. In fact, during certain periods of phonological development, they may be tolerant of homonymous forms because of phonetic or phonotactic limitations within their systems that reduce the potential for contrast. However, there is a trade-off between the simplicity of homonymy and the efficiency of unambiguous communication. When successful communication is significantly affected by too many homonyms, the phonological system is likely to change. If it cannot change (due to SSD), the child may begin to supplement oral communication with gestures or pantomime and/or become frustrated.

From Syllable to Segment

As discussed in earlier chapters, children do not acquire phonology by learning one phoneme at a time and then sticking them together. They first master syllable and word shapes through an extensive period of prelinguistic speech practice (babbling) and then use their most well-learned shapes as the basis for words. As the child's lexicon increases and the amount of homonymy becomes unworkable, reorganizations occur that may trigger the emergence of segmental contrast—the systematic use of speech sounds to differentiate (minimal pair) words (e.g., "hat, cat, sat, rat, bat, pat;" "bush, book, bull;" "piece, pace, puss, pus, pass"). Such contrastive sounds can then be referred to as phonemes. Once segmental contrast enters the picture, the child's variability in the production of segments that contrast with each other may decrease (Rice, 1996). In other words, children may produce (contrastive) phonemes more consistently than other sounds.

Timmy (Vihman et al., 1994), whose speech was considered previously, is a case in point. His words and babble were so similar that they were difficult to distinguish for a period of almost 6 months. At 10 to 11 months, he produced one monosyllabic word shape, [bɑ]. As he began to talk, he used this syllable in the presence of balls, blocks, and boxes and to imitate other [b] words, such as "basket, bell, boat, book, button," and by 15 months, "bird, brush, bunny, baa." From 11 months on, he used another favorite word shape [kɑkɑ], usually in disyllabic form, to refer to "kitty, quack-quack, car, duck, key, Teddy." Because of the phonotactic (word length) as well as phonetic contrast between the two word forms, they do not form a true minimal pair. Thus, it cannot be said that Timmy really had two consonant phonemes, although admittedly he did appear to be categorizing words as either labial or not. Rather, he had two production patterns. His overuse of these two simple patterns was extremely limiting to the amount of contrast that was possible within his lexicon. As a result, he had an extremely high level of homonymy.

At 14 to 15 months, a change occurred as Timmy began to be creative with his [C+ɑ] syllable pattern. He appeared to select consonantal features from target words and attach them to his favorite vowel [ɑ] in a productive manner. "Eye" (phonetically similar to [ɑj] in adult English), for instance, became [jɑ], and [βɑ][3] was used for words containing consonants with labial contact and/or frication ("Ruth, fire, flies, flowers, plum"). Forms such as [nɑ] for "nose" and [mɑ] for "moo" and "moon" followed. At this point, then, Timmy could be said to have a clear set of minimal pairs. Because they served to differentiate these minimal pairs, the consonants /b, j, β, n/ could now be described as phonemes (i.e., phones functioning to create contrast) within Timmy's phonological system. However, there was still no vowel contrast whatsoever in his vowel system, as one single element cannot contrast with itself.

A similar lack of contrast can be seen when we consider the nouns in the lexicon of Holly, a 28-month-old with CAS (Velleman, 1994). Holly's sets of homonymous words at 2;4 were the following:

[b] nouns (bunny, bear, bird, baby (whispered), bell, pig (with gesture), Bert):

[bijə, bɛə, bɪʊ]

Other nouns (tree, kitty, coffee, and others with non-labial initial consonants; often unglossable[4]): [tʰ, tˢ, dɪ], coronal (alveo-palatal) click.

[3] [β] is a voiced bilabial fricative.

[4] Not able to be interpreted as a certain word.

As with Timmy's words, Holly's nouns appeared to be based upon two favorite word shapes that were overused. In Holly's case, each of these word shapes had a few variants, but these were interchanged in a nonsystematic manner; they were not contrastive. It cannot be said that Holly had the phonemes /b/ and /t/ at that point, as these consonants were inseparable from their word shapes; her word forms were somewhat vaguely specified articulatory gestures rather than true sequences of consonants and vowels. Some words (especially within the [b] noun class) were disambiguated slightly using vocal or gestural cues; for example, "baby" was whispered, and "pig" was accompanied by a gesture. Therefore, contrast appears to have been intended. Despite this, Holly's intelligibility was severely affected by her limited phonetic and phonotactic repertoires.

As the child's phonological system emerges, segmental contrast may be available to a limited extent but with templates continuing to play a role. Such is the case of Alice (Vihman, 1992; Vihman et al., 1994). At 15 months, she produced a convincing set of minimal pairs, but the contrast lay in the initial consonants only, as shown in Table 7-9. Although she did produce a variety of other word shapes, this palatalized form was clearly a favorite. Its ease of production for her may have facilitated her development of initial phonemic contrasts in words of this and similar structures. By holding the rest of the word form constant, she may have been more able to experiment with and master the initial phoneme contrasts.

Both Timmy and Alice appeared to develop segmental contrasts in initial position first, but this isn't necessarily always the case. Molly, whose phonology was studied by Vihman and Velleman (1989), appeared to focus more on final position. She demonstrated word-final production patterns for both nasals and voiceless obstruents (stops and fricatives). The chronology of the emergence of word-final nasal segments in her speech was as follows.

At 1;0.26 (1 year, 0 months, and 26 days), Molly first attempted words that had a nasal in final position in the adult form, "bang, balloon, button." However, although "bang" was produced with a final nasal, the others were not. In fact, no

TABLE 7-9 Alice's Initial Minimal Pairs

blanket	[bɑji]
bottle	[pɑji]
mommy	[mɑji]
dolly	[dɑji]
daddy	[tɑji]
(good)night	[nɑji]

From Vihman, M. M. (1992). Early syllables and the construction of phonology. In C. A. Ferguson, L. Menn, & C. Stoel-Gammon (Eds.), *Phonological development: Models, research, implications.* Timonium, MD: York Press; Vihman, M. M., Velleman, S. L., & McCune, L. (1994). How abstract is child phonology? Towards an integration of linguistic and psychological approaches. In M. Yavas (Ed.), *First and second language phonology* (pp. 9–44). San Diego, CA: Singular Press.

TABLE 7-10 Molly's Endings for "Bang"

[bæ:]
[bæʔ]
[bæ̃k]
[bæ:ŋ]
[bæ:ɪn]
[bæ:ini]
[bæŋ^{ŋ}i]

From Vihman, M. M., & Velleman, S. L. (1989). Phonological reorganization: A case study. *Language and Speech, 32*, 149–170.

consistent production pattern was discernible across these three words:

bang [bɑɪŋ][5]

balloon [bɣɛʰ][6]

button [bʌʔ]

At 1;1.8, Molly imitated "down" using a final velar nasal in keeping with her production pattern for "bang" as [tæŋ] as though she were trying out an established pattern on a new word. She also experimented with a wide variety of different endings for "bang," as shown in Table 7-10. This would appear to represent regression on her part, but it is in fact progress, because she was moving toward a more mature system.

Following this experimental period, Molly appeared to settle on the (C)VN:V[7] (e.g., [bæŋ:i]) pattern as her preferred way of producing nasal-final words. This pattern appeared to have the advantage of making the final nasals more salient by placing them in medial syllable-onset position (before a vowel). By one month later (1;2.20), Molly was even restructuring other word types in accordance with her newly established word recipe. Some words with medial nasals in the adult form and eventually (at 1;3.24) even one word with a target *initial* nasal ("Nicky") were pronounced in this way. Some examples are given in Table 7-11.

Molly's focus on a pattern for producing final nasals in medial syllable-onset position actually reduced the contrast within her system in one respect. Molly's mother noticed that "button," "balloon," "banana," and "bunny" had become indistinguishable, as they were now all produced as [pʌn:ə] or [pɑn:ə]. This may have seemed to her mother like regression. However, the use of this production pattern increased the contrast within Molly's system in another sense by providing an easy frame for producing final consonants so that the contrast between, for example, [n] and [m], could be maintained. Furthermore, at the same time as her final nasal production pattern became evident, a final obstruent pattern

[5]Note that transcriptions in examples taken from Vihman and Velleman (1989) are somewhat simplified for clarity.

[6]"Baby gamma," [ɣ], is an upper mid-back unrounded vowel (Pullum & Ladusaw, 1986).

[7]Colon (:) indicates a prolonged sound.

TABLE 7-11 Molly's Final Nasal Pattern at 1;3.24

button	[pɑnə]
round	[hɑnʌ]
around	[wɑnə]
Ernie	[hʌnə]
Brian	[pɑnə]
down	[tænə]
Grandma	[næmʌ]
hand	[hɑnɛ]
bang	[pɑnə]
green	[kɣni]
in	[ɪni]
name	[nɛmi]
Nicky	[ɪnni]

From Vihman, M. M., & Velleman, S. L. (1989). Phonological reorganization: A case study. *Language and Speech, 32*, 149–170.

was also emerging. This pattern, illustrated in Table 7-12, also appeared to be based upon making final consonants as salient as possible, in this case by appending either a final vowel (as she had done for nasals) or a very strong aspirate release ([^{h}]), or both.

As a result of these two patterns, Molly's segmental contrasts in final position were quite clear. Note that her contrasts still were not all parallel to the contrasts of the adult system, however. For instance, "tock"/"clock" was not a minimal pair in her speech at that time, although "click"/"clock" and "block"/"clock" were.

Thus, children with similar phonetic repertoires may use the phones available to them in different ways, such as achieving contrast in initial position, as Alice did, versus final position, as Molly did. (See Ingram [1996] for further discussion of this point.)

TABLE 7-12 Molly's Final Obstruent Pattern

glasses	[kɑk^{h}i]
red	[wɑt^{h}]
book	[p^{h}ʊk^{h}]
house	[hɑʊt^{h}]
that	[tɑt^{h}]
Ruth	[hʌt^{h}]
oink	[hok^{h}]
peek	[pik^{h}]
pig	[p^{h}ɪk^{h}]
stuck	[k^{h}ɑk^{h}]
walk	[wɑk^{h}ə]
work	[hʌk^{h}]
tock	[t^{h}ɑk^{h}i]
block	[p^{h}ɑk^{h}]
click	[k^{h}ɪk^{h}]
clock	[k^{h}ɑk^{h}]

From Vihman, M. M., & Velleman, S. L. (1989). Phonological reorganization: A case study. *Language and Speech, 32*, 149–170.

Key Concept: Variability Isn't Always Bad

The differences between variety (resulting from the size of the phonetic inventory and the number of combinations of consonants and vowels in syllables that the child uses) and variability (inconsistency) were addressed in Chapter 6. The point was made that variability tends to interfere with communicative effectiveness, because it makes it harder for the listener to determine the speaker's message.

Here we see an additional nuance: Despite the challenges it engenders, variability is not always a negative. It may be a sign of:

(a) Poor motor planning, motor control, or mental representations, resulting in inconsistent productions of words, or
(b) The fact that a system that has been stable is no longer functioning adequately and needs to change without, yet, a new pattern having been established. As highlighted within dynamic systems theory (Thelen & Smith, 1994; Van Lieshout, 2004) and by Menn and colleagues (as in Menn, Schmidt, & Nicholas, 2013), instability of this sort is progress toward a new, more mature state.

These two situations call for very different therapeutic interventions.

Functional Load

Functional load (the role of the sound in maintaining contrast within the language; see Chapter 2) is another critical factor, both in determining children's order of acquisition and in determining their intelligibility. For example, [ð] (as in "the, these, those, there, then..." as well as "either, other" and "breathe, bathe") is used frequently in English but rarely in contexts in which it conveys important communicative meaning. It is also a fairly quiet sound that differs little acoustically from [v]. These factors no doubt contribute to its late acquisition among English learners. Similarly, despite the fact that geminate (lengthened) medial consonants are more frequent in Welsh, by the time they are combining words into short phrases, Finnish children produce more such geminates. This is hypothesized to be due to the fact that Welsh geminates are predictable, while those in Finnish are contrastive—that is, they serve to differentiate key early vocabulary words (Menn & Vihman, 2011). Thus, they have a higher functional load and are a higher priority for communicative efficacy. Stokes and Surendran (2005) estimated that functional

TABLE 7-13 Mike's High Functional Load for Alveolars

balls	[dɑ]
dish	[dɪ]
fast	[dæ]
got	[dɑ]
hat	[næ]
mask	[næ]
right	[nɑ]
stand	[dɑ]
sun	[dɑ], [dɑn]
tent	[dɛ]

From Pollock, K. E. (1983). Individual preferences: Case study of a phonologically delayed child. *Topics in Language Disorders, 3*, 1–23.

load accounted for 55% of the variance in the ages of emergence of consonants among seven children learning English.[8] Those consonants with the highest functional loads tended to be mastered first.

For a child with small consonant or vowel repertoires (or both), certain segments may have very high functional loads, as illustrated by Pollock (1983) and in Table 7-13. Her participant, Mike, was quite unintelligible because of the high functional loads of [d], [n], and [ɑ] in his speech. Mike's many resulting homonyms no doubt made him very difficult to understand.

Grunwell's (1982) Martin, whose speech sample is given in Table 7-14, demonstrated a similarly high functional load as a result of his patterns of substituting other fricatives and affricates with [f] and of coalescing all consonant clusters to [f]. The workload of this one consonant [f] was enormous, and listeners were not able to determine which of the many possible targets were intended in specific cases.

Accuracy Versus Contrast

It is important to note that the development of contrast does not necessarily depend upon the accurate production of each phoneme or allophone that is relevant to that contrast. Neither Timmy nor Alice, for example, produced their words in an adult-like manner. Yet, both had sets of minimal pairs by 14 to 15 months, and therefore, they did achieve a kind of segmental contrast within the contexts of their own phonological systems.

Bedore, Leonard, and Gandour (1994) provide an example of a child who maintained sound class contrast in

TABLE 7-14 Martin's High Functional Load for [f]

cheese	[fi]
chimney	[fɪmni]
drinking	[fɪnʔɪn]
farm	[fɑm]
feather	[fɛvə]
flag	[fɑv]
flower	[fɑʊə]
juice	[fuʔ]
sandwiches	[fɑmwɪʔɪ]
scissors	[fɪvə]
ship	[fɪp]
sleeping	[fiʔm]
strawberries	[fɔbɛɹi]
string	[fɪn, fɪm]
sugar	[fʊvə]
swimming	[fɪmɪn]
thread	[fɛv]
thumb	[fʌm]
train	[feɪm]
tree	[fi]

From Grunwell, P. (1982). *Clinical phonology.* Rockville, MD: Aspen.

a very unusual way. This child, "C," a 4-year-old monolingual English speaker, produced dental clicks ([ǀ]) in place of all sibilants ([s, z, ʃ, ʒ]). These clicks, which are produced by flattening the anterior portion of the tongue behind the teeth to create suction, were sometimes combined with stops by this child in order to represent affricates (e.g., [dǀ] for [dʒ])—just as stops are usually combined with fricatives to form affricates. Furthermore, C used clicks to mark morphologically important fricatives: third person singular, possessives, and noun plurals were all indicated with a click. Some examples are given in Table 7-15.

This child was able to produce sibilants when cues were provided, and she began to produce them all in an adult-like manner after a very brief period of intervention (four sessions) focused only on /s/. The authors note that click had been a favorite sound of C's since her earliest word productions and that dental clicks have similar noise spectra as sibilants.

TABLE 7-15 C's Use of Clicks

some	[ǀəm]	stove	[ǀov]
this	[ðɪǀ]	snake	[ǀneɪk]
upside-down	[əǀɑɪdɑʊn]	schoolbus	[kulbəǀ]
shark	[ǀɑɚk]	treasures	[twɛǀɚǀ]
touch	[təǀ]	jelly	[ǀɛwi]
bridge	[bwɪdǀ]		

From Bedore, L. M., Leonard, L. B., & Gandour, J. (1994). The substitution of a click for sibilants: A case study. *Clinical Linguistics & Phonetics, 8*, 283–293.

[8]Note, however, that frequency was the best predictor of emergence for children learning Cantonese. For accuracy of production, articulatory complexity was the best predictor in English, and frequency was the best predictor in Dutch. Thus, frequency, articulatory complexity, and functional load are all important factors in early phonological development, but the importance of these factors varies from outcome measure to outcome measure, from language to language, and—most likely, though this was not examined by Stokes and Surendran (2005)—from child to child.

They also speculate that using a click rather than stops to substitute for sibilants avoided the problem of increasing the functional loads of [t] and [d]. However, using one phone (click) to substitute for an entire sound class must have been diminishingly effective for a child whose vocabulary was likely to have been growing at a rapid rate. This may account, in part, for her extremely rapid learning once her attention was focused through therapy on the appropriate production patterns.

Another striking case of contrast without articulatory accuracy was reported by Howard (1993). She described a child with cleft palate, Rachel, whose phonetic repertoire included very few standard English phones. Phones that she could produce in an adult-like manner were restricted to [m, b, f, θ, w, j, ʔ]. The other phones that Rachel used are considered "deviant" by English speakers. They included non-English places of articulation (e.g., uvular and pharyngeal) and manners of articulation (e.g., ingressive airflow) as well as non-English combinations of features (e.g., voiced velar glide, labiodental nasal).

Despite these very odd phonetic characteristics, Rachel enjoyed a "high level of intelligibility," and she was "exceptionally resistant to therapy" (Howard, 1993, p. 300). Upon investigation, it was determined that this child's phonotactic repertoire was adult-like. She was able to produce even three-element consonant clusters with three consonants—albeit very inaccurately. Furthermore, she was using her unusual set of phones to signal most contrasts within English phonology. She was particularly successful at maintaining the nasal–oral contrast and the continuant contrasts (stops versus fricatives versus affricates). For example, she contrasted nasal versus oral stops by using a uvular nasal for the former and a glottal plosive (combined with place of articulation cues, such as lip closure) for the latter. She contrasted stops versus fricatives by achieving complete closure somewhere in the vocal tract for stops and achieving friction somewhere for fricatives. In addition, she distinguished stops from affricates by using a sequence of closures for the affricate, in keeping with English phonology. Neither the stops nor the affricates were produced in a form that closely resembled adult articulation of such contrasts, as illustrated below:

tap [ʔæʔ^h]

jam [ʔjæm]

However, affricates were produced as conjunctions of two consonantal elements, as in typical English.

Place and voicing contrasts were less successfully maintained, but evidence was found to indicate that Rachel was attempting to make these distinctions as well. The alveo-palatal contrast from the English fricative series (e.g., s/ʃ) was signaled using labialization to mark palatals. This tendency mirrors the lip-rounding that typically accompanies production of palatal fricatives, resulting in /s/-/ʃ/ minimal pairs being expressed via very non-English consonant phones:

Sue [ç̃u] shoe [ç̃^{w}u][9]

sock [ç̃ɒʔ^h] shop [ç̃^{w}jɒp^h]

Thus, Rachel successfully maintained contrasts between appropriate English phonological categories while using few of the appropriate articulatory characteristics of the phonemes/sound classes in question. Howard speculates that Rachel's resistance to therapy resulted from her reluctance to dismantle a complex system of contrasts that was, after all, working for her. Intervention in such cases must be designed in such a way as to do as little damage to the functioning aspects of the system as possible while gradually replacing the "deviant" elements with more appropriate ones. Unfortunately, Howard does not indicate how (or, indeed, whether) this was achieved in Rachel's case.

In any case, Rachel is a perfect example of a child who has managed to maintain most of the contrasts within the language without being able to produce a number of the phonemes with which they are usually maintained. One could say that she exhibited a phonetic disorder in the absence of a phonological disorder.

Heselwood (1997) provides a similar example of an adult who was severely dysfluent. This patient used a voiced nasal click to represent sonorants and a non-nasal click to represent obstruents. With these substitutions, he was able to maintain all of the contrasts expected in adult English.

Summary

Early and delayed/disordered phonologies may exhibit a certain amount of tension between reliance on well-practiced word patterns or favorite sounds and the need for contrast. Some children manage to communicate with very little contrast (and therefore, a high degree of homonymy) for periods of time. However, as their vocabularies grow, new solutions must be sought to increase the potential for contrast, or they will be unintelligible. Some children's—and adults'—unusual solutions may increase contrast in a manner that largely parallels but does not match the normal adult phonology.

Phonemes and Allophones: Surface and Underlying Representations in Child Phonology

To say that two phones (speech sounds) contrast in a child's speech—or in a language—is to say that those two phones are phonemes in that language (as indicated by writing them using slashes / /): they function to differentiate word meanings. Recall that some phonemes are pronounced in different ways in different contexts, such as the English voiceless stop phonemes /p/, /t/, /k/, which are aspirated in initial but

[9] [ç̃] represents a voiceless palatal fricative—[ç]—with audible nasal escape. [ç̃^{w}] is the labialized version of the same (Duckworth, Allen, Hardcastle, & Ball, 1990).

typically not in final position: [pʰæt], [tʰæp], [kʰæt], and [tʰæk]. These aspirated phones are allophones (as indicated by writing them in brackets: [pʰ], [tʰ], [kʰ]) of these phonemes /p, t, k/, in complementary distribution (i.e., predictably occurring in distinct word positions). Other allophones are in free variation (i.e., are interchangeable or occur for non-linguistic reasons), such as unreleased [t̚], which may or may not occur in word-final position. The allophones that we produce are at the "surface" articulatory level. The phonemes that they represent—our abstract mental representations of the speech sounds of our language—are at the "underlying" representational level.

The issue of children's underlying representations has generated much intellectual heat in the past (beginning with papers such as Braine, 1974, 1976; Macken, 1979; Moskowitz, 1975; Smith, 1973; Stampe, 1969), and it will undoubtedly continue to do so for some time to come. The focus here will be on those aspects of the debate that bear most directly on actual clinical practice.

The fundamental question to be posed is "What do children know, and when do they know it?" That is, are children's mental representations the same as those of adults, from the onset of word production? Another possibility is that the child's underlying form of the word is the adult's phonetic form—in other words, the child initially thinks that every allophone is a phoneme. Alternatively, the child's production target may be an incomplete or incorrect version of the adult word. If children do store the full adult phonemic or phonetic forms of words in their recognition (perception) memories, do they store them less accurately in their production lexicons? Or is the word accurately stored in one location only, with "output rules" that turn an accurate perceptually based memory into an inaccurately produced word? Or is each word simply stored in the way that the child produces it—errors and all?

A few studies of children's discrimination (speech sound perception) have shown a relationship between non-adult perception and non-adult production of specific, acoustically difficult contrasts. That is, children who do not do well at producing certain contrasts also perform poorly at discriminating those same contrasts (e.g., /f/ versus /θ/; Velleman, 1988). They appear to be unaware that the adult phonemes are supposed to contrast. Although misperception likely does not account for the majority of children's phonological simplifications, Wolfe, Presley, and Mesaris (2003) demonstrated that children with poorer discrimination of error sounds make slower progress on remediation of those same sounds. In turn, poor production skills predict poorer phonological awareness skills, which suggests that the accuracy and completeness of the child's understanding of the phonological system has repercussions not only for the quality of their speech but also for later literacy skills (McDowell, Lonigan, & Goldstein, 2007). Nijland (2009) found that both children classified as having phonological disorders and children with a diagnosis of CAS demonstrated speech perception deficits. Interestingly, the children with phonological disorders only demonstrated "higher-order" perception difficulties (e.g., deficits in phonological awareness, such as rhyming), while those with CAS had difficulty with lower-order tasks (e.g., discrimination between two non-words) as well as higher-order perception tasks.

Young and disordered children often distort the adult forms of words in significant manners, including cases that seem extreme, such as **migration** or **metathesis** across intervening elements (including [uz] for "zoo" from Leonard and McGregor, 1991; [gɑbi] for "buggy" from Berman, 1977), cases that are quite rare in adult phonology. Fee (1991), Fikkert (1991), Lleó (1992), Macken (1993), McDonough and Myers (1991), Menn and Matthei (1992), Ohala (1991), Velleman (1992), Vihman and colleagues (1994), and others have proposed that young and/or disordered children, regardless of what they may be capable of perceiving, may have simplified phonological output representations of words. In other words, their production plans may be simpler than their perceptual abilities would suggest. For example, children who have a preferred production template (perhaps reflecting a former favorite babble pattern) at any given time may seem to ignore a reasonable amount of perceived word-specific information. Such children may use the phonetic and/or phonotactic patterns that they have established as production templates rather than the actual adult form of the word, even if they "know" at some level how the word should sound.

In fact, in some cases, one can be reasonably sure that a child is choosing (subconsciously, of course) not to use the proper adult form of the word. Recall Mickey (see Chapter 6), who learned her own name early on but pronounced it as [didi]. Even at the point at which she was able to accurately produce the word "monkey," she persisted in calling herself [didi]. However, she would respond angrily if others mispronounced her name; she expected everyone else to call her "Mickey." In other cases, a child's earlier fairly accurate word forms may appear to regress as the words come to conform more closely to one another. For example, Molly's apparent regression (discussed previously) as she forced previously more accurate words into her production template illustrates that children may choose not to use information that they have in planning their productions of words. The form of this apparently unused information about the word (e.g., whether these early relatively accurate word forms are stored as unanalyzed wholes) is unknown. Similarly, it has not been determined whether such information is still available somewhere in the learner's brain to assist in discriminating that word from others, or whether it is filtered completely out of the incoming auditory signal.

One group of researchers, including Elbert, Gierut, Dinnsen, and Weismer, instituted a program of research aimed at identifying children's phonological knowledge:

in other words, the information about the word that is available to the child's speech production planning mechanism. Their clinical research demonstrates that this factor may predict learning curves and improvement resulting from phonological intervention. Specifically, Dinnsen and Elbert (1984); Elbert, Dinnsen, and Powell (1984); and Gierut (1985) showed that children make the most progress on aspects of adult phonologies about which they have the most knowledge.

"Phonological Knowledge" Versus "Phonological Awareness"

It is important to distinguish phonological knowledge from phonological awareness. The phrase "phonological knowledge" is used to refer to evidence that a child is using two different phones contrastively in her speech. For example, if a child uses the minimal pair words "Pooh" and "boo" with different meanings, we can infer that she knows that /p/ and /b/ are different phonemes in her language. However, we would not expect her to be able to comment on that fact.

In contrast, the phrase "phonological awareness" is used to refer to conscious awareness of the sounds and sound structures (syllable and word shapes) of the language. This includes tasks such as rhyming, identifying initial and final consonants (e.g., "What's the first sound in 'boat?'"), deletion ("If you take the [b] off of the word 'boat,' what's left?"), and even reversal (e.g., "What's 'sick' backward?").

Unfortunately, it is impossible to directly assess a child's phonological knowledge; we can't see into their minds. This information must be inferred either from the child's phonemic perception (determined via discrimination testing, a sometimes challenging process) or from the child's production patterns. Elbert and Gierut (1986) and their colleagues opted for the second of these routes, using a variety of different means for identifying the child's use of phonemic contrasts and inferring the child's knowledge of these contrasts. First, one determines the child's phonetic repertoire, including the distribution requirements that operate on this repertoire. For instance, consider a child who uses fricatives and voiceless stops only in final position, voiced stops only in syllable-initial (word-initial or word-medial) positions, and no liquids in any words. This information makes it possible to determine which of these sounds are used contrastively by the child. If the child uses fricatives only in final position, then a fricative-stop phoneme contrast is not possible in syllable-initial position. But if stops are also used in final position, then contrast may be possible there. For example, words like "fan" and "pan" or "puffy" and "puppy" would not sound different in the youngster's speech, but "puff" and "pup" would. Thus, it would be appropriate to say that the child has some limited knowledge of fricatives; minimal pairs in final position indicate that fricatives are phonemes in this position.

In contrast, if voiced stops are used in syllable-initial position only, and voiceless stops in postvocalic final position only, then no voiced–voiceless stop contrast is possible: "pick," "pig," and "big" would all be pronounced [bɪk]; "picky," "piggy," and "biggie" would all be pronounced [bɪgi]. Voiced and voiceless stops would be said to be in complementary distribution in this case. For this child, they are allophones rather than phonemes with respect to each other because they do not contrast with each other, and the appearance of each is predictable based on word position. If no evidence of a contrast ever occurs, it is less likely that the child has any phonological knowledge of that contrast. In this hypothetical case, liquids may be neither phonemes nor allophones for this youngster because they simply do not occur in the child's speech at all.

Another clue to the nature of a child's underlying representations may stem from his attempted productions of clusters. Recall that English voiceless stops in initial position are aspirated—produced with a long delay between the release of the consonant (the burst) and the onset of the vowel (voicing). As such, they exemplify the "voiceless unaspirated" type of voicing: [t^{h}ɑp] ("top"). In contrast, voiceless stops following /s/ in English are released at about the same time as the vowel begins; from a universal phonetic perspective, they are "voiceless unaspirated"—with a similar voicing lag to that between the release of a voiced stop and the onset of the following vowel: [st$^=$ɑp]. Thus, when children produce words such as "stop" without the initial [s] and we perceive "dop," it is incorrect to say that they have voiced the initial /t/. In fact, they have merely maintained the appropriate voicing for that allophone of /t/, as it would be pronounced if the [s] had also been produced. A child who pronounces "stop" as [t$^=$ɑp] (to our ears, "dop") and "top" as [t^{h}ɑp] is actually correctly maintaining a contrast between the two words (albeit in an immature way). It is the child who produces both "stop" and "top" as [t^{h}ɑp] who has not maintained the English voicing contrast. The former child knows that the two situations are different and therefore has more phonological knowledge of the presence and impact of initial /s/ than the latter.

Sometimes, a contrast can be discovered that is not immediately evident from the child's typical productions. For example, a child who produces both "pig" and "pick" as [pɪ] may appear to have no knowledge of final voicing contrasts—or even of final consonants at all. Yet, if the same child pronounces "piggie" as [pɪgi] and "picky" as [pɪki], then it is inferred that she must know that there is a final consonant in "pig" and that it is voiced, even though she does not pronounce it as such. In syllable-initial medial position, at least, /g/ and /k/ contrast and are thus phonemes for that child. For this reason, Elbert and Gierut (1986) advocated

TABLE 7-16 Nathan's Use of [d] and [n] (Hypothetical)

doggie	[dɔdi]
cookie	[dʊdi]
go	[do]
Mom	[nɑn]
more	[nod]
no	[no]
butter	[dʌdʌd]
bye	[dɑɪ]
pig	[dɪd]
shoe	[du]
feather	[dɛdʊd]
sing	[dɪn]
string	[dɪn]
blue	[du]
basket	[dædæ]
monster	[nʌnʌ]
first	[dɪd]

searching for minimal pairs in a variety of phonological and morphological contexts ("piggie" as well as "pig," "digging" as well as "dig," etc.). In one study (Barlow, 1996), children with more knowledge produced less variable forms of target sounds. However, in other studies, such as Velleman (1988), children's variability initially increased when they became aware of a phonemic contrast (specifically, /f/ versus /θ/).

Some examples should help to clarify the issues of phonemes and allophones in children's phonological systems. First, consider the data in Table 7-16 from a hypothetical child called "Nathan." Looking at Nathan's use of [d] and [n], one can see that he uses them contrastively. Both phones occur in all word positions and before the same vowels. Furthermore, there are minimal pairs in all word positions:

[do]—[no] ("go" versus "no" and "more")

[dʌdʌ]—[nʌnʌ] ("butter" versus "monster")

[dɪd]—[dɪn] ("pig" versus "sing")

The phones [n] and [d] differentiate words in Nathan's system. If one is substituted for another, it will make a different word. Therefore, "n" and "d" are separate phonemes for Nathan, and slashes are used to indicate this: /n/, /d/. Similarly, Nathan uses a variety of vowel phones, and many of these are contrastive, as in:

[dɔdi]—[dʊdi] ("doggie" versus "cookie")

[dʌdʌ]—[dædæ] ("butter" versus "basket")

These vowels are separate phonemes for Nathan because they function to add contrast to his system, and slash notation is used to indicate this: /ɔ/, /ʊ/, /ʌ/, /æ/.

Sometimes a child is able to produce both members of a phonotactic or phonetic contrast pair, but only inconsistently

TABLE 7-17 Jacob's Harmony

[dædum, gɑkɑ, dædæ, dɑitɑ, gigʌ, didi, dejdɑ]	"thank you"
[geikʌ, dedɑ]	"Jacob"

From Menn, L. (1978). Phonological units in beginning speech. In A. Bell & J. B. Hooper (Eds.), *Syllables and segments* (pp. 157–171). Amsterdam, The Netherlands: North-Holland Publishing Co.

with no predictable phonological pattern. The phones that are involved in this type of variability are typically referred to as allophones in free variation, as discussed in Chapter 2 with respect to adult phonologies. For example, Menn's (1978) Jacob produced variant forms of each word with different (usually harmonized) consonants in different productions, shown in Table 7-17. For Jacob, [d] and [g] are clearly not distinct phonemes. They vary randomly with each other. Although the two consonants in one word will typically agree in place of articulation (although not always, according to Menn), it is not predictable whether that place of articulation will be alveolar or velar in any given production of the word. Therefore, [d] and [g] are allophones in free variation for Jacob at this stage.

Other children's patterns may appear similar at first glance but differ in important ways. Consider the data from Bleile (1991) in Table 7-18. Initially, one may expect there to be d/g minimal pairs within this set, but there are only vowel minimal pairs (e.g., di—du, go—gæ). When one looks more closely, it is evident that [d] and [g] are allophones in complementary distribution. Specifically, [d] occurs before high vowels (since it requires the tongue tip to be up) and [g] before lower vowels (since the tongue *tip* is typically lower for [g], although the tongue dorsum is higher). As Bleile points out, the vowels are actually providing the only contrast.

A strong note of caution is necessary here. Acoustic studies, such as those of Kornfeld (1971); Macken and Barton (1980); Weismer, Dinnsen, and Elbert (1981); and Velleman (1988), have demonstrated that some children who appear to demonstrate either a lack of contrast or a pattern of allophones may in fact be maintaining a phonemic contrast

TABLE 7-18 Consonant-Vowel Interactions

tea	[di]
toe	[go]
go	[go]
goose	[du]
key	[di]
train	[gæŋ]
dress	[gə]
dog	[gæ]
clue	[du]
cloud	[gæ]

Data from Bleile, K. M. (1991). *Child phonology: A book of exercises for students.* San Diego, CA: Singular Pub Group.

but not well enough. That is, the child may be differentiating words articulatorily by producing two sounds or sound classes contrastively within words. However, due to motor limitations, the child may produce the sounds or sound classes in such a way that the difference is not perceived by adult English speakers (except, in some cases, by parents or speech-language pathologists who are accustomed to the individual child's speech).

In the three examples described by Weismer and colleagues (1981), final stops were omitted from all words. If no final stops are present, then of course the voicing contrast cannot be preserved in final position—or can it? Two of the three children Weismer and colleagues studied actually lengthened the vowels in words that should have had final *voiced* stops only. They produced words such as "cab" with prolonged vowels ([kæ:]) and words such as "cap" with shorter ones ([kæ]). Although most American English speakers actually do tend to produce longer vowels before voiced than voiceless stops, listeners expect to hear the final consonant as well, so these children had not previously been given credit for maintaining this contrast. Yet, participants in this study actually were contrasting voiced versus voiceless final consonants in a sense by way of the preceding vowels. This strategy parallels that used by English speakers to maintain the contrast between word pairs such as "ladder" and "latter" (['læ:ɾɚ] and ['læɾɚ]), discussed in Chapter 2. It also parallels patterns demonstrated by speakers of AAE, a dialect in which production of final consonants is often optional. Even if the consonants are absent, AAE speakers produce longer vowels before target voiced consonants (e.g., "cap" [kæ]/"cab" [kæ:]) and nasalized vowels before target nasal consonants (e.g., "pad" [pæ:]/"pan" [pæ̃:]) (Moran, 1993; Stockman & Vaughn-Cooke, 1989).

Kornfeld (1971) reported a similar finding for children who were labeled as "gliders." That is, they appeared to be producing [w] for adult /ɹ/ and /l/. Kornfeld found acoustic differences between their attempted glides (/w/) and their attempted liquids (/l/, /ɹ/), even though all three sounded the same to the adult ear. Thus, these children were presumably attempting to differentiate /w/ from the liquids, but were unable to do so in a manner that could be detected by listeners. Velleman (1988) found a similar pattern among some children who appeared to be substituting [θ] for /s/ but not for children who substituted [f] for /θ/.

From the most functional point of view, the children in these studies were still neutralizing the contrasts in question because the articulatory distinctions that they were making could not be perceived and therefore did not make the children any more intelligible. However, prognosis for improvement is considered to be far better for children who are producing a contrast at any level (perceptible or not) than for children who are apparently unaware that there is a distinction to be made. Articulatory attempts at phonological contrast provide one more piece of evidence about the child's phonological knowledge that is predictive of outcome (Dinnsen & Elbert, 1984; Elbert et al., 1984; Gierut, 1985; see discussion above). In fact, many other studies have demonstrated that children can discriminate many pairs of error phonemes (i.e., that their substitutions of those phonemes for each other are not due to a lack of recognition of minimal pairs formed with those phonemes).

TABLE 7-19 Child Partial Neutralization (Hypothetical)

go	[doʊ]
dough	[doʊ]
coat	[tot]
duck	[dʌk]
tuck	[tʌk]
egg	[ɛk]
dad	[dæt]
hat	[hæt]
quack	[twæk]
dog	[dɔk]
good	[dʊt]
bad	[bæt]
bat	[bæt]
back	[bæk]

Just like adult phonologies, child phonologies may include pairs of sounds (or sound classes) that are in contrast in some contexts but neutralized in others. Often, voicing is the contrast that is **partially neutralized** in child speech just as it is in German (as discussed in Chapter 2). Consider the sample in Table 7-19. Considering initial position, one can see that voiced and voiceless stops do contrast there as they do in adult English. Minimal pair contrasts such as "duck" versus "tuck" are maintained. However, in final position, all consonants are devoiced. There is no contrast in the child's productions of "bad" versus "bat." Therefore, the voicing contrast is neutralized in final position only in this child's phonology just as it is in German. Similarly, the child neutralizes the velar–alveolar contrast in initial position (such that "dough" and "go" sound identical) but preserves it in final position (such that "bat" and "back" are a minimal pair).

Summary

Phonemes are minimal speech sound units that convey a lexical meaning difference between two words. They help us to distinguish one word from another. Pairs of sounds that are not in contrast with one another may be allophones in free variation (random occurrence of one or the other) or allophones in complementary distribution (predictable occurrence of one or the other). The contrastive use of two different phones—whether the contrast is phonetically adult-like or not—is an important indicator of phonological knowledge, which may be a predictor of progress in therapy.

Persistent Speech Sound Disorders

This chapter has focused thus far primarily on young children with or without speech sound disorders/delays. The speech disorders classification scheme devised by Shriberg and colleagues (e.g., Shriberg, Austin, Lewis, McSweeny, & Wilson, 1997a; Shriberg, Austin, Lewis, McSweeny, & Wilson, 1997b; Shriberg, Fourakis, et al., 2010) includes a category for children whose speech sound errors persist beyond 8 years of age. The prevalence of such persistent speech sound disorders has been estimated to be approximately 1% to 5% of children 9 years old and beyond (Preston & Koenig, 2011). Their errors most often consist of distortions of liquids (especially /ɹ/) and of sibilant fricatives (especially /s/) but may also include omissions and substitutions (Felsenfeld, Broen, & McGue, 1994; Shriberg et al., 1997b). Those whose speech deficits persist the most significantly tend to share the following features in comparison to those whose problems resolve to a greater extent: male, lower socioeconomic status, lower IQ, and weak non-word repetition skills (Wren, 2015). In addition, children with persistent SSD tend to have slower speech rates than typically developing peers when producing target words embedded in phrases, though not in conversational speech (Flipsen, 2003). They may also have poorer language, phonological awareness skills, and literacy skills (Farquharson, 2015; Flipsen, 2003; Preston & Edwards, 2009). Even in adulthood, up to 50% of people with moderate to severe articulation difficulties in childhood ("multiple sound substitutions and omissions that had not resolved by the end of first grade" per Felsenfeld et al., 1994, p. 1343) may continue to produce residual errors. These residual errors may be socially stigmatized (Shriberg, Fourakis, et al., 2010).

Phones and Phonemes in Children with Specific Syndromes

Certain types of disorders or even specific syndromes may be associated with particular patterns of speech sound errors. As noted in Chapter 3, dysarthria often results in speech sound imprecision or distortions (Chen & Stevens, 2001; Tomik et al., 1999). Syndromes associated with low tone, such as Down syndrome (DS) and Williams syndrome (WS), often result in this type of distorted speech. These distortions are typically consistent. That is, similar distortions occur whenever the child attempts to produce the same sound regardless of context. The correct phoneme is articulated, but imprecisely. For children with DS, vowels as well as consonants often require protracted learning processes, with higher than age-appropriate levels of speech sound errors in both adults and children. These errors are both developmental (i.e., typical of younger children without speech sound disorders) and atypical (i.e., disordered). Place of articulation errors for stops and fricatives, as well as vowel errors, have significant impacts on functional contrast (Bunton et al., 2007; Kent & Vorperian, 2013). Children with WS have particular difficulty with sibilants (/s, z, ʃ, ʧ, ʒ, ʤ/) and approximants (/l, w, j, ɹ/) (Huffman, Velleman, & Mervis, 2012a, 2012b).

The consistent distortions that are reported for children with dysarthria are in contrast to the "distorted substitutions" that are sometimes reported for children with CAS (Shriberg et al., 2010b; Shriberg, 2013). In the latter case, the child substitutes one phoneme for another, but the substitution may be imprecise as well. It is not clear whether this results from inaccurate representations, inaccurate retrieval, inaccurate motor planning, insufficient self-monitoring, or, most likely, some combination of these. Children with CAS may demonstrate substitutions, omissions, and distortions that are similar to those of children with more "garden variety" SSD, but they also produce atypical errors, and as noted above, vowels are an area of particular difficulty (ASHA, 2007). As noted before, CAS is most often "idiopathic" (i.e., the cause is unknown), but symptoms of CAS also may accompany certain genetic syndromes (including Down syndrome as described by Rupela & Manjula, 2007; Rupela & Manjula, 2010; and Rupela, Manjula, & Velleman, 2010; velocardiofacial syndrome [microdeletion of chromosome 22q11.2], as described by Kummer, Lee, Stutz, Maroney, and Brandt, 2007; and 7q11.23 duplication syndrome, as described by Velleman & Mervis, 2011) as well as perinatal strokes and other neurologic conditions.

Children with autism spectrum disorders (ASD) often present with speech sound disorders. Even among those with high-functioning autism or Asperger syndrome, a higher proportion exhibit speech sound disorders than in neurotypical populations. Estimates of the frequency of speech delay/disorder among children with ASD range from 12% to 33% (Shriberg, Paul, Black, & van Santen, 2011; Rapin, Dunn, Allen, Stevens, & Fein, 2009; Cleland, Gibbon, Peppe, O'Hare, & Rutherford, 2010). Of the studies reviewed by Shriberg and colleagues (2011), 64% reported increased prevalence of SSD among children with ASD diagnoses. Their errors include developmental patterns, atypical patterns (such as initial consonant deletion), and distortions, according to Cleland and team (2010). Symptoms of CAS may occur (Velleman et al., 2009).

EXERCISE 7-2

Phonological Contrast in SSDs

ASSESSMENT

This chapter has covered many different aspects of children's acquisition of sounds. These include the following:

- Phonetic inventories: the sounds produced, regardless of target
- Phonetic accuracy: the ability to produce given consonants and vowels correctly
- Contrast: the use of sounds to achieve successful communication

Recall that there are two primary approaches to phonological evaluation: independent analysis, in which the child's consonant and vowel repertoires are considered as such with respect to their quantity and diversity independently of the target words, and relational analysis, in which the child's productions are compared to the adult targets in order to generate a list of errors. We consider the assessment of each of these aspects from independent and relational perspectives below.

Assessment of Phonetic Repertoires

Children's inventories of spoken phones—regardless of the targets, if any—are typically assessed based on a spontaneous speech sample. For independent analysis, the meaningfulness of the utterances (i.e., whether a given vocalization sounds like an adult word) is not the focus. The primary concern is what sounds the child produces in a variety of phonetic contexts (e.g., initial position, before a high vowel). However, there are several factors to consider. Some children avoid sounds that they know they find difficult, thus reducing the size of the inventory based on spontaneous speech. Additionally, first words are often phonetically simpler than late babbles. Thus, it may prove useful to differentiate vocalizations that are believed to be word attempts versus those that are not in order to be able to compare the child's repertoire of sounds in words versus her repertoire in babble.

The ideal source of a phonetic repertoire is a speech sample of half an hour or longer—at least 100 utterances. This is often not a possibility in clinical settings, where the time for collecting, transcribing, and analyzing such a sample is not available. Furthermore, spontaneous speech allows the child the luxury of avoiding difficult sounds. Another possibility is to use an articulation test as a means of eliciting a wider variety of sounds from a wider variety of contexts. Unfortunately, although more comprehensive articulation tests can ensure that all phonemes within a given language are sampled, such tests cannot be long enough to test all phonemes in all contexts. Eisenberg and Hitchcock (2010) propose that to truly assess children's mastery of phones, they must be elicited in words that are carefully controlled to rule out extraneous factors such as the effects of consonant harmony and complex stress patterns. Their criteria are described in more depth later in this chapter. On the other hand, a test that met the Eisenberg and Hitchcock guidelines would not assess the child's ability to produce sounds in more challenging contexts, such as multisyllabic words and unstressed syllables. Thus, neither a speech sample alone nor an articulation test alone can capture all that we want to know about a child's phonetic inventory. A speech sample supplemented by an articulation test or a word elicitation procedure would be most appropriate for obtaining representative consonant and vowel inventories.

Once a speech sample has been obtained and transcribed, notations can be made on consonant and vowel inventories, provided here for English as Forms 7-1 and 7-2. These forms are laid out in a manner that is intended to facilitate identification of gappy or asymmetrical systems to facilitate goal selection. Note that the term "medial" here references intervocalic consonants (such as [n] in "winnow"); elements from consonant sequences between two vowels (such as [n] or [d] from "window") should not be included here. In most cases, these "medial" consonants will be syllable initial (['wɪ.no]) although some may be shared between the two syllables (as in "warren" ['wɑɚ-ən]). In the latter case, the rhotic will be listed on the vowel chart as a rhotic diphthong, but a note can be added to the consonant chart.

These forms can be used in various ways. Most simply, the SLP can just circle those sounds that the child was observed to produce during the assessment. Recall that this is independent analysis, so it does not matter whether the child's production is the same as the adult production. The question to be answered is "Which speech sounds is this child capable of producing?" and not "Does this child produce speech sounds correctly?" The individual SLP can determine the criterion for mastery depending upon the size of the sample and level of confidence in the data collected. Note that "mastery" does not mean the youngster necessarily produces the phone accurately (i.e., in the appropriate words). It merely identifies those sounds that she consistently produces. In most cases, three occurrences in an assessment session (or set of sessions) in which the child produced at least 100 words, or two occurrences in at least 50 words if more cannot be obtained, are recommended as appropriate criteria for determining that a certain consonant or vowel has been mastered. Those phones that are never produced should be X'd out. The others (which are neither circled nor X'd out) will be assumed to be emerging in the child's speech. If desired, the numbers of occurrences of each of these emerging sounds can be indicated with a raised numeral.

Only consonant singletons should be counted for this form. Consonants that occur in clusters will appear on a later form, as these require more refined motor speech skills. Similarly, elements of diphthongs do not count in the single vowel portion of the vowel form. Thus, for example, [ɔ] and [ɪ] would not be counted if the child said [ɔɪ]; this would count as a production of [ɔɪ] only. Note also that [ɹ] is not listed in final position on the consonant inventory as [ɚ] is considered (by this author, as by many other phonologists) to be a **rhotic vowel** (as in [kɑɚ] "car" and [biɚd] "beard") and is therefore listed on Form 7-2. This phone should be credited as a consonant in medial position only where it is a syllable onset (e.g., in the word [mə.'ɹun][10] "maroon"), not where it is vocalic (e.g., in the word ['mɝ.dɚ] "murder"). In some cases, as in "purring" (['pɝɪŋ]), a rhotic vowel serves both roles. As noted previously, in these cases, it should be listed on the

[10]Note that the period represents a syllable boundary here.

Form 7-1

Name: Age:
Date: Examiner:
Source of sample: Size of sample:

CONSONANT REPERTOIRE

Note: Phones circled are "mastered" (i.e., occurred at least _____ times in that position in any context, whether correct or not). Phones X'd out did not occur in any context.

INITIAL:	lab	interd	alv	pal	velar	glott	Other/Notes:
STOPS	b		d		g		
	p		t		k		
NASALS	m		n				
GLIDES	w			j			
FRICATIVES	v	ð	z	ʒ			
	f	θ	s	ʃ		h	
AFFRICATES				tʃ, dʃ			
LIQUIDS			l	ɹ			

MEDIAL:	lab	interd	alv	pal	velar	glott	Other/Notes:
STOPS	b		d		g		
	p		t		k	ʔ	
NASALS	m		n		ŋ		
GLIDES	w			j			
FRICATIVES	v	ð	z	ʒ			
	f	θ	s	ʃ		h	
AFFRICATES				tʃ, dʒ			
LIQUIDS			l	ɹ			

FINAL:	lab	interd	alv	pal	velar	glott	Other/Notes:
STOPS	b		d		g		
	p		t		k	ʔ	
NASALS	m		n		ŋ		
FRICATIVES	v	ð	z	ʒ			
	f	θ	s	ʃ			
AFFRICATES				tʃ, dʒ			
LIQUIDS			l				

Note: [ɹ] is not listed in final position as [ɚ] is a rhotic *vowel*. Medially, [ɹ] should be counted only where it is consonantal (e.g., "around"), not vocalic (e.g., "bird").

Form 7-2

Name: Age:
Date: Examiner:
Source of sample: Size of sample:

VOWEL REPERTOIRE

Note: Phones circled are "mastered" (i.e., occurred at least _____ times in any context, whether correct or not). Phones X'd out did not occur in any context.

SIMPLE VOWELS			
	front	**central**	**back**
high			
tense	i		u
lax	ɪ		ʊ
mid			
tense	e		o
lax	ɛ		ɔ
low	æ	ʌ, ə	ɑ
DIPHTHONGS			
			ɔɪ
			ɑɪ
			ɑʊ
RHOTIC VOWELS			
	front	**central**	**back**
high			
	iɚ		uɚ
mid			
	ɛɚ		ɔɚ
low			
		ɝ, ɚ	ɑɚ

TABLE 7-20 APP-R Data from Jonathan, Aged 5;6

bæəs	basket	dɑ̃	nose
bot^{h}	boats	bes	page
dæ	candle	ɛbɪ	(air)plane
de	chair	win	queen
gɑʊbɔɪʔæt^{h}	cowboy hat	wɑk^{h}	rock
de	crayons	sæ dʌs	Santa Claus
bi	three	du dɑ	screwdriver
bæk	black	sdu	shoe
ji	green	wɑɪ	slide
jɑjo	yellow	nok	smoke
fɛbʊ	feather	nɛt^{h}	snake
fɪʃ	fish	dʌp	soap
væ:	flower	bu	spoon
fɔk	fork	gɛ	square
dæ	glasses	s:tɑ	star
dʌf	glove	wi	string
gʌm	gum	wɛ:ə	sweater
hæ	hanger	dɛvɪdi	television
hɑs:	horse	ʌm	thumb
ɑs du	ice cubes	bɛbʌʃ	toothbrush
jʌp dʌt	jump rope	dʌk^{h}	truck
vif	leaf	ve	vase
mæs	mask	wɑ	watch
mɑʊ	mouth	jɑjo	yo-yo
mugi mæt^{h}	music box	jip	zipper

vowel chart, but a note should be added to the consonant chart.

A speech sample obtained through the administration of the *Assessment of Phonological Processes—Revised* (Hodson, 1986; precursor to the Hodson Assessment of Phonological Patterns—3, Hodson, 2004) to Jonathan, a 5.5-year-old with CAS, is given in Table 7-20. This sample is used to illustrate completing the vowel and consonant inventory forms in Examples 7-1 and 7-2. Recall that this is an *independent* analysis. In other words, Jonathan's consonant and vowel productions are not compared to the consonants and vowels of the target words. Errors are not the focus. Rather, the purpose is to identify those consonants and vowels that Jonathan actually does produce. This informs the clinician about the status of his phonetic repertoire and about accidental and systematic gaps within his system. In this way, specific remediation goals can be identified.

This sample is small and is based upon the APP-R words, which are slightly more heavily weighted to clusters. However, more singleton consonants are available for analysis from Jonathan's productions as he reduces most clusters (and in independent analysis, the targets are irrelevant). Trends observed in this analysis could be confirmed through additional sampling procedures in therapy.

Clearly, Jonathan has a limited repertoire of mastered consonants, although there are several more that he produces occasionally. Because the form is laid out by place and manner of production, it's fairly easy to see that he has several systematic gaps: No voiceless stops occur in syllable-initial positions (whether word-initial or word-medial), and no voiced stops occur in final position. Very few fricatives are in evidence, especially voiced fricatives. Jonathan appears to have a preference for bilabials in syllable-initial positions but not in final position. Some of the gap sounds appear to be emerging and could be encouraged through therapy—[n] and [s] in initial position, [p] and [f] in final position. Other gaps that Jonathan's speech-language pathologist might hope to fill in include [z] in initial position, since he has other alveolars and other fricatives in that position. The bilabials seem to be emerging together in final position. If [j] or [v] do indeed continue to develop in syllable-initial word-medial position, the clinician should be able to facilitate the accompanying glide [w] (since bilabial is already established for [b]) and the accompanying fricatives [s] and/or [z] (since alveolar is already established for [d]) in that position as well. If [m] does continue to develop in final position, [n] and [ŋ] should not be far behind, given that the alveolar feature is already established for [t] and [s] and the velar feature is already established for [k]. In general, it is encouraging that various nasals and fricatives appear to be emerging in all positions. These sound classes are likely to become established without an extreme amount of effort.

Jonathan's repertoire of simple vowels is less limited. The infrequent occurrence of [ʊ] and [ɔ] in his speech may well be due to their scanty presence within the APP-R words (and within English in general). However, the APP-R did include an appropriate number of target rhotic vowels and diphthongs, none of which were produced by this child. This represents a systematic gap in his vowel inventory.

In summary, a phonetic repertoire laid out by place and manner of articulation can help us to identify systematic versus accidental gaps in the child's consonant and vowel inventories. These, in turn, will facilitate intervention planning.

Another example is provided using the sample from Marvin, a 21-month-old with hypotonia (low muscle tone), given in Table 7-21, to examine the babble repertoire of a prelinguistic child, as shown in Examples 7-3 and 7-4. Note that essentially identical babble forms that Marvin produced several times are not listed repeatedly in the table. Also, given the smaller size of the sample, two occurrences are used as the criterion for mastery in this case. Further observation will be used to confirm these findings.

Example 7-1

Name: *Jonathan* | Age: *5;6*
Date: | Examiner: *SLV*
Source of sample: *APP-R* | Size of sample: *50 words*

CONSONANT REPERTOIRE

Note: Phones circled are "mastered" (i.e., occurred at least _3_ times in that position in any context, whether correct or not). Phones X'd out did not occur in any context.

INITIAL:	lab	interd	alv	pal	velar	glott	Other/Notes:
STOPS	(b)		(d)		(g)		
	~~p~~		~~t~~		~~k~~		
NASALS	(m)		n^2				
GLIDES	(w)			(j)			
FRICATIVES	(v)	~~ð~~	~~z~~	~~ʒ~~			
	(f)	~~θ~~	s^1	~~ʃ~~		h^2	
AFFRICATES				~~tʃ~~, ~~dʒ~~			
LIQUIDS			~~l~~	~~ɹ~~			
MEDIAL:	lab	interd	alv	pal	velar	glott	Other/Notes:
STOPS	(b)		(d)		g^1		
	~~p~~		~~t~~		~~k~~	ʔ^1	
NASALS	m^1		~~n~~		~~ŋ~~		
GLIDES	~~w~~			j^2			
FRICATIVES	v^1	~~ð~~	~~z~~	~~ʒ~~			
	(f)	~~θ~~	~~s~~	~~ʃ~~		~~h~~	
AFFRICATES				tʃ, ~~dʒ~~			
LIQUIDS			~~l~~	~~ɹ~~			
FINAL:	lab	interd	alv	pal	velar	glott	Other/Notes:
STOPS	~~b~~		~~d~~		~~g~~		
	p^2		(t)		(k)	~~ʔ~~	
NASALS	m^1		~~n~~		~~ŋ~~		
FRICATIVES	~~v~~	~~ð~~	~~z~~	~~ʒ~~			
	f^2	~~θ~~	(s)	ʃ^2			
AFFRICATES				~~tʃ~~, ~~dʒ~~			
LIQUIDS			~~l~~				

Note: [ɹ] is not listed in final position as [ɚ] is a rhotic *vowel*. Medially, [ɹ] should be counted only where it is consonantal (e.g., "around"), not vocalic (e.g., "bird").

Example 7-2

Name: *Jonathan*	Age: *5;6*
Date:	Examiner: *SLV*
Source of sample: *APP-R*	Size of sample: *50 words*

VOWEL REPERTOIRE

Note: Phones circled are "mastered" (i.e., occurred at least _3_ times in any context, whether correct or not). Phones X'd out did not occur in any context.

SIMPLE VOWELS			
	front	**central**	**back**
high			
tense	(i)		(u)
lax	(ɪ)		ʊ^{1}
mid			
tense	(e)		(o)
lax	(ɛ)		ɔ^{1}
low	(æ)	(ʌ), (ə)	(ɑ)
DIPHTHONGS			
			ɔɪ^{1}
			ɑɪ^{1}
			ɑʊ^{2}
RHOTIC VOWELS			
	front	**central**	**back**
high			
	~~iɚ~~		~~uɚ~~
mid			
	~~ɛɚ~~		~~ɔɚ~~
low			
		~~ɝ~~, ~~ɚ~~	~~ɑɚ~~

TABLE 7-21 Babble Sample from Marvin at 21 Months

ʃugɑgɑ
gɪgɪ
tʰɪtʰɪ
r::: (alveolar trill)
dɪdɪ
x:: (voiceless velar fricative)
ɪdɛwəwʊ
i:dʊjɛdʊɪdə
kədʌwɛ:
ɑʊkə
dɪʊkə
hɑɪdʊ
dʊɪ
dɑxəgɑʊgə
gəgədədə
β::: (voiced bilabial fricative)
æ::
kwɪkəkʰɪkə
kətʰɪtʰɪkətʰɪ
dʊkdʊkə
ktʃə
ɑɣɑɪgəgəgɑgə (ɣ: voiced velar fricative)
dʊkə
ɑdʊdʊkə

Again, the systematic layout of the forms helps us to see that Marvin produces voiced and voiceless alveolar and velar stops in his babble, with the syllable-initial medial labio-velar glide [w]. No other labials are noted and no nasals; these limitations are somewhat unusual and should be monitored. Various non-English fricatives are used, especially as isolated consonants, which is not uncommon in babble. They have been added to the form in the appropriate locations. The total lack of final consonants is of no concern at this speech stage, although of course it does constitute somewhat of a delay for Marvin's chronologic age. When he begins to produce adult-based words (with stimulation provided in therapy, as described in Chapter 6, later in this chapter, and in Chapter 8), his phonetic repertoire will be expected to expand to include more consonant types and his phonotactic repertoire to include more word shapes.

Marvin's vowel repertoire is spread across the oral cavity, with front, back, high, and low vowels all occurring. The frequent occurrence of lax vowels and infrequent occurrence of tense vowels is probably a result of his low oral muscle tone. Occasional diphthongs are also in evidence. Rhotic diphthongs are not expected at this age or this stage. In therapy, motor speech activities will address his low oral tone. For example, tense vowels ([i, e, u, o]) will be modeled in play contexts (e.g., "oh!" for surprising events, "ooh" for something pretty, "Whee!" for sliding) in an attempt to stimulate his motivation and ability to achieve the lingual muscle tone required for such vowels.

EXERCISE 7-3

Assessment of Phonetic Development

Relational Analysis of Speech Sounds

It is important to know what sounds a child is producing regardless of target, but of course to be a successful communicator, the child must be able to use these sounds meaningfully. Listeners will have difficulty understanding if the correct phones are not used. Thus, accuracy of production must be determined.

At the macrolevel, it is useful to know how accurate, overall, children of given ages should be expected to be. The percent consonants correct metric developed by Shriberg and colleagues serves this function. In its most recent incarnation (Shriberg et al., 1997a), "Percent Consonants Correct—Revised" (PCC-R) is calculated by dividing the total number of consonants that a child produced correctly by the total number of consonants attempted, in a conversational speech sample:

$$\frac{\text{No. of consonant tokens produced correctly}}{\text{Total no. of consonant tokens produced}}$$

In this revised version of the PCC measure, distortions are counted as "correct." Reference data calculated using this formula indicate that children who are typically developing produce 94% of the consonants that they attempt correctly by their fourth year of life (i.e., between 3;0 and 3;11), as shown in Table 7-22 based on Austin and Shriberg (1997). These data are very useful, as the full norms compare children by sex and by speech status (TD versus speech delayed) as well as by age. PCC-R has been demonstrated to be correlated with severity and to differentiate children with typical speech, including those whose speech had been delayed or disordered but is now age appropriate, from those with ongoing speech deficits (Shriberg & Kwaitkowski, 1990; Shriberg et al., 1997a, 1997b).

TABLE 7-22 Austin and Shriberg (1997) Percent Consonants Correct-Revised Norms

Age	Typically Developing PCC-R	Speech Delayed PCC-R
3;0–3;11	94	69
4;0–4;11	93	73
5;0–5;11	94	71
6;0–6;11	95	73
7;0–7;11	97	73
8;0–8;11	97	69
9;0–11;11	98	93

Example 7-3

Name: *Marvin* Age: *21 mos.*

Date: Examiner: *SLV*

Source of sample: *babble sample* Size of sample: *50 babbles*

CONSONANT REPERTOIRE

Note: Phones circled are "mastered" (i.e., occurred at least _ 2 _ times in that position in any context, whether correct or not). Phones X'd out did not occur in any context.

INITIAL:	lab	interd	alv	pal	velar	glott	Other/Notes:
STOPS	~~b~~		(d)		(g)		*C's in isolation:*
	~~p~~		t[1]		(k)		[ɹ, x, β]
NASALS	~~m~~		~~n~~				
GLIDES	~~w~~			~~j~~			
FRICATIVES	~~v~~	~~ð~~	~~z~~	~~ʒ~~			
	~~f~~	~~θ~~	~~s~~	ʃ[1]		h[1]	
AFFRICATES				~~tʃ~~, ~~dʒ~~			
LIQUIDS			~~l~~	~~ɹ~~			

MEDIAL:	lab	interd	alv	pal	velar	glott	Other/Notes:
STOPS	~~b~~		(d)		(g)		
	~~p~~		(t)		(k)	(ʔ)	
NASALS	~~m~~		~~n~~		~~ŋ~~		
GLIDES	(w)			j[1]			
FRICATIVES	~~v~~	~~ð~~	~~z~~	~~ʒ~~	ɣ[1]		
	~~f~~	~~θ~~	~~s~~	~~ʃ~~		~~h~~	
AFFRICATES				~~tʃ~~, ~~dʒ~~			
LIQUIDS			~~l~~	~~ɹ~~			

FINAL:	lab	interd	alv	pal	velar	glott	Other/Notes:
STOPS	~~b~~		~~d~~		~~g~~		
	~~p~~		~~t~~		~~k~~	~~ʔ~~	
NASALS	~~m~~		~~n~~		~~ŋ~~		
FRICATIVES	~~v~~	~~ð~~	~~z~~	~~ʒ~~	ɣ[1]		
	~~f~~	~~θ~~	~~s~~	~~ʃ~~			
AFFRICATES				~~tʃ~~, ~~dʒ~~			
LIQUIDS			~~l~~				

Note: [ɹ] is not listed in final position as [ɚ] is a rhotic *vowel.* Medially, [ɹ] should be counted only where it is consonantal (e.g., "around"), not vocalic (e.g., "bird").

Example 7-4

Name: *Marvin* Age: *21 mos.*

Date: Examiner: *SLV*

Source of sample: *babble sample* Size of sample: *50 babbles*

VOWEL REPERTOIRE

Note: Phones circled are "mastered" (i.e., occurred at least __*2*__ times in any context, whether correct or not). Phones X'd out did not occur in any context.

SIMPLE VOWELS			
	front	central	back
high			
tense	i[1]		u[1]
lax	(ɪ)		(ʊ)
mid			
tense	~~e~~		~~o~~
lax	(ɛ)		~~ɔ~~
low	æ[1]	(ʌ),(ə)	(ɑ)
DIPHTHONGS			
			~~ɔɪ~~
			(ɑɪ)
			(ɑʊ)
RHOTIC VOWELS			
	front	central	back
high			
	~~iɚ~~		~~uɚ~~
mid			
	~~ɛɚ~~		~~ɔɚ~~
low			
		~~ɝ~~, ~~ɚ~~	ɑɚ

In fact, this measure has been used frequently in research studies as an index of severity. For example, Ambrose and colleagues (2014) used PCC-R to demonstrate that 2-year-olds with hearing loss have deficient consonant production in comparison to their TD peers. Other studies have used PCC or PCC-R to estimate the impact of speech sound disorders on later literacy skills (Peterson, Pennington, Shriberg, & Boada, 2009; Preston & Edwards, 2010) with mixed results.

Data for Percent Vowels Correct—Revised (PVC-R) are also available in this Waisman Center technical report. Austin and Shriberg's (1997) data show that by the time that they are 3 years old (3;0–3;11), typically developing children are producing approximately 98% of English vowels correctly. Those with speech sound disorders are 88.5% accurate on vowels at this age. The Percent Vowels Correct—Revised (PVC-R) data for typically developing versus speech-delayed children are given below in Table 7-23. Note, however, that children with CAS are likely to have higher vowel error rates (ASHA, 2007).

PCC-R and PVC-R tell us how often the child's production is wrong. However, they don't tell us how "off" the child's production was (e.g., was it a substitution or an omission? If a substitution, was it a predictable error, such [f] for /θ/? or something bizarre like [k] for /ɹ/?). It also does not indicate how systematic the child's errors were nor the impact of the word position on the child's accuracy. Finally, because it's based on counting incorrect consonants, only errors that occur in intelligible words can be counted: if we don't know the target word, we don't know which sounds within the word were correct. In this sense, unintelligible words are "free"—the child's score is not decreased by their presence in the sample.

The impact of these limitations to this measure can be striking in some cases. Two recordings of one child followed clinically for several years by Velleman and colleagues were used in a study by Shriberg, Aram, and Kwiatkowski (1997). This child's speech progressed over a three-year period from being highly unintelligible and restricted to only monosyllabic words with open syllables (no final consonants) to quite intelligible multisyllabic words with clusters and final consonants, although there were still many errors (e.g., "bastet ball"). Because PCC-R is based only on segmental accuracy in intelligible words—not syllable or word shapes—and with no way to take the percentage of words that are intelligible into account—this child's PCC-R remained very low with very little change throughout this time period. Shriberg, Aram, and colleagues (1997) drew the conclusion that "Child 7/14 made virtually no gains in his speech development during a three-year period, as shown by his PCC at five years four months (79.3%) and again at eight years five months (78.3%)" (p. 316). His therapists, his family, and his teachers saw the situation very differently! Thus, while PCC-R is valuable for estimating the severity of a child's speech difficulties, its limitations must also be kept in mind. It should not be used to the exclusion of other measures.

The majority of single-word articulation tests that are on the market provide related but more detailed information; they identify a child's errors via the traditional substitution, omission, distortion analysis (**SODA**). Most such tests use pictures to elicit the client's production of a variety of consonants, mostly in initial, medial, and final positions (often including medial consonant sequences as well as singleton syllable-initial medial consonants). The majority also assess some clusters. A few include vowels. Many provide the means for testing stimulability (i.e., whether the child can produce the word when additional cues, such as one or multiple auditory models, visual models, or tactile cues, are provided).

These tests have several positive features: the pictures are typically colorful, engaging, and age appropriate; the words are selected to include "all phonemes" of English (though certainly not all allophones), usually in at least two word positions; the words are known so the examiner is not faced with unintelligible words that cannot be used for SODA analysis; systematic forms are provided for data collection; only certain phonemes in each word have to be scored; the IPA form of the target word is often provided to make the examiner's job even easier; and norms are included so that the child's performance can be compared with a reasonable amount of confidence to that of other children of the same age. Due to the possibility of avoidance in spontaneous speech, standardized tests are more likely to elicit more complex word forms (Masterson, Bernhardt, & Hofheinz, 2005). As such, single-word articulation tests clearly have many appropriate uses.

TABLE 7-23 Austin and Shriberg (1997) Percent Vowels Correct—Revised Norms

Age Range	Typically Developing	Speech Delayed
3;0–3;11	98.0	88.5
4;0–4;11	98.4	94.8
5;0–5;11	98.7	94.2
6;0–6;11	99.1	91.8
7;0–7;11	99.4	93.4
8;0–8;11	99.6	86.5

COMMON *Confusion*

PREPOSITIONS MATTER!

When talking or writing about substitutions, be careful about preposition use. "For" and "with" have very different implications in this context:

- "He substitutes **x** for **y**" means /y/ is the target and [x] is what the child produces.
- "He substitutes **x** with **y**" means /x/ is the target and [y] is what the child produces.

It is common for SLPs to use the notation "x/y" to indicate that [x] is substituted for /y/ (i.e., /y/ is the target but the child says [x]).

However, there are also important limitations to single-word articulation tests. For example, children's productions of single words are often quite different than their productions in spontaneous speech, especially if the words are imitated (Dyson & Robinson, 1987; Walker, Archibald, Cherniak, & Fish, 1992). Not surprisingly, this holds for children with phonological disorders as well as typically developing children and for those whose first language is Spanish as well as those who speak English (Goldstein, Fabiano, & Iglesias, 2004). In fact, even productions of nouns (the main stimuli on single-word articulation tasks) versus verbs (more common in speech samples) tend to differ (Camarata & Schwartz, 1985), with verbs being less accurate and more variable. Thus, it is worthwhile to elicit and analyze both single words and conversational speech whenever possible.

Disadvantages of standardized articulation tests also include the fact that picture naming is a common task in mainstream American culture, but not so in many other cultures including some American cultures (e.g., Hispanic, African American; Peña & Quinn, 1997). Children's speech in elicited contexts such as picture naming may be quite different from spontaneous verbal interactions, especially if the former is an unfamiliar activity.

For children for whom the task is not alien, accuracy in single-word production may be far better than in phrase- or sentence-level utterances due to the reduction of other demands (e.g., syntax, semantics). Well-established sounds may be more accurate in spontaneous speech, while sounds that are emerging may be more accurate on articulation tests (Morrison & Shriberg, 1992). On the other hand, articulation tests elicit the production of the more complex targets that are likely to be emerging, which the child can avoid during spontaneous speech, sometimes resulting in higher accuracy in conversational speech (Masterson et al., 2005).

Many articulation tests purport to provide a sufficient sample of consonant and vowel sounds in a variety of contexts. As noted above, Eisenberg and Hitchcock (2010) refuted this in a study in which they carried out an analysis of 11 frequently used articulation/phonology tests. Their criteria were based on the concept that target words must be carefully phonetically controlled in order to minimize contextual factors that might mask the child's ability to produce the sound. In other words, they propose that all factors that might make it more challenging for the child to produce the target consonant or vowel be avoided in order to see how well the child can produce the desired sound under the best possible phonetic conditions. These criteria are given in Table 7-24. They include stipulations that the target words must be monosyllabic or at least in stressed syllables if the words are disyllabic and that the target sounds must occur in non-harmonic contexts (avoiding words such as "cake" and "puppy"). They also suggest that the target sounds must be sampled in different phonetic contexts (e.g., consonants before two different vowels, vowels in two different words) in order to verify that the child can produce them in varied contexts. To be comprehensive, word positions should include syllable initial position within words (e.g., [d] in "window"), syllable final position within words (e.g., [n] in

What Factors Should Be Considered in Selecting a Single-Word Articulation Test?

- *Appropriateness to the client, especially the age level of the words and illustrations, but also the length of time required to administer the test*
- *Appropriateness to the purpose, including:*
    - *Comprehensiveness: Are vowels as well as consonants tested? Consonants in syllable-initial medial position? A good variety of clusters? Contextual effects (coarticulation)? Multisyllabic words?*
    - *Reliability and validity*
    - *Normative data and standardization, including norming on the population from which the child comes*
    - *Analyses facilitated, such as stimulability, spontaneous versus imitated production, single-word versus elicited sentences, etc.*
- *Appropriateness to the clinician: Does the clinician have the knowledge and skills necessary to administer, score, and interpret the test?*

TABLE 7-24 Criteria for Phonetically Controlled Articulation Tests

Target Segments	Minimally Challenging Contexts
Word-initial consonants	Singleton (not in a cluster) Monosyllabic or bisyllabic word If bisyllabic, target is in initial stressed syllable Non-harmonic (all consonants different)
Word-final consonants	Singleton (not in a cluster) Monosyllabic or bisyllabic word If bisyllabic, target is in final stressed syllable Non-harmonic (all consonants different) Monomorphemic (target is not in a separate morpheme, such as "s" in plurals)
Vowels	Monosyllabic or bisyllabic word If bisyllabic, target is in initial stressed syllable Not before a liquid consonant

Adapted from Eisenberg, S. L., & Hitchcock, E. R. (2010). Using standardized tests to inventory consonant and vowel production: A comparison of 11 tests of articulation and phonology. *Language, Speech, and Hearing Services in Schools, 41*, 488–503.

"window"), true intervocalic position (e.g., [n] in "winnow"), and various possible positions within various possible clusters (including, e.g., initial position in initial clusters, such as the [s] in "string," medial position in medial clusters, such as the [s] in "hamster," and final position in final clusters, such as the [s] in "hearts") as well as the more commonly studied initial and final word positions. The tests that they analyzed and their core characteristics are given in Table 7-25. Eisenberg and Hitchcock did not find a single test that adequately sampled the sounds of English according to their guidelines. They reported that the Bankson-Bernthal Test of Phonology (Bankson & Bernthal, 1990) had the best coverage of initial and final consonants. The most phonetically controlled, comprehensive tests for vowels were the Fisher-Logemann Test of Articulation Competence (Fisher & Logemann, 1971), the Smit-Hand Articulation and Phonology Evaluation (Smit & Hand, 1992), and the Templin-Darley Tests of Articulation (Templin & Darley, 1968).

It must be noted that Eisenberg and Hitchcock (2010) are using a very specific definition of "mastery" of a speech sound. This raises the question of whether a child can be considered to have mastered a sound if he cannot produce it in unstressed syllables, in harmonized contexts, etc. This issue is by no means resolved within our field. In any case, if the question is whether the child can produce a certain phone under the simplest possible conditions, Eisenberg and Hitchcock's criteria can guide the SLP to choosing what those conditions should be.

From a clinical point of view, studies of the extent to which single-word elicitation (as in articulation testing) and conversational elicitation (as in speech sampling) yield the same clinical results vary, with some researchers concluding that articulation tests "yield neither typical nor optimal measures of speech performance" (Morrison & Shriberg, 1992, p. 259) and others that "a single-word task tailored to some extent to the client's phonological system gives sufficient and representative information for phonological evaluation" (Masterson et al., 2005, p. 229). Most studies report variation among children in this respect (McLeod, Hand, Rosenthal, & Hayes, 1994).

A further limitation of articulation tests of this sort is that they focus solely on the child's error patterns: What is he doing wrong? As in the case of Menn and team's (2009) "Ellie," a child may produce a consonant such as [ʃ] but never when the target is /ʃ/. An articulation test would highlight the fact that /ʃ/ was never produced correctly, but miss the fact that the child actually is able to produce this sound in non-target contexts. Independent analysis complements such testing by identifying the phones produced, regardless of the target. Thus, while standardized tests of articulation definitely have their uses, especially for identifying the presence of an SSD, the administration of such a test should not be mistaken for having carried out a thorough assessment of the child's phonology.

In addition, sometimes, the administration of a test is not a possibility due to child factors, such as age, attention span, or behavioral profile, or to site factors such as the availability of standardized testing materials in the appropriate language(s).

TABLE 7-25 Core Characteristics of 11 Popular Single-Word Articulation/Phonology Tests

Test	Norm Referenced?	Word Positions	Vowels Tested?	No. of Words
AAPS-3	Yes	Initial final	Yes	46
BBTOP	Yes	Initial final	No	81
CAAP	Yes	Initial final	No	44
DEAP	Yes	Initial final	Yes	30
FLTA	No	Initial medial final	Yes	104
GFTA-2 and KLPA-2	Yes	Initial medial final	No	53
HAPP-3	Yes	N/A	Yes	50
PAT-3	Yes	Initial medial final	Yes	77
SHAPE	Yes	Initial final	No	81
SPAT-II	Yes	Initial medial final	No	45
TDTA	Yes	Initial medial final	Yes	141

AAPS-3: Arizona Articulation Proficiency Scale, 3rd Edition (Fudala, 2000).
BBTOP: Bankson-Bernthal Test of Phonology (Bankson & Bernthal, 1990).
CAAP: Clinical Assessment of Articulation and Phonology (Secord, Donohoe, & Johnson, 2002).
DEAP: Diagnostic Evaluation of Articulation and Phonology (Dodd, Hua, Crosbie, Holm, & Ozanne, 2006).
FLTA: Fisher-Logemann Test of Articulation (Fisher & Logemann, 1971).
GFTA-2: Goldman-Fristoe Test of Articulation, 2nd Edition (Goldman & Fristoe, 2000).
KLPA-2: Khan-Lewis Phonological Analysis, 2nd Edition (Khan & Lewis, 2002)—Uses same stimuli as GFTA-2, so they were considered together.
HAPP-3: Hodson Assessment of Phonological Patterns, 3rd Edition (Hodson, 2004).
PAT-3: Photo Articulation Test, 3rd Edition (Lippke, Dickey, Selmar, & Soder, 1997).
SHAPE: Smit-Hand Articulation and Phonology Evaluation (Smit & Hand, 1992).
SPAT-II: Structured Photographic Articulation Test, 2nd Edition (Dawson & Tattersall, 2001).
TDTA: Templin-Darley Tests of Articulation (Templin & Darley, 1968).
Adapted from Eisenberg, S. L., & Hitchcock, E. R. (2010). Using standardized tests to inventory consonant and vowel production: A comparison of 11 tests of articulation and phonology. *Language, Speech, and Hearing Services in Schools, 41*, 488–503.

In an attempt to develop a summary statistic representing a child's ability to produce a variety of sounds correctly, Ingram (2002) developed the phonological mean length of utterance (PMLU) measure as described in Chapter 5. This statistic is calculated by counting the number of consonants produced in a word (whether they are distinct from each other or not—e.g., "mommy" [mɑmi] would be counted as having two consonants) and then adding an additional point per consonant that was produced correctly. A further measure involves dividing the child's PMLU points by the PMLU of the target word (i.e., the number of points one would get if the word were produced with 100% accuracy), yielding the "proportion of whole-word proximity" (PWP). The point system does not take the phonotactic complexity of the word into account, however. Stoel-Gammon (2010) proposed the "Word Complexity Measure," which reflects the difficulty of the structures (clusters, multisyllabic words, etc.) as well as the consonants that the child produces. Such measures, which are applicable to bilingual as well as monolingual children (Burrows & Goldstein, 2010), may give an overview score that can be used to summarize a child's phonological status, but they are not intended to facilitate specific treatment planning. Far more detail is necessary for the latter purpose.

When appropriate, forms similar to Forms 7-1 and 7-2 from the beginning of this chapter, renumbered as Forms 7-3 and 7-4, can be used as tools for this more detailed relational phonetic/phonemic analysis. In this case, the phonemes of adult English are listed on the forms. The clinician should write the actual phone produced above or beside the phoneme listed for each consonant and vowel sound in the language. Multiple substitutions should be listed in order of frequency of occurrence with the most frequent substitutions listed first.

Correct productions may be listed or not as appropriate to the situation. In cases in which the child sometimes produces the correct form but sometimes substitutes, it is helpful to list the occurrences of the correct form. If this is done, the clinician will know upon looking at the form later that the correct phone was produced and with what relative frequency. For example, "$v^{b,v,w}$" would indicate that the child most often substituted [b] for /v/, next most often produced it correctly, and least often substituted [w]. It's even better to list the frequencies of each substitution, for example, "$v^{b6,v2,w1}$" ([b] substitution six times, correct [v] production two times, [w] substitution once).

In Example 7-5, the substituted consonant phones of the hypothetical child called Johnny Stopper are listed in italics; the same is done for Johnny's vowels in Example 7-6. As in analyzing the child's phonetic repertoire, these forms are then scrutinized for gaps in sound classes. Such gaps may occur either with respect to which sounds are produced correctly (e.g., velars never produced correctly) or with respect to which sounds are attempted (e.g., velars never attempted). Phones that occur often as substitutes for adult phonemes are also appropriate candidates for functional load analysis, as described further.

What's with All the &#^% Forms?

School systems often require that standardized tests be given so that scores can be used to determine the presence or absence of an SSD. However, as noted above, these tests are really only appropriate for identification, not for thorough assessment. The forms provided here allow for more in-depth assessment. In addition, in some cases, especially for independent analysis, there is no test that will yield the necessary information. Both the independent analysis forms and the substitution forms in this section can be used for spontaneous speech samples.

Secondly, repertoires in spontaneous speech may be quite different than those in single-word naming tasks, especially if imitation is used, as described previously.

Finally, carrying out detailed analyses "by hand" will help you to develop instincts about what's going on in children's phonologies. Once you have used the forms a few times, you will no longer need to use all of them for every child. The instincts that you will have developed will serve you in good stead for determining which forms for which clients at which times to use in the future based on areas of greatest need. What you will have learned from using the forms will also deepen your insight into what is going on in a disordered phonology even if you only give a standardized single-word articulation test. You will notice more than the test is designed to highlight.

The better you understand the phonological deficits of the children with whom you work, the more appropriate and efficient your remediation goals and strategies will be.

Assessment of Phonemes

As with all other aspects of a child's phonology, there are two ways to analyze and assess the contrast in a child's phonological system: independent analysis and relational analysis. To assess contrast independently, sources of contrast within the child's own word forms must be identified without consideration for the target forms. For example, if [b] and [β] function to differentiate words within the child's system, they will be considered to be contrastive phonemes within that system, regardless of the fact that they are not distinct phonemes in adult English. If the adult homonyms "bear" and "bare" are produced distinctly by the child as [bɛ] and [βɛ], for instance, then these two words will be considered to be minimal pairs within that child's system, with child phonemes /b/ and /β/, even though those words are homonyms for adult English speakers. Regardless of their status in the ambient language, they are contrastive for the child.

To assess contrast relationally, the contrasts produced by the child are compared directly to those of the adult language to see if the child has the same phonemic system—system of contrasts among consonants and vowels—as in the ambient language. This is typically done indirectly, by determining

Form 7-3

Name: Age:
Date: Examiner:
Source of sample: Size of sample:

CONSONANT PHONEME SUBSTITUTIONS
(RELATIONAL ANALYSIS)

Indicate substitutions beside (presumed) target phonemes (e.g., f^b). Phonemes X'd out were not attempted in this sample. Ø indicates the sound was omitted.

INITIAL:	**lab**	**interd**	**alv**	**pal**	**velar**	**glott**	**Other/Notes:**
STOPS	b		d		g		
	p		t		k		
NASALS	m		n				
GLIDES	w			j			
FRICATIVES	v	ð	z	ʒ			
	f	θ	s	ʃ		h	
AFFRICATES				tʃ, dʒ			
LIQUIDS			l	ɹ			
MEDIAL:	**lab**	**interd**	**alv**	**pal**	**velar**	**glott**	**Other/Notes:**
STOPS	b		d		g		
	p		t		k	ʔ	
NASALS	m		n		ŋ		
GLIDES	w			j			
FRICATIVES	v	ð	z	ʒ			
	f	θ	s	ʃ		h	
AFFRICATES				tʃ, dʒ			
LIQUIDS			l	ɹ			
FINAL:	**lab**	**interd**	**alv**	**pal**	**velar**	**glott**	**Other/Notes:**
STOPS	b		d		g		
	p		t		k	ʔ	
NASALS	m		n		ŋ		
FRICATIVES	v	ð	z	ʒ			
	f	θ	s	ʃ			
AFFRICATES				tʃ, dʒ			
LIQUIDS			l				

Note: [ɹ] not listed in final position as [ɚ] is a rhotic vowel. Medially, [ɹ] should be counted only where it is consonantal ("around"), not vocalic ("bird").

Form 7-4

Name: Age:
Date: Examiner:
Source of sample: Size of sample:

VOWEL PHONEME SUBSTITUTIONS (RELATIONAL ANALYSIS)

Indicate substitutions beside (presumed) target phonemes (e.g., $ʊ^{ə}$). X out any Phonemes not attempted.

SIMPLE VOWELS			
	front	**central**	**back**
high			
tense	i		u
lax	ɪ		ʊ
mid			
tense	e		o
lax	ɛ		ɔ
low			
lax	æ	ʌ,ə	ɑ
DIPHTHONGS			
			ɔɪ
			ɑɪ
			ɑʊ
RHOTIC VOWELS			
	front	**central**	**back**
high			
	ɪɚ		uɚ
mid			
	ɛɚ		ɔɚ
low			
		ɚ, ɝ	ɑɚ

Example 7-5

Name: *Johnny Stopper* Age: *4;10*
Date: *8/8/98* Examiner: *SLV*
Source of sample: *free play* Size of sample: *150 words*

CONSONANT PHONEME SUBSTITUTIONS
(RELATIONAL ANALYSIS)

Indicate substitutions beside (presumed) target phonemes (e.g., f^{b}). X indicates that Phonemes were not attempted in this sample. Ø indicates the sound was omitted.

INITIAL:	lab	interd	alv	pal	velar	glott	Other/Notes:
STOPS	b		d		g^{d3}		
	p		t		k^{t1}		
NASALS	m		n				
GLIDES	w			j			
FRICATIVES	v^{b1}	ð^{d1}	z^{d2}	X (ʒ)			
	f^{p4}	θ^{t3}	s^{t7}	ʃ^{t3}		h	
AFFRICATES				tʃ^{t2}, dʒ^{d1}			
LIQUIDS			l^{w1,j1}	ɹ^{w4}			
MEDIAL:	lab	interd	alv	pal	velar	glott	Other/Notes:
STOPS	b		d		g^{d2}		
	p		t		k^{t3,k1}	X (ʔ)	
NASALS	m		n		ŋ^{n4}		
GLIDES	w			j			
FRICATIVES	v^{b1}	ð^{d1}	z^{d3}	ʒ^{d1}			
	f^{p4}	θ^{t2}	s^{t6}	ʃ^{t1}		h	
AFFRICATES				tʃ^{t1}, dʒ^{d1}			
LIQUIDS			l^{w2,j1}	X (ɹ)			
FINAL:	lab	interd	alv	pal	velar	glott	Other/Notes:
STOPS	b		d		g^{d4}		
	p		t		k^{t3,k1}	X (ʔ)	
NASALS	m		n		ŋ^{n8}		
FRICATIVES	v^{b1}	ð^{d1}	z^{d5}	X (ʒ)			
	f^{p3}	θ^{t1}	s^{t6}	ʃ^{t2}			
AFFRICATES				tʃ^{t1}, dʒ^{d1}			
LIQUIDS			l^{ʊ5}				

Note: [ɹ] is not listed in final position as [ɚ] is a rhotic vowel. Medially, [ɹ] should be counted only where it is consonantal ("around"), not vocalic ("bird").

Example 7-6

Name: *Johnny Stopper* Age: *4;10*

Date: *8/8/98* Examiner: *SLV*

Source of sample: *free play* Size of sample: *150 words*

VOWEL PHONEME SUBSTITUTIONS (RELATIONAL ANALYSIS)

Indicate substitutions beside (presumed) target phonemes (e.g., ʊ^{ə}). X out any Phonemes not attempted.

SIMPLE VOWELS			
	front	**central**	**back**
high			
tense	i		u
lax	ɪ		ʊ
mid			
tense	e		o
lax	ɛ		ɔ
low			
lax	æ	ʌ,ə	ɑ
DIPHTHONGS			
			ɔɪ^{ɔ1,ɪ1}
			ɑɪ^{ɑ2,ɪ2}
			ɑʊ^{ɑ2,ʊ1}
RHOTIC VOWELS			
	front	**central**	**back**
high			
	~~iɚ~~		~~ʊɚ~~
mid			
	~~ɛɚ~~		~~ɔɚ~~
low			
		~~ɝ~~, ~~ɚ~~	~~ɑɚ~~

whether the child pronounces words correctly, thereby maintaining adult contrasts.

These two different approaches are reviewed below.

Independent Analysis of Contrast

Many types of contrast can be assessed by extending the analysis of the data organized via procedures that have already been discussed. For example, Forms 7-1 and 7-2, "Consonant Repertoires" and "Vowel Repertoires," which facilitate the identification of the child's phonetic repertoires, are useful for answering questions about whether the child produces potentially contrastive sounds or sound classes. Therefore, a first look for contrastive sound classes may be made using Forms 7-1 and 7-2. Sound classes that are missing from the phonetic inventory clearly are not available for such functional communication purposes. For example, if the child lacks fricatives in all positions, then fricatives clearly are not available to contrast with other consonant phonemes. The same holds for individual phonemes; for instance, if [s] is not ever produced, then it does not participate in phonemic contrasts.

Another important aspect of contrast that can be gleaned from these phonetic inventory forms is the occurrence of contrast across positions. It is common for children to have restrictions on which sound classes occur in which word positions. Some questions that are often useful in this respect include the following:

- Voicing: Is the child able to contrast voiced elements with voiceless elements at the same position in the word? For example, do both voiced and voiceless stops occur in initial position? Final position? If, for instance, all voiced stops occur only in initial position while voiceless stops occur only in final position (as often happens in very young children's speech), there is no possibility that they will contrast with each other.
- Fricatives, nasals: Do fricatives, nasals, and stops occur in the same word positions? In some children's repertoires, fricatives and/or nasals will occur in final position only with oral stops occurring in all but final position. Again, there is no possibility of contrast if two or three sound types do not show up in the same places.
- Velar consonants: Do all places of articulation occur in all word positions? It is not unusual for a child to produce velars in final position only. Other places of articulation may occur in all positions (in which case there is the possibility of contrast with velars only in final position—partial neutralization) or may occur in all except final position (in which case there is no possibility for contrast with velars, as the place of articulation features are in complementary distribution).

Any sound classes that have restricted distributions of these types will participate in a limited number of contrasts.

Another simple speech sample contrast analysis strategy is to search for minimal pairs and other phonetically similar words within the speech sample collected from the child. Minimal pairs easily identify a child's phonemes. As noted above, if the adult homonyms "bear" and "bare" are produced distinctly by the child as [bɛ] and [βɛ], for instance, then these two words will be considered to be minimal pairs within that child's system, with child phonemes /b/ and /β/.

However, in a small sample (e.g., 200 words or less), one would not expect to find very many minimal pairs. Fortunately, word pairs that differ by only two rather than one segment (**near-minimal pairs**) can often be found. Examples of such near-minimal pairs could include "strike/swipe, Parker/Harper, and pray/clay" as evidence that [k] and [p] are in contrast, for instance. Although one near-minimal pair is insufficient evidence of contrast, phones that occur in several such near-contrastive pairs (as do [k] and [p] in these examples) are highly likely to be separate phonemes in the child's system.

Let us consider again the data from Molly at 14 to 15 months. Molly tended to focus on final position and many of her words had very similar endings. There are several minimal pairs or near-minimal pairs within her speech sample, as illustrated in Table 7-26.

The occurrence of these pairs makes it clear that Molly is using several different consonants (e.g., [p] versus [w]; [p^{h}] versus [k^{h}]; [t] versus [w]) and vowels (e.g., [ɑ] versus [ɪ] versus [ʊ]; [ɑʊ] versus [ʌ]; [æ] versus [ɛ], etc.) contrastively. Therefore, each of these phones probably functions as a distinct phoneme within her system. Note that aspirated versus unaspirated stops (e.g., [k^{h}] versus [k]) may also be contrastive even though they are not distinct phonemes in adult English; further data would confirm or disconfirm this possibility.

If minimal pair (or near-minimal pair) words are difficult to locate, minimal pair syllables can also be sought in a child who (unlike Molly) does produce varied bisyllabic words. For example, if the child says [bɑdʊ] for "bottle" and [dɑdi] for "daddy," the two initial syllables of these words provide some evidence for a b/d contrast—[bɑ] versus [dɑ]. Similarly, the two final syllables—[dʊ] versus [di]—support an ʊ/i contrast. Of course, minimal pair syllables, like near-minimal pair words, provide less convincing evidence of the phonemic status of the relevant phones. Multiple examples of these types would be required. Form 7-5 provides a framework for listing all of

TABLE 7-26 Molly's Minimal Pairs

Minimal Pairs	Near-Minimal Pairs
[pɑnə], [wɑnə]	[hɑnʌ], [hʌnə]
[hɑnʌ], [hɑnɛ]	[næmʌ], [nɛmi]
[p^{h}ɑk^{h}], [k^{h}ɑk^{h}]	[pik^{h}], [p^{h}ɪk^{h}]
[k^{h}ɑk^{h}], [k^{h}ɪk^{h}]	[tɑt^{h}], [t^{h}ɑk^{h}i]
[p^{h}ʊk^{h}], [p^{h}ɪk^{h}], [p^{h}ɑk^{h}]	[kɑk^{h}i], [k^{h}ɑk^{h}]
[tɑt^{h}], [wɑt^{h}]	
[k^{h}ɪk^{h}], [p^{h}ɪk^{h}]	
[hɑʊt^{h}], [hʌt^{h}]	

From Vihman, M. M., & Velleman, S. L. (1989). Phonological reorganization: A case study. *Language and Speech*, *32*, 149–170.

Form 7-5

Name: Age:
Date: Examiner:
Source of sample: Size of sample:

WORD AND SYLLABLE CONTRASTS

Contrast	Minimal Pair Words	Minimal Pair Syllables	Near-Minimal Pairs
Example: b - k	bi - ki *bee - key*	bebi - mʌŋki *baby - monkey*	bæt - kæp *bat - cap*

Example 7-7

Name: *Christine* Age: 5;4
Date: Examiner: *SLV*
Source of sample: *spontaneous conversation* Size of sample: 55 *words*

WORD AND SYLLABLE CONTRASTS

Contrast	Minimal Pair Words	Minimal Pair Syllables	Near-Minimal Pairs
i - ɑɪ	mi - mɑɪ *me - mommy*		
i - ʌ - æ- u	di - dʌ - dæ - du *see-stuff-that-too*		
s - p - m	ʌs - ʌp - ʌm *us - up - home*		
w - m	wɑɪ - mɑɪ *why - mommy*		
j - m ɛ - æ			jɛs - mæs *yes - mask*
n - m		næsdi - mæs *nasty - mask*	

these types of contrast systematically, such that minimal pairs, near-minimal pairs, and syllable minimal pairs that provide evidence for the same contrast can be listed in one row. Data are filled in on this form for a hypothetical child named Christine in Example 7-7.

As is typical in a small speech sample, there are only a few minimal pairs, near-minimal pairs, and minimal pair syllables in Christine's speech. Note that she has several contrasts and potential contrasts with [m]; /m/ is likely a well-established phoneme in her system. The vowels [i] and [æ] also participate in two contrasts/potential contrasts each and are therefore probable phonemes.

Relational Analysis of Phonemes

The forms used above to identify substitutions (Forms 7-3 and 7-4) can also be used to analyze the contrast available within a child's phonological system. It is evident from Johnny Stopper's data in Examples 7-5 and 7-6 that this child lacks the following sound class contrasts: fricative–stop, liquid–glide, velar–alveolar, rhotic–nonrhotic vowel, and simple vowel/diphthong.[11] However, the fact that /k/ is sometimes produced as [k] in medial and final position (indicated by the fact that both [t] and [k] are listed there) indicates that the velar–alveolar contrast may be emerging. Therefore, this contrast would be an appropriate goal for remediation.

Note that the variants of each assumed target phoneme are listed; presumably, these are the allophones of that phoneme. For instance, Johnny's phoneme /k/ has the allophone [t] in all positions and the additional allophone [k] in medial and final positions. Since it is not predictable (as far as can be determined from the form) which will occur in medial and final positions, these allophones are considered to be in partially free variation. His /l/ phoneme has the allophones [j] and [w] prevocalically, in initial and medial position, that are in free variation with each other. In final position, [ʊ] occurs. Because the environment (position of occurrence) of the [ʊ] allophone is predictable (final position), [ʊ] is considered to be in complementary distribution with the other two allophones of /l/ ([j] and [w]).

Another important question that can be addressed using this type of relational analysis is whether the child is avoiding any adult phonemes. If velars, for instance, are never attempted, this has important implications for remediation. In order to avoid attempting words containing velars (but not other places of articulation), the child must be able to discriminate velars from other places of articulation. Furthermore, avoidance indicates the child's awareness that this sound class is a difficult one (for him or her). Although the avoidance of a sound

[11] In fact, Johnny may not even be aware of some of these contrasts. This is one of the drawbacks of relational analysis; it assumes that the child is fully aware of adult word forms and that the child's speech production target is the adult form. In reality, we cannot be sure of the child's underlying representation without more in-depth analysis of his phonology, preferably including discrimination probing and/or acoustic analysis of the contrasts in question.

class (or a phoneme) may have an important impact on the child's communication (since words that contain those sounds will not even be attempted), the clinician should recognize that resistance will undoubtedly occur if and when the child is pressed to produce avoided sounds (Schwartz & Leonard, 1982; Schwartz, Leonard, Frome-Loeb, & Swanson, 1987).

In the case of Johnny Stopper, rhotic diphthongs are never attempted. Johnny clearly avoids words that include such vowels, although he does attempt words with [ɚ]. The speech-language pathologist who works with Johnny should be aware of this in choosing target words for other sounds (e.g., "lair" would not be a good target word for the production of [l], as Johnny would be reluctant to attempt such a word). His willingness to at least attempt [ɚ] may be a window into this sound class if the production of rhotic vowels is targeted in therapy. Johnny's lack of attempts at [ʒ] in initial and final position is not of concern, as this phoneme is quite rare in the language, so few opportunities are available for its production in a speech sample. Furthermore, it would be a low priority for therapy even if it were a phoneme with which he had difficulty.

In short, segmental contrast can be determined by identifying potentially contrastive sound classes within the child's speech, by identifying minimal and near-minimal pairs or minimal syllables in the child's speech, and by considering the child's substitutions for assumed target phonemes.

Other Evidence of Contrast

Grunwell (1985) and Ingram (1981) suggest looking for homonyms in children's productive vocabularies as an indication that certain types of contrast may be missing. An appropriate worksheet can easily be created for those children for whom it appears appropriate, simply by listing word shapes and meanings under two headings. This was illustrated in Table 7-8 above for Joan (Ingram, 1981). Data from Holly (Velleman, 1994), the child with CAS who was described above, are repeated here in Table 7-27. Note that this is not a relational analysis, as the target (adult) forms are not compared to the child forms; only the target *meanings* are relevant.

The important information to be gleaned from this exercise is that Holly (in this case) has at least two sets of homonymic forms, each of which represents a wide phonetic variety of up to seven target words. Furthermore, in each case, the homonymic form includes two or more allomorphs (e.g., "bunny" may be pronounced as [bijə], [bɛə], or [bɪʊ]). Clearly, this will reduce her intelligibility significantly. The fact that she is using paralinguistic cues (whisper, gesture) to help to distinguish her homonyms indicates that she is aware of the inefficiency of her speech for communication purposes.

TABLE 7-27 Molly's Homonyms

Child Forms	Meanings
[bija,bɛə, bɪʊ]	bunny, bear, bird, baby (whispered), bell, pig (with gesture), Bert
[tʰ, tˢ, dɪ], coronal click	tree, kitty, coffee

TABLE 7-28 Molly's Variability

Child Meanings	Child Forms
bunny	[bijə, bɛə, bɪʊ]
tree	[tʰ, tˢ, dɪ], coronal click

The converse of homonymy is variability. In contrast to homonymy, in which one form has many meanings, when variability occurs, one meaning corresponds to many forms. In this case also, a meaning-form table can be helpful to summarize such situations, as shown with some of the same data for Holly in Table 7-28. Note that the same child may demonstrate both variability and homonymy, thereby drastically lowering her intelligibility.

For relational analysis of child phones that have high functional loads, as suggested by Grunwell (1985), a self-created worksheet is also appropriate. This can easily be done by taking the information from Forms 7-3 and 7-4, described previously for noting substitutions. Simply list each child phone in one column and the adult phonemes to which it appears to correspond in another. A third column can be used for the specific environments (positions) in which the substitution occurs. As an example, Martin's [f] and [v] (described above, from Grunwell, 1982) are listed in Table 7-29, along with all of the adult phonemes that they represent—most fricatives and affricates, clusters with fricatives and affricates, some stops, some liquids, and some stop + liquid clusters. This simple chart clearly confirms the clinician's suspicions that Martin is using labiodental fricatives for far too wide a variety of functions; they have a high functional load.

Summary

Standardized articulation tests and speech sample independent analysis forms are both options for identifying the child's functional contrastive use of speech sounds. Word forms elicited using articulation or process test pictures can be used for both purposes, but it is preferable to elicit a speech sample either instead of or as well as using single-word naming productions alone. The additional information about contrast that can be determined from a speech sample includes functional loads, homonymy, and preferred patterns.

EXERCISE 7-4

Contrast Assessment

TABLE 7-29 Martin's Substitutions

Child Phone	Assumed Target Phonemes	Restrictions/ Environments
[f]	/f/	Initial position
	/f/ clusters	Initial position
	Other fricatives, affricates	Initial position
	Clusters with fricatives	Initial position
	Clusters with affricates	Initial position
	Stop + /ɹ/ clusters	Initial position; infrequent
[v]	Non-labial stops	Medial, final positions
	Voiced fricatives	Medial position
	Voiced affricate /dʒ/	Final position
	/l/	Medial position

From Grunwell, P. (1985). *Phonological Assessment of Child Speech (PACS)*. Scarborough, ON: Nelson Thomson Learning.

IMPLICATIONS FOR REMEDIATION

Introduction

There are many factors to consider when selecting treatment approaches for children's speech sound production. The most basic question is whether to treat phonetically or phonemically—motorically or linguistically—or both. This requires deciding whether the child's difficulty results from sensory–motor or linguistic deficits, *or both*. In some cases, this appears to be an easy question, but it may be more subtle than it appears. Recall the case of Rachel, the child with cleft palate described by Howard (1993). Clearly, atypical structures and the resulting physiologic differences were at least the major sources of her SSD. Yet, she was very intelligible and also very resistant to therapy because her atypical system was largely working for her to achieve the contrast necessary for successful communication. For this reason, a contrast-based (phonemic) therapy strategy would most likely have been far more appropriate for her than the phonetic (motoric) approach that had been unable to create change in her system.

Of course, this is not to say that phonetic therapy approaches are never appropriate. A variety of the available phonetic approaches have been shown to be effective intervention strategies for some children. They are described below and summarized in the top of Table 7-30.

Phonetic Therapy Approaches

More traditional types of phonetic therapy, dating back to Van Riper (1939) and even before, focus on speech production of specific sounds, usually consonants. This often includes emphasis on placement, instructing the child explicitly as to where the articulators should be placed, what movements are required, etc. Typically, child-friendly terminology is used, such as referring to voiceless consonants as "quiet sounds," the alveolar ridge as "the bump behind your teeth," etc. This type of therapy traditionally progresses from producing the sound in isolation to syllables, to short words, to more complex words, to phrases, and so on. This may be preceded by **ear training** (i.e., sound identification training), in which the child is asked first to identify the sound when it is heard (e.g., "when you hear a snake sound [sː], point to the picture of the snake"), then to discriminate words in which the sound is produced correctly versus those in which it is produced in error ("Did I say that right?"). Note that this type of discrimination is different from both phonemic discrimination (differentiating minimal pairs) and phonemic awareness (the ability to consciously reflect upon or manipulate the sounds in words, as in rhyming). This phonetic approach (with or without ear training) is almost always used for a child who has one sound in error and that error is a distortion, as in the case of a lisp or a somewhat glided /ɹ/.

In a retrospective review of 73 intervention cases, Shriberg and Kwaitkowski (1990) identified auditory discrimination as one factor that seemed to yield better outcomes than others, but when further analyses were carried out, it appeared that these benefits were actually attributable to the use of self-monitoring procedures within the session. However, this study grouped together all children receiving therapy for SSD over a period of many years. The use of perceptual training was clarified in a study by Wolfe and colleagues (2003). They demonstrated that sound identification training of this sort was helpful for children who had poor perceptual skills for identifying the target sound at the beginning of treatment. For children who could already identify and discriminate the target sound, it made no difference. Children with poor identification of the target sound who did not receive ear training benefited less from production training alone, but on the other hand, production training did have some impact on the children's ability to identify the sound perceptually.

A typical therapy session using this traditional approach might include the following:

1. The child is asked to listen to the SLP's productions of words containing the target sound—some correct, some incorrect (with an attempt to produce the same errors as the child). The child judges whether each production is accurate or not ("Did I say it right?").
2. The child is given explicit instruction on how to articulate the target sounds (e.g., "Put your tongue on the bump behind your teeth.").
3. The child is asked to label pictures using words that contain the target sound. Feedback may include knowledge of performance ("your tongue was in the right place") or knowledge of acoustic results ("that didn't sound right").
4. Additional cues, such as pictures of articulatory postures or labels for target productions (e.g., "Make a snake sound"), are provided as needed.

TABLE 7-30

	Nature of SSD	Typical Treatment Approach(es)
Phonetic Focus	• Single sound in error; residual SSD (e.g., lisp, distorted /ɹ/)	• Traditional placement therapy

	• Sensory-motor deficit; unstimulable	• Phonetic therapy with hierarchy of cues
		  • PROMPT
		  • DTTC
		  • Dynamic treatment
		• Motor learning principles (Chapter 5)
		• Self-monitoring

	• Inability to discriminate correct/incorrect	• Auditory discrimination (ear training)
Linguistic Focus	• High level of lexical variability (same word produced different ways)	• Core vocabulary

	• Lack of phonemic discrimination (perception of minimal pairs)	• Naturalistic therapy with feigned confusion
		• Receptive contrast therapy
		  • Minimal pairs: target vs. substitute
		  • Minimal pairs: two target sounds
		  • Maximal pairs
		  • Multiple oppositions
		  • Nonsense words or real words
		  • Metaphon

	• Lack of phonemic distinction (production of minimal pairs)	• Naturalistic therapy with feigned confusion
		• Production contrast therapy
		  • Minimal pairs: target vs. substitute
		  • Minimal pairs: two target sounds
		  • Maximal pairs
		  • Multiple oppositions
		  • Nonsense words or real words
		  • Metaphon

	• Lack of phonemic awareness as well as SSD	• Combination of speech production and phonemic awareness therapy (e.g., Metaphon, LiPS)

Such a session might include drill and/or drill play formats based on motor learning principles.

Gestural or tactile cues, such as those advocated within the PROMPT approach (Hayden & Square, 1994), may be used to supplement verbal descriptions and pictures as cues to proper articulator placement (place of articulation) or movement (manner of articulation). PROMPT is a system of tactile cues used to stimulate the child's awareness and coordination of relevant motor systems for speech production (e.g., touching the lips for labial sounds or the side of the nose for nasals). Through a hierarchy of linguistic difficulty levels (ranging from producing the sound in isolation to producing it within a word within a sentence during a storytelling activity), the systematic use of cues is also depicted in the intervention portion of the Scaffolding Scale of Stimulability (Glaspey & Stoel-Gammon, 2005) discussed in Chapter 5. A 21-point hierarchical scale of different types of cues (ranging from none to a combination of verbal instruction, models, prolongation, and/or tactile cues) and of different linguistic environments (from producing the sound in isolation to within a story context) is provided for in-depth documentation of the client's ability level prior to and throughout therapy.

A variety of cues are also incorporated into the systematic use of concurrent production (clinician and child speaking the target words together), followed by direct imitation, delayed imitation, then elicited speech that is key to another motoric intervention program, Dynamic Tactile and Temporal Cueing (DTTC), developed from integral stimulation by Strand (reported, e.g., by Strand & Skinder, 1999). (See Chapter 5, especially Fig. 5-5.) Although the details of these approaches differ, they all share the systematic provision of carefully selected levels of motoric and/or linguistic difficulty with supports (e.g., cues, simultaneous productions) that are gradually withdrawn as they cease to be necessary for the child. In all cases, backtracking—returning to a simpler level and/or adding support back in—is highly recommended when needed.

These motor approaches may also be supplemented by programs such as the Secord Contextual Articulation Tests (S-CAT) (Secord & Shine, 1997) that assess the phonetic contexts in which the child is best able to produce the target sound. For example, although many people instinctively assume that clusters are always more difficult than singletons, some children are able to produce [s] more accurately in homorganic clusters such as st- and sn- because the second element of the cluster is produced at the same place of articulation as the [s], thus guiding the tongue to the appropriate placement. Similarly, when targeting consonants in final position, a phrase may be useful for creating the appropriate context, such as "bus tires" for placement of [s] in the scenario just described.

Factors that Impact Phonetic Therapy Outcomes

A variety of factors may impact the success of intervention that is focused on the improvement of the production of specific sounds. Some of these are extrinsic to the child, in other words, relating to the universal or language-specific nature of the target sounds or to the therapy context or procedure. Others are intrinsic to the child, in other words, relating to her learning style, imitation ability, and other strengths and weaknesses. These are described below and summarized in Figure 7-1.

Extrinsic Factors

The usual order of acquisition of speech sounds in typically developing children might appear to be the default order for therapy goals as well. However, there are important limitations to this assumption. First of all, such orders are determined via averaging the levels of accuracy of large groups of children. It could be that no single child in such a study actually exemplified the order exhibited by the group as a whole when all individual differences are thus smoothed out. Secondly, individual children with SSDs do not necessarily acquire sounds in the same order as that of typically developing children. Those with CAS, in particular, are renowned for following unusual phonetic developmental paths. Finally, research has demonstrated the importance of several other factors in predicting therapy outcomes.

For example, phonetic universals must be taken into account in treatment planning. First of all, those sounds that are most universal generally (the unmarked ones) can be assumed to be perceptually or articulatorily (or both) easier than those that are rare. Markedness has been shown to be at least somewhat predictive of order of acquisition of vowels, singleton consonants, and consonant clusters (Bernhardt & Stoel-Gammon, 1996). Thus, the phonologies of children who acquire many marked sounds instead of unmarked sounds first (such as some children with CAS) may be considered atypical.

Secondly, as described above, the kinds of sound repertoires that tend to occur in languages with smaller consonant or vowel inventories than English may occur in early stages of the development of English phonology. Systems of this sort should be cause for less concern than systems that do not conform to universal tendencies.

It is widely accepted that within-class generalization is common; that is, treating one member of a class (such as [s] as a fricative) may result in progress on other members of the same sound class (such as other fricatives). Research has been contradictory with respect to whether more across-class generalization occurs as a result of targeting more challenging targets (e.g., systematic gaps or more complex/marked features of which the child has no phonological knowledge) versus less challenging targets (e.g., sounds that the child sometimes produces correctly or accidental gaps). For example, Miccio and Powell (2010) suggest targeting phones in the most difficult word positions rather than in word positions that are developmentally earlier or in which the child is sometimes accurate. Other studies have focused on whether targeting sounds that are more complex in more abstract respects is more beneficial. For example, Gierut and colleagues have proposed that the most complex sounds be targeted first, with complexity being tested variously in different research projects as reflecting later development according to norms (Gierut et al., 1996) or to universal markedness (Tyler & Figurski, 1994). For example, Tyler and Figurski (1994)

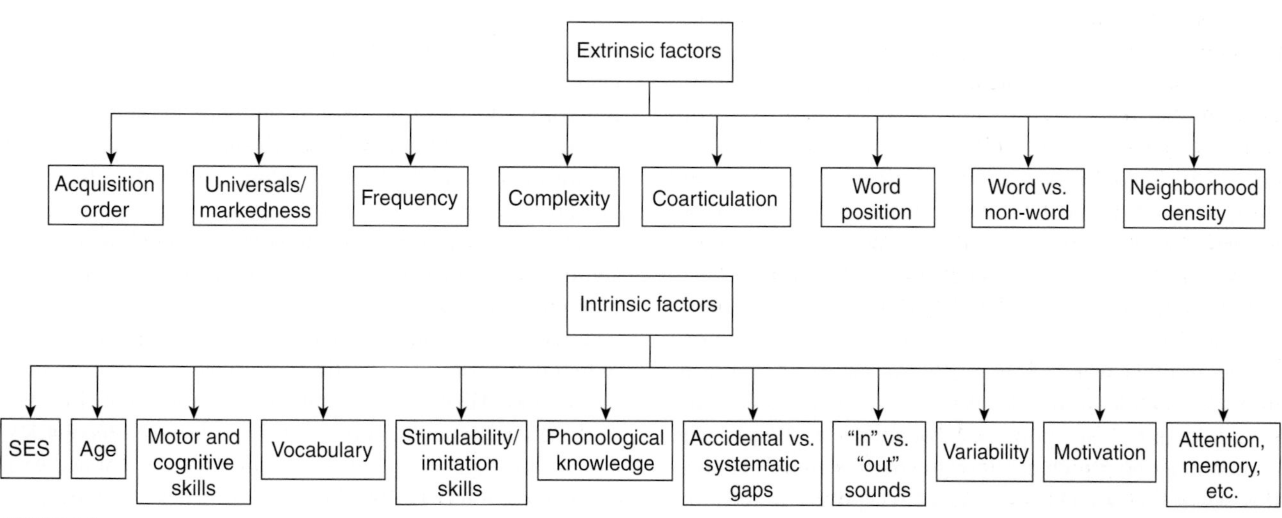

FIGURE 7-1.

selected targets from the most mature level of Dinnsen and colleagues' (1990) phonetic hierarchy (Table 7-2). The child who was treated for the most marked sounds (i.e., those at the most complex level) demonstrated more across-class generalization to more untreated sounds than did the one who was treated for a sound that would normally have been deemed more developmentally appropriate. Gierut (2007) has proposed that when more complex sounds are treated, less complex sounds are also acquired "for free."

However, Rvachew and Nowak (2001) identified flaws in the studies that purport to have demonstrated an advantage to targeting more complex targets. In their much larger and more rigorous study of 48 children, those participants who received direct treatment for earlier-developing sounds made more progress on their targets than did matched participants who received direct treatment for later-developing sounds. There was no difference in amounts of generalization to other targets between the groups. Furthermore, in a retrospective study of 60 children, Gierut, Morrisette, and Ziemer (2010) themselves reported that the participants demonstrated more generalization to treated sounds than untreated sounds; in other words, there was little across-class generalization that occurred "for free." Thus, the current best answer to the question of whether efficacy, including generalization to untreated sounds, is enhanced by targeting later, more complex phonemes rather than earlier-developing ones appears to be "no."

Several studies have noted that the frequency of occurrence of sounds or words in the ambient language has a positive impact on order of acquisition in typically developing children. Morrisette and Gierut (2002) demonstrated that the same is true for children with SSD. In their study of eight children with functional phonological delays, both immediate generalization and long-term generalization—both to the same sounds and to sounds within the same class—were better when higher-frequency words were used as stimuli. With low-frequency stimuli (i.e., words that are not commonly used in the language), the children learned the target sounds but did not generalize them, although they did generalize to some extent to untreated sounds in other sound classes. This represents a challenge: Sometimes, the most picturable word with a certain sound in a certain position is not a common one. Many children have learned words such as "vase" and "leap" from their "artick" cards, but this learning may not generalize as well as learning based on more common words.

Morrisette and Gierut (2002) also studied a related factor, neighborhood density. Recall that neighborhood density is a measure of how many words are similar to the target word—in other words, how many minimal pairs and near-minimal pairs a word has. "Neighbors" of the word "cup" would include "cap, pup, cut," for example. Words with denser neighborhoods are thought to face more competition when they are being processed receptively or retrieved for production; many similar words could be accidentally triggered instead of the target word. Thus, adults recognize lower-density words faster and more accurately; they also produce them faster and more accurately. Morrisette and Gierut (2002) found that slightly more generalization occurred when low-density words were targeted in speech therapy than when high-density words were, but the effect of density was much less than the effect of frequency.

Another factor that has recently been identified as having a therapeutic impact is the use of words versus non-words in therapy. Gierut and colleagues (e.g., Gierut et al., 2010; Gierut & Morrisette, 2010) have demonstrated that children treated using non-words made similar or better progress than did those treated with real-word stimuli. This progress included generalization to other portions of the child's phonological system as well as improvement in the production of the target sounds. The benefits of this approach may result from circumventing children's pre-existing incorrect motor programs or incorrect underlying representations. Note, however, that for some children, communicative efficacy must be taken into consideration; for children with extremely small intelligible expressive vocabularies, expanding the number of intelligible words that they can produce may take precedence initially. Practicing meaningless forms will not increase communicative efficacy, at least not over the short term.

Finally, in a retrospective review of 73 SSD intervention cases, Shriberg and Kwiatkowski (1990) identified the incorporation of self-monitoring within the therapy session as the factor that was the most related to the child's generalization. As emphasized within the DIVA model of motor performance, self-monitoring and self-evaluation encourage the development of internal feedforward and feedback processes, and these internal mechanisms lead to better generalization than external feedback can. This reinforces the notion that SLP feedback should not always be immediate and constant; allowing time and opportunities for self-evaluation facilitates the child's learning.

Child-Specific Intrinsic Factors

Dodd and colleagues (Holm & Dodd, 1999b; Dodd & Bradford, 2000; Crosbie, Holm, & Dodd, 2005) have shown that the choice of therapy approach should depend upon the nature of the child's disorder. Most specifically, they have demonstrated the value of a core vocabulary approach for children with severe SSD characterized by high levels of variability of the type in which the same word is pronounced in different manners upon different occasions, in different contexts, etc. Recall that this approach consists of selecting a set of highly functional words that are drilled to maximize their consistency. All of those who interact with the child are alerted to these goals and encouraged to provide social feedback—communication success for better productions, feigned confusion for less accurate productions—in order to make it clear to the child that consistency matters. Absolute accuracy is not necessary; in many cases, the key players decide what level of accuracy will be accepted for each word with an emphasis on the various words being produced distinctly so that contrast is achieved. Presumably, this treatment assists the child in forming either more reliable, more clearly specified motor programs or more reliable or more clearly specified underlying representations of words—or possibly both.

A set of case studies by Dodd and colleagues (Crosbie et al., 2005; Dodd & Bradford, 2000; Holm & Dodd, 1999a) indicates that children who do not make progress using other strategies are more successful when this core vocabulary approach is taken first. Once their speech has become more consistent, the children then benefit from other approaches, suggesting that they have learned how to create and retain more clearly specified motor programs and/or phonemic representations of words, as well as acquiring more reliable motor programs for those specific words. Unfortunately, subjects have not been clearly differentiated in these studies between those who are inconsistent within repeated productions of the same word in a series, which is differentially diagnostic of CAS (ASHA, 2007), versus those who are inconsistent in their production of the same sound in different words, the same sound in different word positions, or the same word from one time to the next. The latter two types of inconsistency may also be found in children with CAS as well as in children with other SSDs. More research in this area is clearly warranted.

In the meantime, the Consistency Index developed by Tyler (2002) is helpful for determining how many different ways the child has of producing each target phoneme. This is adapted for the purposes of this book as Form 7-6, with its usage illustrated in Example 7-8 with data from a hypothetical child named Elias. Target phonemes are listed in the far left column. Different ways of producing the sound—including both correct productions of the target and omissions—are then listed by word position. The smaller the consistency average, the more consistent the child's speech patterns. For example, a child who averages only one substitution per phoneme (consistency average = 1.0) is very consistent; a child who averages three substitutions per phoneme (consistency average = 3.0) is not. The more different ways a given phoneme is produced by a child, the harder that child will be to understand. For example, a child who produces /s/ variously as [f], [θ], and [ʃ]—three different ways of producing the same phoneme, none of which is correct—is likely be less intelligible than one who consistently produces /s/ as [t] even though the various fricative substitutions may be considered to be more mature, in a sense.

Note that Elias has multiple substitutions for four different target phonemes. Some target phonemes are produced differently depending upon the context (e.g., /s/); others have the same substitutes regardless of context (e.g., /ʃ/). The additional complication that [s] is sometimes substituted for /ʃ/ while also [ʃ] is sometimes substituted for /s/ likely renders his speech quite unintelligible.

Stimulability has long been a factor tested by speech-language pathologists before selecting therapy goals (Lof, 1996). This refers to the degree to which the child can approximate the target sound under various circumstances (e.g., with various levels of auditory, visual, or tactile cueing; with explicit feedback). Miccio, Elbert, and Forrest (1999) have confirmed that stimulable sounds (versus unstimulable sounds) are most likely to change when targeted in therapy; they are also most likely to change even if they are not directly treated, however. Gierut, Elbert, and Dinnsen (1987) also reported more progress among children who received treatment for stimulable targets (i.e., targets for which they had more "productive phonological knowledge," p. 462). Similarly, Powell, Elbert, and Dinnsen (1991) reported that children who were stimulable for [ɹ] were more likely to make progress when therapy targeted that sound than children who were non-stimulable at the beginning of treatment. Rvachew, Rafaat, and Martin (1999) and Rvachew (2005) reported that children with SSDs were more likely to benefit from therapy for sounds for which they were stimulable if they also demonstrated good speech discrimination of those sounds. Furthermore, in their studies, a combination of phonetic and speech perception treatment facilitated the development of sounds that were previously either unstimulable, poorly perceived, or both.

Lof (1996) investigated the stimulation conditions that are most likely to result in improved productions. The extrinsic factor that appeared to make the most reliable difference was the visibility of the sound (e.g., labials are highly visible but velars are much more difficult to see). Significantly related intrinsic factors included the age and socioeconomic status of the child (with older, higher-SES children benefitting more) and the child's overall imitation ability.

The tendency for all sound systems to be orderly, using the features that are relevant within the language to their maximum and being more receptive to new sounds that fill in accidental rather than systematic gaps, is reflected in children's sound systems as well. Speech-language pathologists can capitalize on this in choosing remediation targets. It is possible that intervention chosen to fill in accidental gaps first using all possible combinations of existing features within the child's system may result in more rapid progress. For instance, it seems likely that a child who already accurately produces at least one velar (e.g., [ŋ]), some stops (e.g., [b, p, d]), and some voiced consonants (e.g., [b, d, z]) will learn [g] more rapidly than will one who lacks one or more of these features (dorsal/velar, noncontinuance/stop, voicing). However, this hypothesis has not been tested scientifically.

In 1982, Schwartz and Leonard demonstrated that individual children are more likely to attempt new words if the

Form 7-6

Name: Age:
Date: Examiner:
Source of sample: Size of sample:

Consistency Index (adapted from Tyler, 2002)

Target phoneme	Production Types (Correct, Substituted, Omitted)			Total # of different productions for that phoneme
	Initial productions	Medial productions	Final productions	

Total number of production types ÷ total number of phonemes attempted = consistency average

Note: Production types that occur in multiple word positions only count once. For example, if a child substitutes [t] for /k/ in initial, medial, and final positions, only one production type is counted in the right-most column, because that one substitution is consistent across all word positions. Production types that occur within consonant clusters are counted in the same manner as singleton consonants.

Example 7-8

Name: *Elias (hypothetical)* Age: *6;7*
Date: *12-12-13* Examiner: *SLV*
Source of sample: *play* Size of sample: *100 words*

Consistency Index (based on Tyler, 2002)

Target phoneme	Production Types (Correct, Substituted, Omitted)			Total # of different productions for that phoneme
	Initial substitutions	Medial substitutions	Final substitutions	
/s/	[f], [s]	[θ], [s]	[ʃ], ∅	5
/ʃ/	[ʃ], [s]	[ʃ], [s]	[ʃ], [s]	2
/ɹ/	[w]	[w]	[ʊ]	2
/l/	[w]	[j]	[ʊ]	3

Total number of prroduction types ÷ total number of phonemes attempted = consistency average

Note: Production types that occur in multiple word positions only count once. For example,if a child substitutes [t] for /k/ in initial, medial, and final positions, only one production type is counted in the right-most column, because that one substitution is consistent across all word positions. Production types that occur within consonant clusters are counted in the same manner as singleton consonants.

words share the phonological characteristics of the youngsters' existing individual lexicons. The children more often tried to say these "in" words in imitation, and they learned to use them spontaneously in fewer sessions than it took for them to learn the "out" words that did not fit their current systems. Schwartz and colleagues (1987) extended this finding, demonstrating that words that contain consonants that the child has attempted but never produced correctly are attempted and learned as reluctantly as out words that contain consonants that the child has never attempted. Only those words that contain sounds that the child has already successfully produced are attempted earlier and more successfully. Of course, limiting therapy targets to sounds that the child can already produce is not likely to result in much change in the child's intelligibility. One discouraging implication of this study is that we will encounter resistance if our therapy approaches push our clients to expand their phonetic repertoires, a challenge SLPs confront every day. However, Schwartz and team (1987) did report that children with SSD are less impacted by "in" versus "out" words than are children who are typically developing.

Unfortunately, this study has not been extended to examine words with in and out *features*. However, it seems likely that child phonologies will be more receptive to sounds that include only—or mostly—features that they have already mastered rather than sounds that include features that they have not successfully produced. The former type of sounds would fill accidental gaps. It has been the author's experience that addressing such accidental gaps is easier than attempting to add systematic gap elements, which do not fit within the child's existing system. This might provide a means of expanding children's phonetic repertoires to sounds that they have not produced accurately but that include elements that are already present in their systems.

The argument can and has been made that those sounds that are most likely to be acquired are the least in need of treatment and that clinical energy is better spent on more challenging targets. For this reason, Miccio and Elbert (1996) and Miccio (2005) proposed focusing primarily on sounds that are not stimulable, although stimulable sounds were also included in therapy sessions so that the clients could experience some success. In this program, non-stimulable sounds were associated with gestures (e.g., a sliding gesture for [s]) and/or characters (such as a snake for [s]) to make them "come alive" for the children as they were modeled. Imitation was not required, but the activities were designed to be engaging enough to inspire the children to attempt the sounds. Once the sounds became stimulable, they began to emerge more naturally within the clients' speech.

Goal Attack Strategies

As noted in Chapter 5, once a set of therapy goals has been selected, there remain additional decisions to be made about how such goals should be addressed. For example, will therapy target single sounds one by one (training narrow) or classes of sounds united by some manner, place, or voicing feature (e.g., fricatives, velars) (training broad)? Targeting classes of segments is more effective for children with many sounds in error than treating sounds one by one (see much more discussion of this in Chapter 9). The debate about the value of targeting more complex items with potential generalization to less complex items also applies here: Is it more efficient to target the most marked items within a class (e.g., /ʒ / or /θ/, if the goal is to improve fricative production) or to target the segments that are developmentally earlier (e.g., /f/, /ʃ/)? Similarly, is the most effective manner to improve an entire sound class to treat certain representative items from that class, or to treat the entire class at once? As discussed in Chapter 5, there are pros and cons of each of these. As noted there and in Chapter 9, there is evidence to suggest that addressing a whole natural sound class at once with a variety of exemplars is most effective for many children.

Summary

Both intrinsic factors, such as stimulability, and extrinsic factors, such as the markedness of a potential target sound, have been shown or proposed to impact the progress of phonetic therapy. Goal attack strategies also must be selected.

Contrast Remediation Approaches

Dodd and McIntosh (2008) explored the question of whether the primary cause of SSDs is sensory–motor or cognitive–linguistic. That is, are children with SSD typically unable to program or execute the production of the sounds with which they struggle, are they unable to perceptually process speech sounds, or is the source of their disorder a lack of understanding of the linguistic system to which they have been exposed? Their SSD and control participants, none of whom had neurologic or cognitive deficits, completed tasks challenging (1) their abilities to match syllables spoken by speakers on two video monitors, including some items for which the video and audio did not match as in the "McGurk effect" (e.g., video for [bɑ] but audio for [gɑ]); (2) their oral–motor skills (as tested using isolated and sequenced non-speech movements such as protruding the tongue) and motor speech skills (as tested, e.g., using diadochokinesis such as the repetition of the phrase "pat-a-cake"); and (3) their abilities to generate, use, and flexibly change rules, such as learning from rewards (e.g., computer animations) to initially match items on a computer screen based on color and then switching to a shape-matching strategy without explicit instructions being given. Dodd and McIntosh (2008) found no group differences on the speech perception and non-speech oromotor tasks. The typically developing (TD) children did better on the diadochokinesis task, but the difference was based only on the accuracy of the SSD group's production of the target [k] in "pat-a-cake;" rate and fluency of production did not differ by group. The SSD group had significantly more difficulty with the rule-learning tasks than did the TD group; their ability to shift perspective when the rules changed was especially impaired. Based on their findings, Dodd and McIntosh (2008) suggest that there is more often a cognitive–linguistic basis for SSD than a sensory–motor basis. This suggests that focusing our intervention efforts on the phonological system—the system of contrasts and patterns within the language—rather than on articulation per se is likely to pay off, at least for the majority of clients with SSDs. A variety of linguistic approaches are described below and summarized in the bottom of Table 7-30.

Whatever the source, a child whose phonology does not allow for sufficient contrast will not be able to communicate effectively. "Sufficient" contrast is difficult to define, as it depends in large part upon the child's communicative needs. Vocabulary size, mental age, familiarity of listeners, and motivation are just a few of the factors that determine the necessary amount of contrast. Unintelligibility (especially as reported by very familiar listeners, such as parents) and the frustration levels of the child and his significant others are key indicators of insufficient contrast.

What then, do children need to learn about phonological contrast, and how can we teach it? An initial question to ask is whether receptive as well as expressive contrast training is needed. Referring back to the hypothetical Elias, whose consistency patterns were shown in Example 7-8, we see that his patterns of substitution for /s/ and /ʃ/ are different (though overlapping). This may indicate that Elias is beginning to be aware that these are two different phonemes in English but has not yet figured out how to pronounce them differently. A similar argument could be made about his /ɹ/ and /l/ substitutions. Thus, Elias appears to be an excellent candidate for speech discrimination testing to see if he does indeed perceive [s] versus [ʃ] (e.g., "Sue" versus "shoe," "mess" versus "mesh") and [ɹ] versus [l] (e.g., "rock" versus "lock," "pray" versus "play") as different. Recall that Wolfe and colleagues (2003) demonstrated that children with poorer discrimination of error sounds make slower progress on remediation of those same sounds. In their study, production training did improve perception of target sounds to some extent, but combined perception and production training led to greater gains for children with low discrimination scores. Thus, the results of discrimination testing will determine whether perception as well as production contrast therapy would be appropriate for Elias.

In contrast treatment, whether it is receptive or expressive or both, the conceptual level rather than the sensory–motor level of speech is the focus. The goal is to highlight feature contrasts and to emphasize the need for communicative efficacy rather than to induce perfect pronunciation. For this reason, some clinical researchers advocate a naturalistic approach to this therapy. Camarata (1993, 1995), for example, suggested that therapy should be based upon conversation during natural activities with no imitative prompts or direct motor training. Thus, the SLP may load the room with words that require accurate production of the target sounds then feign incomprehension if the child substitutes within a word. This type of confusion can be used, it is believed, to trigger change in a disordered phonological system. For instance, this author was able to teach one child the value of correctly producing velars by consistently imitating his own production of his cat's name—"Dumb-ball" rather than "Gumball"—and commenting on how stupid his pet must be to have warranted such a name. The child quickly learned to say [g] in spirited defense of what he claimed was a very smart cat. However, it is not easy to arrange many such situations in a naturalistic setting.

The most traditional form of contrast therapy is minimal pairs therapy, in which minimal pairs are presented to the child in a systematic manner to spark the realization that contrast is vital to effective communication. In a typical therapy session, for example, the child and the SLP might play "Fish" with minimal pair cards ("ring"—"wing," "ride"—"wide," etc.). If the child fails to pronounce the target word correctly, he or she does not receive the card that may be needed to complete a set. In the purest form of minimal pairs therapy, no knowledge of performance comments would be made about the child's articulation of the target sound. Only knowledge of results would be provided via communication failure. The cause of that failure would remain implicit for the child to surmise.

Many variations on this basic type of contrast therapy have been proposed. Some of these relate to which and how many phonemes are contrasted; others depend upon the exact nature of the therapy activities. One example of the latter consists of beginning therapy with perceptual discrimination tasks; the client is asked only to point to pictures or objects representing the chosen minimal pairs, not to produce them. The assumption of this preliminary step is that there is no use in practicing the production of a sound until the child is aware of the role of that sound—as a contrastive phoneme—in the language.

The choice of which and how many phonemes to contrast is a complex one. In the first versions of this therapy approach, the target phoneme was contrasted to its substitute; for example, a child who glided /ɹ/ would be asked to discriminate (perceptually) or distinguish (articulatorily) between "ring" and "wing" and other similar word pairs. Williams' (2000) multiple oppositions approach is based on the premise that children with multiple phonemes collapsed into one (e.g., /s/, /ʃ/, /z/, /tʃ/, and /dʒ/ all pronounced as [d]) should be given activities in which minimal pairs encompass all of these substitutions. Such a broad approach, Williams argues, addresses the entire error pattern at one time and is therefore more likely to induce more widespread change in the child's phonological system.

Gierut (1989) proposed that instead of contrasting the target phoneme with its substitute, it would be easier to call the child's attention to the target by contrasting it to a very different sound: maximal pairs. For example, a client who substituted [f] for /s/ might engage in activities designed to contrast /s/ with a maximally different phoneme, /m/.

In a study of three 4- to 5-year-old children with phonological delays/disorders, Gierut (1991) contrasted the traditional contrast approach to yet another therapy strategy. In the typical minimal pairs approach, the child was presented with nonsense words that were minimal pairs that would result from the child's substitutions, such as the nonsense words "dode" ([dod]) and "thode" [ðod] for a child who substituted [d] for /ð/. The nonsense words were presented in a story context so that they acquired meaning for the child. In the other treatment, the focus was on two target sounds, neither of which was in the child's production inventory before therapy (e.g., /tʃ/ and /dʒ/)—and therefore, neither of which was a substitute for the other. Again, nonsense words containing the new sounds were presented in story contexts, but in this condition, minimal pairs were not used. Gierut reported greater progress with this latter approach than when the target was contrasted with its substitute in the minimal pair approach. However, the study was not balanced in the sense that the target sounds in the homonymous (minimal pair) approach were interdental fricatives (/ð, θ/) for all three children, and more acoustically salient strident sounds (/s, z, ʃ, tʃ, dʒ/) with much higher functional loads in English were used for the other treatment condition. This weakness and the fact that only three children were included in the study limits the generalizability of this research.

A typical contrast therapy session, regardless of how the set of phonemes was chosen, might follow the following format:

1. A situation is set up in which the child needs to communicate a particular word. For example, the child and SLP play Fish using minimal pair picture cards, and the child needs to ask for the card depicting "catch" (perhaps a drawing of a girl catching a fish), not the one depicting "cat." If the client says "cat," she is given the wrong card. When she expresses dismay, a comment may be made about which one she asked for ("You didn't ask for 'catch.' You asked for 'cat,' so that's what I gave you.")
2. Phonetic and acoustic feedback are not given. Feedback is knowledge of communication results: Did the listener understand the target word?

The Metaphon approach of Howell and Dean (1994) takes a different tack of explicitly training the child to consciously recognize contrasts, including real-world concrete opposites such as "long" and "short," then generalizing this training to sound contrasts that the child needed to learn (e.g., [s] is long; [t] is short). In the years since their original proposal, other studies (such as Moriarty & Gillon, 2006) have validated the efficacy of combining metaphonological awareness training with speech production training, demonstrating that clients make progress in both areas when they are addressed together in therapy. Another approach that also incorporates phonological awareness with some phonetic components is provided by the *Lindamood® Phoneme Sequencing Program for Reading, Spelling, and Speech* (third edition) **LiPS** program (Lindamood & Lindamood, 1998). In this program, children are taught to categorize speech sounds according to their articulatory characteristics (such as the "lip poppers" [p] and [b], which are "brothers" because they differ only in voicing). They are then trained to associate the articulations of the sounds with their characteristics, their letters, and their letter names. Given that children whose speech production does not normalize by age 6 are at higher risk for literacy difficulties (Nathan, Stackhouse, Goulandris, & Snowling, 2004; Raitano, Pennington, Tunnick, Boada, & Shriberg, 2004), incorporating phonological awareness training into speech therapy from an early age has construct validity.

Summary/Implications

Phonetic therapy approaches emphasize accurate production of speech sounds at different levels of linguistic complexity (syllable, word, phrase, etc.). Contrast therapy approaches focus on the functional roles of phonemes for maximizing communicative efficacy. The former is grounded in sensory–motor aspects of speech; the latter is grounded in the abstract cognitive–linguistic system. However, phonetic and phonemic/contrast therapy should not be seen as polar opposites, a dichotomous choice to be made. Some studies have suggested that making a sound stimulable may have an impact on the child's phonological system as well as on the sensory–motor system (Miccio, Elbert, & Forrest, 1999; Tyler & Macrae, 2010). Furthermore, Saben and Ingham (1991) demonstrated that some children benefit from phonetic therapy strategies such as imitation and placement cues being incorporated into contrast (minimal pair) therapy. Thus, eclectic approaches that marry the two perspectives may be optimal for some children.

EXERCISE 7-5

Phone/Phoneme Intervention

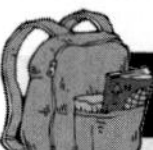

KEY TAKE-HOME MESSAGES

1. Physiology (as reflected in phonetic universals), the ambient language, and child-specific preferences all impact the progression of speech sound development.
2. During assessment, it is important to look for signs that the child has phonological knowledge of a contrast even if that contrast is not detectable in the child's production.
3. A combination of relational analysis (such as administration of a standardized test) and independent analysis (phonetic repertoires and contrast) is ideal for developing a true understanding of a child's speech sound system and therefore developing appropriate intervention goals.
4. Phonetic (motoric) and phonemic (linguistic) approaches to speech sound therapy are each appropriate in different intervention circumstances; sometimes the best approach is a combination of the two.

CHAPTER 7

Phones and Phonemes Review

Exercise 7-1

Multiple choice. Choose the best answer.

1. Which of the following consonant repertoires is most likely to be found in a typically developing English-learning child in initial position?
   a. ɹ, l, θ, ð, ʒ
   b. ŋ, k, g, j, p, t
   c. f, s, ʃ, tʃ, h
   d. m, n, w, b, d, h
2. Which of the following vowel repertoires is most likely to be found in a typically developing English-learning child?
   a. e, o, ə
   b. ɪ, ɛ, ʊ
   c. u, ɑ, i
   d. o, u, æ
3. Independent analysis focuses on:
   a. actual productions regardless of targets.
   b. targets regardless of actual productions.
   c. norm-referenced acquisition.
   d. articulatory inaccuracies.
4. Phonetic acquisition is typically more advanced in:
   a. girls than boys.
   b. children with smaller vocabularies.
   c. children learning AAE than those learning GAE.
   d. children with SSD.
5. In phonological acquisition models (e.g., Dinnsen, 1992) as well as in studies of English-speaking children (e.g., Stoel-Gammon, 1985):
   a. voiceless stops are learned before voiced stops.
   b. voiced stops are learned before voiceless stops.
   c. nasals are learned before glides.
   d. fricatives are learned before nasals.
6. When learning new phones, children tend to:
   a. acquire consonants and vowels that have features they're already using.
   b. master salient diphthongs before lax vowels.
   c. be affected more by ease of perception than ease of production.
   d. be unaffected by the frequency of phones in their language(s).

Exercise 7-2

A. *Answer the following questions using the data in Table 7-13.*

1. Are [d] and [n] different phonemes for Mike? Justify your answer.
2. Are [ɑ] and [æ] different phonemes for Mike? Justify your answer.

B. *Use the sample below in combination with the sample from Table 7-14 to explore contrast in the speech of Martin (Grunwell, 1982) by answering the following questions.*

1. What fricatives are included in Martin's phonetic repertoire?
2. Which of these fricatives are phonemes for Martin (i.e., in contrast with each other)? Explain.
3. Is voicing a contrastive feature in Martin's speech at this time? Justify your answer.

Bridge [bɪv]
Pig [bɪv]
Cage [geɪv]
Color [kʊvə]
Finger [fɪnvə]
Red [ʊɛv]

Exercise 7-3

A. *Using the transcript provided below, determine Lacie's consonant and vowel repertoires (using the forms). Then answer the questions.*

Note: *Glosses* are not provided because this is independent analysis; targets are irrelevant.

1. Based upon the number of consonants in her inventory, what would you guess is Lacie's age if she were typically developing?
2. What sound classes does Lacie produce?
3. Based upon the actual consonants and vowels in Lacie's inventories, does she appear to be typically developing? Why or why not?
4. What are Lacie's relative strengths? Relative weaknesses?

'bɑðɑ ɑʊʔ
'dædæ dɛʊ
θɑ æʔ
'ɛzə dɪp
fɑ ðɑ
'æðɪ ðʌ
θʌ 'nɑnɑ
'ɑðə ɑɪ
'ɱɑɱɑ fi
ɱæ 'ɱuɱu
ðɑɪt fɑɪ
i wɑ
'dɑðə ju
ðɑɪ oʔ
nɑɪt ɑʊp
du ðɑ
nɑ dɪ
ə'vɑnɑ 'ðiði
'ðɑðɑ dʌ
ɑɪt jɑ
'woʊwoʊ 'jɑjo
'ɪhɪ 'æzæ
dæ wi
'dɛdo vɪ
nɑʊ ðʌ

KEY: [ɱ] is a voiced labiodental nasal.

B. Consider Timmy's phonetic development over time, shown below (from Vihman et al., 1994). Does he add consonants in a systematic manner? Specifically:

1. Identify accidental gaps in Timmy's speech at particular ages. What happens to those gaps in the time periods that follow?
2. Identify systematic gaps in Timmy's speech at particular ages. What happens to those gaps in the time periods that follow?

Age (mo.)		**Phonetic Repertoire**			
		LABIAL	ALVEOLAR	VELAR	GLOTTAL
9-10	STOP	b			
11-13	STOP				
	vd	b			
	vl			k	
14	STOP				
	vd	b			
	vl			k	
	GLIDE		j		
15	STOP				
	vd	b	ɟ		
	vl			k	
	NASAL		n		
	GLIDE		j		
	FRIC/AFF/APPROX.				
	vd	β			
15.5	STOP				
	vd	b			
	vl			k	
	NASAL	m	n		
	GLIDE		j		
	FRIC/AFF/APPROX.				
	vd	β	ɟ		
16	STOP				
	vd	b	ɟ		
	vl		t	k	
	NASAL	m	n		
	GLIDE		j		
	FRIC/AFF/APPROX.				
	vd	β			
16.5	STOP				
	vd	b	ɟ		
	vl		t	k	
	NASAL	m	n		
	GLIDE	w	j		
	FRIC/AFF/APPROX.				
	vd	β			

Key:

β voiced labial fricative

ɟ voiced palatal plosive

Exercise 7-4

A. Essay questions.

1. Based on the information in this chapter, if you were to design a speech sound test, which of the test feature choices listed below would you prioritize? Justify your choices using information from this chapter and other sources.
   - Singletons versus clusters
   - Consonants versus vowels
   - Initial versus medial versus final position
   - Monosyllabic versus multisyllabic words
   - Single words versus phrases versus sentences
   - Sound-by-sound errors versus error patterns
2. Amy, age 5, produces eight different consonants and five vowels. However, her consonant repertoire (1) does not include any stops or glides and (2) is used apparently randomly with two types of inconsistency: the same target consonant is produced in different ways in different words, and the same target consonant is produced in different ways in the same word on different occasions. The consonants that she can say are not necessarily produced correctly; for example, she produces [f] but not when it is the target consonant.

   May, Amy's twin sister, produces four different consonants and five vowels. When the target word contains a consonant or vowel that she can produce, she produces it accurately. That is, she matches the target whenever possible. Her substitutions are completely predictable, regardless of the word or word position.

   Which of the twins has the more severe phonological disorder? Which is likely to be more intelligible? Which is likely to make more rapid progress in therapy?

   Use information from this chapter and other sources to justify your answers.

B. Case study question.

Consider Lacie's productions again, this time with glosses provided (below).

1. What sound classes does Lacie produce accurately? Which sound classes are distorted? Which are substituted? Assume, for simplicity's sake, that substitutions of a single consonant for a cluster are just that (i.e., that the consonants in the cluster are merged into one).
2. Are there contrasts within Lacie's speech? Identify her phonemes, and justify your answers.
3. Identify homonymy and variability within Lacie's speech.
4. What are the major impediments to intelligibility (i.e., effective communication) in Lacie's speech?

Production	Target Word
1. 'bɑðɑ	basket
2. ɑʊʔ	boats
3. 'dædæ	candle
4. dɛʊ	chair
5. θɑ	clouds
6. æʔ	cowboy hat
7. 'ɛzə	feather
8. dɪp	fish
9. fɑ	flower
10. ðɑ	fork
11. 'æðɪ	glasses
12. ðʌ	glove
13. θʌ	gum
14. 'nɑnɑ	hanger
15. 'ɑðə	horsie
16. ɑɪ	ice (cubes)
17. 'ŋɑŋɑ	jumping
18. fi	leaf
19. ŋæ	mask
20. 'ŋuŋu	music box
21. ðɑɪt	page
22. fɑɪ	plane
23. i	queen
24. wɑ	rock
25. 'dɑðə	screwdriver
26. ju	shoe
27. ðɑɪ	slide
28. oʔ	smoke
29. nɑɪt	snake
30. ɑʊp	soap
31. du	spoon
32. ðɑ	square
33. nɑ	star
34. dɪ	string
35. ə'vɑnɑ	swimming
36. 'ðiði	television
37. 'ðɑðɑ	toothbrush
38. dʌ	truck
39. ɑɪt	vase
40. jɑ	watch
41. 'woʊwoʊ	yoyo
42. 'jɑjo	yoyo
43. 'ɪhɪ	zipper
44. 'æzæ	crayons
45. dæ	black

46. wi	green
47. 'dɛdo	yellow
48. vɪ	three
49. nɑʊ	nose
50. ðʌ	mouth

KEY: [ɱ] is a voiced labiodental nasal

Exercise 7-5

Use the data from Martin (Tables 7-14 and 7-29) to answer the following questions.

1. Use two different approaches (e.g., based upon universals versus development versus complexity) to goal selection to identify appropriate sounds or sound classes to address next in therapy for Martin. Justify your choices.
2. Develop four therapy lesson plans for one of the goals you selected above for Martin: one using a traditional phonetic/articulatory approach, one using a contextually based approach, one using a contrast approach, and one using a phonological awareness approach.

References

Ambrose, S. E., Berry, L. M. U., Walker, E. A., Harrison, M., Oleson, J., & Moeller, M. P. (2014). Speech sound production in 2-year-olds who are hard of hearing. *American Journal of Speech Language Pathology, 23*, 91–104.

ASHA. (2007). *Childhood Apraxia of Speech [Technical Report]*. Rockville Pike, MD: American Speech-Language-Hearing Association.

Austin, D., & Shriberg, L. D. (1997). *Lifespan reference data for ten measures of articulation competence using the speech disorders classification system (SDCS), Phonology Technical Reports*. Madison, WI: Waisman Center, University of Wisconsin-Madison. Available at: http://www.waisman.wisc.edu/phonology/techreports/TREP3_REV.PDF

Bankson, N. W., & Bernthal, J. E. (1990). *Bankson-Bernthal Test of Phonology*. Chicago, IL: Riverside.

Barlow, J. A. (1996). Variability and phonological knowledge. In T. W. Powell (Ed.), *Pathologies of speech and language: Contributions of clinical phonetics and linguistics* (pp. 125–133). New Orleans, LA: International Clinical Phonetics Association.

Bedore, L. M., Leonard, L. B., & Gandour, J. (1994). The substitution of a click for sibilants: A case study. *Clinical Linguistics & Phonetics, 8*, 283–293.

Berman, R. A. (1977). Natural phonological processes at the one-word stage. *Lingua, 43*, 1–21.

Bernhardt, B. M., & Stoel-Gammon, C. (1996). Underspecification and markedness in normal and disordered phonological development. In C. E. Johnson & J. H. V. Gilbert (Eds.), *Children's language, Vol. 9*. (pp. 33–54). Mahwah, NJ: Lawrence Erlbaum Associates.

Bleile, K. M. (1991). *Child phonology: A book of exercises for students*. San Diego, CA: Singular Pub Group.

de Boysson-Bardies, B., Sagart, L., Halle, P., & Durand, C. (1986). Acoustic investigation of cross-linguistic variability in babbling. In B. Lindblom & R. Zetterstrom (Eds.), *Precursors of early speech*. New York, NY: Stockton Press.

Braine, M. D. S. (1974). On what might constitute learnable phonology. *Language, 50*(2), 270–299.

Braine, M. D. (1976). Review of N. V. Smith, *The acquisition of phonology*. *Language, 52*, 489–498.

Bunton, K., Leddy, M., & Miller, J. (2007). Phonetic intelligibility testing in adults with Down syndrome. *Down Syndrome Research and Practice, 12*(1), 1–4.

Burrows, L., & Goldstein, B. (2010). Whole word measures in bilingual children with speech sound disorders. *Clinical Linguistics & Phonetics, 24*(4–5), 357–368.

Camarata, S. (1993). The application of naturalistic conversation training to speech production in children with speech disabilities. *Journal of Applied Behavior Analysis, 26*(2), 173–182.

Camarata, S. M. (1995). A rationale for naturalistic speech intelligibility intervention. In M. E. Fey, J. Windson, & S. F. Warren (Eds.), *Language intervention: Preschool through the elementary years* (pp. 63–84). Baltimore, MD: Paul H. Brookes Publishing Co.

Camarata, S. M., & Schwartz, R. G. (1985). Production of object words and action words: Evidence for a relationship between phonology and semantics. *Journal of Speech and Hearing Research, 28*, 323–330.

Cataño, L., Barlow, J. A., & Moyna, M. (2009). Phonetic inventory complexity in the acquisition of Spanish: A retrospective, typological study. *Clinical Linguistics & Phonetics, 23*, 446–472.

Chen, H., & Stevens, K. N. (2001). An acoustical study of the fricative /s/ in the speech of individuals with dysarthria. *Journal of Speech, Language, and Hearing Research, 44*(6), 1300–1314.

Cleland, J., Gibbon, F. E., Peppe, S. J. E., O'Hare, A., & Rutherford, M. (2010). Phonetic and phonological errors in children with high functioning autism and Asperger syndrome. *International Journal of Speech-Language Pathology, 12*(1), 69–76.

Crosbie, S., Holm, A., & Dodd, B. (2005). Intervention for children with severe speech disorder: A comparison of two approaches. *International Journal of Language and Communication Disorders, 40*(4), 467–491.

Dawson, J., & Tattersall, P. (2001). *Structured Photographic Articulation Test* (2nd ed.) DeKalb, IL: Janelle Publications.

Dinnsen D. A. (1992). Variation in developing and fully developed phonologies. In C. A. Ferguson, L. Menn, & C. Stoel-Gammon (Eds.), *Phonological development: Models, research, implications* (pp. 191–210). Timonium, MD: York Press.

Dinnsen D. A., & Elbert, M. (1984). On the relationship between phonology and learning. In M. Elbert, D. A. Dinnsen, & G. Weismer (Eds.). *Phonological theory and the misarticulating child* (ASHA Monographs No. 22, pp. 59–68). Rockville, MD: American Speech-Language-Hearing Association.

Dinnsen, D. A., Chin, S. B., Elbert, M., & Powell, T. W. (1990). Some constraints on functionally disordered phonologies: Phonetic inventories and phonotactics. *Journal of Speech, Language, and Hearing Research, 33*(1), 28–37.

Dodd, B., & Bradford, A. (2000). A comparison of three therapy methods for children with different types of developmental phonological disorder. *International Journal of Language & Communication Disorders, 35*(2), 189–209.

Dodd, B., Huo, Z., Crosbie, S., Holm, A., & Ozanne, A. (2006). *Diagnostic Evaluation of Articulation and Phonology*. Upper Saddle River, NJ: Pearson.

Dodd, B., & McIntosh, B. (2008). The input processing, cognitive linguistic and oro-motor skills of children with speech difficulty. *International Journal of Speech-Language Pathology, 10*(3), 169–178.

Duckworth, M., Allen, G., Hardcastle, W., & Ball, M. J. (1990). Extensions to the International Phonetic Alphabet for the transcription of atypical speech. *Clinical Linguistics & Phonetics, 4*, 273–280.

Dyson, A. (1988). Phonetic inventories of 2- and 3-year-old children. *Journal of Speech and Hearing Disorders, 53*, 89–93.

Dyson, A. T., & Robinson, T. W. (1987). The effect of phonological analysis procedure on the selection of potential remediation targets. *Language, Speech, and Hearing Services in Schools, 18*, 364–377.

Eisenberg, S. L., & Hitchcock, E. R. (2010). Using standardized tests to inventory consonant and vowel production: A comparison of 11 tests of articulation and phonology. *Language, Speech, and Hearing Services in Schools, 41*, 488–503.

Elbert, M., & Gierut, J. (1986). *Handbook of clinical phonology: Approaches to assessment and treatment.* San Diego, CA: College-Hill Press.

Elbert, M., Dinnsen, D., & Powell, T. (1984). On the prediction of phonologic generalization learning patterns. *Journal of Speech and Hearing Disorders, 49*, 309–317.

Fabiano-Smith, L., & Goldstein, B. (2010a). Early-. middle-, and late-developing sounds in monolingual and bilingual children: An exploratory investigation. *American Journal of Speech-Language Pathology, 19*, 66–77.

Fabiano-Smith, L., & Goldstein, B. (2010b). Phonological acquisition in bilingual Spanish-English speaking children. *Journal of Speech, Language, and Hearing Research, 53*, 160–178.

Farquharson, K. (2015). After dismissal: Examining the language, literacy, and cognitive skills of children with remediated speech sound disorders. *Perspectives on School-Based Issues, 16*, 50–59.

Fasolo, M., Majorano, M., & D'odorico, L. (2008). Babbling and first words in children with slow expressive language development. *Clinical Linguistics & Phonetics, 22*, 83–94.

Fee, E. J. (1991). *Underspecification, parameters, and the acquisition of vowels* (doctoral dissertation). Vancouver, BC: University of British Columbia.

Felsenfeld, S., Broen, P. A., & McGue, M. (1994). A 28-year follow-up of adults with a history of moderate phonological disorder. *Journal of Speech and Hearing Research, 37*, 1341–1353.

Fikkert, P. (1991). *Well-formedness conditions in child phonology: A look at metathesis.* Paper presented at the Crossing Boundaries: Formal and Functional Determinants of Language Acquisition. Tubingen, Germany: University of Tubingen.

Fisher, H. B., & Logemann, J. A. (1971). *Fisher-Logemann Test of Articulation Competence.* Iowa City, IA: Houghton Mifflin.

Flipsen, P. (2003). Articulation rate and speech-sound normalization failure. *Journal of Speech, Language, and Hearing Research, 46*, 724–737.

Fudala, J. B. (2000). *Arizona Articulation Proficiency Scale* (3rd ed). Los Angeles, CA: Western Psychological Services.

Gierut, J. A. (1985). *On the relationship between phonological knowledge and generalization learning in misarticulating children* (doctoral dissertation). Bloomington, IN: Indiana University.

Gierut, J. A. (1989). Maximal opposition approach to phonological treatment. *Journal of Speech and Hearing Disorders, 54*(1), 9–19.

Gierut, J. (1991). Homonymy in phonological change. *Clinical Linguistics & Phonetics, 5*(2), 119–137.

Gierut, J. A. (2007). Phonological complexity and language learnability. *American Journal of Speech-Language Pathology, 16*, 6–17.

Gierut, J. A., Elbert, M., & Dinnsen, D. A. (1987). A functional analysis of phonological knowledge and generalization learning in misarticulating children. *Journal of Speech and Hearing Research, 30*, 462–479.

Gierut, J., & Morrisette, M. (2010). Phonological learning and lexicality of treated stimuli. *Clinical Linguistics & Phonetics, 24*(2), 122–140.

Gierut, J., Morrisette, M. L., Hughes, M. T., & Rowland, S. (1996). Phonological treatment efficacy and developmental norms. *Language, Speech, and Hearing Services in Schools, 27*, 215–230.

Gierut, J. A., Morrisette, M. L., & Ziemer, S. M. (2010). Nonwords and generalization in children with phonological disorders. *American Journal of Speech-Language Pathology, 19*, 167–177.

Gierut, J. A., Simmerman, C. L., & Neumann, H. J. (1994). Phonemic structures of delayed phonological systems. *Journal of Child Language, 21*(2), 291–316.

Gildersleeve-Neumann, C., Kester, E. S., Davis, B. L., & Peña, E. D. (2008). English speech sound development in preschool-aged children from bilingual English–Spanish environments. *Language, Speech and Hearing Services in Schools, 39*, 314–328.

Glaspey, A., & Stoel-Gammon, C. (2005). Dynamic assessment in phonological disorders: The scaffolding scale of stimulability. *Topics in Language Disorders, 25*(3), 220–230.

Goldstein, B., Fabiano, L., & Iglesias, A. (2004). Spontaneous and imitated productions in Spanish-speaking children with phonological disorders. *Language, Speech, and Hearing Services in Schools, 35*, 5–15.

Goldman, R., & Fristoe, M. (2000). *Goldman-Fristoe Test of Articulation—Second edition (GFTA-2).* Bloomington, MN: Pearson Assessments.

Goodell, E. W., & Studdert-Kennedy, M. (1991). Articulatory organization of early words: From syllable to phoneme. In *Proceedings of the XIIth International Congress of Phonetic Sciences* (pp. 166–169). Aix-en-Provence, France: Universite de Provence.

Grunwell, P. (1985). *Phonological Assessment of Child Speech (PACS).* Scarborough, ON: Nelson Thomson Learning.

Grunwell, P. (1982). *Clinical phonology.* Rockville, MD: Aspen.

Hayden, D. A., & Square, P. A. (1994). Motor speech treatment hierarchy: A systems approach. *Clinics in Communication Disorders, 4*, 162–174.

Heselwood, B. (1997). A case of nasal clicks for target sonorants: A feature geometry account. *Clinical Linguistics & Phonetics, 11*(1), 43–61.

Hodson, B. (1986). *The Assessment of Phonological Processes—Revised.* Austin, TX: Pro-Ed.

Hodson, B. W. (2004). *Hodson Assessment of Phonological Patterns (HAPP-3)* (3rd ed). East Moline, IL: LinguiSystems.

Holm, A., & Dodd, B. (1999a). Differential diagnosis of phonological disorder in two bilingual children acquiring Italian and English. *Clinical Linguistics & Phonetics, 13*(2), 113–129.

Holm, A., & Dodd, B. (1999b). An intervention case study of a bilingual child with phonological disorder. *Child Language Teaching and Therapy, 15*(2), 139–158.

Howard, S. J. (1993). Articulatory constraints on a phonological system: A case study of cleft palate speech. *Clinical Linguistics & Phonetics, 7*(4), 299–317.

Howell, J., & Dean, E. (1994). *Treating phonological disorders in children: Metaphon-theory to practice* (2nd ed.). London, UK: Whurr Publishers Ltd.

Huffman, M. J., Velleman, S. L., & Mervis, C. B. (2012a). *Relations among speech and intellectual abilities in children with Williams syndrome.* Paper presented at the Williams Syndrome Association, Boston.

Huffman, M. J., Velleman, S. L., & Mervis, C. B. (2012b). *Relations between motor speech skill and single-word accuracy in children with Williams syndrome.* Paper presented at the International Clinical Phonetics and Linguistics Association, Cork, Ireland.

Ingram, D. (1975). Surface contrast in children's speech. *Journal of Child Language, 2*(2), 287–292.

Ingram, D. (1981). *Procedures for the phonological analysis of children's language.* Baltimore, MD: University Park Press.

Ingram, D. (1985). On children's homonyms. *Journal of Child Language, 12*(3), 671–680.

Ingram, D. (1996). Some observations on feature assignment. In B. Bernhardt, J. Gilbert, & D. Ingram (Eds.), *Proceedings of the UBC international conference on phonological acquisition* (pp. 53–61). Somerville, MA: Cascadilla Press.

Ingram, D. (2002). The measurement of whole-word productions. *Journal of Child Language, 29*(4), 713–733.

Kent, R. D. (1992). The biology of phonological development. In C. A. Ferguson, L. Menn, & C. Stoel-Gammon (Eds.), *Phonological development: Models, research, implications*. Timonium, MD: York Press.

Kent, R. D. (1997) Gestural phonology: Basic concepts and applications in speech-language pathology. In M. J. Ball & R. D. Kent (Eds.), *The new phonologies: Developments in clinical linguistics* (pp. 247–268). San Diego, CA: Singular.

Kent, R. D., & Bauer, H. R. (1985). Vocalizations of one-year-olds. *Journal of Child Language, 12*, 491–526.

Kent, R. D., & Vorperian, H. K. (2013). Speech impairment in Down syndrome: A review. *Journal of Speech, Language, and Hearing Research, 56*, 178–210.

Khan, L. M., & Lewis, N. P. (2002). *Khan-Lewis Phonological Analysis* (2nd ed). Circle Pines, MN: American Guidance Service, Inc.

Kim, M., & Stoel-Gammon, C. (2011). Phonological development of word-initial Korean obstruents in your Korean children. *Journal of Child Language, 38*, 316–340.

Kornfeld, J. R. (1971). *Theoretical issues in child phonology*. Paper presented at the Seventh Regional Meeting of the Chicago Linguistic Society, Chicago, IL.

Kummer, A. W., Lee, L., Stutz, L. S., Maroney, A., & Brandt, J. W. (2007). The prevalence of apraxia characteristics in patients with velocardiofacial syndrome as compared with other cleft populations. *Cleft Palate-Craniofacial Journal, 44*(2), 175–181.

Leonard, L. B., & McGregor, K. K. (1991). Unusual phonological patterns and their underlying representations: A case study. *Journal of Child Language, 18*(2), 261–272.

Lindamood, P., & Lindamood, P. (1998). *Lindamood® Phoneme sequencing program for reading, spelling, and speech* (3rd ed). San Luis Obispo, CA: Gander Educational Publishing.

Lindblom, B. (1992). Phonological units as adaptive emergents of lexical development. In C. Ferguson, L. Menn, & C. Stoel-Gammon, (Eds.), *Phonological development: Models, research, implications* (pp. 131–163). Timonium, MD: York Press.

Lindblom, B., Krull, D., & Stark, J. (1993). Phonetic systems and phonological development. In B. de Boysson-Bardies, S. de Schonen, P. Jusczyk, P. MacNeilage, & J. Morton (Eds.), *Developmental neurocognition: Speech and face processing in the first year of life*. The Netherlands: Kluwer Academic Publishers.

Lippke, B. A., Dickey, S. E., Selmar, J. W., & Soder, A. L. (1997). *Photo Articulation Test* (3rd ed). Austin, TX: PRO-ED.

Lleó, C. (1990). Homonymy and reduplication: On the extended availability of two strategies in phonological acquisition. *Journal of Child Language, 17*(2), 267–278.

Lleó, C. (1992). *A parametrical view of harmony and reduplication processes in child phonology*. Hamburg, Germany: University of Hamburg. Unpublished Manuscript.

Locke, J. L. (1983). *Phonological acquisition and change*. New York, NY: Academic Press.

Lof, G. L. (1996). Factors associated with speech-sound stimulability. *Journal of Communication Disorders, 29*(4), 255–278.

Macken, M. A. (1979). Developmental reorganization of phonology: A hierarchy of basic units of acquisition. *Lingua, 49*, 11–49.

Macken, M. (1993). Developmental changes in the acquisition of phonology. In B. de Boysson-Bardies, S. de Schonen, P. Jusczyk, P. MacNeilage, & J. Morton (Eds.), *Changes in speech and face processing in infancy: A glimpse at developmental mechanisms of cognition* (pp. 435–449). Dordrecht, The Netherlands: Kluwer.

Macken, M. A., & Barton, D. (1980). The acquisition of the voicing contrast in English: A study of voice onset time in word-initial stop consonants. *Journal of Child Language, 7*, 41–74.

Masterson, J. J., Bernhardt, B. H., & Hofheinz, M. K. (2005). A comparison of single words and conversational speech in phonological evaluation. *American Journal of Speech-Language Pathology, 14*, 229–241.

McDonough, J., & Myers, S. (1991). *Consonant harmony and planar segregation in child language*. Los Angeles, CA: UCLA and Austin, TX: University of Texas. Unpublished Manuscript.

McDowell, K. D., Lonigan, C., & Goldstein, H. (2007). Relations among socioeconomic status, age, and predictors of phonological awareness. *Journal of Speech, Language, and Hearing Research, 50*, 1079–1092.

McIntosh, B., & Dodd, B. J. (2008). Two-year-olds' phonological acquisition: Normative data. *International Journal of Speech-Language Pathology, 10*(6), 460–469.

McLeod, S., Hand, L., Rosenthal, J. B., & Hayes, B. (1994). The effect of sampling condition on children's productions of consonant clusters. *Journal of Speech and Hearing Research, 37*, 868–882.

Menn, L. (1978). Phonological units in beginning speech. In A. Bell & J. B. Hooper (Eds.), *Syllables and segments* (pp. 157–171). Amsterdam, The Netherlands: North-Holland Publishing Co.

Menn, L., & Matthei, E. (1992). The "two-lexicon" account of child phonology: Looking back, looking ahead. In C. Ferguson, L. Menn, & C. Stoel-Gammon (Eds.), *Phonological development: Models, research, implications*. Timonium, MD: York Press, Inc.

Menn, L., Schmidt, E., & Nicholas, B. (2009). Conspiracy and sabotage in the acquisition of phonology: Dense data undermine existing theories, provide scaffolding for a new one. *Language Sciences, 31*(2–3), 285–304.

Menn, L., Schmidt, E., & Nicholas, B. (2013). Challenges to theories, charges to a model: The linked-attractor model of phonological development. In M. M. Vihman & T. Keren-Portnoy (Eds.), *The emergence of phonology: Whole-word approaches and cross-linguistic evidence* (pp. 460–502). Cambridge, UK: Cambridge University Press.

Menn, L., & Vihman, M. M. (2011). Features in child phonology: Inherent, emergent, or artefacts of analysis? In N. Clements & R. Ridouane (Eds.), *Where do phonological features come from? Cognitive, physical and developmental bases of distinctive speech categories*. Amsterdam, The Netherlands: John Benjamins.

Miccio, A. W. (2005). A treatment program for enhancing stimulability. In A. G. Kamhi & K. Pollock (Eds.), *Phonological disorders in children: Clinical decision-making in assessment and intervention* (pp. 163–173). Baltimore, MD: Paul H. Brookes.

Miccio, A. W., & Elbert, M. (1996). Enhancing stimulability: A treatment program. *Journal of Communication Disorders, 29*(4), 335–351.

Miccio, A. W., Elbert, M., & Forrest, K. (1999). The relationship between stimulability and phonological acquisition in children with normally developing and disordered phonologies. *American Journal of Speech-Language Pathology, 8*(4), 347–363.

Miccio, A. W., & Ingrisano, D. R. (2000). The acquisition of fricatives and affricates: Evidence from a disordered phonological system. *American Journal of Speech-Language Pathology, 9*(3), 214–229.

Miccio, A. W., & Powell, T. W. (2010). Triangulating speech sound generalization. *Clinical Linguistics & Phonetics, 24*(4–5), 311–322.

Moriarty, B. C., & Gillon, G. T. (2006). Phonological awareness intervention for children with childhood apraxia of speech. *International Journal of Language and Communication Disorders, 41*(6), 713–734.

Morrisette, M. L., & Gierut, J. A. (2002). Lexical organization and phonological change in treatment. *Journal of Speech, Language, and Hearing Research, 45*, 143–159.

Moskowitz, B. A. (1975). The acquisition of fricatives: A study in phonetics and phonology. *Journal of Phonetics, 3*, 141–150. http://eric.ed.gov/?id=EJ124316

Moran, M. J. (1993). Final consonant deletion in African American children speaking Black English: A closer look. *Language, Speech, and Hearing Services in Schools, 24*, 161–166.

Morrison, J. A., & Shriberg, L. D. (1992). Articulation testing versus conversational speech sampling. *Journal of Speech and Hearing Research, 35*, 259–273.

Munson, B., Edwards, J., & Beckman, M. E. (2005). Phonological knowledge in typical and atypical speech-sound development. *Topics in Language Disorders, 25*(3), 190–206.

Nathan, L., Stackhouse, J., Goulandris, N., & Snowling, M. (2004). The development of early literacy skills among children with speech difficulties: A test of the "critical age hypothesis." *Journal of Speech, Language, and Hearing Research*, *47*(2), 377–391.

Nelson, K. (1981). Individual differences in language development: Implications for development and language. *Developmental Psychology*, *17*(2), 170–187.

Nijland, L. (2009). Speech perception in children with speech output disorders. *Clinical Linguistics & Phonetics*, *23*(3), 222–239.

Ohala, J. J. (1991). The integration of phonetics and phonology. In *Proceedings of the XIIth International Congress of Phonetic Sciences, Aix-en-Provence, France*, *1*, 1–16.

Otomo, K., & Stoel-Gammon, C. (1992). The acquisition of unrounded vowels in English. *Journal of Speech and Hearing Research*, *35*(3), 604–616.

Pearson, B. Z., Velleman, S. L., Bryant, T. J., & Charko, T. (2009). Phonological milestones for African American English-speaking children learning Mainstream American English as a second dialect. *Language, Speech, and Hearing Services in Schools*, *40*, 229–244.

Peña, E. D., & Quinn, R. (1997). Task familiarity: Effects on the test performance of Puerto Rican and African American children. *Language, Speech, and Hearing Services in Schools*, *28*, 323–332.

Peters, A. M. (1977). Language learning strategies: Does the whole equal the sum of the parts? *Language*, *53*(3), 560–573.

Peterson, R. L., Pennington, B. F., Shriberg, L. D., & Boada, R. (2009). What influences literacy outcome in children with speech sound disorder? *Journal of Speech, Language, and Hearing Research*, *52*, 1175–1188.

Powell, T. W., Elbert, M., & Dinnsen, D. A. (1991). Stimulability as a factor in the phonological generalization of misarticulating preschool children. *Journal of Speech and Hearing Research*, *34*(6), 1318–1328.

Pollock, K. E. (1983). Individual preferences: Case study of a phonologically delayed child. *Topics in Language Disorders*, *3*, 1–23.

Pollock, K. E., & Hall, P. K. (1991). An analysis of the vowel misarticulations of five children with developmental apraxia of speech. *Clinical Linguistics & Phonetics*, *5*(3), 207–224.

Pollock, K. E., & Keiser, N. J. (1990). An examination of vowel errors in phonologically disordered children. *Clinical Linguistics & Phonetics*, *4*(2), 161–178.

Preston, J. L., & Edwards, M. L. (2009). Speed and accuracy of rapid speech output by adolescents with residual speech sound errors including rhotics. *Clinical Linguistics & Phonetics*, *23*(4), 301–318.

Preston, J., & Edwards, M. L. (2010). Phonological awareness and types of sound errors in preschoolers with speech sound disorders. *Journal of Speech, Language, and Hearing Research*, *53*, 44–60.

Preston, J. L., & Koenig, L. L. (2011). Phonetic variability in residual speech sound disorders: Exploration of subtypes. *Topics in Language Disorders*, *31*(2), 168–184.

Pullum, G. K., & Ladusaw, W. A. (1986). *Phonetic symbol guide*. Chicago, IL: The University of Chicago Press.

Pye, C., Ingram, D., & List, H. (1987). A comparison of initial consonant acquisition in English and Quiche. In K. E. Nelson & A. Van Kleek (Eds.), *Children's Language* (*Vol. 6*). Hillsdale, NJ: Erlbaum.

Raitano, N. A., Pennington, B. F., Tunick, R. A., Boada, R., & Shriberg, L. D. (2004). Pre-literacy skills of subgroups of children with speech sound disorders. *Journal of Child Psychology and Psychiatry*, *45*(4), 821–835.

Rapin, I., Dunn, M. A., Allen, D. A., Stevens, M. C., & Fein, D. (2009). Subtypes of language disorders in school-age children with autism. *Developmental Neuropsychology*, *34*(1), 66–84.

Rice, K. (1996). Default variability: The coronal-velar relationship. *Natural Language and Linguistic Theory*, *14*(3), 493–543.

Robb, M. P., & Bleile, K. M. (1994). Consonant inventories of young children from 8 to 25 months. *Clinical Linguistics & Phonetics*, *8*(4), 295–320.

Rupela, V., & Manjula, R. (2007). Phonotactic patterns in the speech of children with Down syndrome. *Clinical Linguistics & Phonetics*, *21*(8), 605–622.

Rupela, V., & Manjula, R. (2010). Diadochokinetic assessment in persons with Down syndrome. *Asia Pacific Journal of Speech, Language, and Hearing*, *13*(2), 109–120.

Rupela, V., Manjula, R., & Velleman, S. L. (2010). Phonological processes in Kannada-speaking adolescents with Down syndrome. *Clinical Linguistics & Phonetics*, *24*(6), 431–450.

Rvachew, S. (2005). Stimulability and treatment success. *Topics in Language Disorders*, *25*(3), 207–219.

Rvachew, S., & Nowak, M. (2001). The effect of target-selection strategy on phonological learning. *Journal of Speech, Language, and Hearing Research*, *44*(3), 610–623.

Rvachew, S., Rafaat, S., & Martin, M. (1999). Stimulability, speech perception skills, and the treatment of phonological disorders. *American Journal of Speech-Language Pathology*, *8*, 33–43.

Saben, C. B., & Ingham, R. J. (1991). The effects of minimal pairs treatment on the speech sound production of two children with phonological disorders. *Journal of Speech and Hearing Research*, *34*, 1023–1040.

Schwartz, R. G., & Leonard, L. B. (1982). Do children pick and choose? An examination of phonological selection and avoidance in early lexical acquisition. *Journal of Child Language*, *9*, 319–336.

Schwartz, R. G., Leonard, L. B., Frome Loeb, D. M., & Swanson, L. A. (1987). Attempted sounds are sometimes not: An expanded view of phonological selection and avoidance. *Journal of Child Language*, *14*(3), 411–418.

Secord, W. A., Donohoe, J., & Johnson, C. (2002). *Clinical assessment of articulation and phonology*. Greenville, SC: Super Duper.

Secord, W. A., & Shine, R. E. (1997). *Secord Contextual Articulation Tests (S-CAT)*. Sedona, AZ: Red Rock Educational Publications.

Selby, J. C., Robb, M. P., & Gilbert, H. R. (2000). Normal vowel articulations between 15 and 36 months of age. *Clinical Linguistics & Phonetics*, *14*(4), 255–265.

Shriberg, L. D. (2013). *State of the art in CAS diagnostic marker research*. Paper presented at the Childhood Apraxia of Speech Research Symposium, Atlanta, GA.

Shriberg, L. D., Aram, D. M., & Kwiatkowski, J. (1997). Developmental apraxia of speech: III. A subtype marked by inappropriate stress. *Journal of Speech, Language, and Hearing Research*, *40*(2), 313–337.

Shriberg, L. D., Austin, D., Lewis, B. A., McSweeny, J. L., & Wilson, D. L. (1997a). The percentage of consonants correct (PCC) metric: Extensions and reliability data. *Journal of Speech, Language, and Hearing Research*, *40*, 708–722.

Shriberg, L. D., Austin, D., Lewis, B. A., McSweeny, J. L., & Wilson, D. L. (1997b). The speech disorders classification system (SDCS): Extensions and lifespan reference data. *Journal of Speech, Language, and Hearing Research*, *40*, 723–740.

Shriberg, L. D., Fourakis, M., Hall, S. D., Karlsson, H. B., Lohmeier, H. L., McSweeny, J. L., . . . Wilson, D. L. (2010). Extensions to the speech disorders classification system (SDCS). *Clinical Linguistics & Phonetics*, *24*(10), 795–824.

Shriberg, L. D., Jakielski, K. J., & Strand, E. A. (2010). *Diagnostic markers of childhood apraxia of speech*. Paper presented at the American Speech-Language-Hearing Association National Convention, Philadelphia, PA.

Shriberg, L. D., & Kwaitkowski, J. (1990). Self-monitoring and generalization in preschool speech-delayed children. *Language, Speech, and Hearing Services in Schools*, *21*, 157–170.

Shriberg, L. D., Paul, R., Black, L. M., & van Santen, J. P. (2011). The hypothesis of apraxia of speech in children with autism spectrum disorder. *Journal of Autism and Developmental Disorders*, *41*(4), 405–426.

Smit, A. B., Hand, L., Freilinger, J. J., Bernthal, J. E., & Bird, A. (1990). The Iowa articulation norms project and its Nebraska replication. *Journal of Speech and Hearing Disorders*, *55*(4), 779–798.

Smit, A. B., & Hand, L. (1992). *Smit-Hand Articulation and Phonology Evaluation*. Los Angeles, CA: Eastern Psychological Services.

Smith, N. V. (1973). *The acquisition of phonology: A case study*. Cambridge, UK: Cambridge University Press.

Stampe, D. (1969). The acquisition of phonetic representation. *Papers from the 5th Regional Meeting of the Chicago Linguistic Society*, 443–454.

Stockman, I., & Vaughn-Cooke, F. B. (1989). Addressing new questions about Black children's language. In R. W. Fasold & D. Schriffin (Eds.), *Language change and variation* (pp. 275–300). Amsterdam, The Netherlands: John Benjamins.

Stoel-Gammon, C. (1985). Phonetic inventories, 15–24 months: A longitudinal study. *Journal of Speech and Hearing Research*, *28*(4), 505–512.

Stoel-Gammon, C. (1987). Phonological skills of 2-year-olds. *Language, Speech, and Hearing Services in Schools*, *18*, 323–329.

Stoel-Gammon, C. (2010). The Word Complexity Measure: Description and application to developmental phonology and disorders. *Clinical Linguistics & Phonetics*, *24*(4–5), 271–282.

Stoel-Gammon, C., & Herrington, P. B. (1990). Vowel systems of normally developing and phonologically disordered children. *Clinical Linguistics & Phonetics*, *4*(2), 145–160.

Stokes, S., Lau, J. T.-K., & Ciocca, V. (2002). The interaction of ambient frequency and feature complexity in the diphthong errors of children with phonological disorders. *Journal of Speech, Language, and Hearing Research*, *45*, 1188–1201.

Stokes, S. F., & Surendran, D. (2005). Articulatory complexity, ambient frequency, and functional load as predictors of consonant development in children. *Journal of Speech, Language, and Hearing Research*, *48*(3), 577–591.

Strand, E. A., & Skinder, A. (1999). Treatment of developmental apraxia of speech: Integral stimulation methods. In A. J. Caruso & E. A. Strand (Eds.), *Clinical management of motor speech disorders in children* (pp. 109–148). New York, NY: Thieme.

Studdert-Kennedy, M., & Goodell, E. W. (1992). Gestures, features and segments in early child speech. *Haskins Laboratories Status Report on Speech Research, SR-111/112*, 89–102. Available at: http://www.haskins.yale.edu/sr/sr111/sr111_06.pdf

Templin, M. C., & Darley, F. L. (1968). *The Templin-Darley Tests of Articulation*. Iowa City, IA: University of Iowa Press.

Thelen, E., & Smith, L. B. (1994). *A dynamic systems approach to the development of cognition and action*. Cambridge, MA: MIT Press.

Tomik, B., Krupinski, J., Glodzik-Sobanska, L., Bala-Slodowska, M., Wszolek, W., Kusiak M., & Lechwacka, A. (1999). Acoustic analysis of dysarthria profile in ALS patients. *Journal of the Neurological Sciences*, *169*(1–2), 35–42.

Tyler, A. A., & Figurski, G. R. (1994). Phonetic inventory changes after treating distinctions along an implicational hierarchy. *Clinical Linguistics & Phonetics*, *8*(2), 91–107.

Tyler, A. A. (2002). Language-based intervention for phonological disorders. *Seminars in Speech and Language*, *23*(1), 69–82.

Tyler, A. A., & Macrae, T. (2010). Stimulability: Relationships to other characteristics of children's phonological systems. *Clinical Linguistics & Phonetics*, *24*(4–5), 300–310.

Van Lieshout, P. H. H. M. (2004). Dynamical systems theory and its application in speech. In B. Maassen, R. D. Kent, H. F. M. Peters, P. H. H. M. van Lieshout, & W. Hulstijn (Eds.), *Speech motor control in normal and disordered speech* (pp. 51–81). Oxford, UK: Oxford University Press.

Van Riper, C. (1939). *Speech correction: Principles and methods*. Englewood Cliffs, NH: Prentice-Hall.

Velleman, S. L. (1988). The role of linguistic perception in later phonological development. *Journal of Applied Psycholinguistics*, *9*, 221–236.

Velleman, S. (1992). *A nonlinear model of harmony and metathesis*. Paper presented at the Linguistic Society of America, Philadelphia, PA.

Velleman, S. L. (1994). The interaction of phonetics and phonology in developmental verbal dyspraxia: Two case studies. *Clinics in Communication Disorders*, *4*(1), 67–78.

Velleman, S. L., Andrianopoulos, M. V., Boucher, M., Perkins, J., Averback, K. E., Currier, A., . . . Van Emmerik, R. (2009). Motor speech disorders in children with autism. In R. Paul & P. Flipsen (Eds.), *Speech sound disorders in children: In honor of Lawrence D. Shriberg* (pp. 141–180). San Diego, CA: Plural.

Velleman, S., Huntley, R., & Lasker, J. (1991). *Is it DVD or is it phonological disorder?* Atlanta, GA: American Speech-Language Hearing Association.

Velleman, S. L., & Mervis, C. B. (2011). Children with 7q11.23 Duplication syndrome: Speech, language, cognitive, and behavioral characteristics and their implications for intervention. *Perspectives on Language Learning and Education*, *18*(3), 108–116.

Velleman, S. L., & Pearson, B. Z. (2010). Differentiating speech sound disorders from phonological dialect differences: Implications for assessment and intervention. *Topics in Language Disorders*, *30*(3), 176–188.

Velten, J. (1943). The growth of phonemic and lexical patterns in infant language. *Language*, *19*, 281–292.

Vihman, M. M. (1981). Phonology and the development of the lexicon: Evidence from children's errors. *Journal of Child Language*, *8*(2), 239–264.

Vihman, M. M. (1992). Early syllables and the construction of phonology. In C. A. Ferguson, L. Menn, & C. Stoel-Gammon (Eds.), *Phonological development: Models, research, implications*. Timonium, MD: York Press.

Vihman, M. M., Macken, M. A., Miller, R., Simmons, H., & Miller, J. (1985). From babbling to speech: A re-assessment of the continuity issue. *Language*, *61*(2), 397–445.

Vihman, M. M., & Velleman, S. L. (1989). Phonological reorganization: A case study. *Language and Speech*, *32*, 149–170.

Vihman, M. M., Velleman, S. L., & McCune, L. (1994). How abstract is child phonology? Towards an integration of linguistic and psychological approaches. In M. Yavas (Ed.), *First and second language phonology* (pp. 9–44). San Diego, CA: Singular Press.

Walker, J. F., Archibald, L. M. D., Cherniak, S. R., & Fish, V. G. (1992). Articulation rate in 3- and 5-year-old children. *Journal of Speech and Hearing Research*, *35*, 4–13.

Weismer, G., Dinnsen, D. A., & Elbert, M. (1981). A study of the voicing distinction associated with omitted, word-final stops. *Journal of Speech and Hearing Disorders*, *46*, 320–328.

Williams, A. L. (2000). Multiple oppositions: Theoretical foundations for an alternative contrastive intervention approach. *American Journal of Speech-Language Pathology*, *9*(4), 282–288.

Wolfe, V., Presley, C., & Mesaris, J. (2003). The importance of sound identification training in phonological intervention. *American Journal of Speech-Language Pathology*, *12*(3), 282–288.

Wren, Y. (2015). "He'll grow out of it soon—Won't he?"—The characteristics of older children's speech when they do—and don't—grow out of it. *Perspectives on School-Based Issues*, *16*, 25–36.

CHAPTER 8

The Phonological Framework

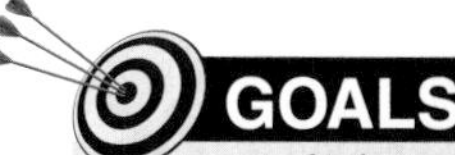

GOALS of This Chapter

1. Review the impacts of phonotactic limitations on child speech production.
2. Describe approaches to assessment of phonotactics.
3. Describe approaches to treatment of phonotactics.

I
it
sit
spit
spite
sprite
spritely
spriteliness
unspriteliness
unspritelinesses
....

Jonah, a 7-year-old, has been denied school speech-language services because he has "reached age-appropriate articulatory developmental milestones" for his age; he produces all stops, nasals, glides, liquids (with a distorted /ɹ/), fricatives except interdentals (and distorted /s/), and affricates. Yet, he is unintelligible. Analyses of his spontaneous speech reveal that he produces few final consonants, clusters, or words of more than two syllables in length. Is his phonology actually age appropriate? What can be done to improve his intelligibility?

PREPARATION

As we have seen, long before an infant speaks—or even understands—a single word, she begins to develop expectations through implicit learning about the phonological framework of her language. This framework includes both the prosody (the topic of Chapter 10) and the syllable and word structures of the language (phonotactics). These distributional, phonotactic characteristics of the language or languages to which the child is exposed include patterns of co-occurrence (i.e., which syllables or segments are likely to follow each other). For instance, 10-month-olds prefer sequences of consonants and vowels from their own languages (Gerken & Zamuner, 2004) and are more likely to respond to pairs of syllables as if they are words if the abutting medial consonants are more commonly found in the language in that position (such as the [ŋk] of "monkey" versus the [pt] of "reptile") (Morgan, 1996). These detailed infant expectations about the phonological framework to which they have been exposed lay the groundwork for producing consonants and vowels in language-appropriate structures: syllables, words, phrases, and beyond.

IMPORTANCE OF ANALYZING CHILD SPEECH AT THE SYLLABLE LEVEL AND ABOVE

Since Waterson's pivotal 1971 paper on this topic, the critical significance of syllable-level and word-level analysis for describing and explaining child—and adult—phonologies has been increasingly recognized. Ingram (1978) lists four main reasons for focusing on syllable and word structure in child phonologies:

1. Some phonological patterns, such as consonant cluster reduction and final consonant omission, function primarily to simplify syllables.
2. Other patterns, such as unstressed syllable deletion and reduplication (repetition of the same syllable, as in "booboo"), operate only on entire words.
3. The development of many segments differs according to their placements within the syllable or word (e.g., velars often develop first in final position).
4. Segmental complexity (the difficulty and variety of sounds within the word) interacts with syllabic complexity (the shape of the syllable) and triggers word-level patterns (such as harmony, to be described below). As segmental complexity increases, syllabic complexity may decrease and vice versa. In other words, the child may be able to produce either difficult sounds or difficult word shapes but not both within the same word. For example, Macken's (1978) Spanish-speaking participant "J" at 2;1 initially produced the word "silla" with a fricative in a monosyllabic word form ([ʃɑ]). As she expanded her word shapes to include two-syllable words at 2;2, she resorted to simpler phonetic forms of the word ([kɪjɑ] or [tɪ:jɑ]). This trade-off between phonetics and phonotactics was an apparent regression phonetically (see Chapter 6). Eventually, at 2;3, she was able to combine the increased phonotactic complexity (two syllables) with increased phonetic complexity (fricative) into [ʃɪ:jɑ].

Many child phonologists feel that very early phonology, at least, is exclusively word or syllable based and that children's early phonological systems do not refer to the segmental level at all. Furthermore, it is well documented that clients of any age generalize their learning much better when sounds are targeted at the syllable or word levels rather than in isolation. Although the impacts of phonotactic factors typically become far more subtle as children approach school age, many aspects of the phonological context significantly affect children's ability to produce speech sounds. For example, the consonantal accuracy of typically developing children between the ages of 2 and 3 years is apparently not affected by the stress pattern of the word, though syllable deletion patterns are (Schwartz & Goffman, 1995). However, segmental accuracy is lower in weak (unstressed) syllables among 4-year-olds who are typically developing and in 5- to 6-year-olds with speech–language impairment (SLI) (Goffman, Gerken, & Lucchesi, 2007). In Childhood Apraxia of Speech (CAS), and perhaps in other speech sound disorders (SSDs) as well, phonotactic accuracy, phonotactic complexity, and phonotactic frequency determine phonetic accuracy. That is, segments are most accurate in words that are also produced phonotactically correctly, especially if the words have simple structures that are frequent in the language the child speaks (Jacks, Marquardt, & Davis, 2006). In short, focusing solely on the child's production of segments can severely limit our understanding of those factors that impact their accuracy. Without understanding these factors, appropriate intervention goals and strategies cannot be selected.

Summary

Syllables and words are at least as important in child phonology as individual segments or phonemes.

CHILD PHONOTACTIC LIMITATIONS

Children—whether they have SSDs or not—often have more restrictions on their syllable and word shapes than the language that they are learning. This becomes a problem when their limitations on syllable and word shapes are very persistent or extremely restrictive while their vocabularies continue to grow. Examples of restrictions on phonological structures and strategies that some learners use in response to those restrictions are provided in the following sections.

Number of Syllables in a Word

English-speaking children are especially partial to monosyllabic words, probably due to the fact that English words tend to be short in comparison to those of other languages. However, Stoel-Gammon (1987) found that 79% of 34 children at the age of 24 months used CVCV words at least some of the time; 67% used two-syllable words ending in a final consonant (CVCVC). The most common response to a preference for short words among English-learning children is to omit unstressed syllables, yielding forms like [ˈnænə] for "banana," [waʊn] for "around," and [ˈɛfɪn] for "elephant." Word-stress patterns have an influence on this tendency, as will be discussed in Chapter 10.

It may seem obvious to English speakers that monosyllabic words are easier than are longer words, but this is, in fact, not the case for speakers of many other languages. Two-syllable words are more common in many other languages than monosyllabic words are, unlike in English, and children's production patterns reflect that. For example, in Kannada (a Dravidian language spoken in southern India), children produce three-syllable and even longer words before they learn the relatively few monosyllabic words in the language (Rupela & Manjula, 2006).

Vowel as Syllable Nucleus

Most children include a vocalic nucleus in every syllable with the exception of certain English words that allow a liquid or nasal to serve as a nucleus (e.g., the final syllables in "little" [lɪɾl̩] and "button" [bʌʔn̩]). In addition, there are a few motherese sound effects that some children may treat as words (e.g., "shh," "mmm"). Some children with disorders, especially CAS, may exhibit particular difficulty in building consonant + vowel syllables. These children may use an unusually high number of words that consist of a single consonant without a vowel nucleus or of a single vowel without a consonant onset.

Inclusion of Consonant Onset

Fikkert (1994), Demuth and Fee (1995), Demuth (1996), and Fee (1996) have proposed CV as the **core syllable** with which all children begin phonological acquisition. Like some adult languages, some young children epenthesize (add) consonants at the beginnings of vowel-initial words (e.g., "up" pronounced as [bʌp]). Other children may use other strategies, such as metathesis—reversing the order of segments within the word—to ensure the presence of an onset (e.g., "up" pronounced as [pʌ]). For example, Gnanadesikan (1996) describes a child, Gita, who avoided vowel-initial syllables in medial positions of words by moving the final consonant into the middle of the word. Thus, "going" was pronounced as [gonə] and "lion" as [jɑni]. Stemberger (1988) reported that his daughter used **resyllabification**, in which the coda of a word in a phrase was used as the onset of the next word in order to avoid vowel-initial words, as in "get up and go" being produced as [dɑ tʌ pi:n doʊ].

However, this tendency for children to prefer syllables with onsets is far from an absolute universal. Omissions of initial consonants, or even additions of vowels before initial consonants, are not unusual in children learning languages in which the first syllable is unstressed, such as French and Spanish (Vihman, Nakai, & DePaolis, 2006) and Portuguese (Freitas, 1996). Velleman and Vihman (2002a, 2002b) provide several examples of English-learning as well as French-learning children who not only produce vowel-initial words as such but also omit initial consonants or add vowels before them (e.g., "apple" as [ɑpi], *poupee* "doll" as [ɑpʊ], *merci "thank you"* as [ɛsih], "water" as [əwɑwɪ], *balle* "ball" as [ɑbɑ]). Finnish-, Welsh-, and Japanese-learning children may also omit initial consonants. This has been hypothesized to be due to their heightened attention on word-medial consonants because that is the position in which highly salient geminates (prolonged "double" consonants) occur. Initial consonant deletion has also been reported in typically developing children learning Hindi and Estonian (Vihman & Velleman, 2000a, 2000b; Vihman & Croft, 2007).

Open Versus Closed Syllables

Many children enter into word production with only **open** CV and V **syllables**, although this too is dependent to some extent on the language(s) to which they have been exposed. Grunwell (1982) concluded that **closed syllables** typically don't emerge until the English-learning child is producing 8 to 11 different consonants, at about 2 to 2.5 years of age. In contrast, Vihman (personal communication cited by Menn, Schmidt, & Nicholas, 2008) estimates that about 40% of English learners are "CVC kids" (p. 288) who begin producing final consonants fairly early. According to Stoel-Gammon (1987), 100% of 2-year-olds produce CV syllables, and 97% produce CVC syllables at least some of the time. Branigan (1976) states that "...monosyllables are the first structures to be closed and ... this operation occurs simultaneous with the production of bisyllables" (p. 128). Redford and Gildersleeve-Neumann (2009) report that even 3-year-olds are able to increase the frequency at which they release final consonants in CVC words—thereby making them clearer to the listener—when they are encouraged to talk "like an adult."

Demuth and Fee (1995) and Fee (1996) noted that two-syllable words and final consonants often appear to develop nearly simultaneously. Thus, children may expand their word shapes in both ways at the same time—to include a second syllable and to include a final consonant on monosyllables. The co-occurrence of these two different phonotactic expansions suggests that they may result from some underlying development that facilitates both.

Interestingly, children are more likely to include final consonants after lax vowels than after tense vowels or diphthongs. For example, the final [p] is more likely to be preserved in "pip" [pɪp] than in "peep" [pip] or "pipe" [pɑɪp]. This likely reflects the child's (implicit) knowledge that **light syllables** such as [pɪ], [pɛ], and [pʊ] are not allowed in English (Kehoe & Stoel-Gammon, 2001; Demuth, Culbertson, & Alter, 2006). It is not known whether this tendency to close syllables in order to make them appropriately **heavy** occurs in children with disorders as well as in young children who are typically developing.

Other studies have also shown that typically developing children are more likely to produce codas in CVC words when the onset + vowel sequence is a frequent one (i.e., when the word has high phonotactic probability). Thus, for example, the final [d] is more likely to be preserved in a nonsense word like [nɑɪd] (where [nɑɪ] is a relatively common C+V sequence: "night, nine, knife," etc.) than in [mɔɪd] (where [mɔɪ] begins far fewer common words: "moist, moil.."??) (Zamuner, Gerken, & Hammond, 2004).

This result is consistent with the more general finding that words that contain more frequent sequences of sounds (i.e., sequences with higher phonotactic frequency) are learned more quickly by typically developing children (Storkel, 2001, 2003)—with respect to associating the sound sequence with a particular meaning, not with respect to producing every phoneme in the word accurately. However, a word of caution is necessary here: It appears that children with SSDs actually learn words (i.e., associate the forms of words with their meanings) when the words contain uncommon sequences of sounds more rapidly than they do words with higher phonotactic frequency levels (Storkel, 2004). In other words, children who are typically developing seem to find it easier to remember words with expected sequences of sounds while those with SSD rely on distinctive sound sequences to help them remember new words. The impact on the pronunciations of the words is not clear from the study though.

It is well established that syllable closure constraints often persist beyond age expectations in children with SSDs. Metathesis, the interchange of elements within a word, may be motivated by restrictions on final consonants (Velleman, 1996). Attempts to produce consonants only in initial position may result in productions such as [pʌ] for "up," [fɔ] for "off," or [gɛ] for "egg." When complicated by omissions within the word due also to the child's SSD, these forms can be quite confusing, such as the use of [kʌ] for "stuck." An SLP who does not consider phonotactic factors would not understand such a child's errors and would therefore be unable to develop appropriate goals and strategies for addressing them.

Consonant Clusters

Many children have phonotactic limitations against all or most clusters in any position, especially early in their phonological development. Stoel-Gammon (1987) reports 58% of 24-month-olds use at least some initial two-element consonant clusters, 48% use some such clusters in final position, and 30% use some in medial position. Similarly, McLeod, van Doorn, and Reed (2001a) found typical ranges of one to two clusters in Australian 26-month-olds (mean 2.3), 7 to 17 in 31-month-olds (mean 6.9), 9 to 21 in 35-month-olds (mean 9.3), and 8 to 19 in 39-month-olds (mean 10.8). In both studies, many of these clusters were incorrect, and there was considerable variation among the children with respect to which clusters they produced. The researchers stress that progress during this early time period may be better represented by an increasing number and variety of clusters produced rather than an increase in accuracy. Although research and intervention have tended to focus more heavily on initial position, McLeod, van Doorn, and Reed (2001b) summarize past research demonstrating that in English and also some other languages as different as Telugu and Spanish, final clusters tend to emerge before initial ones, though some children demonstrate the opposite pattern. This has been confirmed for German, Dutch, and English in other studies (respectively, Lleó & Prinz, 1996; Levelt, Schiller, & Levelt, 2000; Kirk & Demuth, 2005).

Children with reduced intelligibility often lack consonant clusters in their speech (Grunwell, 1981; Hodson & Paden, 1981; Stoel-Gammon & Stone, 1991). According to McLeod, van Doorn, and Reed (1997), the typical sequence of cluster development in children with SSD is "word-final nasal clusters, followed by word-initial two-element stop clusters, word-initial two element fricative clusters and finally word-initial three-element fricative + stop clusters" (p. 100):

final nasal + stop > initial stop + glide / liquid
> initial fricative + glide / liquid
> initial /s/ + stop + glide / liquid

They stress that word shapes, syllable shapes, and the actual constituents of the cluster (the consonants of which it is composed) can each have marked impacts on the child's production of that cluster. This is another example of some aspects of phonotactics impacting each other.

The simplifications that children with SSD—and young children—use to avoid clusters that are too difficult for them to produce may include omissions, coalescence (mergers of sounds), epenthesis (additions of sounds), metathesis (interchanges of sounds), and migration (movements of sounds) (as discussed further below). These structural changes to clusters may be more likely in conversational speech rather than in single-word productions (McLeod, Hand, Rosenthal, & Hayes, 1994). As they gradually become able to produce clusters in a more adult-like fashion, children increasingly produce the correct number of consonants in roughly the correct order, but they substitute simpler constituents for more complex ones (e.g., substituting pw- for pɹ- or -nt for -ns) (McLeod et al., 2001b).

Restrictions on consonant clusters include not only limits on the number of adjacent consonants and the locations of clusters but also co-occurrences of particular consonants with each other. According to Grunwell (1981, 1997), initial obstruent + approximant clusters (such as pl-, dr-, kw-, etc.) are acquired between 2;6 and 4;0. She indicates that initial consonant clusters composed of /s/ + another consonant are mastered slightly later, between 3;0 and 4;0. McLeod and colleagues (2001a, 2001b) also reported that the earliest clusters produced were often Cw- clusters, including some that do not occur in adult English (e.g., pw- and bw-). In contrast, they also found that initial clusters with /l/ and /s/ were the earliest to be produced correctly, with nasal clusters (such as -mp) produced correctly first in final position. Similar findings for English word-initial cluster development of typically developing children by Smit, Hand, Freilinger, Bernthal, and Bird (1990) and Chin and Dinnsen (1992) are summarized in Table 8-1. More detail, including gender differences, is provided by Smit, Hand, Freilinger, Bernthal, and Bird (1990), given in Table 8-2.

TABLE 8-1 Acquisition of Initial Clusters

Cluster Type	Approximate Age of Acquisition
stop+[w]	4;0
stop+[l], fl-	5;6
[s] + stop, nasal, glide, or liquid; stop + [ɹ] and fɹ-	6;0
three elements; θɹ-	7;0–9;0

From Smit, A. B., Hand, L., Freilinger, J. J., Bernthal, J. E., & Bird, A. (1990). The Iowa articulation norms project and its Nebraska replication. *Journal of Speech and Hearing Disorders, 55*(4), 779–798; and Chin, S., & Dinnsen, D. (1992). Consonant clusters in disordered speech: Constraints and correspondence patterns. *Journal of Child Language, 19*, 259–285.

TABLE 8-2 Ages at Which 75% of Children Produce Initial Clusters Accurately

Cluster	Age of 75% Acquisition (Years;Months)	
	Females	Males
tw-	3;6	3;6
kw-	3;6	3;6
pl-	4;0	5;6
bl-	4;0	5;0
kl-	4;0	5;6
sp-	4;6	5;0
st-	4;6	5;0
sk-	4;6	6;0
sw-	4;6	6;0
gl-	4;6	4;6
fl-	4;6	5;6
kɹ-	4;6	5;6
skw-	4;6	7;0
sm-	5;6	7;0
sn-	5;6	5;0
sl-	6;0	7;0
pɹ-	6;0	5;6
bɹ-	6;0	6;0
tɹ-	6;0	5;6
dɹ-	6;0	5;0
gɹ-	6;0	5;6
fɹ-	6;0	5;6
spl-	6;0	7;0
θɹ-	7;0	7;0
spɹ-	8;0	8;0
stɹ-	8;0	8;0
skɹ-	8;0	8;0

Adapted from Smit, A. B., Hand, L., Freilinger, J. J., Bernthal, J. E., & Bird, A. (1990). The Iowa articulation norms project and its Nebraska replication. *Journal of Speech and Hearing Disorders*, *55*(4), 779–798.

Recall the sonority hierarchy (from Chapter 2), a ranking of least to most open segments, roughly:

Most sonorant:	vowels
	glides
	liquids
	nasals
	fricatives
	affricates
Least sonorant:	stops

This hypothesis includes the generalization that the most sonorant segments (e.g., vowels) tend to occur in the middle of the word with segments of decreasing sonority toward the edges so that the least sonorant segments (e.g., stops) are at word boundaries. This helps to cue the listener that one word has ended and the next is beginning. Clusters in the languages of the world tend to follow this generalization with the least sonorant consonants such as stops at the beginnings of initial clusters and at the ends of final clusters. Thus, a typical CCVCC word that followed the hierarchy would have the following shape:

$$\left\{\begin{matrix}\text{stop}\\\text{fricative}\end{matrix}\right\}\left\{\begin{matrix}\text{liquid}\\\text{nasal}\\\text{glide}\end{matrix}\right\}\{\text{vowel}\}\left\{\begin{matrix}\text{liquid}\\\text{nasal}\\\text{glide}\end{matrix}\right\}\left\{\begin{matrix}\text{stop}\\\text{fricative}\end{matrix}\right\}$$

However, in English and some other languages, this hierarchy is sometimes violated in initial clusters beginning with [s] (e.g., sp-, st-, sk- in which the slightly more sonorous [s] precedes the less sonorous stops) and final clusters ending in [s] (e.g., -ps, -ts, -ks).

These clusters that violate the sonority hierarchy are therefore universally marked. As a result, one might expect them to be more difficult than less-marked clusters. However, the tables above illustrate that the English clusters that violate the sonority hierarchy ([s] + stop) typically are not acquired later than other [s] clusters by English-learning children. This has been confirmed for at least one child with a phonological disorder by Klopfenstein and Ball (2010). Thus, exposure to an ambient language that violates sonority appears to be enough to override universal human physiologically based trends in cluster production, at least in some languages.

Articulatory ease explains word position preferences as well as cluster preferences according to Kirk and Demuth (2005). They report that children acquire stop+/s/ and nasal+/z/ final clusters (as in "pots" and "pans") earlier than the parallel /s/+stop and /s/+nasal-initial clusters (as in "stop" and "snake") and also earlier than nasal+stop and /s/+stop final clusters (as in "bump" and "fast"). After testing several alternative hypotheses, they conclude that sonority, frequency, or morphology cannot account for these findings. They infer that ease of articulation is the determining factor, at least among their 12 participants. The aspects of ease of articulation that they propose as explanatory include the tendency for /s/ to be learned earlier and pronounced more accurately in word-final position, the difficulty of coordinating the raising/lowering of the velum that is required for producing a nasal+stop cluster, and a preference for clusters in which a change of place of articulation is not required (e.g., sn- preferred over sm-).

Thus, clusters present complex problems for young children and those with SSD; they are hard in many respects. Avoidance is one option that some youngsters choose—to simply refuse to attempt words with difficult target clusters. Several other options are also available.

Omission (often called "cluster reduction") occurs when one or more elements of the cluster are not produced at all (e.g., [pɑt] or [bɑt] for "spot"). Ingram (1976) indicates that children typically go through an initial stage in which neither member of the cluster is preserved, then another in which they preserve only one member of the cluster. Lleó and Prinz (1996) confirm the latter pattern for German-speaking and Spanish-speaking children as well. But which member of the cluster is preserved? Some studies have shown that consonant cluster preservation patterns are predicted by markedness. Bleile (1995) states that the earliest acquired consonant (which is typically the least marked one) will remain when others are omitted. Both Ingram (1989) and Chin and Dinnsen (1992) suggest that the marked member of a two-element cluster is more likely to be omitted than is the unmarked member. Thus, children tend to omit the first element, [s], in [s] + stop clusters (e.g., [tɑp] for "stop," [dɛk] for "desk"). In contrast, they omit the second element, the liquid, in word-initial stop + liquid clusters (e.g., [gɑk] for "clock"). Although some English-speaking children may delete the unmarked member of a cluster while preserving the marked member, this is rare and brief according to Ingram (1989).

Pater and Barlow (2003) report that some children may violate sonority principles in their cluster production patterns because of avoidance of certain consonant features (such as fricative or dorsal [i.e., velar]). In their study of two typically developing children and one with a speech sound disorder, they showed that sonority factors can be overridden by other considerations. For example, sonority would predict that a child who cannot produce clusters would delete the [l] from a kl- cluster in order to have a maximum sonority difference between the initial consonant and the vowel (i.e., [k] is more different in sonority from a vowel than [l] is). However, children who avoid velars would most likely delete the velar instead.

The language of exposure may make a difference in cluster production patterns as well. For example, Lleó and Prinz (1996) report different error patterns for different language groups. For target initial stop + sonorant consonant clusters, for instance, German-speaking children preserve the stop while Spanish-speaking children preserve the sonorant. The same holds true of syllable-initial obstruent + sonorant clusters in medial position. Lukaszewicz (2007) reports data from a Polish-speaking child whose reduction of onset clusters mostly respected sonority. In some respects, however, this child also demonstrated both a preference for respecting language-specific patterns over universal patterns and adherence to some idiosyncratic cluster production patterns. Thus, language-specific factors, universal factors such as sonority and markedness, and even child-specific preferences may all play a role in the child's development of clusters in various word positions.

In addition to omission of one (or more) consonant(s) from a cluster, young, delayed, or disordered children may also opt to coalesce the sequence of consonants, to separate them by inserting a schwa, or to move one of them in order to avoid producing the cluster. When coalescence occurs, the elements of the cluster are phonetically merged, and one phone that is a combination of features from the original phones is produced. For instance, the child might say [fɑt] for "spot." In this case, the [f] is a combination of the frication of the [s] plus the labiality of the [p]. Other children attempt to produce [s] + nasal clusters by combining the voicelessness of the [s] with the nasality of the nasal, yielding a voiceless nasal. Thus, a word such as "snake" is pronounced as [n̥eɪk].

Once a child has devised a coalescence pattern for some clusters, she may apply it to other clusters, whether it actually represents a coalescence of those other clusters or not. For example, [f] substitutes for a variety of clusters in many children's speech, especially children with SSD. The example in Table 8-3 from Grunwell (1982) of a 6-year-old named Martin is typical. Martin initially used [f] as a coalescence of /s/ plus /w/ for sw- clusters. The labiality of the /w/ combined with the frication of the /s/ to yield [f]. His production of /ɹ/ as [w] may have influenced him to extend this pattern to clusters with /ɹ/ such as stɹ- (treating /ɹ/ in the same way as /w/). However, eventually the pattern of coalescing clusters to [f] was also extended to other clusters with /s/, such as sl-. It was also extended to other clusters with /ɹ/, such as θɹ -, dɹ-, and tɹ-. As a result, [f] ended up with a huge functional load, substituting for the majority of target clusters, a difficult situation for listeners.

Another strategy for avoiding consonant clusters is the use of epenthesis. Epenthesis involves the insertion of a vowel between the consonants in the cluster (e.g., [bəlu] for "blue," [səpɑt] for "spot"). For some reason, this is more common in the speech of foreigners than it is in children's speech. However, overeager speech-language pathologists or parents, who encourage the child to pronounce each element of the cluster separately and then attempt to blend them together, can sometimes inadvertently encourage a child with SSD to use this pattern. Some children with severe SSD or with CAS may come up with this strategy on their own, especially if they are literate and therefore aware of both elements of the cluster. Other children speak so slowly that it sounds as though they are epenthesizing vowels between consonants or even extra consonants within clusters. Recall that producing extra material is not always more difficult; for example, many Americans pronounce the word "hamster" as [hæmpstɚ] because a nasal + fricative intersyllabic combination is challenging.

Sometimes, the order rather than the number of consonants is problematic for the child developing a system. In this case, the child may resort to changing the order. A stereotypical example of simply reversing the order of two consonants,

TABLE 8-3 Martin's Coalescence of Clusters

string	[fɪn, fɪm]
strawberries	[fɔbɛɹi]
swimming	[fɪmɪn]
thread	[fɛv]
tree	[fi]
sleeping	[fiʔm]
drinking	[fɪnʔɪn]

From Grunwell, P. (1982). *Clinical phonology.* Rockville, MD: Aspen.

which also occurs in some dialects of American English (e.g., African American English), is metathesis of -sk- to -ks- as in [ækst] for "asked" and [bæksɪt] for "basket."

Some children move one element of a cluster completely away from the other element, sometimes even crossing over a vowel. For instance, a child might say [kus] for "school" (Leonard & McGregor, 1991). This is migration—one element has moved to a different word position but without trading places with another segment. This demonstrates again the importance of syllable-level analysis. One cannot hope to describe such a pattern without reference to the syllable or word as a whole. Describing the pattern of saying [kus] for "school" as deletion of /s/ plus substitution of [s] for /l/ is an inappropriate explanation of what's actually going on.

In some cases, other factors can cause a child to produce consonant clusters unnecessarily. The same child described above (Leonard and McGregor, 1991), "W," for example, had a strong preference for fricatives to occur in final rather than initial position. As seen in Table 8-4, she moved them to coda position even when the result was a coda cluster such as –ps or even a non-English combination such as -nf.

It is important to note that between-word sequences of consonants may also be restricted in a child's phonological system, resulting in either a coda consonant or an onset consonant being omitted when the target contains both, as in "big dog" produced as [bɪ dɔg] or [bɪgɔg] by a child who usually produces both codas and onsets in single-word productions. Similarly, clusters may be reduced in either onset or coda position when two words are juxtaposed (e.g., "best friend" produced as [bɛs fɹɛn] or [bɛst fɛn]) even if such clusters would not be reduced by the child in single-word contexts (Stemberger, 1988; Howard, 2004, 2007; Klein & Liu-Shea, 2009).

In short, individual children's consonant cluster repertoires will be determined by many different phonotactic factors, such as word position and the number of consonants allowed in a row, and by phonetic factors such as sonority, the universal markedness of specific consonants or consonant features (typically reflecting ease of articulation), language-specific markedness (i.e., frequency and/or functional load), and even child-specific markedness (Chin & Dinnsen, 1992; McLeod, van Doorn, & Reed, 1997).

TABLE 8-4 W's Fricative Migration

fall	[ɑf]
fine	[ɑɪnf]
school	[kus]
soup	[ups]
zoo	[uz]
sheep	[ips]
shoe	[us]

From Leonard, L. B., & McGregor, K. K. (1991). Unusual phonological patterns and their underlying representations: A case study. *Journal of Child Language, 18*(2), 261–272.

Inclusion of Sequences of Vowels

As noted in Chapter 7, children—including those with SSD and especially those with CAS—have particular difficulty with diphthongs (Pollock & Keiser, 1990; Pollock & Hall, 1991). Of the 15 subjects in the Pollock and Keiser (1990) study, 14 made errors on diphthongs, and 19% of the total vowel errors that the children made were diphthong reductions. However, in 9% of cases, the children diphthongized simple vowels, and some diphthongs were substituted with other diphthongs (e.g., [ɔɪ] replaced with [oʊ]), so the picture is not as simple as one might hope.

Vowel sequences can also occur across word boundaries. Recall that some languages use deletion (e.g., English contractions such as "I'm") or epenthesis (e.g., [go w̲ɑn] for "go on") to avoid two vowels in a row. Stemberger (1988) gives one example of a child who omitted a final vowel before a word beginning with another vowel. In this case, his daughter, Gwendolyn, produced "How about him?" (/hɑu əˈbɑʊt hɪm/) as [hɑʊ bɑ tʰɪm]. (Note that the [t] of "about" was used as an onset to the word "him," which had lost its /h/, in this case.)

Variation within the Word: Reduplication and Harmony

Some children are not limited so much with respect to the structure of the syllable or the word per se but with respect to the contents of those structures. It may be too difficult for a learner to produce two different consonants within the same word, for example, or even two different syllables within the same word. Reduplication and harmony are frequent responses to such limitations on variety within the word.

Reduplication occurs when a whole syllable is repeated; harmony allows slightly more variety within the word, with either the consonants or the vowels being produced alike. They occur as original creations as well as in words children learn from baby talk ("mama," "boo-boo," "dydee" [ˈdɑɪdi] for "diaper," and the like). Some examples of one child's consonant harmony, vowel harmony, and reduplication provided by Menn[1] (1978) are shown in Tables 8-5 through 8-7.

TABLE 8-5 Child Consonant Harmony

doggie	[dʌdi]
diaper	[bɑpi]
thank you	[gɛgo], [dɛ:do:]
tractor	[gogi]

Based upon Menn, L. (1978). Phonological units in beginning speech. In A. Bell & J. B. Hooper (Eds.), *Syllables and segments* (pp. 157–171). Amsterdam, The Netherlands: North-Holland Publishing Co.

[1]Menn's transcriptions have been changed slightly to conform more closely to IPA.

TABLE 8-6 Child Vowel Harmony

baby	[bibi], [bɑbɑ], [bæbæɪ]
hammer	[hæʰmæ]
tractor	[ʔsætæ]

Based upon Menn, L. (1978). Phonological units in beginning speech. In A. Bell & J. B. Hooper (Eds.), *Syllables and segments* (pp. 157–171). Amsterdam, The Netherlands: North-Holland Publishing Co.

Note that, in this child's phonology, consonant harmony applies to all places of articulation. Describing his productions as segmental substitution patterns would require the claim that he both moves velar consonants forward (to both alveolar and labial placements) and moves alveolar consonants back (to a velar placement). This could seem like a confusing pattern, but in fact the child is following a very simple rule: "Don't ever change place of articulation within the same word." However, note that it is not possible to predict, based on these data alone, which consonant "wins" in his speech when there are two different places of articulation in the word.

Schwartz, Leonard, Wilcox, and Folger (1980) report that reduplication appears to have two motivations in the phonologies of typically developing children. Many of the reduplicating children in their study only produced reduplicated multisyllabic forms, indicating that reduplication may have been a means for them to increase the number of syllables in the word without having to increase its segmental difficulty. A few of their participants also appeared to be using reduplication as a strategy for avoiding the use of final consonants. Similarly, children with SSD may resort to reduplication (e.g., [popo] for "police") in order to produce disyllabic or multisyllabic words at a time when they cannot vary consonants within such words (Leonard, Miller, & Brown, 1980).

Both Vihman (1978) and Lleó (1990) document that older children may continue to use reduplication or harmony as an entry into producing longer words without having to produce more complex series of segments. For example, Lleó's trilingual (German–Catalan–Spanish) participant Laura produced *bicicleta* "bicycle" as [blɛˈblɛka] and [blɛˈblɛtsa], reduplicating the first syllable, before learning to pronounce it correctly. Again, similar strategies may be found in the phonologies of children with SSD (Leonard et al., 1980). Of the 25 instances of consonant harmony that their eight participants with SSD produced, 19 appeared to result from avoidance of a consonant or cluster that was not yet in the child's repertoire. These included both monosyllabic words (e.g., [kʌk] for "truck") and longer ones (e.g., [ˈgɑgəˌgɔ] for "Santa Claus").

TABLE 8-7 Child Reduplication

down	[doʊdoʊ]
around	[wæwæ]
handle	[hɑhɑ]

Based upon Menn, L. (1978). Phonological units in beginning speech. In A. Bell & J. B. Hooper (Eds.), *Syllables and segments* (pp. 157–171). Amsterdam, The Netherlands: North-Holland Publishing Co.

Stoel-Gammon (1996) illustrates that word position has an impact on the frequency and development of harmony. For example, velars are more strongly associated with final position, and therefore, velar harmony is more likely to occur if the triggering velar is in this word position (e.g., velar harmony is more likely in "bag" than in "gab"). She says that velars in initial position are more likely to be substituted with an alveolar (fronted; see Chapter 9) than to cause harmony. Her findings emphasize again the importance of considering the whole word when analyzing harmony patterns.

Sometimes, it is not only the whole word but the whole phrase that matters in triggering harmony. Klein and Liu-Shea (2009) report that, very rarely, consonant harmony occurs between words as in "take maybe one" pronounced as [**tep** mebi wʌn] by a child who could produce "take" correctly in a single-word utterance. Velleman (2003a) gives a similar example of a 2.5-year-old child with CAS who was able to say the word "dog" beginning with [d] when it was alone, but her production of the phrase "dog boo-boo" was [bu bubu]. Similarly, the word "not" accommodated to its context: "Not in" was [ĩ ɪn] while "not out" was [aʊ̃ aʊ].

Consonant–Vowel Assimilation

As noted in Chapter 6, Davis, MacNeilage, and colleagues (e.g., Davis & MacNeilage, 1990; MacNeilage & Davis, 2000; Kern & Davis, 2009) have demonstrated a strong consonant–vowel interdependency for many children from a variety of languages during the babbling and early word periods. These children showed a strong tendency to produce high front vowels such as [i, ɪ] (both correctly and in error) in the context of coronal (alveo-palatal) consonants such as [t, d, n], high back vowels such as [u, ʊ] with velar consonants such as [k, g], and mid and low vowels ([ʌ, ə, ɑ]) with labial consonants such as [p, b, m]. These tendencies have a strong articulatory basis. High front vowels and coronal consonants both involve raising the tongue tip near/to the alveo-palatal region. High back vowels and velar consonants are formed by bunching the posterior body of the tongue upward toward the velum. Neutral and low vowels as well as labial consonants are dependent upon mandibular positioning only (i.e., the tongue remains in a neutral position).

Vihman (1992) tested this hypothesis using babbled syllables (and some very early words) from children exposed to American English, French, Swedish, and Japanese. None of the associations found by Davis and MacNeilage (1990) was universal in these children. However, the majority showed a positive association between labials and central vowels. About half showed a positive association between alveolars and front vowels, and two-thirds of the children who used both velars and back vowels showed a positive association between them. For each comparison, some children showed a negative association (e.g., a tendency to use labials with other vowels). Vihman emphasizes "the strong role played by the individual child" (p. 405) at this transition point between babble and words and suggests that stronger consonant–vowel associations might be found in earlier babble. Similarly, Lleó (1996) used data from Spanish-speaking children to illustrate that some children demonstrate frequent consonant–vowel interactions in early words while others exhibit interactions among consonants only or vowels only (i.e., consonant or vowel harmony). Thus, individual children may not demonstrate these general patterns.

This connection between vowels and consonants in some children is in keeping with Stoel-Gammon's earlier (Stoel-Gammon, 1983) report that coronal consonants tend to be produced (both correctly and in error) with high front vowels. For instance, one child she studied, Daniel, produced "bubble," "bottle," "ball," and "balloon" with initial [b] but "bye-bye" as [dɑɪdɑɪ] and "baby" as [didi]. "Pee-pee," "Big Bird," and "beep-beep" were also produced with an initial [d] (as were words that begin with [d] in the adult form). Thus, the child used [d] whenever the vowel was a high front one, even if the target consonant was /b/.

Several interesting examples of such interactions from Dutch children are given by Levelt (1992). One child (Elke), for instance, attempted to produce the Dutch word "schoen," which means "shoe" and is pronounced by adults as [sχun]. Elke's pronunciation was [pum]. Why did she produce both the initial and final consonants as labial? None of the target consonants in this word are labial; where did this place of articulation come from? Levelt claims that it must have been spread from the vowel, which is [round] (or [labial]).

This type of pattern has also been documented occasionally in children with disorders. It was observed by this author in a nearly 4-year-old child with CAS who pronounced "baby" as either [didi] or [bɑbɑ]. She could not produce either [bi] or [dɑ] in any context (Velleman, 1994). Williams and Dinnsen (1987) have also documented such a case in a child with a phonological disorder.

Smith (1973) illustrated a case of consonant–vowel assimilation later in phonological development. The child that he studied, Amahl, demonstrated vowelization of final /l/, a common pattern among English-speaking children. Often, adult final /l/ is produced as [ʊ] or [u] in children's speech. In Amahl's case, alveolars became velar (i.e., back) before the resulting [u]s, as shown in Table 8-8. Without considering the effect of the vowels, there would be no way to explain why this backing of alveolars only happened before [u]. In other word-medial contexts, alveolars remained alveolar. Clearly, these alveolar consonants were affected by the place of articulation of the following vowels. They became velar before the back vowel [u].[2] Stoel-Gammon (1996) provides data from other children also demonstrating that vowel place of articulation may have an impact on velar harmony.

TABLE 8-8 **Amahl's Consonant-Vowel Assimilation**

pedal	[bɛgu]
lazy	[de:di:]
beetle	[bi:gu]
horses	[ɔ:tid]
bottle	[bɔgu]
sometimes	[fʌmtɑɪmd]

From Smith, N. V. (1973). *The Acquisition of phonology: A case study.* Cambridge, UK: Cambridge University Press.

Distribution Requirements

Many authors have explored children's preferences for certain features in certain positions. Some, such as Edwards (1996), Macken (1996), and Velleman (1996), have stressed the importance of edges of words in this regard. That is, these preferences tend to occur in either initial or final position not (syllable-initial intervocalic) medial position. Default consonants, in contrast, tend to occur in medial position (Priestly, 1977; Stemberger, 1993; Velleman, 1996). Recall that these are consonants for which the child (or the language) shows a preference, frequently using them to substitute for other consonants. Often, these are unmarked sounds or those that are easier for the individual toddler. Some examples are given in Table 8-9.

Some very young or very disordered children may have very simple distribution restrictions, such as allowing voiced consonants only in initial position and voiceless consonants only in final position. This is a kind of assimilation; initial consonants are voiced before vowels (which are voiced), and final consonants are voiceless before the end of the word (at which point voicing stops because the child ceases to talk). Grunwell (1982) provides an example, excerpted here as Table 8-10.

Another child, nicknamed Lasan, was unable to produce an adult-like voiceless/voiced contrast. In initial position, he produced all stops and fricatives as voiced. However, he used a very unusual strategy for preserving this contrast in final position; he aspirated final voiceless consonants (e.g., [vitʰ]

TABLE 8-9 **Medial Consonant Defaults**

Christopher (English; Priestly, 1977)	
dragon	[dajak, dajan]
coaster	[kajoʊs]
Laurent (French; Vihman, 1993)	
chapeau	[bobo, bolo]
la brosse	[pəla]

[2] There are further complications in Amahl's case that will not be considered here.

TABLE 8-10 Child Voicing Constraints

pig	[bɪt]
big	[bɪt]
fork	[bɔt]
Bob	[bɑp]
soup	[dup]
talk	[dɔt]
dog	[dɑt]
cot	[dɑt]
cup	[dəp]
shed	[dɛt]

From Grunwell, P. (1982). *Clinical phonology*. Rockville, MD: Aspen.

for "feet") and added a nasal after final voiced ones (e.g., [vidn̩] for "feed") (Fey & Gandour, 1982). In this way, he was able to produce the correct voicing even though it was at the cost of adding a syllable consonant in final position.

Another common pattern is for stops to occur in initial position, while fricatives occur in final position (Farwell, 1977; Fikkert, 1994; Dinnsen, 1996; Edwards, 1996). Gildersleeve-Neumann, Davis, and MacNeilage (2000) even reported this tendency in babble. Velars also may occur in final but not initial position in some children's phonological systems (Ingram, 1974). This is related to another frequent requirement that the consonants in the word progress from front to back ("fronting"), so that the more front consonants occur in initial position and the more back consonants occur at the end. In some cases, the child will rearrange the sounds in the word via migration or metathesis in order to achieve the desired pattern of consonants (e.g., "animal" produced as [mænu], "cream" as [miŋ], *café* "coffee" as [pɛtɛk], and *cuiller* "spoon" as [bədək] [Ingram, 1974]). Trying to explain these cases using a SODA analysis would be useless.

Some children have less common distribution requirements, such as Berman's (1977) Shelli, who rearranged words to fit a velar-first pattern (e.g., [gɑbi] for "buggy," [kibi] for "piggie," and [god] for "dog"). These "word recipes" have been studied more systematically by a few investigators, including Macken (1996) and Velleman (1996). Although they are by no means universal (Stoel-Gammon, 1984), restrictions of these types are common in the phonological systems of both typical youngsters and of children with delayed or disordered phonologies.

ASSESSMENT

Essentially, no standardized tests have been designed to assess a child's phonotactic development. Many do include final consonants, clusters, multisyllabic words and the like, but these variables of syllable and word length and complexity are not systematically controlled. The Kaufman Speech Praxis Test for Children (Kaufman, 1995) does consist of imitations of words that vary with respect to their complexity (CV, CVC, CCVC, etc.); however, the scoring is designed to determine the severity of the child's speech problem, not specifically to identify the child's phonotactic maturity. Thus, the best option for the SLP is to elicit a speech sample and then analyze the child's production.

Recall the measures described in Chapter 6 that may help give somewhat of an overview of the child's phonotactic level. In principle, mean babble level (Stoel-Gammon 1989; Smith, Brown-Sweeney, and Stoel-Gammon, 1989) could be used to measure the variety (i.e., lack of reduplication or harmony) in words as well as in babble. Jakielski's (2000) Index of Phonetic Complexity and Stoel-Gammon's Word Complexity Measure (Stoel-Gammon, 2010) both give points for structural complexity (e.g., the presence of clusters) as well as for consonantal maturity (e.g., the use of fricatives as well as stops). Thus, they are hybrid measures of both phonetics and phonotactics that give summary scores of the maturity of either prelinguistic or meaningful speech production. However, much more detail than these measures provide would be needed to actually develop an intervention program.

As we have seen, the aspects of phonotactic patterns that must be considered when assessing a child's phonology for treatment planning include the following:

1. Syllable and word shapes produced by the child, including restrictions on the number of syllables allowed per word, open versus closed syllables, and clusters in various word positions
2. Word-level patterns, such as harmony, assimilation, and reduplication patterns and epenthesis
3. Distribution requirements, including word recipes as a result of which words may be adapted using word-level patterns; recall from Chapter 6 and the introduction to this chapter that these may result in apparent regressions
4. Phrase-level effects—occurrences of any of the above in phrases

These patterns are all of primary importance when assessing a child's phonology, especially if the child is young or her phonology is very delayed. It is vital to consider them together as well as separately. A child who has restrictions only on clusters is much more phonotactically mature than one who also is restricted to one syllable per word. A child without cluster constraints but whose distribution requirements do not allow initial fricatives will not acquire #s-clusters (such as sp-, sn-, sl-, etc.) until she overcomes this distribution requirement. (See Chin & Dinnsen, 1992 and McLeod, van Doorn, & Reed, 1997 for further discussion of this issue.) The reader may well feel overwhelmed by this list; nightmare visions of extremely detailed, time-consuming

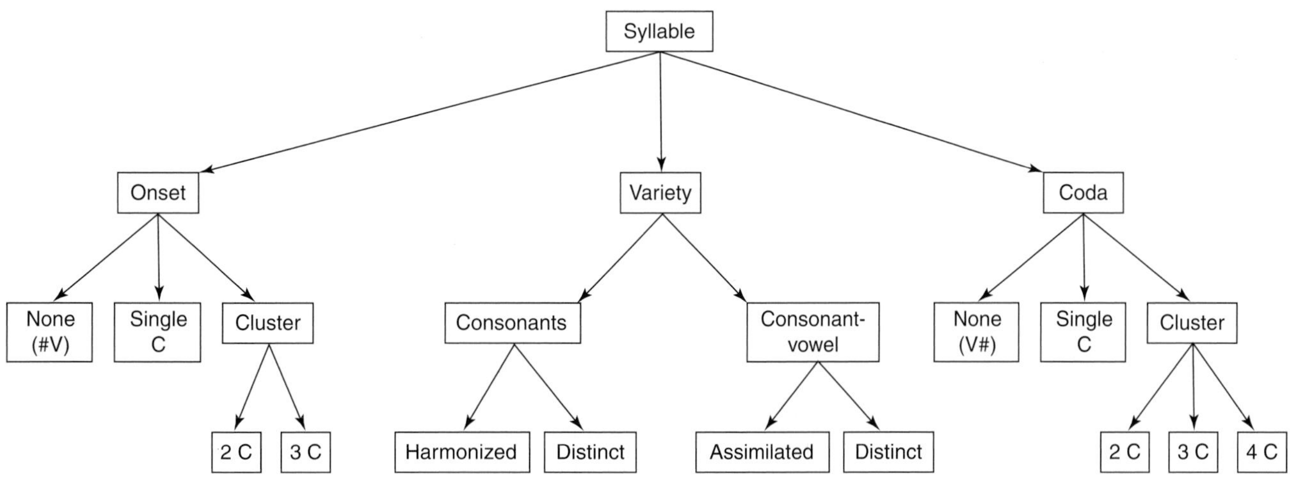

FIGURE 8-1. Syllable-level contrast.

phonological analyses may be appearing. But all of these patterns can be reduced to a single question: Does the child have an appropriate number of phonotactic options given her current communication needs? In other words, does the child produce enough contrastive word shapes?

Phonotactic contrast can be achieved via the following, which are also depicted in Figures 8-1 and 8-2:

Syllable-Level Contrast

- Initial consonant versus initial vowel (i.e., no onset) (e.g., "cup" versus "up")
- Final consonant versus final vowel (i.e., no coda) (closed versus open syllable e.g., "goat" versus "go")
- Clusters versus singleton consonants (e.g., "square" [skwɛɚ] versus "care" [kɛɚ]; "once" [wʌnts] versus "one" [wʌn])
- Syllable variety (harmony and assimilation):
  - Different consonants within the same syllable (e.g., "pot" versus "pop")
  - Consonant–vowel combinations (e.g., baa," "bee," "boo," "bow," "bye," etc.)

Word-Level Contrast

- Word lengths (different numbers of syllables, e.g., "pea" versus "peepee")
- Word variety (e.g., reduplication and harmony)
  - Different consonants within the same word across syllables (e.g., "lady" versus "baby")
  - Different vowels within the same word across syllables (e.g., "lookie" versus "leaky")
  - Different syllables within the same word (e.g., "taboo" versus "boo-boo")
- Order variety (distributional flexibility, e.g., "gum" versus "mug;" "soup" versus "oops")

If they can be found in the child's repertoire, phonotactic minimal pairs such as those listed above can help to identify the structure-based contrasts that the child appears to be making. The more varied the syllable and word shapes the child can control productively, the more contrast will be available to him.

If the phonotactic patterns observed are too restricted and are resulting in many homonyms or are forcing the child to supplement words with gestures, facial expressions, and

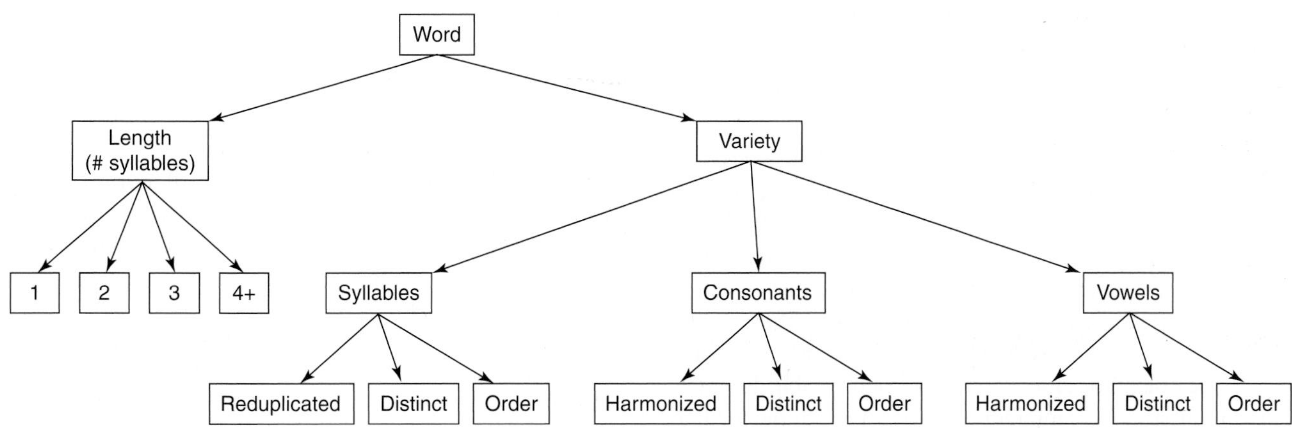

FIGURE 8-2. Word-level contrast.

sound effects, then the child's phonology is non-functional. In that case, the clinician's job is to expand the child's phonotactic possibilities so that more differentiation between words will be possible. If speech-language pathologists understand what phonotactic patterns are and how they can work to restrict or expand the child's phonological possibilities, then they have the information that is needed to facilitate that child's phonological development. In the next section, specific procedures for assessing a child's phonotactic system will be presented.

Assessment Tools

There are two possible levels of analysis for phonotactic assessment: basic word and syllable shapes and syllable/word-level effects (i.e., the presence versus absence of variety within the syllable or word). Often, the former level is not addressed at all by clinicians or by popular assessment tools; whether a final consonant is omitted or substituted, it is simply marked as an error. Many of the assessment tools available that focus on phonological patterns (e.g., processes; see Chapter 9) include syllable/word-level effects within their analyses of phonological patterns. Unfortunately, they often fail to differentiate phonotactically motivated errors (such as an alveolar consonant harmonizing with a velar as in [gɔgi] for "doggie") from phonetically motivated patterns (such as producing all alveolars as velars like [gægi] for "daddy," for instance). These types of tests are typically well-normed, so they can be used to identify children as having a speech sound delay/disorder in comparison to their typically developing peers. But the information that they yield is often insufficient to identify a child's phonological—phonetic, phonemic, *and* phonotactic—strengths and weaknesses.

If quantitative data (standard scores, percentiles, etc.) and/or age norms are not needed, many phonotactic factors can be assessed fairly simply using a speech sample obtained from spontaneous speech, from the administration of a standard articulation or process test, or (preferably) both. Then, worksheets can be used to qualitatively determine the phonotactic patterns used by the child. Any immature or deviant patterns identified can be even more thoroughly quantified later to set baselines in therapy.

Word and Syllable Shapes

Before the child's word and syllable shapes can be analyzed, the child's words (or word-sized utterances, if these do not have meaning) need to be divided into syllables. In doing so, the "maximize onset" rule is applied in most cases. That is, divide the word into syllables in such a way that as many syllables as possible have an onset consonant. Thus, "pepper" [ˈpɛpɚ] would be divided into [pɛ] + [pɚ], not [pɛp] + [ɚ], because in the latter case, the second syllable does not have an initial consonant. Only in cases in which the medial consonant cannot be an onset consonant (e.g., for "singing," [sɪ] + [ŋɪŋ] is not an appropriate syllable division) should this principle be violated. Another important guideline is that, for this form, glottals are not considered true consonants. Therefore, [ʔ] and [h] are ignored. Syllables such as [ʔʌʔ] and [hæ] are considered to be "vowel alone," [hʊp] to be "VC," and so on.

The syllable and word shapes produced by the child, including restrictions on the number of syllables allowed per word, open versus closed syllables, and clusters in various word positions, are simple to assess informally using a list of potential syllable and word shapes and cluster types, such as that provided in Form 8-1: Word and Syllable Shapes. This form, or a similar list that can be self-generated, can be used in three possible ways:

- Quantitatively, indicating percent occurrences for each type
- With approximate frequencies indicated, using terms such as "predominant," "frequent," "occasional," "rare," and "absent" (see further discussion)
- By simply checking off each type that does occur

The simplest option for using this form is to merely check off any pattern that is ever observed. A slightly more time-consuming but far more revealing check-off rule is to check off all forms or types that occur at least three times (or if the speech sample is small, twice) in the child's sample. This reduces the listener error to some extent. Transcribers do tend to "fill in the blanks" sometimes, mentally assuming that missing elements were actually there in the process of interpreting disordered speech. But if the speech-language pathologist transcribes the same element or pattern three times within one speech sample, chances are fairly good that it really did occur.

If the speech-language pathologist has the time to approximate the frequencies of occurrence of each type of syllable or word shape, then the adjectives listed can be circled for this purpose. This method is more precise than the check-off approach, yet less time-consuming than counting and calculating frequencies. The approximate frequencies that correspond to each adjective choice are the following[3]:

- Predominant: 61% or more
- Frequent: 41% to 60%
- Occasional: 16% to 40%
- Rare: 1% to 15%
- Absent: 0% to 0.9%

This approach reduces the clinician's burden from counting every instance of a pattern and figuring its exact percentage of occurrence to rating the approximate frequencies on a five-point scale. However, some people initially feel insecure

[3]The individual clinician is, of course, free to use different frequencies if these appear inappropriate. However, consistency (always using the same frequencies within your own clinical practice) is vital.

about making such estimates. Using the exact counting method a few times typically increases confidence.

The most reliable—and also the most time-consuming—approach to this worksheet is to count each instance of each pattern and then divide the total by the total number of potential occurrences of that pattern. It is important that percentages be based upon the total number of instances of that type of element. For example, the percentage of CV syllables a child produces should be computed by dividing the number of CV syllables produced by the total number of syllables (not words) produced. Similarly, the number of words with CC (consonant cluster) onsets is divided by the total number of potential word onsets (i.e., the total number of words) to identify the percentage of occurrence of initial consonant clusters.

Note that for these analyses, the (presumed) target forms of the words are not considered. Only the child's actual productions are analyzed. In other words, this is an independent phonotactic analysis. Therefore, for example, "total number of syllables" refers to the total number of syllables produced by the child, regardless of the total number that would have been produced by an adult saying the same words (if there are identifiable word targets). The clinician may wish to do a phonotactic relational analysis—comparing the child's actual productions to his or her targets—at some later point. But for the purpose of determining whether or not the child's phonotactic system is functional, analyzing what the child is actually producing is often far more useful.

Some of the relevant formulas can be written as below:

$$\frac{\text{No. of C alone syllables}}{\text{Total no. of syllables}} \times 100 = \%\ \text{C alone syllables}$$

$$\frac{\text{No. of \#CC}}{\text{No. of words}} \times 100 = \%\ \text{initial clusters}$$

$$\frac{\text{No. of monosyllabic words}}{\text{Total no. of words}} \times 100 = \%\ \text{of monosyllabic words}$$

To take a simple example, if a child produced 100 syllables and 50 of them were of the form CV, then her percentage occurrence of CV syllables would be 50%—a frequent level of occurrence.

One question that often arises is that of counting or not counting multiple identical productions of the same word. This decision is left to the individual speech-language pathologist. There are definite advantages to counting every occurrence (token) of each word, in that this strategy increases the amount of data that can be analyzed. Furthermore, if the child often produces multiple identical productions of the same word, this is important to note. However, if one word is produced several times in a very unusual manner (i.e., in a way that is not otherwise typical of that child), then including every production will bias the analysis in an inappropriate direction. In any case, it is important to be consistent. If each production is counted for one analysis, the same approach normally should be used for all analyses of that child's sample.

Consider some sample word and syllable shape data and how it would be entered on the form at each level. The data in Table 8-11, from Vihman and Velleman's (1989) Molly at age 13 months, can be used for this purpose, though it would be better to have a larger sample than only these 32 productions. Example 8-1 illustrates the use of Form 8-1 to identify Molly's syllable types, clusters, and word shapes. Recalling that [h] and [ʔ] are not considered to be true consonants on this form, this analysis yields the following:

- Syllable types: Molly produces quite a few "vowel alone" syllables (20%), though most of them actually do include [h] and/or [ʔ], such as [hæʔ]. Her other productions are composed mostly (55%) of open CV syllables (e.g., the syllables in words like [bɑ], [pɑnə], [gɔgʌ]). However, CVCs (such as [tʌŋ] and the second syllable of [gʊgʊk]) are occasional. VCs (such as [æt^{h}]) are relatively rare (8%). Altogether, 26% of her syllables end in consonants. This would be fairly surprising if her native language were Japanese or even French or Spanish; it is even somewhat on the high side for English.
- Clusters: The only cluster that we can identify is the initial tj- in one production ([tjæŋ], which is actually not a possible word of English). In other words, she has one two-element cluster in initial position.
- Word shapes: Molly produces both one- and two-syllable words quite frequently (44% and 53% of the time, respectively) with only one three-syllable production occurring ([kʊgʊgɔ]).

Making all three levels of analysis available on a single form allows the clinician to become comfortable with the form and the concepts it represents without having to get bogged down in counting and calculating percentages.

TABLE 8-11 Data from Molly at 13 Months

bɑ	box
pɑp^{h}, pɑpʌp, pəp	burp
pɑnə	button
tʌŋ, dæn, dɑŋ::, ʔedɑɪn, dɑʊnə, dænə, tjæŋ	down
gʊgʊk, gʊgɣ, gɔgʌ, gɔgɔ, gʊgʌ, kʊgʊgʌ, kʊkʌ	good girl
hæʔ, hæ^{h}	hat
æt^{h}, hæt, hæt^{h}, hætə̥, hæ	hot
hɑnʌ, hʌni, ænɪ, ænə	round
æp, ɔpə̥	up

NOTES: Transcriptions somewhat simplified.
"::" indicates lengthening (e.g., [ŋ::] is a long drawn-out velar nasal);
[̥] indicates voicelessness (e.g., [ə̥] is a voiceless schwa);
[ɣ] is a uvular trill such as babies make when they coo.
From Vihman, M. M., & Velleman, S. L. (1989). Phonological reorganization: A case study. *Language and Speech*, *32*, 149–170.

Form 8-1

Name:	Age:
Date:	Examiner:
Source of sample:	Size of sample:
Note: C = consonant	predominant: 60-100%
V = vowel	frequent: 40-60%
# = word boundary	occasional: 15-40%

PHONOTACTIC REPERTOIRE
Word and Syllable Shapes

SYLLABLE TYPES

	% or ✓	Frequency Estimate[@]: Circle appropriate word.				
INCOMPLETE:						
C alone	____	predominant	frequent	occasional	rare	absent
V, Vʔ, ʔV	____	predominant	frequent	occasional	rare	absent
OPEN:						
CV	____	predominant	frequent	occasional	rare	absent
CLOSED:						
VC, ʔVC	____	predominant	frequent	occasional	rare	absent
CVC*	____	predominant	frequent	occasional	rare	absent

[@]Out of all syllables.
**Includes CCVC, CVCC, etc.*

CLUSTERS

	% or ✓	Frequency Estimate[+]: Circle appropriate word.				
INITIAL:						
#CC-	____	predominant	frequent	occasional	rare	absent
#CCC-	____	predominant	frequent	occasional	rare	absent
FINAL:						
-CC#	____	predominant	frequent	occasional	rare	absent
-CCC#	____	predominant	frequent	occasional	rare	absent
MEDIAL:						
-CC-	____	predominant	frequent	occasional	rare	absent
-CCC-	____	predominant	frequent	occasional	rare	absent

WORD SHAPES

	% or ✓	Frequency Estimate[+]: Circle appropriate word.				
# OF SYLLABLES:						
1	____	predominant	frequent	occasional	rare	absent
2	____	predominant	frequent	occasional	rare	absent
3	____	predominant	frequent	occasional	rare	absent
4+	____	predominant	frequent	occasional	rare	absent

+ Divided by total # of words

MAXIMUM # OF SYLLABLES PRODUCED IN ANY WORD: ____

Notes:

Example 8-1

Name: *Molly* Age: *13 months*
Date: *2/18/93* Examiner: *SLV*
Source of sample: *play* Size of sample: *32 word tokens*

Note: C = consonant predominant: 60-100%
V = vowel frequent: 40-60%
# = word boundary occasional: 15-40%

PHONOTACTIC REPERTOIRE
Word and Syllable Shapes

SYLLABLE TYPES *51 syllables*

	% or ✓	Frequency Estimate@: Circle appropriate word.				
INCOMPLETE:						
C alone	*0%*	predominant	frequent	occasional	rare	**absent**
V, V?, ?V	*20%*	predominant	frequent	**occasional**	rare	absent
OPEN:						
CV	*55%*	predominant	**frequent**	occasional	rare	absent
CLOSED:						
VC, ?VC	*8%*	predominant	frequent	occasional	**rare**	absent
CVC*	*18%*	predominant	frequent	**occasional**	rare	absent

@Out of all syllables.
**Includes CCVC, CVCC, etc.*

CLUSTERS

	% or ✓	Frequency Estimate+: Circle appropriate word.				
INITIAL:						
#CC-	*3%*	predominant	frequent	occasional	**rare**	absent
#CCC-	*0%*	predominant	frequent	occasional	rare	**absent**
FINAL:						
-CC#	*0%*	predominant	frequent	occasional	rare	**absent**
-CCC#	*0%*	predominant	frequent	occasional	rare	**absent**
MEDIAL:						
-CC-	*0%*	predominant	frequent	occasional	rare	**absent**
-CCC-	*0%*	predominant	frequent	occasional	rare	**absent**

WORD SHAPES

	% or ✓	Frequency Estimate+: Circle appropriate word.				
# OF SYLLABLES:						
1	*44%*	predominant	**frequent**	occasional	rare	absent
2	*53%*	predominant	**frequent**	occasional	rare	absent
3	*3%*	predominant	frequent	occasional	**rare**	absent
4+	*0%*	predominant	frequent	occasional	rare	**absent**

+ Out of all words

MAXIMUM # OF SYLLABLES PRODUCED IN ANY WORD: _*3*_

Notes: *Only #CC was tj- (not American English cluster). Not consistent in # of syllables in attempts at same word (e.g., "good girl" = 2 or 3 syllables; "down" = 1 or 2 syllables). Also not consistent in closing syllables (e.g., "hot" = [hæ] and [hæt]).*

As time permits, more specific data can be gathered on the same form as baselines for children who are to be seen in therapy. With practice, the approximate frequency ratings will become almost as easy and quick to score as simply checking off those patterns that occur. Eventually, the clinician will find that the form has become a mental checklist, and these data can be gathered "online" while conversing with the child.

A holistic type of relational analysis, comparing the child's overall phonotactic repertoire to that of the adult language, is not difficult to do in one's head after a worksheet such as Form 8-1 has been completed. English has multisyllabic words; consonant clusters in initial, medial, and final positions; and both open and closed syllables. Any English-learning child who lacks these has nonadult phonology (which may or may not be age appropriate). However, a clinician may wish to make specific comparisons to establish how the child matches her productions to the adult's (presumed target) word shapes. For instance, a child may produce a closed syllable (of any type) only when the adult syllable ends with a voiceless stop. This is an indication that the child is aware of and able to produce syllable closure, at least in some instances. It identifies an area of phonological knowledge and skill that can be built upon in therapy. These issues of relational analysis and correspondences between child and adult forms will be dealt with in much more detail in Chapter 9.

Consonant Clusters

Form 8-1, discussed previously, identifies whether or not the child produces two-element and/or three-element clusters in initial, medial, or final position. However, it does not provide for detailing which clusters are produced. More specific information about a child's consonant clusters can be tallied using Forms 8-2 and 8-3. Clusters that are observed to occur should be indicated with a checkmark, a number (representing number of occurrences), or a percentage (percent occurrences out of all words produced). Lines representing cluster combinations that do not occur are left blank. Obviously in analyzing the phonology of a child who produces no clusters of any kind or even very few clusters, the clinician will not bother with Forms 8-2 and 8-3. Therefore, it would be a waste of time to use these forms with either of the children discussed above. Neither has more than a few clusters.

Bryan is 3;11 with language and phonological delay and has several clusters as shown in Table 8-12. His clusters are boldfaced to make them easier to identify. The types of clusters that he finds most easy to deal with are clear when his APP-R and CELF-P data are transferred to Forms 8-2 and 8-3, as shown in Examples 8-2 and 8-3.

Of Bryan's 19 initial consonant cluster tokens (nine types), 13 (68%) are fricative + glide including two cluster types that do not typically occur in adult English (fw- and ʃw-). Three others are fricative + stop and two are fricative + nasal. Clearly, Bryan prefers fricative-initial clusters. He is just beginning to branch from fricative + glide to stop + glide (one instance of kj-).

Of Bryan's 16 final clusters, almost a third are -nt, in keeping with Kirk and Demuth's (2003) report that homorganic final clusters emerge first. Overall, 12 final cluster tokens (75%) are nasal initial. Over half of these (7/12, or 58%) are nasal + stop, and the others are nasal + fricative/affricate. There are three stop + fricative clusters (including one instance of -bs, which doesn't normally occur in English), and one fricative plus stop cluster (-sk).

Good options for a clinician who has decided to expand Bryan's repertoire of consonant clusters include focusing

TABLE 8-12 APP-R and CELF-P Data from Bryan, 3;11

ɛɚpeɪnt	(air)plane
bots	boats
fwɪdz	bridge
bʌtɪnz	buttons
feɪənz	crayons
ɑɪsmɪnt	elephant
fwʌv	glove
fint	green
ɑɪs kjubs	ice cubes
sʌmt	jumped
wʌntʃ	lunch
mæsk	mask
owɪndʒ	orange
feɪfaʊnd	playground
su swɑɪbə	screwdriver
sju	shoe
swɑɪd	slide
fwɪŋki	slinky
smok	smoke
sneɪk, seɪnt	snake
spɑɪdə	spider
spunt	spoon
swɛɚ	square
stɑɪ	star
swɪŋ	string
swɛdɚ	sweater
swɪŋ	swing
swi	three
tɑɪmz	times
ʃwʌk	truck
wɑpɪnt	wrapping
swɪpɚ	zipper

Form 8-2

Name:	Age:
Date:	Examiner:
Source of sample:	Size of sample:

INITIAL CONSONANT CLUSTERS

Indicate with ✓, specific # or specific % those clusters that occur in the child's speech. (Note: If the child produces an "illegal" cluster that does not normally occur in English, list it under "other".)

Two-Element Clusters

Obstruent + liquid

pɹ-___	pl-___	pj-___		bɹ-___	bl-___	bj-___	
tɹ-___		tj-___	tw-___	dɹ-___		dj-___	dw-___
kɹ-___	kl-___	kj-___	kw-___	gɹ-___	gl-___	gj-___	gw-___
						mj-___	
						nj-___	
fɹ-___	fl-___	fj-___					
θɹ-___		θj-___	θw-___				
	sl-___	sj-___	sw-___				
ʃɹ-___							
		hj-___					
		vj-___					
		lj-___					

[s] + obstruent

sp-___ st-___ sk-___ sm-___ sn-___

NOTE: The glide [j] occurs far more often in initial clusters in British than in American English.

OTHER:

Three-Element Clusters

spɹ-___	spl-___	spj-__	
stɹ-___		stj-___	
skɹ-___	skl-___	skj-___	skw-___

OTHER:

Form 8-3

Name: Age:
Date: Examiner:
Source of sample: Size of sample:

FINAL CONSONANT CLUSTERS

Indicate with ✓, specific # or specific % those clusters that occur in the child's speech. (Note: If the child produces an "illegal" cluster that does not normally occur in English, list it under "other".)

Two-Element Clusters

NASALS

-mp___ -mt___ -md___ -mf___ -mθ___ -mz___

-nt___ -nd___ -nθ___ -ns___ -ntʃ___ -ndʒ___ -nz___

-ŋk___ -ŋd___ -ŋz___

STOPS

-pt___ -bd___ -pθ___ -ps___ -bz___

-tθ___ -ts___ -dz___

-kt___ -gd___ -ks___ -gz___

FRICATIVES

-ft___ -vd___ -fθ___ -fs___ -vz___

-θt___ -ðd___ -θs___ -ðz___

-sp___ -st___ -sk___ -zd___ -zm___

-ʃt___ -ʒd___

-tʃt___ -dʒd___

LIQUIDS

-lp___ -lt___ -lk___ -ld___ -lm___ -ln___

-lv___ -lf___ -lθ___ -ls___ -ltʃ___ -ldʒ___ -lz___

OTHER:

Three-Element Clusters

-mps___

OTHER:

-nts___ -nst___

-ŋst___ -ŋks___

-lps___ -lts___ -lst___ -lks___

on the emerging initial types (stop + glide), as well as on increasing his frequency of use of /s/ + nasal clusters. In final position, the frequency of nasal + obstruent (stop or fricative) and final stop + [s/z] combinations can be increased. This would be a good time to address regular plurals (and/or possessive and/or third person singular) with Bryan; gains can be made in both phonology and morphology through work on nasal and stop clusters with final [s/z] morphologic markers (targeting words like "pins" [pɪnz] and "pots" [pɑts]). Other nasal + obstruent (e.g., -mp or -mz) clusters would also be promising. In addition, the emergence of final fricative + stop clusters (thus far, in the form of one instance of -sk) can be encouraged. Although they will of course eventually have to be addressed, initial and final clusters with liquids would be a major challenge at this point as Bryan does not produce any such clusters; in fact, target liquids are consistently either omitted or substituted with [w] even in singleton contexts.

Syllable- or Word-Level Patterns

Syllable- or word-level patterns that reduce variety within the word such as harmony and reduplication can also be screened using a simple worksheet that facilitates these analyses, such as Form 8-4. Again, the simplest way to use this form is to merely check off those types of reduplication or harmony that do occur (three times or more) in the child's speech. Or the therapist can indicate an approximate frequency of occurrence of each type ("predominant," "frequent," "occasional," "rare," or "absent"). For more precision, the occurrence of reduplication (or harmony) can be quantified exactly by counting the total number of multisyllabic words and dividing this into the number of reduplicated (or harmonized) words and then multiplying by 100:

$$\frac{\text{No. reduplicated words}}{\text{Total no. of multisyllabic words}} \times 100 = \%\ \text{reduplicated words}$$

To identify reduplication, it is only necessary to know whether the child's multisyllabic words contain the same syllable two or more times as compared to a variety of distinct syllables. For example, [bɑbɑdɑdi] would be considered to be reduplicated even though not all of the syllables are the same.[4] In a CVCVC production, reduplication can be considered to have occurred if the two CVs are the same, even though the first syllable is open and the second is closed. For example, [bɑbɑp] would be considered to be reduplicated.[5]

To identify harmony in multisyllabic words, one must determine whether the child's multisyllabic words contain the same consonant or vowel two or more times in a row as compared to a variety of distinct consonants and vowels. For instance, [bɑbidɑ] would be considered to exemplify consonant harmony even though not all of the consonants are the same and [bɑdɑdi] would be considered to exemplify vowel harmony even though not all of the consonants are the same.[6] Thus, the frequencies of words with harmonized vowels and the frequency of those with harmonized consonants are determined.

$$\frac{\text{No. of harmonized C words}}{\text{Total no. of words with two or more Cs}} \times 100 = \%\ \text{C harmony}$$

$$\frac{\text{No. of harmonized V words}}{\text{Total no. of words with two or more Vs}} \times 100 = \%\ \text{V harmony}$$

Note that no word is counted as both reduplicated and harmonized. If two or more syllables in the vocalization or word are the same, then the word is counted as reduplicated only even though it usually follows that the consonants and vowels are also harmonized. Also, recall that this is independent analysis. Therefore, all words that are reduplicated or harmonized are counted as such, whether the target is reduplicated (e.g., "boo-boo") or harmonized (e.g., "baby") or not. Some children may selectively attempt only or primarily words that are simple in this respect; others may attempt a variety of words but simplify them in these ways. Either way, it is important to know what they are actually producing, regardless of the target.

As the SLP deems appropriate, vowels that differ only in tenseness (e.g., [i] versus [ɪ], [u] versus [ʊ], etc.) may (or may not) be considered identical for the purposes of the reduplication and harmony calculations, especially for children whose phonologies are quite immature or deviant. Consonants may be considered identical if they differ in voicing only, as most young children and children with severe SSD do not have control of voicing. Furthermore, transcription of voicing contrasts is notoriously unreliable. Whichever of these rules the SLP chooses to apply or not, this should be done consistently across children and across time in order for the results to be comparable.

Of course, only multisyllabic words can be used to calculate the frequency of reduplication. Similarly, only words with two or more consonants are used to calculate the frequency of consonant harmony (e.g., "uppy"—[ʌpi]—would not count as a nonharmonized two-syllable word as it only contains one consonant despite being bisyllabic). For parallel reasons, only words with two or more vowels are used to calculate the frequency of vowel harmony.

Unlike reduplication and vowel harmony, consonant harmony can occur in monosyllables (e.g., [gɔg] for "dog," [pup] for "soup") as well as multisyllabic words (e.g., [gɔgi]

[4]The individual examiner may decide to use different rules for determining which utterances are considered to be reduplicated. This is fine as long as the rules are applied consistently.

[5]See Footnote 4.

[6]Again, different rules may be devised and applied consistently if the individual SLP so chooses.

Example 8-2

Name: *Bryan* Age: *3;11*
Date: *5/17/93* Examiner: *SLV*
Source of sample: *APP-R* Size of sample: *75 words (32 with clusters)*

INITIAL CONSONANT CLUSTERS

Indicate with ✓, specific # or specific % those clusters that occur in the child's speech. (Note: If the child produces an "illegal" cluster that does not normally occur in English, list it under "other".)

Number of occurrences

Two-Element Clusters

Obstruent + liquid

pɹ-___ pl-___ pj-___ bɹ-___ bl-___ bj-___

tɹ-___ tj-___ tw-___ dɹ-___ dj-___ dw-___

kɹ-___ kl-___ kj-_*1*_ kw-___ gɹ-___ gl-___ gj-___ gw-___

mj-___

nj-___

fɹ-___ fl-___ fj-___

θɹ-___ θj-___ θw-___

sl-___ sj-_*1*_ sw-_*8*_

ʃɹ-___

hj-___

vj-___

lj-___

[s] + obstruent

sp-_*1*_ st-_*1*_ sk-___ sm-_*1*_ sn-_*1*_

NOTE: The glide [j] occurs far more often in initial clusters in British than in American English.

OTHER: *fw- 3, ʃw- 1*

Three-Element Clusters

spɹ-___ spl-___ spj-__

stɹ-___ stj-___

skɹ-___ skl-___ skj-___ skw-___

OTHER:

Example 8-3

Name: *Bryan* Age: *3;11*
Date: *5/17/93* Examiner: *SLV*
Source of sample: *APP-R* Size of sample: *75 words (32 with clusters in them)*

FINAL CONSONANT CLUSTERS

Indicate with ✓, specific # or specific % those clusters that occur in the child's speech. (Note: If the child produces an "illegal" cluster that does not normally occur in English, list it under "other".)

Two-Element Clusters

NASALS

-mp__ -mt_*1*_ -md__ -mf__ -mθ__ -mz_*1*_

-nt_*5*_ -nd_*1*_ -nθ__ -ns__ -ntʃ_*1*_ -ndʒ_*1*_ -nz_*2*_

-ŋk__ -ŋd__ -ŋz__

STOPS

-pt__ -bd__ -pθ__ -ps__ -bz__

-tθ__ -ts_*1*_ -dz_*1*_

-kt__ -gd__ -ks__ -gz__

FRICATIVES

-ft__ -vd__ -fθ__ -fs__ -vz__

-θt__ -ðd__ -θs__ -ðz__

-sp__ -st__ -sk_*1*_ -zd__ -zm__

-ʃt__ -ʒd__

-tʃt__ -dʒd__

LIQUIDS

-lp__ -lt__ -lk__ -ld__ -lm__ -ln__

-lv__ -lf__ -lθ__ -ls__ -ltʃ__ -ldʒ__ -lz__

OTHER: *-bs 1*

Three-Element Clusters

-mps__ OTHER: *none*

-nts__ -nst__

-ŋst__ -ŋks__

-lps__ -lts__ -lst__ -lks__

Form 8-4

Name: Age:
Date: Examiner:
Source of sample: Size of sample:

PHONOTACTIC REPERTOIRE
Reduplication and Harmony

Note: C = consonant
V = vowel
Reduplication = Same syllable repeated in word (baba, deedee, gogo, etc.)
Harmony = Same C repeated (**g**o**gg**ie, **t**oo**t**ie, etc.) or
same V repeated (d**a**b**a**, b**oo**g**oo**, etc.)
predominant: 60-100%
frequent: 40-60%
occasional: 15-40%

WORDS OF TWO SYLLABLES OR MORE:

% or ✓ Frequency Estimate*: Circle appropriate word.

Reduplicated
Syllables _____ predominant frequent occasional rare absent

Harmonized
Vowels _____ predominant frequent occasional rare absent

Harmonized
Consonants_____ predominant frequent occasional rare absent
**Out of all words with two syllables or more*

MONOSYLLABIC CVC WORDS:

% or ✓ Frequency Estimate+: Circle appropriate word.

Harmonized
Consonants_____ predominant frequent occasional rare absent
+Out of all monosyllabic CVC words

Summary/Notes:

Example 8-4

Name: *Molly* Age: *13 months*
Date: *2/18/93* Examiner: *SLV*

Reduplication and Harmony

C = consonant V = vowel
Reduplication = Same syllable repeated in word (baba, deedee, gogo, etc.)
Harmony = Same C repeated (goggie, tootie, etc.) or
same V repeated (daba, boogoo, etc.)
predominant: 60-100%
frequent: 40-60%
occasional: 15-40%

WORDS OF TWO SYLLABLES OR MORE: *Total: 17*

	% or ✓	Frequency Estimate*: Circle appropriate word.				
Reduplicated syllables	*18%* *(3/17)*	~~predominant~~	~~frequent~~	occasional	~~rare~~	~~absent~~
Harmonized vowels	*0%* *(0/17)*	~~predominant~~	~~frequent~~	~~occasional~~	~~rare~~	absent
Harmonized cons.	*29%* *(5/17)*	~~predominant~~	~~frequent~~	occasional	~~rare~~	~~absent~~

**Out of all words with two syllables or more*

MONOSYLLABIC CVC WORDS: *total: 6*

Harmonized cons.	*33%* *(2/6)*	~~predominant~~	~~frequent~~	occasional	~~rare~~	~~absent~~

+Out of all monosyllabic CVC words
Summary/Notes: 6 VCV, 7 CVCV, 2 CVCVC, 1 CVCVCV, 1 VCVC; 11 bi- or multisyllabic with 2 true C's

for "doggie," [bʌpeɪp] for "cupcake"). To identify harmony in monosyllabic words, it is only necessary to know whether two different consonants occur within the same word. Again, words in which both consonants are identical are counted. For this calculation, the denominator is the total number of CVC words. A space for indicating the frequency of harmonized consonants in monosyllabic words is included toward the bottom of the form.

Using Form 8-4, we can determine the prevalence of reduplication and harmony in Molly's speech (from Table 8-11) at 13 months; the result is shown in Example 8-4. Because we are ignoring voicing, the first two syllables of [kʊgʊgɔ] are considered to contain essentially identical consonants, and the production is classified as reduplicated. This worksheet yields the following results:

- Words of two syllables or more: Most of Molly's words contain syllables that differ in some way; only 16% are reduplicated. The vowels always differ. The consonants are identical (harmonized) 63% of the time in non-reduplicated words with two or more consonants.

- Monosyllables: When two non-glottal consonants are produced within the same one-syllable word, they are different 75% of the time (harmonized 25% of the time).

Thus, we can conclude that Molly has better control of vowel contrasts within a word than of consonant contrasts and that her ability to produce consonant contrasts is slightly better within monosyllabic words. Since Molly produces predominantly open syllables, in two-syllable words, the consonants typically will both be in syllable-initial position (e.g., [dænə]). When the word is a monosyllable, the two consonants in the word must be in syllable-initial and syllable-final position, respectively (e.g., [tʌŋ]). (Since there is only one syllable, they cannot both be in syllable-initial position.) Therefore, Molly appears to be better at distinguishing consonants in different syllable positions than in similar syllable positions. This is a common finding that mirrors the harmony patterns in adult languages.

Consonant–Vowel Dependencies

Assimilation and dissimilation, which refer to adjacent elements becoming more (or less) alike, typically include effects of vowel on consonant or vice versa in young or moderately to severely phonologically delayed children. These are assessed by looking for consonant–vowel dependencies, that is, by determining whether certain consonants are restricted to co-occurrence with certain vowels or vice versa. Form 8-5 addresses this issue. Once again, this form can be used qualitatively by simply indicating with an X or checkmark those combinations that do occur or quantitatively by tallying the frequency with which each combination occurs. If the former strategy is used, looking down the columns of the form makes it easy to see whether there is a good scatter of combinations, indicating that the child does not have consonant–vowel association restrictions, or whether, on the other hand, only certain limited combinations occur.

Given that syllable-initial consonants are more likely to be affected by following vowels than syllable-final consonants are by preceding vowels and that many children with moderate to severe disorders produce primarily open syllables, syllable-final consonants typically are not considered. However, vowel–consonant sequences could be done as well using another copy of the same form if the clinician felt that this was relevant to a particular child's speech. Note also that strictly adjacent consonants and vowels are most likely to affect each other. Therefore, in the case of a cluster, it is the consonant that is beside the vowel that is considered. For example, the word "play" pronounced as [pleɪ] would be counted in the [l] + [e] box, not in the [p] + [e] or in the [l] + [ɪ] box.

For this form, percentages refer to the percent of each type of consonant that co-occurs with each vowel type. Thus, for example, the number of syllables that fall within the labial stop + high front vowel square is divided by the total number of syllables that begin with a labial stop, indicating what percentages of labials co-occur with high front vowels. In other words, percentages are calculated for each row. (One could, of course, calculate the types of vowels that occur with each consonant type instead by dividing by column totals, indicating, for example, what percentage of high front vowels co-occur with labials.)

The results of using this form to assess Molly's word productions (see Table 8-11) are as shown in Example 8-5. These results indicate that:

- Almost all consonants co-occur with the neutral mid central vowels [ə] and [ʌ] (a common finding).
- Only coronal (alveo–palatal) consonants (which require relatively front positioning of the tongue) and glottals (which do not involve the tongue) co-occur with front vowels. This makes sense; vowels and consonants that require anterior positioning of the tongue occur together so that Molly doesn't have to move her tongue much as she transitions from consonant to vowel. Glottals don't require tongue positioning at all, so they don't interfere with the production of front vowels.
- Labial and velar consonants co-occur with back vowels—labials with low back vowels and velars with high back vowels. Physiologically, these patterns also make sense. The transition from a labial consonant into a low back vowel requires only the opening of the jaw. Both velars and mid to high back vowels require the back of the tongue to be raised toward the velum, so that again, minimal tongue movement is required from consonant to vowel within the syllable. These patterns mirror those reported by Davis and MacNeilage (2000).

Thus, Molly appears to have some consonant-vowel preferences. It is important to note, however, that these restrictions aren't absolute in her case. Molly does produce some [dɑ] syllables, demonstrating that she is able and willing to combine tongue and mandible movement for certain productions.

It must be kept in mind that the language to which a child is exposed may be responsible for some biases in consonant-vowel co-occurrences. Also, one could not of course expect to find every possible combination of consonant and vowel in a small sample such as this. Therefore, general patterns rather than co-occurrences of specific consonants with specific vowels are of interest here.

Filling out these forms would have been even faster and simpler if the frequencies had been estimated rather than calculating percentages. Of course, this procedure is far less precise than using percentages, and both are far less precise than the types of in-depth analyses suggested by Ingram (1981) and Grunwell (1985). However, the worksheets included here allow the speech-language pathologist to quickly identify possible areas of concern that can be explored in greater depth if need be in order to establish baselines for treatment.

Form 8-5

Name: Age:
Date: Examiner:
Source of sample: Size of sample

PHONOTACTIC REPERTOIRE
Consonant-Vowel Dependencies

INDICATE (✓ OR %) COMBINATIONS THAT DO OCCUR:

C Type	*V Type* high front (i, ɪ)	mid front (e, ɛ)	low front (æ)	mid central (ə, ʌ)	high back (u, ʊ)	mid back (o, ɔ)	low back (ɑ)
STOPS labial (b, p)							
alveolar (d, t)							
velar (k, g)							
NASALS labial (m)							
alveolar (n)							
GLIDES labial (w)							
palatal (j)							
LIQUID alveolar (l)							
palatal (ɹ)							
FRIC. labial (f, v)							
labio-dental (θ, ð)							
alveolar (s, z)							
palatal (ʃ, ʒ)							
AFFRIC. (tʃ, dʒ)							
GLOTT. (h, ʔ)							

Notes:

Example 8-5

Name: *Molly* Age: *13 months*
Date: *2/18/93* Examiner: *SLV*

PHONOTACTIC REPERTOIRE
Consonant-Vowel Dependencies

INDICATE (✓ OR %) COMBINATIONS THAT <u>DO</u> OCCUR:

C Type / *V Type*	high front (i, ɪ)	mid front (e, ɛ)	low front (æ)	mid central (ə, ʌ)	high back (u, ʊ)	mid back (o, ɔ)	low back (ɑ)
STOPS labial (b, p)				*50%*			*50%*
alveolar (d, t)			*29%*	*29%*			*42%*
velar (k, g)				*28%*	*50%*	*22%*	
NASALS labial (m)							
alveolar (n)	*50%*			*50%*			
GLIDES labial (w)							
palatal (j)			*100% (1 ex.)*				
LIQUID alveolar (l)							
palatal (ɹ)							
FRIC. labial (f, v)							
labio-dental (θ, ð)							
alveolar (s, z)							
palatal (ʃ, ʒ)							
AFFRIC. (tʃ, dʒ)							
GLOTT. (h, ʔ)		*ʔ 100% (1 ex.)*	*h 75%*	*h 12.5%*			*h 12.5%*

Notes: Mid central vowels co-occur with everything. Only alveolars, palatals (both anterior tongue positions) and glottals (no tongue involved) co-occur with front vowels. Mid to high back vowels (tongue back and high) co-occur only with velars. Some alveolar + [ɑ] syllables break the pattern.

In summary, for Molly, if she were older and delayed or disordered rather than simply young, possible intervention targets would include closed syllables, consonant clusters, consonant variety (i.e., decreasing consonant harmony), and consonant-vowel combinations (i.e., decreasing consonant-vowel dependencies).

Analyzing Unintelligible Speech

Many children with SSDs produce large numbers of unintelligible utterances. The typical SLP will perhaps estimate an intelligibility level using one of the strategies discussed in Chapter 4. Few of us do anything more with such productions. However, one can learn a great deal from the analysis of unintelligible forms, looking for commonalities among them. This can assist the speech-language pathologist in determining factors contributing to unintelligibility. For example, if all unintelligible forms are multisyllabic, then it is clear that multisyllabic words should be a target for intervention. Ellen produced the unintelligible utterances shown in Table 8-13 at age 2;3. These words share a heavy reliance on [b] and on reduplication ([bububu, ʌbububibu], etc.). Less obvious is her frequent use of a labial consonant-alveolar consonant alternation ([bɔdə, bidə, bʌdə bʌ bʌdə], etc.). With these apparent preferences in mind, Ellen's intelligible utterances were re-examined and found to exhibit the same patterns. Reduplication and a heavy functional load for labials had already been identified, but Ellen's labial–alveolar consonant alternation was not noticed until these unintelligible forms were examined. It is likely that this combination of preferences significantly reduced the contrasts available within Ellen's production vocabulary and that it was responsible for much of Ellen's unintelligibility. Thus, an early goal for her would focus on increasing her distributional flexibility, such as by targeting alveolar-labial words.

TABLE 8-13 Ellen's Unintelligible Utterances
bidə
bububu
bʌdə bʌ bʌdə
ʌbububibu
ɔdɔtʰ
bʊdɪvʊ
ʌdʌbɑbɑɪ
ɑʔl
bʊdæ
bʌdʊ
bʌnəmɑʊ
bʌdʌmbʌ
bʌdʌ

EXERCISE 8-1

Phonotactic Assessment

INTERVENTION

General Guidelines

Shockingly little information is available about treating phonotactic deficits other than consonant cluster reduction. Furthermore, most treatment materials available to address cluster reduction focus on the consonants within the clusters (e.g., workbooks for "s blends," "r blends," and the like) rather than on the production of a sequence of consonants per se.

The main goal in phonotactic intervention is to expand the child's phonotactic capabilities. The clinician should not strive for segmental accuracy for the sake of segmental accuracy. For example, if a child who produces only open syllables can be taught to close those syllables, the actual consonants that he uses to do so are of secondary importance until the structural goal has been met. To determine a starting point, consider the list of the child's current phonotactic patterns that have been generated using the worksheets provided. Presumably the patterns available are insufficient for effective communication and the child is lacking one, some, or even all of the following structures:

- initial consonants
- final consonants
- multiple syllables within a word
- different syllables within a word
- different consonants within a word
- different vowels within a word
- different consonant-vowel combinations within a syllable
- consonant clusters in initial, medial, and/or final position

There are various considerations in choosing which patterns to target first, but the primary question to ask is:

1. What is preventing this child from producing phonotactically varied words? What syllable or word-level restrictions are most limiting for this child?
   Additional questions include the following:
2. Are any other patterns beginning to emerge in the child's speech? If, for instance, the child is typically restricted to CV word shapes but occasionally says "mama" rather than simply "ma," the speech-language pathologist may be able to capitalize on this alternate word shape by introducing other two-syllable reduplicated CVCV words ("boo-boo, bye-bye, pee-pee, no-no, yoyo," etc.).
3. What new pattern would "buy" the child the most in terms of communicative effectiveness? If, for example, the child is restricted to CV word shapes and therefore

TABLE 8-14 Combining Phonetic/Phonemic and Phonotactic Targets

	Old Segment/Natural Class	New Segment/Natural Class
Old Structure	automaticity	flexibility
New Structure	flexibility	too challenging??

has many CV homonyms (e.g., [mɑ] for "mom," "mad," "mine," "moo," "milk," "money;" [bɑ] for "bottle," "bye-bye," "bike," "bath," "back," "ball;" etc.), either adding final consonants or adding second syllables (as described above) would be helpful in differentiating his words. Homonyms are usually an important clue to determining communicative effectiveness as was discussed in Chapters 6 and 7.

4. What patterns occur first developmentally? All else being equal, two-syllable words or final consonants would usually be targeted before consonant clusters, for instance.
5. Motivation: Which words does the child seem to need? What does she want to express that she cannot? If, for example, the child needs to be able to express her emotions, perhaps CVCs like "mad," "sad," and "bad" could be targeted. If she has many siblings who pick on her verbally, a CVCV insult reply such as "dummy!" could be helpful (Judith Johnston, personal communication).

It is generally considered wise to choose therapy targets that either comprise new segmental material (e.g., fricatives or velars) or that are new phonotactically, not both at once. This is represented in Table 8-14. For a child with CAS, it might be appropriate to focus on the automaticity (production fluency) of segments that she can already produce in syllable or word shapes that she can already produce to firm up the motor plans for those combinations. For other children with SSDs, their challenge points are more likely to lie in the realms of new sounds in mastered structures or mastered sounds in new structures. In many cases, new sounds in new structures may be too challenging. However, in some cases, this approach may be warranted or at least worth a try. For example, given that nasals, velars, and fricatives often (but don't always) emerge first in final position, one might target final nasals for a child who produced neither nasals nor final consonants. This author has addressed fricatives in final position for three children who had a fricative systematic gap and no codas. In all three cases, the clients developed a generic frication sound in final position (typically something in the neighborhood of a voiceless velar fricative [x], which provides lots of tactile feedback) and then differentiated that sound into individual, more appropriate fricatives.[7]

[7]Note that these were not controlled studies. Thus, it is impossible to know what might have happened if alternative goals had been addressed instead.

Similarly, some children are able to produce [s] more accurately when it is in a homorganic cluster than as a singleton. Therefore, in cases in which the child has neither /s/ nor clusters, one might try addressing both together.

Treatment Strategies

Omissions of Syllables and Segments

Moving a child from mostly monosyllables to longer words can often be facilitated by repeating a single syllable (i.e., by using reduplication as a stepping stone to more sophisticated two-syllable word shapes). Counting books can be useful for this: Instead of actually counting, repeat the word labels (e.g., "ball ball ball" for a page where three balls are displayed). Then move on to words in which the target is reduplicated ("boo-boo, bye-bye, pee-pee, mama, papa, no-no, yoyo," etc.).

A lack of initial consonants is typically viewed as the most concerning phonotactic error pattern for children learning English, although as described above, it is developmentally appropriate in some other languages, especially for very young children, to omit onsets. The goal for a child who deletes initial consonants should be that he will include initial consonants, regardless of the accuracy of the consonant itself. The mere presence of any initial consonant is progress toward this goal. Often /h/ (used in simple, emotionally charged words such "hi," "hohoho," "who," "haha," "hey," etc.) is an easy first initial consonant to introduce, given the minimum of articulatory precision that is required to produce it. For children whose production of VC words is better than of CVs, Bernhardt (1994) also suggests using repetitions of the VC to facilitate production of a CVC: "ick-ick-ick" → "kick-kick-kick." This type of strategy is also used in the Nuffield Centre Dyspraxia program (Nuffield Centre, 2004).

A lack of final consonants is far more common than a lack of initial consonants in English. There are several strategies that can be used to remediate this deficit. In choosing goals or objectives, for example, it is important to keep in mind that certain sound classes, specifically velars, nasals, and fricatives, have a tendency to emerge first in final position in some children, as previously noted. Thus, these categories may be appropriate first steps to achieving the production of final consonants. However, once again, the use of any coda consonant should be the goal regardless of phonetic accuracy. Weiner (1981) documented the successful use of minimal pair treatment in which the child was given social credit for a contrast as long as the coda consonant slot was filled (e.g., [nod] was recognized as adequately distinct from [no] in the child's attempt to produce "nose"). He reported that the children studied increased their use of closed syllables, produced final consonants more accurately even though this was not the target of the therapy, and generalized their gains to other final consonants. Both targeting multiple consonants at once and targeting a single consonant and hoping for generalization to other consonants have been shown to be effective for some children (Bernhardt & Gilbert, 1992; Bernhardt, 1994). Bernhardt, Stemberger, and Major (2006) suggest that for children who also omit medial consonants from CVCV words, it may be efficient to target these at the same time as final consonants from CVC words. In both cases, it is a postvocalic C2 that is the goal.

Recall that studies of contextual effects have also yielded important information relative to targeting coda production. For example, children are more likely to produce final consonants in words in which the vowel is lax: [pɪt] "pit" will be more likely to be pronounced completely than [pit] "peat" (Kehoe & Stoel-Gammon, 2001). Similarly, they are more likely to produce final consonants accurately in CVC words in which the initial CV of the word is more common (e.g., [ti] as in "teed, teak, teal, team, teen, teat, teeth, tease" versus [mʊ] as in "mush" [in some dialects only]) (Zamuner, Gerken, & Hammond, 2004).

CLINICAL TIP

To increase the production of final consonants, target CVC words that:

1. have lax vowels.
2. begin with commonly occurring CV combinations.

Bernhardt (1994) suggests using the child's abilities to shape the new closed syllable target form: Ask the child to produce a CVCV word, then gradually fade the second vowel so that what is left is a CVC. Another strategy is to have the child produce the final consonant in a phrase immediately before a word beginning with the same consonant, as in "ba**d d**og" (Secord & Shine, 1997). The onset consonant facilitates the production of the coda. Codas are also facilitated when they precede a vowel-initial word as is the case for the word final [t]s in the phrase "pu**t i**t in," taking advantage of the natural tendency for resyllabification (Stemberger, 1988).

Two final strategies that may be helpful in targeting final consonants rely on interactions between phonetics and phonotactics. One is to introduce codas first in words with consonant harmony—such as "pop, dad, mom, toot, Bob, kick." The decreased phonetic place and manner of articulation demands in such words may make it possible for a child to produce final consonants even though she cannot otherwise do so. Once words with harmony have been mastered, the consonants could be gradually differentiated. Similarly, final consonants that are articulatorily compatible with the preceding vowels—labials with low and central vowels, alveolars with high front vowels, and velars with high back vowels—might be facilitatory. These approaches have not been tested empirically, however.

COMMON *Confusion*

Some people (e.g., Kaufman, 1998, 2001) advocate simplifying word targets for children with significant SSD in order to make those words more accessible to the child. For example, "spaghetti" might be modeled as [ˈgɛɾi] for a child who is still (belatedly) producing a maximum of two syllables or two singleton consonants only (no clusters) per word. *However, this is strongly contraindicated*; the child who hears the word mispronounced will store that target representation (via implicit learning) and have an additional barrier to overcome in order to eventually learn to pronounce it correctly. It is appropriate to accept word approximations (i.e., to respond as if they were produced correctly) from a child, but *the model should always be correct.*

Syllable and Segmental Variety within a Word

For a child who has mastered producing multiple reduplicated syllables but cannot vary those syllables, more change can gradually be introduced into the word, initially by targeting words that differ only with respect to the vowels (i.e., maintaining consonant harmony as in "baby") or only with respect to the consonants (i.e., maintaining vowel harmony as in "teepee"). Velleman (1994, 2003a) has proposed the use of syllable sequencing repetitions of this sort to give children with CAS practice in (1) identifying the current state of the articulators; (2) planning a movement to another state; and (3) returning to the initial state or to yet another state. For example, the client might initially practice repeating [bɑbɑbɑbɑbɑ] and then progress to [bɑbɑbɑbɑbi], [bɑbibɑbi], and finally [bɑbibebobu] or to [bɑbɑbɑbɑdɑ], [bɑdɑdɑbɑdɑ], and finally [bɑdɑgɑbɑgɑdɑ]. In each case, one element is stable and is returned to repeatedly while the other varies. Thus, the sensory-motor system is trained to use both feedforward and feedback.

To "break" consonant harmony or a word recipe (a restricted distribution pattern such as labial-alveolar), the SLP can systematically vary the places of articulation or the manners of articulation of the consonants within a word. For example, "Moving across Syllables" (Kirkpatrick, Stohr, & Kimbrough, 1990) provides materials for systematically practicing different place of articulation patterns such as labial-velar or palatal-interdental in one-, two-, and three-syllable words. In this case, only place of articulation and order are critical to measuring progress; other aspects of the consonants (voicing or manner of articulation) may be incorrect as long as the place pattern is preserved. Alternatively, manner patterns can be practiced for children who have a distribution restriction in that respect (e.g., nasals or fricatives occurring only in final position); unfortunately Kirkpatrick and team don't provide those materials. Table 8-15 was developed to facilitate goal planning and progress monitoring for manner patterns.

TABLE 8-15 **Chart for Planning Manner Sequence Patterns**

First Consonant → ↓ Second Consonant	Stop ptk bdg	Nasal mnŋ	Glide wj	Fricative fθsʃh vðzʒ	Affricate tʃ dʒ	Liquid l ɹ
Stop ptk bdg						
Nasal mnŋ						
Glide wj						
Fricative fθsʃh vðzʒ						
Affricate tʃ dʒ						
Liquid l ɹ						

To help break vowel harmony, it's often helpful to start with words of the form CVCi. As Davis, MacNeilage, and Matyear (2002) reported, children's first non-vowel-harmonized words are often of this form. English baby talk takes advantage of this tendency in many words that provide excellent therapy targets, such as "mommy, daddy, baby, candy, cookie, horsie, piggie, doggie, birdie," etc. As before, the goal is the structure rather than phonetic accuracy: As long as the child produces two different syllables, two different consonants, or two different vowels (depending upon the goal), the precision of those segments is secondary.

Clusters

As noted above, some children may have more difficulty with clusters that violate the sonority hierarchy—for instance, /s/ + stop and stop + /s/ clusters, in which a less sonorous consonant (the stop) is closer to the middle of the word than the more sonorous consonant (the /s/). However, this is by no means universal, at least not among children learning English. Recall also that the assumption that is often made that initial clusters are easier than final clusters may not be true for many children. Homorganic nasal + stop clusters, such as -nt, -mp, and -ŋk are often among the first to be acquired.

Some approaches to treating consonant clusters are more theoretical, and the results may be complex. For example, Gierut and Champion (2001) found that treating three-element clusters (/s/ + stop + liquid/glide; for example, str-) was successful even with some children who didn't have all two-element clusters, with little apparent difference resulting from the specific cluster addressed. Surprisingly, this did not result in generalization to other similar untreated three-element clusters but rather to untreated singleton consonants and two-element clusters. The nature of the generalization to simpler clusters did depend in part on the child's pre-treatment singleton repertoires. Interestingly, there was also generalization to affricates in some children who did not previously have such complex consonants in their repertoires. Gierut and Champion (2001) conclude that what the participants learned, in part, is that onsets can "branch;" they can be more complex than a simple singleton consonant.

As with final consonants, the use of phrases may assist in developing clusters. A child who can produce a final [s] followed by an initial [t], for example, may be able to gradually merge the two:

"mice tough" "mice tough" "mice tough" → "my stuff" ([maɪ ***st****ʌf])*

*"Pete sees" "Pete sees" "Pete sees" → "Pete's E's" ([pi****ts*** *iz])*

The Nuffield Centre Dyspraxia Programme includes other examples of this sort (Nuffield Centre, 2004).

Other considerations for consonant clusters again merge the phonetic with the phonotactic. The elements included in a cluster may facilitate each others' production. For example, as previously noted, some children may be able to produce /s/ more accurately in a cluster right before or after another alveolar sound (e.g., in sn-, st-, -ts, or -ns clusters). Similarly, velars and /ɹ/ may facilitate each other because of their similar places of articulation.

THE PHONOTACTICS OF CHILDHOOD APRAXIA OF SPEECH

CAS appears to differ from other phonological delays/disorders, partly in that it is more specifically a phonotactic disorder. Although children with CAS certainly do have trouble producing various segments in isolation and in words, their major difficulty lies in putting these segments together into smooth, coherent syllables, words, or phrases. That is, their problem lies not as much in hitting the segmental targets (although that may be an issue as well) as in getting smoothly from one segment to the next. As such, special attention must be paid to their phonotactic limitations and possibilities. However, it is important to note that the same phonotactic simplification options described previously are available for children with CAS as for other children with simple phonologies; they just use them more and to older ages (Velleman & Shriberg, 1999).

In a study of two children with CAS, Velleman (1994) identified phonotactic simplifications that are not unknown in other children but that were more extreme in these participants. One child, Marina, aged 3;11 when first evaluated by this author, reduced the complexity of the syllables she produced by relying on certain consonant-vowel combinations. She did not combine alveolars with back-rounded vowels nor labials with high front vowels. Alveolars preferentially combined with vowels produced in the same region, such as [i]. Labials preferentially combined with vowels that did not require tongue-tip articulation, such as [ɑ]. Thus, she was not stimulable for syllables such as [du], [do], or [bi], [mi]. Her productions of "baby" varied between [didi] and [bɑbɑ]. Marina, then, was able to combine consonants and vowels into simple CV syllables only when a minimum of movement was required from consonant to vowel.

Holly, aged 2;4, provided an interesting contrast. She relied to an unusual extent upon non-syllabic isolated consonants and isolated vowels. Some examples of her words are given in Table 8-16. A disturbing number of Holly's words consisted of either consonants alone or vowels alone; she appeared to have difficulty building complete syllables. The few CV syllables that Holly produced were undifferentiated and were overused for a wide variety of words. For example, [bɛ, bijə, bɪʊ] were used interchangeably for "bunny, bear, bird, baby, bell, pig, and Bert" (i.e., all nouns beginning with bilabial stops). Similarly, [dɪ, deɪ, di, dɛ, dɑ, dɔ] were used interchangeably as deictics (i.e., to mean "there, this, that," etc.). These types of patterns are not unknown in other children, but they may be more pervasive or persistent in children with CAS.

TABLE 8-16 Holly's Limited Syllable Shapes

[m:]	food, eat
[tʰ, ts]	tree, kitty, coffee and other non-labial nouns
[ʃ]	sleep
[n]	in
[ɸ]	elephant (voiceless bilabial fricative)
[ɑʊ]	out
[o]	open
[ɑ:]	all gone

From Velleman, S. L. (1994). The interaction of phonetics and phonology in developmental verbal dyspraxia: Two case studies. *Clinics in Communication Disorders, 4*(1), 67–78.

For obvious reasons, motor learning principles are key to intervention in CAS. In fact, approaches such as PROMPT (Hayden, 2006), Strand's DTTC (Strand & Skinder, 1999) and the ReST treatment developed by Murray, McCabe and Ballard (2012) were developed specifically for this population. As described in Chapter 5, these focus on learning to flexibly plan, implement, and monitor motor plans.

EXERCISE 8-2

Phonotactic Intervention

CHAPTER SUMMARY

Phonotactics typically receives short shrift in the literature on child speech sound development and disorders. There are no standardized tests that provide adequate assessment of this aspect of phonology. Yet, many children demonstrate deficits in this area. Furthermore, research has clearly demonstrated that phonotactics and phonetics interact in many ways beyond the obvious point that children often master a sound or sound class in one word position at a time. The ability to produce a variety of consonants and vowels is not sufficient if these segments cannot be combined into the sound structures expected in the ambient language. Although they are not well known, successful remediation techniques are available to expand a client's repertoire of word and syllable shapes, thus markedly increasing his or her communication potential.

KEY TAKE-HOME MESSAGES

1. The ability to produce the phonological structures of one's language is as important to successful communication as the ability to produce its consonants and vowels.
2. Phonetic and phonotactic factors interact throughout phonological development.
3. Phonotactic therapy focuses on production of the target structures regardless of whether the segments are accurate or not.
4. Specific phonotactic remediation strategies and even a few packaged therapy materials are available.

CHAPTER 8

The Phonological Framework Review

Exercise 8-1: Phonetic Assessment

A. *Multiple choice. Choose the best answer.*

1. Phonotactic analysis is important for many reasons, including:
   a. phonotactic factors may impact phonetic accuracy.
   b. phonotactic norms are more reliable.
   c. phonotactic norms are more valid.
   d. phonotactic development is correlated with language development.
2. Children's likelihood of inclusion of an initial consonant is:
   a. an absolute universal.
   b. marked universally.
   c. optional in most languages.
   d. influenced by the ambient language.
3. The sonority hierarchy predicts that:
   a. s + stop initial clusters will develop early.
   b. stops will occur at the edges of words.
   c. only stops will occur word medially.
   d. final consonant clusters will develop later.
4. Reduplication:
   a. is used only by very young or speech-disordered children.
   b. is a red flag for disorder in English.
   c. may be a strategy for producing multisyllables.
   d. typically outranks CV assimilation.
5. A pattern in which all initial consonants are voiced is an example of:
   a. assimilation.
   b. sonority.
   c. homonymy.
   d. regression.
6. Phonotactic contrast includes:
   a. velar versus alveolar place of articulation.
   b. markedness versus sonority.
   c. open versus closed syllables.
   d. coarticulation versus assimilation.
7. Monosyllabic words cannot be examples of:
   a. consonant harmony.
   b. consonant-vowel dependencies.
   c. distribution requirements.
   d. vowel harmony.
8. Unintelligible productions:
   a. should not be analyzed because the target is unknown.
   b. indicate the presence of a disorder rather than a delay.
   c. can provide insight about a child's phonotactic restrictions.
   d. indicate the presence of a delay rather than a disorder.
9. Children are more likely to produce a coda if:
   a. the vowel is tense.
   b. the initial CV is frequent in the language.
   c. phonetic accuracy is required.
   d. the child has no phonological knowledge of final consonants.
10. Phonotactic therapy typically does not include:
   a. phonetic placement cues.
   b. gradual fading of some elements.
   c. using early patterns as a stepping stone.
   d. phrase-level targets.

B. *Case study question.*

Consider Lacie's below transcript again. Use the forms provided in the chapter to determine what types of phonotactic contrast are available in this child's system. What phonotactic contrasts that are typical in English are not yet available to Lacie? Specifically:

- What syllable and word shapes does she produce most often? Never?
- Does she produce clusters? If so, in what word position(s)?
- How frequent are reduplication and harmony in her speech?
- Are consonant–vowel combinations restricted?

Production

1. 'bɑðɑ
2. ɑʊʔ
3. 'dædæ
4. dɛʊ
5. θɑ
6. æʔ
7. 'ɛzə
8. dɪp
9. fɑ
10. ðɑ
11. 'æðɪ
12. ðʌ
13. θʌ
14. 'nɑnɑ
15. 'ɑðə
16. ɑɪ
17. 'ɱɑɱɑ
18. fi
19. ɱæ
20. 'ɱuɱu
21. ðɑɪt
22. fɑɪ
23. i
24. wɑ
25. 'dɑðə
26. ju
27. ðɑɪ
28. oʔ
29. nɑɪt
30. ɑʊp
31. du
32. ðɑ
33. nɑ
34. dɪ
35. ə'vɑnɑ
36. 'ðiði
37. 'ðɑðɑ
38. dʌ
39. ɑɪt
40. jɑ
41. 'woʊwoʊ
42. 'jɑjo
43. 'ɪhɪ
44. 'æzæ
45. dæ
46. wi
47. 'dɛdo
48. vɪ
49. nɑʊ
50. ðʌ

Exercise 8-2: Phonetic Intervention

A. ***Case study questions.***

1. Based on your results in Exercise 8-1, write two phonotactic goals with two objectives each for Lacie. Although speech sound disorders goals are often a mix of phonetic and phonotactic goals (e.g., "will produce fricatives in final position"), for this exercise write *purely phonotactic goals*. In other words, do not refer to specific articulatory or acoustic features or specific consonants or vowels in these goals. Write a rationale for each goal.
   Make` sure that your goals and objectives are measurable (written with behavioral verbs, with quantitative outcomes) and that the objectives are reasonably sized stepping stones toward the goals.
   Identify and justify at least two strategies that you might use to address these goals and objectives.
2. Jonah, a 7-year-old, has been denied school speech-language services because he has "reached age-appropriate articulatory developmental milestones" for his age; he produces all stops, nasals, glides, liquids (with a distorted /ɹ/), fricatives except interdentals (and distorted /s/), and affricates. Yet, he is unintelligible. Analyses of his spontaneous speech reveal that he produces few final consonants, clusters, or words of more than two syllables in length. Is his phonology actually age appropriate? What can be done to improve his intelligibility? Justify your answer using information from this chapter and other resources.

References

Berman, R. A. (1977). Natural phonological processes at the one-word stage. *Lingua, 43*, 1–21.

Bernhardt, B. (1994). Phonological intervention techniques for syllable and word structure development. *Clinics in Communication Disorders, 4*(1), 54–65.

Bernhardt, B. H., & Gilbert, J. (1992). Applying linguistic theory to speech-language pathology: The case for nonlinear phonology. *Clinical Linguistics and Phonetics, 6*(1–2), 123–145.

Bernhardt, B. H., Stemberger, J. P., & Major, E. (2006). General and nonlinear phonological intervention perspectives for a child with a resistant phonological impairment. *International Journal of Speech-Language Pathology, 8*(3), 190–206.

Bleile, K. M. (1995). *Manual of articulation and phonological disorders: Infancy through adulthood.* San Diego, CA: Singular.

Branigan, G. (1976). Syllable structure and the acquisition of consonants: The great conspiracy in word formation. *Journal of Psycholinguistics Research, 5*, 117–133.

Chin, S., & Dinnsen, D. (1992). Consonant clusters in disordered speech: Constraints and correspondence patterns. *Journal of Child Language, 19*, 259–285.

Davis, B. L., & MacNeilage, P. F. (1990). Acquisition of correct vowel production: A quantitative case study. *Journal of Speech and Hearing Research, 33*(1), 16–27.

Davis, B. L., & MacNeilage, P. F. (2000). On the origin of the internal structure of word forms. *Science, 288*, 527–531.

Davis, B., MacNeilage, P., & Matyear, C. L. (2002). Acquisition of serial complexity in speech production: A comparison of phonetic and phonological approaches to first word production. *Phonetica, 59*, 75–107.

Demuth, K. (1996). Alignment, stress and parsing in early phonological words. In B. Bernhardt, J. Gilbert, & D. Ingram (Eds.), *Proceedings of the International Conference on Phonological Acquisition* (pp. 113–124). Somerville, MA: Cascadilla Press.

Demuth, K., Culbertson, J., & Alter, J. (2006). Word-minimality, epenthesis, and coda licensing in the early acquisition of English. *Language and Speech, 49*(2), 137–174.

Demuth, K., & Fee, E. J. (1995). *Minimal words in early phonological development.* Providence, RI and Halifax, NS: Brown University and Dalhousie University. Unpublished Manuscript.

Dinnsen, D. A. (1996). Context effects in the acquisition of fricatives. In B. Bernhardt, J. Gilbert, & D. Ingram (Eds.), *Proceedings of the UBC International Conference on Phonological Acquisition* (pp. 136–148). Somerville, MA: Cascadilla Press.

Edwards, M. L. (1996). *Word position effects in the production of fricatives.* Paper presented at the UBC International Conference on Phonological Acquisition, Vancouver, BC.

Farwell, C. (1977). Some strategies in the early production of fricatives. *Papers and Reports in Child Language Development, 12*, 97–104.

Fee, E. J. (1996). Syllable structure and minimal words. In B. Bernhardt, J. Gilbert, & D. Ingram (Eds.), *Proceedings of the UBC International Conference on Phonological Acquisition* (pp. 85–98). Somerville, MA: Cascadilla Press.

Fey, M. E., & Gandour, J. (1982). Rule discovery in phonological acquisition. *Journal of Child Language, 9*(1), 71–81.

Fikkert, P. (1994). *On the acquisition of prosodic structure.* Dordrecht, The Netherlands: Holland Institute of Generative Linguistics.

Freitas, M. J. (1996). Onsets in early productions. In B. Bernhardt, J. Gilbert, & D. Ingram (Eds.), *Proceedings of the UBC International Conference on Phonological Acquisition* (pp. 76–84). Somerville, MA: Cascadilla Press.

Gerken, L. A., & Zamuner, T. (2004). *Exploring the basis for generalization in language acquisition.* Paper presented at the 9th Conference on Laboratory Phonology, University of Illinois at Urbana-Champaign.

Gierut, J. A., & Champion, A. H. (2001). Syllable onsets II: Three-element clusters in phonological treatment. *Journal of Speech, Language, and Hearing Research, 44*, 886–904.

Gildersleeve-Neumann, C., Davis, B. L., & MacNeilage, P. F. (2000). Contingencies governing the acquisition of fricatives, affricates, and liquids. *Applied Psycholinguistics, 21*, 341–363.

Gnanadesikan, A. E. (1996). Child phonology in optimality theory: Ranking markedness and faithfulness constraints. In A. Stringfellow, D. Cahana-Amitay, E. Hughes, & A. Zukowski (Eds.), *Proceedings of the 20th annual Boston University Conference on Language Development* (Vol. 1, pp. 237–248). Somerville, MA: Cascadilla Press.

Goffman, L., Gerken, L. A., & Lucchesi, J. (2007). Relations between segmental and motor variability in prosodically complex nonword sequences. *Journal of Speech, Language, and Hearing Research, 50*, 444–458.

Grunwell, P. (1981). *The nature of phonological disability in children.* London, UK: Academic Press.

Grunwell, P. (1982). *Clinical phonology.* Rockville, MD: Aspen.

Grunwell, P. (1985). *Phonological Assessment of Child Speech (PACS).* Scarborough, ON: Nelson Thomson Learning.

Grunwell, P. (1997). Developmental phonological disability: Order in disorder. In B. W. Hodson & M. L. Edwards (Eds.), *Perspectives in applied phonology* (pp. 61–103). Gaithersburg, MD: Aspen.

Hayden, D. (2006). The PROMPT model: Use and application for children with mixed phonological-motor impairment. *International Journal of Speech-Language Pathology, 8*(3), 265–281.

Hodson, B. W., & Paden, E. P. (1981). Phonological processes which characterize unintelligible and intelligible speech in early childhood. *Journal of Speech and Hearing Disorders, 46*(4), 369–373.

Howard, S. (2004). Connected speech processes in developmental speech impairment: Observations from an electropalatographic perspective. *Clinical Linguistics and Phonetics, 18*, 407–417.

Howard, S. (2007). English speech acquisition. In S. McLeod (Ed.), *The international guide to speech acquisition* (pp. 188–203). Clifton Park, NY: Thomson Delmar Learning.

Ingram, D. (1974). Fronting in child phonology. *Journal of Child Language, 1*, 233–241.

Ingram, D. (1976). *Phonological disability in children*. New York, NY: Elsevier North Holland, Inc.

Ingram, D. (1978). The role of the syllable in phonological development. In A. Bell & J. B. Hooper (Eds.), *Syllables and segments* (pp. 143–155). Amsterdam, The Netherlands: North Holland.

Ingram, D (1981). *Procedures for the phonological analysis of children's language*. Baltimore, MD: University Park Press.

Ingram, D. (1989). *Phonological disability in children* (2nd ed.). London, UK: Cole and Whurr Ltd.

Jacks, A., Marquardt, T. P., & Davis, B. L. (2006). Consonant and syllable structure patterns in childhood apraxia of speech: Developmental change in three children. *Journal of Communication Disorders, 39*, 424–441.

Jakielski, K. J. (2000). *Quantifying phonetic complexity in words: An experimental index*. Paper presented at the International Child Phonology Conference, University of Northern Iowa, Cedar Falls, IA.

Kaufman, N. (1995). *Kaufman speech praxis test for children*. Detroit, MI: Wayne State University Press.

Kaufman, N. (1998). *Speech praxis treatment kit for children*. Gaylord, MI: Northern Speech Services, Inc.

Kaufman, N. (2001). *Speech praxis treatment kit for children—2*. Gaylord, MI: Northern Speech Services, Inc.

Kehoe, M. M., & Stoel-Gammon, C. (2001). Development of syllable structure in English-speaking children with particular reference to rhymes. *Journal of Child Language, 28*(2), 393–432.

Kern, S., & Davis, B. L. (2009). Emergent complexity in vocal acquisition: Cross-linguistic comparisons of canonical babbling. In I. Chirotan, C. Coupe, E. Marisco, & F. Pellegrino (Eds.), *Approaches to phonological complexity*. Berlin, Germany: Mouton de Gruyter.

Kirk, C., & Demuth, K. (2003). Coda/onset asymmetries in the acquisition of clusters. In B. Beachley, A. Brown, & F. Conlin (Eds.), *Proceedings of the 27th Boston University Conference on Language Development* (pp. 437–448). Somerville, MA: Cascadilla Press.

Kirk, C., & Demuth, K. (2005). Asymmetries in the acquisition of word-initial and word-final consonant clusters. *Journal of Child Language, 32*, 709–734.

Kirkpatrick, J., Stohr, P., & Kimbrough, D. (1990). *Moving across syllables*. Tucson, AZ: Communication Skill Builders.

Klein, H. B., & Liu-Shea, M. (2009). Between-word simplification patterns in the continuous speech of children with speech sound disorders. *Language, Speech, and Hearing Services in the Schools, 40*(1), 17–30.

Klopfenstein, M., & Ball, M. J. (2010). An analysis of the sonority hypothesis and cluster realization in a child with phonological disorder. *Clinical Linguistics & Phonetics, 24*(4–5), 261–270.

Leonard, L. B., & McGregor, K. K. (1991). Unusual phonological patterns and their underlying representations: A case study. *Journal of Child Language, 18*(2), 261–272.

Leonard, L. B., Miller, J. A., & Brown, H. (1980). Consonant and syllable harmony in the speech of language-disordered children. *Journal of Speech and Hearing Disorders, 45*, 336–345.

Levelt, W. J. M. (1992). Accessing words in speech production: Stages, processes and representations. *Cognition, 42*(1–3), 1–22.

Levelt, C., Schiller, N., & Levelt, W. (2000). The acquisition of syllable types. *Language Acquisition, 8*(3), 237–264.

Lleó, C. (1990). Homonymy and reduplication: On the extended availability of two strategies in phonological acquisition. *Journal of Child Language, 17*(2), 267–278.

Lleó, C. (1996). To spread or not to spread: Different styles in the acquisition of Spanish phonology. In B. Bernhardt, J. Gilbert, & D. Ingram (Eds.), *Proceedings of the UBC International Conference on Phonological Acquisition* (pp. 215–228). Somerville, MA: Cascadilla Press.

Lleó, C., & Demuth, K. (1999). Prosodic constraints on the emergence of grammatical morphemes: Crosslinguistic evidence from Germanic and Romance languages. In A. Greenhill, H. Littlefield, & C. Tano (Eds.), *Proceedings of the 23rd Annual Boston University Conference on Language Development* (Vol. 2, pp. 407–418). Boston, MA: Cascadilla Press.

Lleó, C., & Prinz, M. (1996). Consonant clusters in child phonology and the directionality of syllable structure assignment. *Journal of Child Language, 23*(1), 31–56.

Lukaszewicz, B. (2007). Reduction in syllable onsets in the acquisition of Polish: Deletion, coalescence, metathesis, and gemination. *Journal of Child Language, 34*, 53–82.

Macken, M. A. (1978). Permitted complexity in phonological development: One child's acquisition of Spanish consonants. *Lingua, 44*(2/3), 219–253.

Macken, M. A. (1996). Prosodic constraints on features. In B. Bernhardt, J. Gilbert & D. Ingram (Eds.), *Proceedings of the UBC International Conference on Phonological Acquisition* (pp. 159–172). Somerville, MA: Cascadilla Press.

MacNeilage, P. F., & Davis, B. L. (2000). On the origin of internal structure of word forms. *Science, 288*, 527–531.

McLeod, S., Hand, L., Rosenthal, J. B., & Hayes, B. (1994). The effect of sampling condition on children's productions of consonant clusters. *Journal of Speech and Hearing Research, 37*, 868–882.

McLeod, S., van Doorn, J., & Reed, V. A. (1997). Realizations of consonant clusters by children with phonological impairment. *Clinical Linguistics & Phonetics, 11*(2), 85–113.

McLeod, S., van Doorn, J., & Reed, V. A. (2001a). Consonant cluster development in two-year-olds: General trends and individual difference. *Journal of Speech, Language, and Hearing Research, 44*, 1144–1171.

McLeod, S., van Doorn, J., & Reed, V. A. (2001b). Normal acquisition of consonant clusters. *American Journal of Speech-Language Pathology, 10*, 99–110.

Menn, L. (1978). Phonological units in beginning speech. In A. Bell & J. B. Hooper (Eds.), *Syllables and segments* (pp. 157–171). Amsterdam, The Netherlands: North-Holland Publishing Co.

Morgan, J. L. (1996). A rhythmic bias in preverbal speech segmentation. *Journal of Memory and Language, 35*, 666–688.

Murray, E., McCabe, P., & Ballard, K. J. (2012). A comparison of two treatments for childhood apraxia of speech: Methods and treatment protocol for a parallel group randomised control trial. *BMC Pediatrics, 12*, 112–121.

Nuffield Centre (2004). *Nuffield Centre Dyspraxia Programme* (3rd ed.). Windsor, UK: The Miracle Factory. http:\\www.ndp2004.org

Pater, J., & Barlow, J. A. (2003). Constraint conflict in cluster reduction. *Journal of Child Language, 30*(3), 487–526.

Pollock, K. E., & Hall, P. K. (1991). An analysis of the vowel misarticulations of five children with developmental apraxia of speech. *Clinical Linguistics and Phonetics, 5*(3), 207–224.

Pollock, K. E., & Keiser, N. J. (1990). An examination of vowel errors in phonologically disordered children. *Clinical Linguistics and Phonetics, 4*(2), 161–178.

Priestly, T. M. S. (1977). One idiosyncratic strategy in the acquisition of phonology. *Journal of Child Language, 4*(1), 45–66.

Redford, M. A., & Gildersleeve-Neumann, C. (2009). The development of distinct speaking styles in preschool children. *Journal of Speech, Language, and Hearing Research, 52*(1434–1448).

Rupela, V., & Manjula, R. (2006). Phonotactic development in Kannada: Some aspects and future directions. *Language Forum: A Journal of Language and Literature, 32*(1–2), 83–93.

Schwartz, R. G., & Goffman, L. (1995). Metrical patterns of words and production accuracy. *Journal of Speech and Hearing Research, 38*(4), 876–888.

Schwartz, R. G., Leonard, L. B., Wilcox, M. J., & Folger, M. K. (1980). Again and again: Reduplication in child phonology. *Journal of Child Language, 7*(1), 75–87.

Secord, W. A., & Shine, R. E. (1997). *Secord Contextual Articulation Tests (S-CAT)*. Sedona, AZ: Red Rock Educational Publications.

Smit, A. B., Hand, L., Freilinger, J. J., Bernthal, J. E., & Bird, A. (1990). The Iowa articulation norms project and its Nebraska replication. *Journal of Speech and Hearing Disorders, 55*(4), 779–798.

Smith, N. V. (1973). *The Acquisition of phonology: A case study*. Cambridge, UK: Cambridge University Press.

Smith, B. L., Brown-Sweeney, S., & Stoel-Gammon, C. (1989). A quantitative analysis of reduplicated and variegated babbling. *First Language, 9*, 175–190.

Stemberger, J. P. (1988). Between-word processes in child phonology. *Journal of Child Language, 15*(1), 39–61.

Stemberger, J. P. (1993). *Default onsets and constraints in language acquisition*. Minneapolis, MN: University of Minnesota. Unpublished Manuscript.

Stoel-Gammon, C. (1983). Constraints on consonant-vowel sequences in early words. *Journal of Child Language, 10*(2), 455–457.

Stoel-Gammon, C. (1984). Phonological variability in mother-child speech. *Phonetica, 41*, 208–214.

Stoel-Gammon, C. (1987). Phonological skills of 2-year-olds. *Language Speech and Hearing Services in the Schools, 18*, 323–329.

Stoel-Gammon, C. (1989). Prespeech and early speech development of two late talkers. *First Language, 9*, 207–224.

Stoel-Gammon, C. (1996). On the acquisition of velars in English. In B. Bernhardt, J. Gilbert, & D. Ingram (Eds.), *Proceedings of the UBC International Conference of Phonological Acquisition* (pp. 201–214). Somerville, MA: Cascadilla Press.

Stoel-Gammon, C. (2010). The Word Complexity Measure: Description and application to developmental phonology and disorders. *Clinical Linguistics and Phonetics, 24*(4–5), 271–282.

Stoel-Gammon, C., & Stone, J. R. (1991). Assessing phonology in young children. *Clinics in Communication Disorders, 1*(2), 25–39.

Storkel, H. L. (2001). Learning new words: Phonotactic probability in language development. *Journal of Speech, Language, and Hearing Research, 44*, 1321–1337.

Storkel, H. L. (2003). Learning new words II: Phonotactic probability in verb learning. *Journal of Speech, Language, and Hearing Research, 46*(6), 1312–1337.

Storkel, H. L. (2004). The emerging lexicon of children with phonological delays: Phonotactic constraints and probability in acquisition. *Journal of Speech, Language, and Hearing Research, 47*, 1194–1212.

Strand, E. A., & Skinder, A. (1999). Treatment of developmental apraxia of speech: Integral stimulation methods. In A. J. Caruso & E. A. Strand (Eds.), *Clinical management of motor speech disorders in children* (pp. 109–148). New York, NY: Thieme.

Velleman, S. L. (1994). The interaction of phonetics and phonology in developmental verbal dyspraxia: Two case studies. *Clinics in Communication Disorders, 4*(1), 67–78.

Velleman, S. L. (1996). Metathesis highlights feature-by-position constraints. In B. Bernhardt, J. Gilbert, & D. Ingram (Eds.), *Proceedings of the UBC International Conference on Phonological Acquisition* (pp. 173–186). Somerville, MA: Cascadilla Press.

Velleman, S. L. (2003a). *Resource guide for childhood apraxia of speech*. Florence, KY: Cengage.

Velleman, S. L. (2003b). VMPAC and PEPS-C: Effective new tools for differential diagnosis? In L. D. Shriberg & T. F. Campbell (Eds.), *Proceedings of the 2002 Childhood Apraxia of Speech Research Symposium* (pp. 81–88). Carlsbad, CA: The Hendrix Foundation.

Velleman, S. L., & Shriberg, L. D. (1999). Metrical analysis of the speech of children with suspected developmental apraxia of speech and inappropriate stress. *Journal of Speech Language and Hearing Research, 42*(6), 1444–1460.

Velleman, S. L., & Vihman, M. M. (2002a). The emergence of the marked unfaithful. In A. Carpenter, A. Coetzee, & P. De Lacy (Eds.), *University of Massachusetts Occasional Papers in Linguistics, 26: Papers in Optimality Theory II* (pp. 397–419). Amherst, MA: GLSA.

Velleman, S. L., & Vihman, M. M. (2002b). Whole-word phonology and templates: Trap, bootstrap, or some of each? *Language, Speech, and Hearing Services in the Schools, 33*, 9–23.

Vihman, M. M. (1978). Consonant harmony: Its scope and function in child language. In J. H. Greenberg (Ed.), *Universals of human language* (Vol. 2, pp. 281–334). Stanford, CA: Stanford University Press.

Vihman, M. M. (1992). Early syllables and the construction of phonology. In C. A. Ferguson, L. Menn, & C. Stoel-Gammon (Eds.), *Phonological development: Models, research, implications* (pp. 393–422). Timonium, MD: York Press.

Vihman, M. M. (1993). Variable paths to early word production. *Journal of Phonetics, 21*, 61–82.

Vihman, M. M., & Croft, W. (2007). Phonological development: Towards a "radical" templatic phonology. *Linguistics, 45*(4), 683–725.

Vihman, M. M., Nakai, S., & DePaolis, R. A. (2006). Getting the rhythm right: A cross-linguistic study of segmental duration in babbling and first words. In L. Goldstein, D. Whalen & C. Best (Eds.), *Laboratory Phonology 8* (pp. 341–366). New York, NY: Mouton de Gruyter.

Vihman, M. M., & Velleman, S. L. (1989). Phonological reorganization: A case study. *Language and Speech, 32*, 149–170.

Vihman, M. M., & Velleman, S. L. (2000a). The construction of a first phonology. *Phonetica, 57*, 255–266.

Vihman, M. M., & Velleman, S. L. (2000b). Phonetics and the origins of phonology. In N. Burton-Roberts, P. Carr & G. Docherty (Eds.), *Conceptual and empirical foundations of phonology* (pp. 305–339). Oxford, UK: Oxford University Press.

Waterson, N. (1971). Child phonology: A prosodic view. *Journal of Linguistics, 7*, 179–211.

Weiner, F. (1981). Treatment of phonological disability using the method of meaningful minimal contrast: Two case studies. *Journal of Speech and Hearing Disorders, 46*, 97–103.

Williams, A. L., & Dinnsen, D, A. (1987). A problem of allophonic variation in a speech disordered child. *Innovations in Linguistics Education, 5*, 85–90.

Zamuner, T. S., Gerken, L. A., & Hammond, M. (2004). Phonotactic probabilities in young children's speech production. *Journal of Child Language, 31*, 515–536.

CHAPTER 9

Phonological Patterns

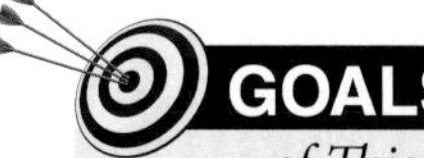

GOALS

of This Chapter

1. Review and critique three theoretical approaches to analyzing phonological patterns in human speech as they apply to child speech sound development and disorders.
2. Describe indepe*dent and relational approaches to assessing error patterns in children's speech.
3. Describe evidence-based treatment approaches to treating error patterns in children's speech.

Wally substitutes p/f, t/θ, t/s, t/ʃ, b/v, d/ð, d/z, d/ʒ[1] *in initial position. He omits /f, s/ from clusters in all word positions. His sleep-language pathologist (SLP) is overwhelmed by the number of goals she will have to address! Isn't there a more efficient way to handle this?*

INTRODUCTION

Research and intuition have confirmed that assessment and intervention of speech sound disorders can be far more efficacious if errors are viewed and treated as patterns rather than as isolated substitutions, omissions, or movements. As discussed in Chapter 2, there are three major perspectives on phonological patterns: rules, processes, and constraints. All three of these approaches reflect the goal of identifying broader patterns within the child's speech. Classes of sounds are examined as well as specific segments; classes of word positions (e.g., syllable final, word initial) are examined as well as specific environments (e.g., following [f]). These strategies facilitate our descriptions of the child's production (and misproduction) of the language. Although there are theoretical differences among the approaches, from a practical standpoint, all three serve this same purpose. Each has both advantages and disadvantages as a means of assessing a child's phonology. The best solution may be to understand all three and use each as appropriate to the specific situation.

In this chapter, the theoretical background, guiding principles, and clinical implications of each of these approaches will be reviewed as they apply to child phonology. Then, relationships among these pattern types will be described using specific clinical examples. Assessment and intervention strategies for each will be presented.

[1]Note that "x/y" is used here, as is common in clinical practice, to indicate that [x] is substituted for /y/.

PHONOLOGICAL PATTERN TYPES

Generative Phonology: Rules

Overview

As reviewed in Chapter 2, generative phonological rules are systematic statements about relationships among phonological elements at different phonological levels. The starting point of the analysis is the underlying mental representation of the word, which is assumed to be the target (but recall from Chapter 7 that this is not always the case). The actual production of the word (the "surface representation") often differs from the mental representation, typically (though not always) in a systematic manner. Some of these alterations are assumed to be phonetically based. In other words, they are seen as articulatory (physiologic) rather than linguistic or cognitive. Other rules are viewed as more abstract linguistic patterns that each language (or speaker) may or may not choose to implement. All share the mutual goals of describing a person's phonological behavior both as generally as possible (referring, for example, to classes of sounds rather than individual phonemes or phones) and as specifically as appropriate (such as identifying particular contexts in which an error occurs).

The assessment and intervention tools that were generated in response to generative phonology focused on identifying and treating errors based on the features that characterize natural classes of sounds (such as continuance, which differentiates stops from fricatives). These tools are no longer in use. Nonetheless, it can be helpful to organize our analyses in these terms by asking oneself:

1. What is the target?
2. What was actually produced?
3. What is the difference between the target and the production (i.e., what is the change)?
4. Under what conditions (in what environments) does this change occur?
5. Are there generalizations that I can make about broader categories of targets, broader categories of changes, or broader categories of contexts?

In rule format, one could write:

$$/\text{target sound or sound class}/ \rightarrow \left[\text{changes}\right] / \text{ in a certain environment or type of environment}$$

Consonant and vowel features and word positions are specified as generally as possible (to indicate, for example, that all fricatives are affected in the same way) but as specifically as necessary (e.g., that the change only occurs after a vowel in final position). Recall the symbols that are used to represent word positions: "#" is used for the edge of a word and "__" for the position of the target sound. Consonant and vowel features are used to describe groups of sounds that share certain characteristics. Thus:

#___ refers to initial position

___# refers to final position

V___V refers to intervocalic/medial position (which is typically syllable initial in English)

#C__ refers to the second element of an initial cluster

__C# refers to the first element of a final cluster

$\#\begin{bmatrix}+\text{ consonantal}\\ +\text{ voice}\end{bmatrix}\begin{bmatrix}+\text{ vocalic}\\ +\text{ tense}\end{bmatrix}$ refers to an initial voiced consonant that precedes a tense vowel, and so on

The commonly used sets of features presented in chapters two and seven are repeated here (in Tables 9-1 and 9-2) for convenience.

For example, since Wally (from the opening case study) produces fricatives as stops in initial position, one could write:

$$\begin{bmatrix}+\text{continuant}\\ -\text{sonorant}\end{bmatrix} \rightarrow [-\text{continuant}] / \#\_\_\_\_$$

Thus, the class of sounds—fricatives, which are continuant but not sonorant—is specified as generally as possible but not more; this pattern does not apply to all consonants, for instance. The use of phonological features (continuant, voiced, front, round, etc.) is critical to achieving the appropriate level of generality. The same is true of the change: only the continuance of the sounds is in error, not any of their other features. Neither voicing nor place of articulation changes in this case (with the exception of some minor place shifts to the closest stop place of articulation). Finally, this pattern always applies in word-initial position but not elsewhere. In sum, this simple rule is both more precise and more general

TABLE 9-1 Feature Specifications for American English Consonants

	p	b	f	v	m	t	d	θ	ð	n	s	z	tʃ	dʒ	ʃ	ʒ	k	g	ŋ	ɹ	l	h	w	j
Syllabic	−	−	−	−	−	−	−	−	−	−	−	−	−	−	−	−	−	−	−	−	−	−	−	−
Consonantal	+	+	+	+	+	+	+	+	+	+	+	+	+	+	+	+	+	+	+	+	+	+	−	−
Sonorant	−	−	−	−	+	−	−	−	−	+	−	−	−	−	−	−	−	−	+	+	+	−	+	+
Nasal	−	−	−	−	+	−	−	−	−	+	−	−	−	−	−	−	−	−	+	−	−	−	−	−
Continuant	−	−	+	+	−	−	−	+	+	−	+	+	−/+	−/+	+	+	−	−	−	+	+	+	+	+
Anterior	+	+	+	+	+	+	+	+	+	+	+	+	−	−	−	−	−	−	−	−	+	−	+	−
Coronal	−	−	−	−	−	+	+	+	+	+	+	+	+	+	+	+	−	−	−	+	+	−	−	+
Strident	−	−	−	−	−	−	−	−	−	−	+	+	+	+	+	+	−	−	−	−	−	−	−	−
Back	−	−	−	−	−	−	−	−	−	−	−	−	−	−	−	−	+	+	+	−	−	−	+	−
High	−	−	−	−	−	−	−	−	−	−	−	−	+	+	+	+	+	+	+	+	−	−	+	+
Low	−	−	−	−	−	−	−	−	−	−	−	−	−	−	−	−	−	−	−	−	−	+	−	−
Voice	−	+	−	+	+	−	+	−	+	+	−	+	−	+	−	+	−	+	+	+	+	−	+	+

TABLE 9-2 Feature Specifications for American English Vowels

	i	ɪ	e	ɛ	æ	ʌ/ə	u	ʊ	o	ɔ	ɑ
Syllabic	+	+	+	+	+	+	+	+	+	+	+
Consonantal	–	–	–	–	–	–	–	–	–	–	–
Sonorant	+	+	+	+	+	+	+	+	+	+	+
Tense	+	–	+	–	–	–	+	–	+	–	–
High	+	+	–	–	–	–	+	+	–	–	–
Low	–	–	–	–	+	–	–	–	–	–	+
Front	+	+	+	+	+	–	–	–	–	–	–
Back	–	–	–	–	–	–	+	+	+	+	+
Round	–	–	–	–	–	–	+	+	+	+	–

Based on Chomsky, N., & Halle, M. (1968). *The sound pattern of English*. New York, NY: Harper & Row.

than the list of Wally's substitutions with which this chapter began: p/f, t/θ, t/s, t/ʃ, b/v, d/ð, d/z, d/ʒ. Furthermore, Wally's SLP now has one goal: teach Wally to produce continuant consonants in initial position. This feels far more achievable.

Clinical Implications

The most critical impact of generative phonology on clinical practice was the new emphasis placed on sound classes, on sound changes, and on phonological environments. A simple table can be made to keep track of these during the phonological analysis process:

Sound/Sound Class	Change	Environment
Affected elements	*Feature difference*	*Position, surrounding sounds*

The difference that was made by this approach at the segmental level can be highlighted using another example. Consider the data from the hypothetical child called Nathan in Table 9-3.

A traditional substitution analysis would yield an extremely long list of consonant substitutions. Based upon these few data only, the report would look something like this:

Initial position: d/b, d/p, d/t, d/k, n/m, d/f, d/s, d/ʃ

Medial position: d/g, d/k, d/s, d/t, d/θ, n/m

Final position: d/g, n/ŋ, d/ɹ

Clusters: d/stɹ-, d/bl-, d/-sk-, n/-nst-, d/-ɹst

This is not very satisfying; it doesn't give us a good sense of what is going on here. It just seems like a big mess. Grouping these substitutions into sound classes in order to write phonological rules is far more helpful:

- All (presumed[2]) target non-nasal consonants are changed to (pronounced as) [d].
- All (presumed) target nasals become [n].

[2]We assume that Nathan is aware of the correct target phoneme, but of course, this may or may not be the case.

TABLE 9-3 Nathan's Use of [d] and [n]

doggie	[dɔdi]
cookie	[dʊdi]
go	[do]
Mom	[nɑn]
more	[nod]
no	[no]
butter	[dʌdʌd]
bye	[dɑɪ]
pig	[dɪd]
shoe	[du]
feather	[dɛdʊd]
sing	[dɪn]
string	[dɪn]
blue	[du]
basket	[dædæ]
monster	[nʌnʌd]
first	[dɪd]

These patterns could be written in rule format as follows:

[-nasal] → [d]

[+nasal] → [n]

Or they could be written in a phonological rule table as shown in Table 9-4. It is not really necessary to specify the environment in this case because this change occurs in all syllable and word positions; the use of the word "everywhere" makes this explicit.

However, a consideration of the features involved leads to the realization that Nathan produces all consonants, regardless of their place of articulation in the adult word, at the alveolar place of articulation. Both [d] and [n] share the place of articulation [+alveolar] (or, more precisely, $\begin{bmatrix}+\text{anterior}\\+\text{coronal}\end{bmatrix}$), and both are considered to be stops ([-continuant]) because the air is stopped in the oral cavity (even though it continues to flow through the nasal cavity, in the case of the nasals). The child does not change nasality features ([-nasal] or [+nasal]). In fact, nasality is the only feature distinction that Nathan consistently maintains. When the adult consonant is nasal, Nathan always produces a nasal; when the target is oral, so is his production. Thus, nasality is not actually relevant to

TABLE 9-4 Phonological Rule Table for Nathan

Sound/Sound Class	Change	Environment
Any non-nasal C	d	*Everywhere*
Any nasal C	n	*Everywhere*

the rule, since it doesn't change. However, all consonants become voiced regardless of their voicing in adult English. With this insight, the rule can be written as follows:

$$\begin{bmatrix}+\text{consonantal}\end{bmatrix} \rightarrow \begin{bmatrix}+\text{anterior}\\+\text{coronal}\\-\text{continuant}\\+\text{voice}\end{bmatrix}$$

or described in the rule table as:

Sound/Sound Class	Change	Environment
Any C	*Noncontinuant voiced alveolar*	*Everywhere*

That is, Nathan produces all consonants as voiced alveolar (nasal *or* oral) stops, in all positions, regardless of surrounding sounds.

Thus, phonological rules can enhance our understanding of sound classes as they are affected by sound changes in certain environments.

Smith's (1973) case of consonant–vowel assimilation later in phonological development, shown in Table 9-5, is another case in point. Smith's son's phonology included a rule of vowelization of final [l]: Amahl ([ˈæməl]) pronounced lateral liquids (i.e., /l/) in final position as [u]. Recall that final [l] is typically velarized or "dark," produced with the tongue backed in a fashion that is more similar to the production of [u]. Thus, this could have been the result either of a misperception of the dark [l] as a vowel or of an inability to produce this vowel-like liquid accurately. In Amahl's speech, alveolars became velar (i.e., back) before the resulting [u]s. This was likely a physiologically based change; [u] is a back vowel, so the consonant assimilated to it. This could have looked like backing (substitution of velars for alveolars), but alveolars remained alveolar in all other contexts. Without considering the effect of the vowels, there would be no way to explain why this velarization of alveolars only happened before [u] and not in other word-medial environments.

Clearly, these alveolar consonants were affected by the place of articulation of the following vowels. The list of sound changes would be as shown in Table 9-6. They could be written in rule format as shown below Table 9-6.

TABLE 9-5 Amahl's Consonant–Vowel Interactions

pedal	[bɛgu]	lazy	[de:di:]
beetle	[bi:gu]	horses	[ɔ:tid]
bottle	[bɔgu]	sometimes	[fʌmtaɪmd]

From Smith, N. V. (1973). *The acquisition of phonology: A case study.* Cambridge, UK: Cambridge University Press.

TABLE 9-6 Phonological Rule Table for Amahl

Sound/Sound Class	Change	Environment
l	u	*Final position*
Alveolar	*Velar (back)*	*Before* [u] *(back vowel)*

From Smith, N. V. (1973). *The acquisition of phonology: A case study.* Cambridge, UK: Cambridge University Press.

$$1.\ \begin{bmatrix}+\text{sonorant}\\+\text{continuant}\\+\text{anterior}\\+\text{coronal}\end{bmatrix} \rightarrow \begin{bmatrix}+\text{vocalic}\\+\text{tense}\\+\text{high}\\+\text{round}\end{bmatrix} /\ \_\_\#$$

$$2.\ \begin{bmatrix}+\text{anterior}\\+\text{coronal}\end{bmatrix} \rightarrow \begin{bmatrix}-\text{anterior}\\-\text{coronal}\\+\text{back}\end{bmatrix} /\ \_\_ \begin{bmatrix}+\text{vocalic}\\+\text{tense}\\+\text{high}\\+\text{round}\end{bmatrix}$$

Note that the rules must be applied in the order in which they are listed. If /l/ had not (yet) changed to [u], then the second rule would not be applicable because its environment (__[u]) would not be present.

Limitations of the Theory

One disadvantage of generative phonology was that it did not facilitate the description of rules affecting an entire syllable, word, or phrase. As described in Chapter 8, such phonotactic patterns are common in the speech of young children and children with SSD. Furthermore, the long lists of features to be remembered and the detailed, abstract notation that gradually developed as the theory of generative phonology was elaborated often seemed way too cumbersome to speech-language pathologists. They wanted an easier way to capture the same generalizations without writing phonological rules. "Natural phonology" provided such a shortcut.

Summary

Generative phonology had an important impact on child phonological theory and also on child phonological intervention. It called attention to the importance of looking for patterns affecting classes of sounds in a systematic manner. Analyses focused on the target sound class, the change (i.e., the features of the sounds that were different when the words were actually pronounced), and the phonetic environments in which the change occurred. However, phonotactic patterns were awkward to describe or explain within this theory. Furthermore, the abstractions and the notational conventions that went along with the theory were not a comfortable fit for clinical practice.

EXERCISE 9-1

Generative Phonology

Natural Phonology: Processes

Overview

As discussed in Chapter 2, the primary insight of natural phonology (Donegan & Stampe, 1979; Stampe, 1972) was the universal phonetic bases of phonology. Proponents of this theory proposed that all phonological patterns—called natural phonological processes in the researchers' model—reflect human physiologic limitations on speech production. For example, the physical difficulty of producing three consonants in a row leads to the tendency among humans to reduce lengthy clusters. This natural process of cluster reduction is seen in the speech of children learning languages such as German and English. Adult speakers of these languages have learned to suppress this process (i.e., to produce such clusters despite their difficulty). Some languages, such as Japanese, avoid temptation by excluding these difficult sequences altogether. In these languages, the cluster reduction process doesn't have to be suppressed because speakers don't have to learn to produce clusters. Thus, each child has to learn to suppress those processes that are not permitted to apply in her language. If the language has many clusters (e.g., German), she must suppress the process of cluster reduction. If the language has many multisyllabic words (e.g., Japanese), she must suppress syllable deletion, and so on. In many cases, the process doesn't have to be completely suppressed. For example, English speakers still do reduce some very long clusters (e.g., we typically omit at least some of the consonants in the phrase "next stop" [nɛ**kst** **st**ɑp]) even though English has a variety of clusters in all positions.

Clinical Implications

From a practical clinical standpoint, the theory of natural phonology provided convenient labels for many of the phonological rules that had been noted in the speech of young TD children and children with SSD. Phonological processes are far easier to refer to either in writing or aloud than are generative rules. As a result, a certain basic set of processes came to be known and agreed upon by most people. However, the principles of the theory—especially the principle of phonetic naturalness—have not always been adhered to. It is just as easy to give process names to phonological rules that do not occur in any language as it is to those that are physiologically "natural." In addition, names that are too general can be confusing. For example, does "backing" refer to producing *any* consonant farther back in the oral cavity (e.g., producing /f/ as [s]) or specifically to producing alveolars as velars? So-called deviant (non-natural) processes have proliferated, and they are not necessarily either phonetically natural or in keeping with universal tendencies.

Some proponents of the theory have attempted to maintain the theoretical rigor of Stampe's original proposal by arguing for a specific set of natural processes and a strict order of naturalness. They suggested that each of the child's error productions should be assigned to one of a small set of only the most natural or basic processes with a predetermined hierarchy of naturalness. The problem with this approach is that different children appear to have different tendencies, many of which are not in keeping with the proposed hierarchies. For example, one child might say [dɔdi] for "doggie" due to consonant harmony while another mispronounces it in the same way due to velar fronting. Thus, categorizing errors in such a rigid manner could result in a loss of insight into some children's speech. Also, many children demonstrate patterns that cannot be described using such a small set of processes (e.g., backing, voicing changes, glottal replacement, and reduplication).

Whatever their viewpoints, most developers of process tests or analyses agree in dividing processes into certain basic types, often referred to as syllable structure processes, assimilation processes, and substitution processes. These are described below.

Syllable Structure Processes

Syllable structure processes are those that affect the shape of the word or the syllable. In other words, they are phonotactic patterns. As such, these processes represent many of the patterns discussed in Chapter 8. Many of these processes result in a reduction in the number of elements within a syllable or word. They include the following:

1. Syllable reduction (also known as unstressed syllable deletion or weak syllable deletion): This process refers to the omission of a syllable that is present in the adult form of the word. As discussed in greater depth in Chapter 10, often the omitted syllable is unstressed, especially in sequences of a weak syllable followed by a strong one (i.e., in iambic words). Of course, in most cases, it is difficult to know for sure whether this syllable is included within the child's underlying representation of the word. Because unstressed syllables have lower salience, some children may not be processing them perceptually as relevant linguistic units. In other words, the child may be ignoring the unstressed syllables because they are not prominent acoustically. Therefore, the term "deletion" may not always be appropriate. The more neutral "omission" may be a more fitting term. In any case, one or more syllables of the adult word form are missing in the productions of children who use syllable reduction.
2. Final consonant deletion: This process occurs when the final consonant of a word is not produced. As noted in Chapter 8, it is sometimes difficult to determine whether the child is unaware of the segment or is aware of the segment but does not produce it. It is important for the clinician to differentiate between words that actually lack a final consonant altogether (e.g., [bʊ] for "book") versus those in which the final consonant has

been glottalized (e.g., [bʊʔ] for "book") or marked in some other way (e.g., with vowel lengthening). In the latter case, the child is demonstrating awareness that the word has a coda, even if he does not know the identity of or perhaps simply cannot produce that particular final consonant. Of course, in many dialects of American English, final /t/ is routinely glottalized; in African American English, this impacts /d/ and sometimes non-alveolars as well.

3. Initial consonant deletion: This process occurs when the initial consonant of a word is not produced. As discussed in Chapter 8, initial consonant deletion is generally considered a "red flag" atypical process for children learning English as a first language; it is one that is neither phonetically natural nor in keeping with phonological universals. Many languages have constraints against word-initial vowels; they require words to begin with consonants. There is no known language that requires words to begin with vowels, as children with initial consonant deletion appear to do. However, recall that children learning languages with geminate medial consonants (Japanese, Finnish) or with word-final stress (French) may demonstrate initial consonant deletion even though they are typically developing (Vihman & Velleman, 2000a, 2000b).
4. Consonant cluster reduction: Consonant cluster reduction involves production of fewer consecutive consonants than are present in the adult form of the word. In some cases, none of the consonants may be produced; in others, two out of three or one out of two may be preserved. Further details about which consonants are most likely to be preserved and at what ages are provided in Chapter 8.
5. Coalescence: As discussed in Chapter 8, coalescence is an alternative strategy for children who have difficulty with clusters. It consists of preserving one or more of the features of each consonant in a cluster, merging these features into one distinct consonant. A common example (illustrated with data from Martin in Chapter 8) is the combination of frication from the [s] and labialization from the [w] in an sw- cluster into a single [f], yielding [fɪmɪŋ] for "swimming," [fit] for "sweet," and so on. When this process occurs, it can sometimes be further generalized by the child, who then produces [f] for a variety of other consonant clusters that may not share features with [f].

   In some cases, coalescence may affect syllables. For example, a child who produces [ˈbænə] for "banana" (/bəˈnænə/) has coalesced the first two syllables of the word, preserving the onset consonant of the first syllable and the vowel of the second.
6. Metathesis, migration: These processes involve movement of elements from their locations within the adult word. In metathesis, elements are interchanged (as in [ækst] for "asked" or [gʌbi] for "buggy"). In migration, one element moves elsewhere, usually due to distribution requirements (as in [nos] for "snow"). One typically developing child who exhibited this process, reported by Leonard and McGregor (1991), was discussed in Chapter 8. She consistently put initial fricative sounds in final position, even when this resulted in final consonant clusters, as shown in Table 9-7 (repeated from Table 8.4).

   Fricatives migrated to final position, apparently to avoid appearing in initial position. Note that this resulted not only in the child unnecessarily producing clusters—which are typically thought of as being difficult—but also in her producing vowel-initial words. This highlights the fact that children's patterns are not always expected based either on universals or on language-specific developmental norms.

TABLE 9-7 Fricative-Final Migration Pattern

fall	[ɑf]
fine	[ɑɪnf]
school	[kus]
soup	[ups]
zoo	[uz]
sheep	[ips]
shoe	[us]

From Leonard, L. B., & McGregor, K. K. (1991). Unusual phonological patterns and their underlying representations: A case study. *Journal of Child Language, 18*(2), 261–272.

Assimilation/Harmony Processes

Assimilation/harmony processes are those in which two elements within the word (or phrase or utterance) become more alike. They typically result in a reduction in articulatory effort, because fewer oral motor transitions need to be made within the word. Contrast within the word is also reduced of course. Recall from Chapter 8 that assimilation occurs when adjacent elements become more alike and harmony when the elements are separated by at least one other element. Assimilation and harmony processes include the following:

1. Consonant or vowel harmony: These processes occur when the consonants (or vowels) within a word become alike or more alike. In child phonological systems, there is often a specific harmony pattern in which all consonants within a word assimilate to a particular feature if it is present anywhere in the word. For example, many children show velar harmony: all consonants within the word become velar if there is a velar anywhere within the word. Often, this is directional: the harmony will change consonants preceding (or following) the velar, but not other consonants.[3]

   The terms **progressive harmony** (also called "left to right" or perseverative harmony, i.e., segments later in

[3]According to Stoel-Gammon (1996), velar harmony occurs most often when the velar is in final position.

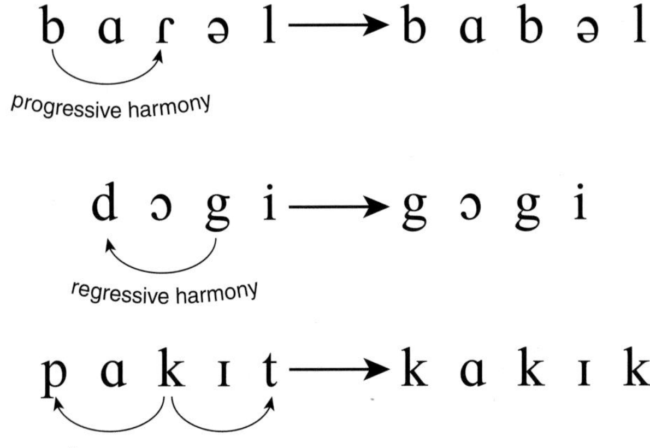

FIGURE 9-1.

the word are affected by earlier ones), **regressive harmony** ("right to left" or anticipatory harmony, i.e., segments earlier in the word are affected by later ones), and **bidirectional harmony** can be used to describe what is happening with respect to the direction of the harmony. For example, [bɑbəl] for "bottle" is an example of progressive labial harmony (the labiality of the initial consonant affecting the medial consonant), [gɔgi] for "doggie" of regressive velar harmony (the velarity of the second consonant affecting the first one), and [kɑkɪk] for "pocket" of bidirectional harmony (velarity spread both "forward" and "back" from the medial consonant). Figure 9-1 illustrates these patterns.

However, in some cases, the harmony affects only certain types of consonants (e.g., coronals, i.e., alveolars or palatals) or vowels (e.g., high vowels). In other words, only one certain type of consonant or vowel may change under the influence of another in addition to the change only operating in one direction or the other. In these instances, the process name is too broad; it is misleading to say that the child has velar harmony, for example, if only alveolars harmonize with velars and this only happens when the alveolar precedes the velar. More specific descriptions should be given in these cases (e.g., "regressive velar harmony affecting alveolars"), reflecting the rule table:

Target	Change	Environment
Alveolar	*Velar*	*Before velar*

Unfortunately, this is usually not done.

2. Reduplication: Reduplication is, in a sense, total harmony. It involves repetition of the same syllable. Examples from Menn (1978) are repeated here:

Down	[doʊdoʊ]
Around	[wæwæ]
Handle	[hɑhɑ]

The process name is quite descriptive, albeit a bit redundant, with appropriate implications about the breadth of its application.

Substitution Processes

Substitution processes are those that result in one element substituting for another when assimilation is *not* the source of the error. They are classified (e.g., by Hodson & Paden, 1991) according to the type of change that occurs:

1. Place changes: The place of articulation of the phoneme changes[4] (i.e., the consonant is produced in a different place of articulation than that of its target). Examples from Hodson and Paden (1991) include the following:
   - Fronting (typically, velars are fronted to alveolar position)
   - Backing (typically, alveolars are backed to velar position)
   - Palatalization (alveolars are palatalized, e.g., /s/ pronounced as [ʃ])
   - Depalatalization (palatals are fronted to alveolar position, e.g., /ʃ/ pronounced as [s] or /tʃ/ as [ts])
   - Place shifts affecting /θ/ (fronting to [f], backing to [s], etc.)

   As these descriptions illustrate, much confusion results from the fact that terms such as "fronting" and "backing" could have many different interpretations. Some people attempt to use them only to refer to very specific changes, while others use them more broadly. It is important to specify the meanings of these terms when using them (e.g., "fronting of /θ/ to [f]"). Making a rule table that specifies the target, the change, and the environment as in generative phonology can be helpful in this respect.
2. Manner changes: The manner of articulation of the phoneme changes. Examples include the following:
   - Stopping (typically, fricatives are stopped at the closest stop place of articulation)
   - Gliding (typically, liquids are produced as glides)
   - Vowelization (vowels substitute for liquids in medial or final position)
   - Affrication (fricatives are partially stopped, yielding, e.g., [tʃu] for "shoe")
   - Deaffrication (affricates are produced either without a stop portion, yielding, e.g., [ʃiz] for "cheese," or without a fricative portion, yielding, e.g., [tiz] for "cheese")

   Again, many variations are possible and must be specified. These include stopping of glides, gliding of fricatives, and affrication of stops. Specification is also necessary in the case of deaffrication to indicate which portion is omitted.
3. Voicing changes: The voicing of the element changes. Typical examples are:
   - Voicing of initial consonants (e.g., [bɪg] for "pig")
   - Devoicing of final consonants (e.g., [pɪk] for "pig")

[4]The use of the word "changes" implies that the child's underlying representation is adult-like, in other words, that the phoneme is changing as it makes its way from underlying to surface levels of the phonology. This is typically assumed by those who advocate natural process analysis but is not assumed to always be true by this author.

- It is important to recall, however, that the apparent voicing of stops that results from cluster reduction in sC- clusters is actually appropriate. Remember that English speakers tend to think of the stops [b, d, g] as voiced, but they are actually voiceless unaspirated, just like stops that follow [s] in a cluster. Thus, the voicing of the "k" in the word "ski" is actually more similar to the voicing of the [g] in "ghee" than to the voicing of the [k] in "key." Thus, a child who is perceived to be producing "ski" as [gi] is guilty of cluster reduction but is *not* really guilty of voicing a voiceless stop.

COMMON *Confusion*

DEPALATALIZATION VERSUS DEAFFRICATION

Students often confuse depalatalization with deaffrication. It is true that if /tʃ/ is produced as [ts] or /dʒ/ is produced as [dz], the result is a sequence of sounds that does not constitute an affricate in English (although both [ts] and [dz] are affricates in some languages). However, it is generally assumed that [ts] and [dz] are still affricates in these cases; the timing of the two consonants is more rapid than would be the case for a -ts or -dz consonant cluster. Therefore, these errors are counted as depalatalization, not deaffrication: the fricative portion is still there but its place of articulation has changed. In contrast, when /tʃ/ is pronounced as [t] or /dʒ/ is pronounced as [d], both depalatalization and deaffrication have occurred. However, when /tʃ/ is pronounced as [ʃ] or /dʒ/ is pronounced as [ʒ], the result is still palatal, so these are examples of deaffrication only.

COMMON *Confusion*

VOWELIZATION VERSUS RHOTIC DIPHTHONG SIMPLIFICATION

There are two frequent errors that occur when a child cannot produce a rhotic diphthong, such as [iɚ], [eɚ], [uɚ], [oɚ], and [ɑɚ].[5] One is that the rhotic portion ([ɚ]) is omitted ([i], [e], [u], [o], and [ɑ]); in this case, diphthong simplification has occurred. The target liquid is not substituted; it is gone. The other is that the rhotic portion is substituted with a vowel, most often a back one ([iʊ], [eʊ], [uə], [oə], and [ɑʊ]). This is vowelization—producing a target liquid as a vowel.

[5]Note: There are many different ways of transcribing these rhotic diphthongs. Specifically:

[iɚ] = [ɪɚ] = [iɹ] = [ɪɹ] = [ir] = [ɪr]
[eɚ]= [ɛɚ] = [eɹ] = [ɛɹ] = [er] = [ɛr]
[uɚ]= [ʊɚ] = [uɹ] = [ʊɹ] = [ur] = [ʊr]
[oɚ]= [ɔɚ] = [oɹ] = [ɔɹ] = [or] = [ɔr]
[ɑɚ]= [aɚ] = [ɑɹ] = [aɹ] = [ɑr] = [ar]

Data on Process Development

Process analysis has been applied to a wide variety of groups, both typical and disordered. McIntosh and Dodd (2008), for instance, reported that the phonological processes that were used by the largest number of 62 two-year-olds (25 to 35 months) were cluster reduction, fronting of fricatives (e.g., /θ/ → [f]), gliding of /ɹ/, and final consonant deletion. In two cases, the frequency of use of the process dropped markedly from 25- to 29-month-olds versus 30- to 35-month-olds; fronting of fricatives dropped from being used by 100% of participants at the earlier age to only 10%, while assimilation dropped from usage by 66% to 10% of participants. Also, the percentage of participants who used a given process wasn't necessarily predictive of the frequency with which those participants demonstrated the process. For example, both stopping and weak syllable deletion were exhibited by 37% of the participants. However, those who did engage in weak syllable deletion did so 83% of the time on average, while those who demonstrated stopping did so only an average of 23% of the time. In other words, the fact that many children exhibited a process did not mean that they exhibited it frequently, and vice versa. These results are shown in Table 9-8.

Roberts, Burchinal, and Footo (1990) analyzed the phonological processes of 145 children ranging in age from 2½ to 8 years of whom 71% were African American. Their family income levels ranged from lower to middle class; over half (60%) of the mothers were single. As shown in Table 9-9, the most common processes across the ages in order of frequency were cluster reduction, gliding of liquids, deaffrication, velar fronting, and stopping. The so-called unusual process of deaffrication occurred more often than the so-called typical processes of velar fronting, stopping, final consonant deletion, and syllable reduction. The authors speculate that trying to divide processes into "typical" and "unusual" may be inappropriate. The only differences in process use by race

TABLE 9-8 Percent Participants and Percent Usage of Phonological Processes by 62 Two-Year-Olds

Process	% Participants Who Used Process	Mean % Use among Users OR Mean # Uses among Users
Cluster reduction	76%	54%
Fronting of fricatives (/θ/ → [f], etc.)	66%	25%
Gliding of /ɹ/	63%	71%
Final consonant deletion	55%	17%
Assimilation	39%	3 uses
Weak syllable deletion	37%	83%
Stopping	37%	23%
Voicing errors	31%	4 uses
Deaffrication	22%	75%
Fronting of velars	18%	5.5 uses

From McIntosh, & Dodd, B. (2008). Two-year-olds' phonological acquisition: Normative data. *International Journal of Speech-Language Pathology, 10*(6), 460–469.

TABLE 9-9 **Phonological Process Use from 2½ to 8 Years**

Process	Percentage Use (with Standard Deviation) by Age in Years							
	2.5	**3**	**3.5**	**4**	**5**	**6**	**7**	**8**
Cluster reduction	68 (21)	42 (26)	25 (21)	15 (21)	10 (16)	7 (12)	3 (8)	3 (6)
Gliding of liquids	25 (17)	12 (13)	8 (9)	5 (9)	5 (9)	3 (8)	1 (6)	1 (3)
Deaffrication*	20 (31)	13 (19)	7 (18)	8 (17)	2 (8)	1 (4)	1 (3)	1 (3)
Velar fronting	18 (17)	8 (12)	6 (11)	3 (5)	2 (4)	1 (3)	0 (1)	0 (1)
Stopping of fricatives	9 (15)	4 (8)	2 (4)	2 (3)	1 (2)	1 (1)	0 (1)	0 (1)
Medial consonant deletion*	7 (6)	5 (5)	3 (3)	3 (3)	2 (3)	2 (3)	1 (2)	1 (2)
Final consonant deletion	6 (7)	8 (11)	5 (8)	3 (7)	2 (3)	3 (5)	1 (3)	1 (3)
Syllable deletion /reduction	3 (3)	2 (5)	1 (3)	1 (2)	1 (2)	0 (1)	0 (1)	0 (1)

*Process designated as "unusual" by Roberts and colleagues (1990).
From Roberts, J. E., Burchinal, M., & Footo, M. M. (1990). Phonological process decline from 2-1/2 to 8 years. *Journal of Communication Disorders, 23*, 205–217.

were a dialect-based tendency for African American children to omit final consonants more often between 2½ and 7 years and to omit medial consonants more often between 2½ and 3½ years. There were no differences by sex.

Similarly, Haelsig and Madison (1986) analyzed the phonological processes of 10 children with no identified speech or language delays or disorders in each of five age groups between 3 and 5 years old. In contrast to Roberts and colleagues (1990), these authors found weak syllable deletion to be among the most common processes throughout this age range, still applying 13% of the time in 5-year-olds (down from 38% in 3-year-olds). Gliding and vowelization of liquids occurred with greater than 20% frequency up through the age of 4 years. Although it occurred with less than 20% frequency by 3½ years, cluster reduction remained the second most frequent process at 5 years (7% occurrence). While glottalization and assimilation (harmony) were frequent among 3-year-olds, they had diminished markedly to about 10% of possible occurrences by 48 months.

Abraham (1989) studied the phonological processes of 13 orally trained children with hearing impairments who were between the ages of 5 and 15 years. The most common processes identified in this group included the two that were predominant in the Haelsig and Madison (1986) study—cluster reduction and gliding/vowelization of liquids. Other frequent processes were deaffrication, final consonant deletion, and stridency deletion (stopping and other substitutions for strident fricatives). The author concluded that the errors of children with hearing impairments are often systematic (rule-based).

Roberts, Long, Malkin, Barnes, Skinner, and colleagues (2005) compared the phonological processes on a single-word test of 50 boys with Fragile X (FX), 32 boys with Down syndrome (DS), and 33 nonverbal mental age-matched boys who were TD. The boys in the disordered groups ranged from preschool to early teen years; the TD boys were 2 to 6 years old. There were no significant differences in their use of substitution processes, although those with DS used these more often (16% of the time) than did those with FX (13%) or who were TD (12%). There were significant differences in their syllable and word structure process use; children with DS used these 15% of the time, while those with FX only used them 5% of the time, and those who were TD used them 3% of the time. Thus, the children with DS had more phonotactic difficulties than the others. The most common substitution processes among all three groups were those affecting fricatives, liquids, and clusters. The most common syllable structure processes among all three groups were cluster reduction and final consonant deletion.

Similarly, Barnes, Roberts, Long, Martin, Berni, and colleagues (2009) compared phonological processes used in the connected speech of 63 boys with Fragile X, 34 boys with Down syndrome, and 45 nonverbal mental age-matched TD boys. Again, the children with Fragile X used syllable structure processes more often than did those who were TD (but not statistically significantly more), but those with Down syndrome used them even more often. Similarly, those with DS used substitution processes significantly more often than did those in the other two groups (who did not differ statistically). Substitution processes were more common than were syllable structure processes in all groups.

Stoel-Gammon (2001) summarized previous studies of the specific phonological processes reported in children with Down syndrome. The most common processes reported included phonotactic patterns such as cluster reduction and final consonant deletion as well as substitution processes such as stopping, deaspiration of initial voiceless stops, gliding and vowelization of liquids, and final consonant devoicing. The children with DS were delayed in their use of these processes in comparison to developmental norms. Rupela, Manjula, and Velleman (2010) confirmed the relatively high incidence of phonological processes among adolescents with Down syndrome who speak a non-Indo-European language spoken in southern India. The most frequent processes of their participants included several that are common among English-learning children, such as cluster reduction, stopping, gliding, and consonant harmony. Others were language specific (e.g., retroflex fronting and degemination), yet still consistent with the processes demonstrated by younger typically developing children.

In contrast, the phonological process use of children with autism spectrum disorders may be quite atypical. Certain processes (e.g., cluster reduction) may persist beyond the expected ages; idiosyncratic processes (such as frication of liquids) may occur that are not expected in typically developing children at any age. Very immature deficits (e.g., apparent inability to produce [m]) may coexist with unexpected strengths (e.g., ability to produce [tʃ]) (Wolk & Giesen, 2000).

In short, children with neurodevelopmental syndromes, including Down syndrome and autism, may exhibit systematic phonotactic or phonetic patterns in their speech. The extent to which such patterns are motorically based versus cognitively based is under debate.

Patterns Have Many Causes

Many people think that the identification of a pattern is the key to differentiating a cognitive–linguistic speech sound disorder from a physiologically based speech sound disorder. But *a physiologic difference can be responsible for a pattern of errors.* A child with a cleft may consistently nasalize oral sounds, demonstrating a "phonological process" that could be referred to as "nasalization." A child with Moebius syndrome may consistently substitute velars for labials, which is an example of "backing." But in these cases, the causes are not cognitive–linguistic; they are due to the cleft and to paralysis of the labial musculature.

Identifying—and treating—error patterns as patterns rather than as individual sounds is an efficacious clinical strategy. As we have seen, pattern-based approaches were initially proposed by people who couched their proposals in terms that came from linguistic theory. Despite these circumstances, we must be careful not to overinterpret the presence of error patterns in a child's speech. Children with physiologically based SSDs may nonetheless demonstrate patterns of errors. In short:

The fact that you can identify a pattern does not tell you whether that pattern is motorically based or cognitively/linguistically based.

Writing Phonological Process Goals

In keeping with the theory of natural phonology, process goals are written in terms of suppressing or decreasing the processes that are deemed inappropriate (Tyler, Edwards, & Saxman, 1987). As stated by Hodson (2011), working on production of a particular phoneme is in this view, "a means to an end rather than the end goal" (p. 16). Typical goals would include the following:

- "Suppress fronting" or, more specifically, "Decrease fronting from 100% to 50% of the time in initial position."
- "Suppress cluster reduction" or, more specifically, "Decrease reduction of s- clusters from 75% to 25% in final position."

Summary

The long-term result of both generative phonology and natural process theory for clinical phonology has been a positive change toward more general statements being made about children's phonologies and toward addressing *classes* of sounds and *patterns* of errors rather than individual segmental substitutions or deletions. Natural process theory provided convenient labels for many of the common phonological patterns seen in the languages of the world and in early or disordered phonologies. The efficiency and clarity of these labels made phonological theory appear far more clinically accessible and increased many clinicians' awareness of phonological patterns. Also, the consideration of syllable structure and harmony processes hastened the interest in patterns affecting whole syllables, words, or even phrases.

However, this shift in perspective has been accompanied by a great deal of confusion about which processes are natural and which are "deviant" and about which processes to address first. Also, the convenient shorthand of process names has not encouraged clinicians to learn to distinguish different children's patterns more specifically (e.g., any instances in which the actual production is more front than is the target are lumped together as "fronting" with little attention to the details). It also has led to a tendency to ignore phonological patterns that do not fit these pre-existing labels (e.g., gliding of fricatives). Ironically, despite their grounding in phonetic naturalness, the easy, even careless use of process labels by a great many people appears to have reduced many clinicians' awareness of the physiologic bases that often underlie phonological patterns. Furthermore, as we shall see below, the theory provides little guidance for prioritizing goals, as many diverse processes may appear to account for one child's phonological profile.

Phonological Avoidance: Constraints

Overview

Recall from Chapter 2 that a markedness constraint is an expression of what is being avoided in the languages of the world or within a particular phonological system. A phonology that included all human speech sounds and structures would not be learnable; therefore, each language has some restrictions. For example, English has a markedness constraint against clicks; they are not included in our phonology, and so they are considered marked. In Optimality Theory, this constraint is abbreviated as *click; the asterisk means "avoid." Constraints may rule out the use of certain sound classes or phonological structures (e.g., clusters, abbreviated *CC), or they may limit the use of such marked segments or structures to certain contexts (e.g., initial position, abbreviated *#CC). Thus, distribution requirements, such as the prohibitions against [ŋ] in initial position (*#ŋ) and [h, w, j] in final position (*h#, *w#, *j#) in English, are additional examples of markedness constraints. As a result of such language-specific constraints, even unimpaired, fluent adult speakers are restricted with respect to which speech sounds and structures are easy for them to produce. They have mastered the challenging aspects of their own phonologies (such as the many fricatives, vowels, and clusters that occur in English) but not the challenging sounds and structures that may be included in other languages.

As reviewed in Chapter 2, languages and individuals (especially children and those with SSDs) may also have constraints against strategies for coping with marked sound classes or structures. In Japanese, clusters (and final consonants) in borrowed words are dealt with by epenthesizing (adding) vowels between the consonants ([nɛkəsɛtu sətɑpu] for "next stop" /nɛkst stɑp/). Deleting consonants is avoided in Japanese because of a faithfulness constraint that says "preserve consonants" (i.e., *ConsonantDeletion). In other words, speakers of this language highly rank the constraint that says consonants must be maintained even if other aspects of the word have to be changed in order to preserve them. Therefore, epenthesis must be used to make that sequence of consonants pronounceable. In English, in contrast, epenthesis is strongly dispreferred (i.e., *Epenthesis). We highly rank the faithfulness constraint that says to avoid adding extra material to our words—in other words, to preserve the segmental structure of the word. Because we cannot epenthesize vowels to separate the consonants in long clusters, instead, we delete some of those consonants to simplify the word ([nɛkstɑp] for "next stop" in casual speech). Thus, these faithfulness constraints tell us in what respects the target word must be maintained and what strategies we can use to try to maintain it in those respects.

Importantly, most of these constraints are not absolute. For example, English speakers do use epenthesis in some cases, such as when trying to deal with some non-English initial clusters (e.g., those in the names of the Congolese cities Nkayi and Mbinda). Furthermore, although we do use deletion to simplify challenging clusters, we obviously don't reduce all clusters to singletons; the constraint against consonant deletion is ranked more highly than the constraint against producing clusters. There is a balance between a strongly ranked faithfulness constraint for preserving clusters (i.e., a faithfulness constraint against deletion), a moderately highly ranked faithfulness constraint against using epenthesis (i.e., against adding material), and a much lower-ranked markedness constraint against clusters that mostly applies to long or unusual ones (e.g., adjoining clusters in phrases, [sf-] as in "sphere"). This balance determines which aspects of a challenging word the speaker produces and how other aspects are approximated.

Developmental and Clinical Implications

Although the germ of the idea has been around for decades in various forms, constraint theory (Optimality Theory) in and of itself is relatively new. Applications to clinical diagnosis and treatment are in their toddlerhood. However, the idea of looking at a child's phonology from the point of view of what that child is *not* doing (i.e., avoiding) rather than what she *is* doing is highly appealing and efficient. There is a much more direct line from constraints, which are the roadblocks within the phonological system, to goals than there is from rules or processes to goals.

In clinical work and studies of speech sound development, markedness constraints correspond to and account for children's error patterns; youngsters who simplify clusters usually do so because of a markedness constraint against sequences of consonants, those who glide usually do so because of a markedness constraint against liquids, and so on. In this sense, Optimality Theory goes beyond identifying patterns; it explains why they occur. Markedness constraints are the sources of the error patterns. As discussed in much more detail below, if we can identify the reason for the error pattern, we can remediate it much more efficiently.

In contrast, identifying faithfulness constraints reminds us to focus on what the child is doing right, which process analysis also does not do. For example, while a child who produces "big" as [bɪ] is indeed failing to produce the final consonant (most likely due to a markedness constraint against codas), she is also being faithful to the initial consonant and to the vowel (Stemberger & Bernhardt, 1997). These are strengths upon which we can build.

Velleman and Vihman (2002) identified the highest-ranked markedness and faithfulness constraints of five young speakers each of English, French, Japanese, and Welsh at the "25-word point" (i.e., at the point at which the child produced 20 to 30 different words within a half-hour recording session). They found that a markedness constraint against syllables without vowels (i.e., against producing syllables with consonantal nuclei) and a faithfulness constraint against deleting or adding vocalic nuclei (i.e., in favor of producing vowel nuclei when they are expected) were the highest-ranked constraints for all four languages. Of course, very few of the targets lacked vowel nuclei (as would be the case for the second syllable of a word like "bottle" [bɑɾl̩], e.g., which has a syllabic liquid as the nucleus of the second syllable), so there were few opportunities for violating the faithfulness constraint in that way. In rare cases, consonant nuclei were changed to vowels (as when /æpl̩/ → [api]) or vocalic nuclei were changed to syllabic consonants (as when /mʌŋki/ → [hm̩mæ]). A markedness constraint against sequences of consonants within the same syllable (i.e., against producing clusters) was also highly ranked in all languages.

However, other rankings were language specific. For example, faithfulness to the presence or absence of onset consonants (i.e., neither deleting nor adding initial consonants) was very highly ranked in English, in which stress most often falls on the first syllable of the word. In other languages, this constraint was ranked lower; in other words, the children were less careful about matching the occurrence of onset consonants (probably because French has consistent stress on the final syllable, and both Welsh and Japanese have long "geminate" consonants in medial position, both of which attract the child's attention to later in the word rather than the beginning of the word, as argued by Vihman and Velleman [2000a, 2000b]). Faithfulness to geminates (producing them where called for and not where not) was highly ranked in Japanese but essentially irrelevant to the other languages. A markedness constraint against codas was much higher ranked in Japanese and French (which have extremely few and relatively few codas, respectively) than in English and Welsh (both of which have many words with a wide variety of final consonants). In short, many of the children's highest-ranked constraints matched those of the languages to which they were being exposed.

Velleman and Vihman (2002) concluded that both markedness and faithfulness constraints are already present in children's early words. Some of these constraints are ranked based upon universal constraint rankings (e.g., preferring vowels as syllabic nuclei, avoiding clusters) and others reflect language-specific preferences (e.g., avoiding versus preserving codas and preserving geminates). The latter result from the finding mentioned many times within this book—that children are sensitive to frequencies of occurrence of specific sounds, sound classes, and phonotactic structures within the languages to which they are exposed. The authors deduce that:

there are two ways in which accommodation to these statistical tendencies of the adult language could occur:

- *the child's productions become statistically more like the language's frequencies because the child's productions become more and more faithful to individual target words, or*
- *the child's productions become statistically more like the language's frequencies in general, without becoming more faithful to individual target words. (p. 407)*

They found evidence for both in this study. Both can be clinical goals—to increase the child's use of some sound or structure that she is avoiding in general (i.e., with progress measured with respect to frequency of use of the avoided sound or structure, whether it is used correctly or not), or to increase the child's correct use of that sound or structure (i.e., with progress measured with respect to how often words with the target sound or structure are pronounced correctly). Obviously, the latter is the ultimate goal, but sometimes, a more general intermediate goal is appropriate.

TABLE 9-10 Hypothetical Initial Consonant Cluster Simplifications (Reduction and Coalescence)

Target	Production
truck	[tʌk]
plate	[pet]
spoon	[fun]
smile	[faɪʊ]

Interactions among various markedness and faithfulness constraints can help us understand child patterns in ways that phonological processes cannot. For example, a child might have a pattern of simplifying some initial clusters via reduction (i.e., deleting one of the elements) but coalescing others (i.e., merging some features from each consonant into a single consonant). Examples from a hypothetical child given in Table 9-10 show that stop+liquid clusters are simplified by deleting the liquid, while fricative+stop clusters are coalesced to [f].

How can we account for these varying outcomes? A process analysis would tell us simply that the child was exhibiting both cluster reduction and coalescence; this is unrevealing. In Optimality Theory, we would first identify a markedness constraint against clusters in initial position. Another markedness constraint against liquids accounts for the deletion of the /ɹ/ in "truck" and the /l/ in "plate" as well as the vowelization of the /l/ in "smile." In addition, there must be faithfulness constraints that say "if there's a fricative, keep the frication" and "if there's a stop or nasal, keep its place of articulation." In order to preserve these features, the child must coalesce them into one consonant that is different in some ways from either member of the cluster. This set of constraints gives us important information: The child is aware of some of the features of both consonants in sp- and sm- clusters. This may indicate that he (1) differentiates fricatives from consonants with other manners of articulation, (2) differentiates labial and alveolar places of articulation from each other, and (3) has some knowledge of clusters. The latter suggests that he might be able to learn to pronounce initial clusters composed of earlier-developing consonants, such as tw-. Furthermore, as he improves his skills at producing singleton liquids, liquid clusters may emerge "for free" or with minimal intervention. More examples of this sort are provided later in this chapter.

An example from Pater (2004) also illustrates constraint interaction. This child, Trevor, produced "garage" (/gəˈɹɑdʒ/[6]) as [gɑdʒ]; the weak syllable was deleted but its

[6]/gəˈɹɑʒ/ in many American English dialects.

TABLE 9-11 Dylan's Syllable and Word Codas

Target	Production
gum	[gʌm]
sun	[dʌn]
song	[dɑŋ]
all	[ʔɑl, ʔɑː]
tooth	[tʰuː]
cake	[kʰeɪʔ]
eight	[ʔeɪ]
bed	[bɛɪ]
big	[bɪː]
snake	[neɪə]
bath	[bæʔ]
tub	[pʰʌː]
dive	[pɑɪ]
chipmunk	[pʰɪʔmʌŋ]
candle	[kʰændəʊ]
meatball	[miʔbɑl]
baseball	[beɪʔbɔ]
dollhouse	[dɑlhaʊ]
numbers	[bʌmbə]
finger	[bɪŋgɛə]

From Bernhardt, B., & Stemberger, J. P. (1998). *Handbook of phonological development: From the perspective of constraint-based nonlinear phonology.* San Diego, CA: Academic Press.

onset consonant was preserved. Importantly, this indicates that Trevor was aware of at least some aspects (the initial consonant) of that weak syllable. Possible constraints, in order of priority (ranking), include the following:

Preserve onsets (or perhaps, preserve stop onsets): Don't delete initial consonants/initial stops.

*Initial weak syllable: Avoid word-initial weak syllables.

And possibly also:

*/ɹ/: Avoid /ɹ/.

Given that Trevor appeared to be aware of the initial weak syllables that he was deleting (or at least of some aspects of them), a goal of teaching him to produce what he has been avoiding—initial weak syllables—would be appropriate.

Bernhardt and Stemberger (1998) provide another interesting case of markedness constraints interacting with faithfulness constraints that reflect the child's phonological knowledge. This boy, Dylan, had strong restrictions on both syllable-final and word-final consonants. Nasals were allowed in either type of final position, and word-final or syllable-final /l/ was occasionally correct, but most other coda consonants were either deleted or replaced by [ʔ]. Sample data are provided in Table 9-11. Dylan's markedness constraints therefore included a highly ranked phonotactic constraint against codas (at both the syllable level and the word level), which was overridden only by a strong faithfulness constraint that required preservation of nasals and an emerging faithfulness constraint for preserving /l/. However, although other codas were not produced, there were various types of evidence showing Dylan was aware of them; in many cases, he "marked the spot" where the coda should be by lengthening the vowel, adding a vowel offset, or producing a glottal stop. In two cases ("tub" and "dive"), he moved the coda place of articulation (labial) to the onset position of the word. We can express this as a general faithfulness constraint such as "preserve coda"—something needs to be kept, but that something is unspecified and may vary from word to word. The information that Dylan had this faithfulness constraint was important for planning intervention; it was not necessary to carry out perception/receptive intervention activities to make him aware of the presence of codas. In fact, the researchers report that therapy with an initial goal to increase Dylan's use of final /p, k/ in VC and CVC words was quite successful.

Limitations of Optimality Theory

The limitations of constraint theory include that it is still under development and that, because it is actively being researched by many linguists, the details of the theory are in a state of constant change. In a way, this is a good thing; newer theories are better equipped to handle the complexities of child phonological development, including atypical development and disorders. But it can be frustrating to try to keep up. Furthermore, this approach has just begun to be accepted in our field. Therefore, it is challenging for a practicing SLP to remain up to date on this approach or to find either literature or tools tailored to its use with clinical populations. Fortunately, that is changing as constraints are being embraced more widely by SLPs.

Furthermore, some of the formal aspects of this model, like those of the generative phonology and natural phonology (phonological processes) models, are based upon assumptions that do not match the behavior of real children learning to talk in the real world. That is, these theories were developed to portray an efficient, linear, systematic process of speech acquisition with as much universality and consistency from child to child and language to language as possible. For this reason, these models fail to appropriately capture the highly individualistic, variable, piecemeal, meandering paths that youngsters follow, complete with "U-shaped curves" (i.e., regressions), exceptions, and idiosyncratic patterns (Menn, Schmidt, & Nicholas, 2013; Vihman, 2014).

Nevertheless, the application of some of the key tenets of constraint theory to child speech sound disorders is insightful and useful: Identify what it is that the child is avoiding (markedness constraints) and what she is preserving (faithfulness constraints). Build on the sound classes and structures to which the client is faithful in order to increase her use of those that are marked within her phonological system.

Summary

Constraint theory facilitates the expression of more basic phonological truths by considering which phonological possibilities do not occur in the (child's) phonology versus those that are preferred. The use of this approach can permit the clinician to write more general goals that address the heart of the problem rather than skirting the issue. However, it has not yet been either fully developed or systematically applied to clinical populations.

RELATIONSHIPS AMONG PATTERN TYPES

One aspect of faithfulness constraints is simply that certain elements or structures are preserved (i.e., they are produced as specified in the target word). Other faithfulness constraints, however, are what may be referred to as **repair strategies**, such as deletion, epenthesis, coalescence, etc. These tell us the answer to the question: when faced with the possible violation of one or more markedness constraints (e.g., the need to produce a cluster), what do the speakers do about it? Consistent preferences for particular repairs are evident in different languages and among different children. In a way, the fact that a repair strategy is used by a speaker is the information that is needed to determine that there is a constraint in that child's speech. The contrapositive[7] of the principle "If it ain't broke, don't fix it" implies that if somebody tried to fix it, she must have thought it was broken. Thus, if speakers use a repair strategy (such as deletion of one consonant from a cluster), then they must consider the form to need fixing for some reason (e.g., it contains a cluster against which they have a markedness constraint). If elements of clusters were never deleted, for example, then there would be no basis for the claim that English has a constraint (albeit a weak one) against clusters.

It is not difficult to see that these constraint repair strategies are the same as the rules discussed in generative phonology and the processes discussed in natural phonology. A child demonstrates stopping of fricatives or cluster reduction because he has a constraint against fricatives or against clusters. Thus, constraint theory does not contradict the patterns identified within these earlier perspectives. Instead, it focuses primarily on the reasons why these rules or processes occur and secondarily on the rules or processes themselves. Within this perspective, rules or processes are pointers to some limitation within the phonological system that the speaker is attempting to circumvent. For example, careful consideration of Nathan's long list of processes reveals his underlying constraint against any non-alveolar consonants. This constraint is the heart of the matter; the many processes he uses are his superficial attempts to cope with the constraint.

It is also important to keep in mind the focus of each approach. Specifically, generative rules and natural phonology have been used clinically to compare child productions to adult productions in order to identify error patterns. Phonological processes, the patterns with which most speech-language pathologists are most familiar, have been used exclusively for relational analysis. The child's production is compared to the adult production of the word and the difference is described as a process. For example, if the child says [dɔ] for "dog," this is noted as an instance of final consonant deletion. The function of the process is comparative only. This highlights the respects in which the child's system is deficient in comparison to an adult English phonological system but does not clarify the manner of functioning of the child's system itself.

Constraints are used to describe the child's own system as well as to compare it to the adult norm. They describe patterns that are not preferred in the child's system—those that do not occur or occur only rarely. For example, a constraint against final consonants (*C#) is actually far more general than either a phonological rule or a process label (final consonant deletion) would be. It will account not only for cases in which the child fails to produce final consonants at all but also for other strategies that the child might choose that could allow him or her to be more faithful to the adult representation without producing a consonant in final position. For example, Molly (Vihman & Velleman 1989), previously discussed in Chapters 6, 7, and 8, went through a stage in which she produced words idiosyncratically, including some words with correct final consonants. After systematizing her phonology, however, she ceased to produce final consonants in final position. Instead, she added a vocalic offset to final obstruents and nasals (vowel epenthesis in final position). This allowed her to produce the adult final consonants somewhere in the word without actually producing consonants *in final position* in her own word forms. This pattern is illustrated in Table 9-12.

TABLE 9-12 Molly's Vocalic Offsets

Target	Production
bang	[pɑn^{n}ə]
around	[wɑnə]
Brian	[pɑnə]
down	[tænə]
clock	[kɑkkɪ]
teeth	[tɪtt^{h}i̥]
peek	[pekxe]
squeak	[k^{h}ʊk^{h}ʌ]
tick	[tɪt^{h}ə]

Note: ^{h} indicates aspiration.
̥ indicates partial voicelessness.
From Vihman, M. M., & Velleman, S. L. (1989). Phonological reorganization: A case study. *Language and Speech*, *32*, 149–170.

[7]For further information about contrapositives, see D. Velleman (2006).

Thus, Molly had the same markedness constraint as a child who uses final consonant deletion to avoid final consonants, but her repair strategy for coping with the *C# constraint differed. Her faithfulness constraint said "Preserve final consonants." To maintain them without producing them in final position, she resorted to adding a vowel. Thinking through her errors as constraints helps us see not only what she is avoiding but also what she is preserving. The fact that she is preserving the final consonants (albeit by making them non-final due to epenthesis) highlights her faithfulness constraint, which tells us that she has phonological knowledge of these codas. She knows that they are there, but she also knows that she cannot produce them.

This example highlights the importance of the flexibility and changeability of constraint priority orders within constraint theory. It is expected that the priority order of constraints within a certain phonological system (that of a language, of a dialect, or of an individual child) might change over time. In other words, a constraint with effects that are prominent at one time might cease to have a visible impact on the phonology at another time as other constraints become more important. This is a useful viewpoint with respect to Molly's phonology. The constraint against final consonants was not weighted heavily at an extremely early stage in her phonology,[8] as she omitted some final consonants but produced others. But avoiding codas was prioritized shortly after she systematized her phonology. Her phonological response to this constraint was to epenthesize vowels in final position in order to preserve the final consonants without having to produce them as such.

In other cases, the same child might omit final consonants part of the time but use epenthesis, migration, or some other strategy another part of the time, all with the same purpose of avoiding final consonants. Several processes or rules would have to be identified to account for these strategies. Unlike a phonological process or rule, the simple constraint "*C#" (no final consonants) will cover all of those cases. It is a direct and explicit statement about the child's phonological limitations rather than about her strategies for dealing with those limitations. The accompanying faithfulness constraints tell us upon what strengths we can build as we remediate the problem.

As such, the constraints provide a more direct route to determining therapy goals. In Molly's case, the appropriate goal (if she were delayed or disordered rather than merely young) would clearly be to increase production of consonants in final position. This would be facilitated by our understanding that Molly knows that the final consonants are there and that she prioritizes producing them. Once her phonology will tolerate final consonants in final position, she will no longer need to use the epenthesis strategy (or any other strategy) to cope with adult final consonants. Note that the goal for Molly *could not* have been "decrease final consonant deletion" because she did not delete final consonants; she merely buried them within the word. If we had addressed the goal "reduce epenthesis," she might have resorted to deletion or some sort of substitution as an alternative strategy.

[8]Or more likely, phonological constraints were irrelevant before phonological systematization.

TABLE 9-13 Constraints on Stop and Fricative Occurrence

Target	Production
cap	[kæf]
fish	[pɪʃ]
stupid	[tufɪz]
dog	[dɔɣ]

Note: [ɣ] is a voiced velar fricative.

Other children's constraints may refer to specific phonetic features. For example, a child may have constraints on where fricatives versus stops can occur, as shown in the data in Table 9-13. This (hypothetical) child uses only stops in initial position and only fricatives in medial and final position. This complementary distribution situation can be written as the following markedness constraints:

$$*\#\begin{bmatrix}+\text{continuant}\\ -\text{sonorant}\end{bmatrix}$$

*V[−continuant]

These constraints state that continuant nonsonorant sounds (fricatives) may not occur in initial position and that noncontinuant sounds (stops) may not occur after vowels (in medial or final position). The child's faithfulness constraints are that she preserves place of articulation and voicing; these do not change. We can build upon this fact and also the fact that she is capable of producing both fricatives and stops—just not in all positions. Again, the therapy goals are clear: to break down the markedness constraints so that stops and fricatives are in contrast instead of in complementary distribution. In other words, the goal is to encourage the child to do exactly what the constraint states that she currently avoids doing:

- Produce fricatives in initial position
- Produce stops in other positions

Since she is not using these consonant types in a contrastive manner (they are in complementary distribution), minimal pairs therapy or some other type of contrast therapy would be appropriate in this case.

The constraints do not actually tell us how the child accommodates her phonological limitations. She happens to stop initial fricatives and fricate medial and final stops. However, this information is actually largely irrelevant to setting therapy goals. If the child becomes able to produce initial fricatives and medial and final stops, the stopping and the frication will cease. If the stopping and frication are eliminated without the ability to produce initial fricatives and medial and final stops, new strategies (processes) could crop up to help her continue to avoid these productions. She might begin to delete or affricate initial fricatives or glide medial or final stops, for example. If process therapy results in new inappropriate strategies replacing the old inappropriate strategies, then the clinician will have to start from scratch, eliminating the new processes.

Another case in which constraints may have broader explanatory value than processes or rules is that of consonant clusters. Again, children whose phonological systems do not include the possibility of consonant clusters have many options for dealing with this problem. Cluster reduction is one possibility, but coalescence (e.g., [fɪm] for "swim"), migration (e.g., [nos] for "snow"), and epenthesis of a vowel between the two consonants (e.g., [bəlu] for "blue") are also common strategies. A list of four different processes or phonological rules affecting clusters may daunt the clinician: The child demonstrates cluster reduction, coalescence, migration, and epenthesis—which process should I work on first? A constraint sums up the situation very concisely: *CC. The goal is now clear: facilitate production of two consecutive consonants. This will have the consequence of reducing all of the child's strategies, thereby decreasing the incidence of all of the processes: cluster reduction, coalescence, migration, and epenthesis. Thus, the question of which process to address first becomes moot.

Considering the faithfulness constraints of the child who does not produce clusters can also be helpful. Does she preserve both consonants (*Delete) by moving them around or by epenthesizing a vowel in between? Then we know she has knowledge of both of them. Does she preserve some features of each via coalescence? Then we know she is aware of those particular features at least. These are strengths upon which we can build.

Constraints may also render goal-setting clear in cases in which a child is using a less common process, or using a common process in an unusual manner. The example given above from Leonard and McGregor (1991), in which the child, W, moved all initial fricatives to final position, is a case in point. Migration of fricatives to final position is not likely to be found in the typical phonological processes therapy kit. Rephrasing of the pattern into constraint form renders it far less formidable:

$$*\#\begin{bmatrix}+\text{continuant}\\-\text{sonorant}\end{bmatrix}$$

The constraint simply states that fricatives are not produced in initial position. Although the constraint isn't specific with respect to this child's strategy for avoiding initial fricatives (it doesn't tell us that they migrate to final position), that information is actually irrelevant for setting therapy goals. Simply reducing W's use of migration might only induce her to use some other equally inappropriate strategy, such as stopping, gliding, or omission of initial fricatives. But facilitating her production of fricatives in initial position—directly addressing the constraint itself—will cause the child to discontinue the use of this inappropriate strategy because it will no longer be needed. We are aided by our knowledge that she is not deleting the fricatives; her faithfulness constraint of preserving them tells us that she knows that they do belong somewhere in the word.

TABLE 9-14 Child 142's Harmony and Deaffrication Patterns

Target	Production
ducks	[gʌks]
dog	[gɔg]
tiger	[kaɪgoʊ]
ticket	[kɪkɪt]
chin	[tɪn]
chew	[tu]
jump	[dʌmp]
jeep	[dip]
cheek	[kik]
chicken	[kɪkɪn]
jacket	[gækət*]

From Dinnsen, D. A. (2008). A typology of opacity effects in acquisition. In D. A. Dinnsen & J. A. Gierut (Eds.), *Optimailty theory, phonological acquisition, and disorders* (pp. 121–176). Oakville, CT: Equinox Publishing/DBBC.
*Note that the final /t/ in "jacket" is not harmonized because it does not *precede* a velar.

A few researchers have reported intervention success resulting from selecting goals based upon constraints. Dinnsen's (2008) case of constraints interacting in an interesting manner is one example. His 4-year-old research participant, referred to as "Child 142," exhibited velar harmony when an alveolar consonant preceded a velar in the word. At the same time, 142 also deaffricated affricates, reducing them to the alveolar stop portion of the affricate (/tʃ/ → [t]; /dʒ/ → [d]). Those "derived" alveolars were affected by velar harmony just like target alveolars were. These patterns are shown in Table 9-14. Thus, four markedness constraint factors were operating:

1. A phonotactic constraint that prohibited two different consonants in a word if the first was an alveolar and the second was a velar, which could be written as follows:

$$*\begin{bmatrix}+\text{anterior}\\+\text{coronal}\end{bmatrix}\begin{bmatrix}+\text{vocalic}\end{bmatrix}\begin{bmatrix}-\text{anterior}\\-\text{coronal}\\+\text{back}\end{bmatrix}\left(\begin{bmatrix}+\text{vocalic}\end{bmatrix}\right)$$

   Note that the parentheses indicate that the second vowel is optional; the constraint applies to both CVC and CVCV words.

2. A ranking of two phonetic faithfulness constraints: Preserving velars given higher priority than preserving

alveolars (so that if one consonant's place of articulation had to be changed in order to accommodate the first constraint, above, it would be the velar one that was preserved):

$$\text{preserve place}\begin{bmatrix}-\text{anterior}\\-\text{coronal}\\+\text{back}\end{bmatrix} > \text{preserve place}\begin{bmatrix}+\text{anterior}\\+\text{coronal}\end{bmatrix}$$

3. A phonetic markedness constraint against affricates (in initial position):

$$*\#\begin{bmatrix}+\text{continuant}\\-\text{continuant}\end{bmatrix}$$

4. A faithfulness constraint to preserve [−continuant] (so that the stop portions of affricates would be maintained).

Therapy focusing on the production of words with an alveolar–velar pattern (i.e., focusing on producing the sequence that the child was avoiding) was successful in eliminating the constraint against this pattern; alveolars were then produced correctly even if there was a velar later in the word. Interestingly, while the constraint against affricates persisted, the child continued to demonstrate velar harmony in the words with an affricate in initial position followed by a velar. In other words, "ticket" was now produced correctly, but "chicken" was still [kɪkɪn]. This suggests (to this author, although apparently not to Dinnsen [2008]) that the child may have mis-stored these affricate-initial words in his mental representations as beginning with velar stops. In any case, once the markedness constraint against affricates was moved to a lower ranking and 142 began producing affricates correctly in other words (i.e., words without velars), he also produced them correctly in words with velars (Dinnsen, 2008).

Dinnsen and Farris-Trimble (2008) discuss intervention aimed at remediating an even odder set of constraints based upon a case published by Leonard and Brown (1984). This 3-year-old girl, nicknamed "T," had an unusual phonotactic markedness constraint against words ending in vowels. Recall that CV is the universal "canonical" syllable; some languages do not even allow codas. While English does allow codas, it also includes many words that are vowel-final. Thus, T's constraint was quite idiosyncratic. While preferring codas, she was also very picky about which consonants could serve as codas—only labial stops and [s] were allowed in that position. Thus, in addition to her odd markedness constraint against word-final vowels, she also had a faithfulness constraint that preserved /p, b, m/ in final position and a markedness constraint against any other coda other than [s]. Some of her data are given in Table 9-15. Leonard and Brown (1984) used the information about both T's avoidance strategies (markedness constraints) and her faithfulness constraints in their choice of intervention goals, successfully adding final [f] (because she was faithful to some fricatives and also to labials in coda position) followed by final [d] (because she was faithful to some voiced stops in coda position) to her repertoire. Even though words ending in open syllables were not explicitly targeted in therapy, the child gradually began producing them as intervention progressed.

TABLE 9-15 T's Final Consonant Constraint Pattern

Target	Production
cup	[kʌp]
home	[hom]
Gabe	[gɑb]
Matt	[mæs]
dog	[dɔs]
girl	[gɜs]
two	[tus]
eye	[ɑs]
boy	[bɔs]
go	[gɔs]

From Leonard, L. B., & Brown, B. L. (1984). Nature and boundaries of phonologic categories: A case study of an unusual phonologic pattern in a language-impaired child. *The Journal of Speech and Hearing Disorders, 49,* 419–428; Cited in Dinnsen, D. A., & Farris-Trimble, A. W. (2008). An unusual error pattern reconsidered. In D. A. Dinnsen & J. A. Gierut (Eds.), *Optimailty theory, phonological acquisition, and disorders* (pp. 177–204). Oakville, CT: Equinox Publishing/DBBC.

Summary

Rules and processes can be seen as the strategies that children (and languages) use to cope with words that would otherwise violate their phonological markedness constraints. In the case of children with SSDs, the markedness constraint is the more basic statement of the actual impediment to functional phonology. The rules and processes may help highlight the limits of the child's phonological system, or they may obscure them. This is especially true if the clinician focuses only on relational analysis—comparing the child's productions to the adult target words. Independent analysis of the child's system, especially of elements or structures that are or are not permitted within the system, is necessary in conjunction with relational analysis, in order to accurately identify the actual source of the difficulty. The process of identifying the child's markedness and faithfulness constraints incorporates both independent and relational analysis to highlight what the child is avoiding and what knowledge and priorities he brings to word production.

Clinical Implications

It has already been stated that constraints are more directly related to therapy goals than are rules and processes. As discussed above, it is more important to note, for example, that a child has no fricatives in her phonology than to know what she does about it (deletion, stopping, gliding, cluster reduction, etc.). The ultimate goal is to eliminate the inappropriate constraints (e.g., to get the child to produce fricatives). Simply eliminating one process or rule (e.g., deletion of fricatives) may well lead to the use of another rule or process (e.g., stopping) that achieves the same purpose (i.e., satisfies the same markedness constraint, no fricatives).

EXERCISE 9-2

Processes and Constraints

ASSESSMENT

Generative Phonological Rules

No currently commercially available tools focus on phonological rule analysis. This approach is primarily important as a reminder that a full phonological analysis of a child requires that we consider all components of the child's error patterns:

- The target sound class or structure (e.g., fricatives, liquids, final consonants, clusters)
- The actual output
- The difference between these two
- The context(s) in which this difference occurs

Phonological Processes

Many commercial tests are available for the identification of processes in a child's speech. Some of these are norm-referenced. Similar selection criteria apply here as to "articulation" tests:

- How many consonant classes are assessed?
- How many vowel classes are assessed?
- How many clusters are assessed?
- In which/how many positions?
- Are multisyllabic words included?
- Are varied stress patterns included?

Several difficult balances have to be struck: Ideally, a wide variety of sound classes should be tested in a wide variety of contexts including clusters and multisyllabic words with varied stress patterns as well as in simpler contexts (such as those advocated by Eisenberg & Hitchcock [2010], for articulation tests). Simple contexts will assess the child's ability to arrive at the correct articulatory position under ideal circumstances; more complex contexts will reveal the phonological strategies that he uses when challenged. Both types of information are key to selecting an appropriate intervention approach. However, to be this comprehensive, a test would have to be far more extensive than is feasible to administer and score.

A similar issue relates to the use of spontaneous speech versus single-word tests for process analysis. Dyson and Robinson (1987) compared process analyses of spontaneous speech versus single-word productions of five children with SSD. The processes that were identified in spontaneous speech only were initial and final consonant deletion, but some of these were due to the nature of casual conversational speech (e.g., omission of /h/ in initial position). In contrast, some processes were not identified in spontaneous speech because the children did not attempt relevant words, such as words with consonant clusters. Thus, there is a trade-off. The ideal solution is to do both—administer a standardized test and analyze a spontaneous speech sample and then compare the two.

Another difficult balance is that of the number of processes that are available for scoring. Tests such as the Bankson-Bernthal Test of Phonology (Bankson & Bernthal, 1990) are easier to score in the sense that a small number of processes are considered and the potential errors that relate to each are pre-transcribed. The administrator can simply select the error from the choices available. However, this can prevent the SLP from discovering the pattern that the child is using because it is not one of the choices on the score form. On the opposite extreme, the Hodson Assessment of Phonological Patterns (HAPP-3; Hodson, 2004) provides a lengthy list of processes to consider for each error, although only a subset of them are used to calculate the child's actual standard score. Some substitutions and even some omissions can be scored or identified in multiple categories (e.g., /sneɪk/ → [neɪk] counts as both cluster reduction and a "sibilant deficiency"). This can be confusing and overwhelming for the inexperienced user, as it requires the examiner to determine which analysis of the errors is most appropriate. This is the cost of providing flexibility of interpretation, which more limited tests do not allow.

If formal testing is not required or to supplement it using a speech sample, Form 9-1 can be used. This form includes a list of common processes and allows the user to indicate which of these occur in a particular child's speech. Alternatively, Form 9-2, which provides a clinician-generated overview of the child's processes, will provide more flexibility albeit less structure. This form allows the user to list those processes that have been noted in the child's speech with frequency indicated.

A process analysis of Nathan's speech (from the sample in Table 9-3) using these forms would be likely to yield the following list of processes:

Fronting (of velars)

Backing (of labials)

Initial consonant voicing

Stopping of fricatives

Stopping of liquids

Consonant cluster reduction

Consonant harmony (alveolar)

Reduplication

These are listed on Forms 9-1 and 9-2 as Examples 9-1 and 9-2 for illustration.

While these terms may be less intimidating than the phonological rules generated for Nathan earlier, they are also clearly less general as more of them are needed to describe the same phonological patterns.

Form 9-1

Name: Age:
Date: Examiner:
Source of sample: Size of sample:

PROCESS SUMMARY

PROCESS **Type/Context/Example/Frequency**

Syllable/Word Structure
Syllable Reduction from iambics
other (describe)
Final Consonant Deletion
Initial Consonant Deletion
Cluster Reduction
Liquid clusters
/s/ clusters
other (describe)
Coalescence (describe)
Metathesis/Migration (describe)
Epenthesis (describe)
Other syllable structure
Harmony/Assimilation
Reduplication
Harmony (specify feature)

Other syllable/word structure
Substitution
Fronting (specify)

Backing (specify)
Palatalization
Depalatalization
Stopping (specify)

Gliding of /l/
of /ɹ/
Vowelization of /l/
of [ɝ] and/or [ɚ]
Affrication
Deaffrication
Voicing (specify)

Denasalization
Vowel deviations
Other substitutions

Comments:

Form 9-2

Name:
Date:
Source of sample:

Age:
Examiner:
Size of sample:

PROCESS ANALYSIS

Process Type	**Target** (Phoneme/Sound Class)	**Process(es)**	**Frequency**
EXAMPLE: substitution	*all fricatives*	*stopping*	*predominant*

Comments:

Example 9-1

Name: *Nathan* Examiner: *SLV*

Source of sample: *hypothetical* Size of sample: *18 words*

PROCESS SUMMARY

PROCESS	**CONTEXT/EXAMPLE/FREQUENCY**
SYLLABLE STRUCTURE	
Syllable Reduction	
Final Consonant Deletion	
Initial Consonant Deletion	
Cluster Reduction:	
liquid clusters	[du] *for 'blue'; 100%*
/s/ clusters	[dɪn] *for 'string'; 100%*
other	
Coalescence	
Metathesis/Migration	
HARMONY/ASSIMILATION	
Harmony: *(Specify feature which is harmonized, e.g., velar, high, etc.)*	
Consonant	*alveolar e.g.,* [dɔdi] *for 'doggie'; 100%*
Vowel	
Reduplication	*e.g.,* [dʌdʌd] *for 'butter'; 3/7 (43% of 2-syllable words)*
SUBSTITUTION:	
Fronting	
velar	*to alveolar e.g.,* [dʊdi] *for 'cookie'*
/ʃ/ → [s]	
/θ/ → [f]	
Backing	
alveolar to velar	
other	*labial to alveolar e.g.,* [daɪ] *for 'bye'*
Palatalization	
Depalatalization	
θ Place Changes	
Other place changes	
Stopping	
all fricatives	*e.g.,* [du] *for 'shoe'; 100%*
/v ð z tʃ dʒ/ only	
other	*liquids, e.g.,* [nʌnʌd] *for 'monster'; 100%*
Gliding	
/l/	
/ɹ/	
Vowelization	
/l/	
/ɚ, ɝ/	
Affrication	
Deaffrication	
Voicing	
voice initial consonants	*e.g.,* [dʊdi] *for 'cookie'*
devoice final consonants	
other voice changes	*voice final* C's, *e.g.,* [dædæd] *for 'basket'*

Example 9-2

Name: *Nathan* Examiner: *SLV*
Source of sample: *hypothetical* Size of sample: *18 words*

PROCESS ANALYSIS

Process Type	Adult Phoneme/ Sound Class	Process(es)	Frequency
syllable structure	*all CC*	*CC reduction - first C omitted*	*100%*
harmony	*Non-alveolars*	*C harmony (alveolar)*	*100%*
substitution	*velars*	*fronting (to alveolar)*	*100%*
	labials	*backing (to alveolar)*	*100%*
	fricatives	*stopping*	*100%*
	liquids	*stopping*	*100%*
	all consonants	*voicing*	*100%*

Of all of these, the one process that seems to describe the largest number of Nathan's words is alveolar consonant harmony. This appears to be quite appropriate for words such as "butter" ([dʌdʌ]) and "feather" ([dɛdʊ]). However, alveolar consonant harmony can't account for words like "go" ([do]), "more" ([no]), "bye" ([daɪ]), "shoe" ([du]), and "blue" ([du]). There is no one process that will cover all of these patterns. A variety of processes seem to be responsible for Nathan's productions of these words. Furthermore, some of the processes appear to be contradictory. For example, fronting and backing both occurred in Nathan's speech. The clinician is left with a long list of processes to address in therapy and little idea of where to start.

Of course, Nathan is a hypothetical child, and the data were selected on purpose to illustrate the possible disadvantages of traditional procedures such as substitution analysis, generative analysis, and process analysis. However, the general problems identified here are common results of process analysis, especially the findings of an overabundance of processes to treat and contradictory processes operating within the same child's speech.

A similar real-life case is provided by Bernhardt and Stemberger (1998). Although he did produce some other consonants in some contexts, this 5-year-old child, Colin, had [g] as his default consonant, as shown in Table 9-16. A process analysis would identify backing, stopping of fricatives and liquids, cluster reduction, voicing, devoicing, and denasalization, among others. It is very challenging to know what to do first when confronted with process analysis results of this sort. A follow-up constraint analysis would indicate a strong (although not absolute) markedness constraint against any non-velar, non-oral, or non-stop consonant. Therapy focusing (in part) on introducing $\begin{bmatrix}+\text{anterior}\\+\text{coronal}\end{bmatrix}$ (i.e., alveolar) stops was successful.

Constraints

Again, no commercially available tests focused on identifying phonological constraints exist. As discussed in the prior section, identifying the processes that a child is using via a standardized process test (or a do-it-yourself process analysis such as Forms 9-1 and 9-2 based upon a speech sample) can be the first step toward identifying her constraints. The question to be posed is "Why is this child using these processes?" Specifically, what common goals are reached through the use of these processes that might relate to:

1. Avoiding difficult elements or structures—in other words, markedness constraints (e.g., omission and substitution of velars in various positions; cluster reduction, migration, and epenthesis)?
2. Preserving certain features, elements, or structures even at the cost of others—in other words, faithfulness constraints (e.g., epenthesis of vowels between the two consonants in a cluster so as to avoid deleting either consonant, preserving some features of each consonant in a cluster by coalescing them into one consonant, such as /sw/ → [f] /#____)?

Put more simply, (1) "What is this child avoiding doing?" and (2) "What is she doing right?" In most cases, the constraints are *what* the child is avoiding, and the processes (or rules) are *how*.

Once identified, the child's constraints, divided into word and syllable structure versus feature constraints, can be organized using Form 9-3, as illustrated for Nathan in Example 9-3.

On this form, the subscripts indicate whether two elements are the same or different. For example, C_1VC_1V indicates that the two consonants are the same (harmonized); C_1VC_2V indicates that they are different. The symbol σ represents a syllable; thus, $\sigma_1\sigma_2$ indicates two different (non-reduplicated) syllables. Note that phonotactic constraints are listed on the first page, while the second page is available for listing phonetic/feature constraints.

Reconsidering Nathan's phonology from this perspective, it is clear that the most general possible description of what's actually non-functional about this child's phonology is a simple statement about his *phonetic* repertoire: He has only two consonants—[d] and [n]—and he uses them everywhere! Various processes or rules conspire to substitute these two consonants for everything. From an efficiency point of view, however, the actual processes involved are far less important to our intervention planning than is this simple phonetic generalization. His markedness constraint is: Avoid everything except alveolar (oral or nasal) stops.

This generalization can be written using a generative phonological rule as discussed above. However, the use of this rule implies that Nathan has all consonant features in his underlying representations. That is, the rule is based upon the assumption that complete information about each adult word is stored in Nathan's mental lexicon. Many child phonologists feel uncomfortable about this type of claim. It is felt that the child is only likely to store those features that are salient and useful phonologically to him at any given time. It is possible to circumvent this issue and to arrive at

TABLE 9-16 **Colin's Default Consonant**

Target	Production
daddy	[gɑhi]
snow	[gɑ:]
laugh	[gaʊ]
thumb	[gɑ:ʔ]
Santa Claus	[gɑgɑgɑk]
radio	[gɑhɑ]

From Bernhardt, B., & Stemberger, J. P. (1998). *Handbook of phonological development: From the perspective of constraint-based nonlinear phonology.* San Diego: Academic Press.

Form 9-3, p. 1

Name: Age:
Date: Examiner:
Source of sample: Size of sample:

CONSTRAINT SUMMARY:
What is the child NOT doing?

Use √ or indicate frequency (%). Make appropriate specifications/comments. All sequences of Cs and Vs are assumed to be within the same word.

KEY:
C: consonant V: vowel
#: word boundary σ: syllable (e.g., σσ = disyllabic word)
x_1x_2: x_1 and x_2 are different from each other
*: not allowed (e.g., *C# - constraint against final consonants)

I. Phonotactic Constraints:

Constraint	Age Equivalence	Restrictions/Comments
Syllable shapes	Expected up to age	
_____*C#	3;0	
_____*#C	not expected	
_____*#CC	4;0	
_____*CC#	4;0	
_____*VCCV		
Word shapes		
_____*#σσ#	2;0	
_____*#σσσ#		
Harmony/Assimilation		
_____*$\sigma_1\sigma_2$	2;0	
_____*C_1VC_2V	2;0	
_____*C_1VC_2	2;0	
_____*CV_1CV_2	2;0	

Comments:

Form 9-3, p. 2

Name: Age:
Date: Examiner:
Source of sample: Size of sample:

CONSTRAINT SUMMARY, CONT.:
What is the child NOT doing?

Specific Feature Constraints

Restricted Feature	**Restricted Word Position**	**Comments, etc.**
EXAMPLES: *velar* *fricatives*	 *final* *all*	 *omitted* *stopped*

Comments:

Example 9-3, p.1

Name: *Nathan* Examiner: *SLV*
Source of sample: *hypothetical* Size of sample: *18 words*

SUMMARY: PHONOLOGICAL CONSTRAINTS

Use √ or indicate frequency of occurrence (with %). Make appropriate specifications/comments.
All sequences of Cs and Vs are assumed to be within the same word.

NOTE: C: consonant
V: vowel
#: word boundary
σ: syllable (e.g., σσ = disyllabic word)
$x_1 x_2$: x_1 and x_2 are different from each other

I. Phonotactic Constraints:

Constraint	Age Equivalence*	Restrictions/Comments
Syllable shapes	*Expected up to:*	
*C#_____	*3;0*	
*#C_____	*not expected*	
*#CC_____	*4;0*	*no clusters*
*VCCV_____		*no clusters*
*CC#_____		*no clusters*
Word shapes		
*#σσ#_____	*2;0*	
*#σσσ#_____		
Harmony/Assimilation		
*$\sigma_1 \sigma_2$_____	*2;0*	*occasional apparent reduplication*
*$C_1 V C_2 V$_____	*2;0*	*occasional apparent harmony*
*$C_1 V C_2$_____	*2;0*	*occasional apparent harmony*
*$C V_1 C V_2$_____	*2;0*	

Comments: *Feature constraints result in apparent reduplication and harmony.*

*Age equivalences are approximate. They are based upon Grunwell (1985); Chin and Dinnsen (1992); Smit et al. (1990); Stoel-Gammon (1987). "Not expected" indicates a constraint

Example 9-3, p.2

Name: *Nathan* Examiner: *SLV*
Source of sample: *hypothetical* Size of sample: *18 words*

SUMMARY: PHONOLOGICAL CONSTRAINTS (cont.)

II. Specific Feature Restrictions:

Restricted Feature	Restricted Word Position	Comments, etc.
non-alveolar	*no non-alveolars anywhere ever*	
continuant (fricative, liquid, glide)	*no continuants anywhere ever*	

a far simpler and more goal-related statement of Nathan's problem by using a constraint rather than a rule. Nathan's markedness constraint is: $*\begin{bmatrix} -\text{coronal} \\ -\text{anterior} \\ +\text{consonantal} \end{bmatrix}$

This constraint indicates that non-alveolar consonants (i.e., consonants that are not both [+coronal] and [+anterior]) are not allowed. Stating simply that Nathan has this constraint implies no assumptions about his underlying representations. It is *only* a statement that he does not produce non-alveolar consonants. It is therefore a claim about his *output forms* only. Information about other places of articulation may or may not be stored in his underlying representation, but the output form is really the only information available to us.

As discussed in the section on phonological rules above, Nathan has a constraint against continuant consonants (fricatives, liquids, and glides) as well. He produces only oral ([d]) and nasal ([n]) stops. This constraint is also fairly simple:

$$*\left[+\text{continuant}\right]$$

This states that he does not produce continuant consonants. Note that this is a separate constraint. If the list of features in the first constraint were simply increased, the constraint would have a meaning that is actually too specific. That is,

$$*\begin{bmatrix} -\text{coronal} \\ -\text{anterior} \\ +\text{continuant} \\ +\text{consonantal} \end{bmatrix}$$

means that non-alveolar continuants are not allowed. It implies that non-alveolar stops would occur, which they do not in this (hypothetical) child's speech.

Nathan's constraint against consonant clusters can also be written simply as *CC. These constraints are simple and pervasive—three general principles that summarize his entire phonological profile: no non-alveolars, no continuants, and no clusters.

Nathan has one faithfulness constraint as well: If the consonant is oral, keep it oral; if it is nasal, keep it nasal. In other words, preserve nasality status. This is a strength upon which his SLP can build in therapy.

Simple statements about constraints clarify the issue of where to intervene. There is no need to choose among all of those processes or rules that may be attributable to this child. All that is needed is to persuade Nathan to weaken his constraints. Our clinical goals will be as follows:

1. Nathan will produce non-alveolar consonants (i.e., he will de-rank his constraint against them).
2. Nathan will produce continuant consonants (i.e., he will de-rank his constraint against them).
3. Nathan will produce consonant clusters (i.e., he will de-rank his constraint against them).

At this point, *which* non-alveolar consonants or continuant consonants or consonant clusters he will produce is a fairly minor question, as is the issue of word position. *Anything* other than [d] or [n] in *any* word position (initial, medial, or final) would represent a significant breakthrough and would be likely to trigger massive changes in Nathan's phonology as a whole. Production of any cluster would also signal significant progress, although the only possibility with his current consonant repertoire is syllable-final -nd. (The medial intervocalic consonant sequence -nd- would also constitute significant progress.) If Nathan appears to be stimulable for any particular class of consonants and/or any particular word position—even if it be [θ] in final clusters (as in the words "warmth" or "breadth"), a developmentally unexpected direction—then a more specific short-term objective will have emerged.

INTERVENTION CONCEPTS

The most important conclusion that can be drawn from what is now decades of research about phonological patterns in children with SSD is this: addressing speech sound disorders sound class by sound class and pattern by pattern instead of sound by sound is far more efficacious. If a pattern can be identified (*regardless of whether its source is motoric or cognitive–linguistic*), in the vast majority of cases, it should be treated as such. There are many further factors that can be considered as one is planning exactly how to do this in particular cases, however.

Where to Begin

Dyson and Robinson (1987) recommend using the following criteria in selecting which goals to target based on process analysis. (Note: constraint equivalencies are given in parentheses, where appropriate)

1. Frequency of occurrence: Target more frequent processes (i.e., constraints with wider, more pervasive impacts).
2. Impact on intelligibility: Target patterns that affect intelligibility the most.
3. Optionality: Target optional patterns (i.e., constraints that are sometimes violated).
4. In phonetic inventory or emerging: Target patterns that affect sounds that are stimulable (perhaps in other word positions).
5. Developmental order: Target earlier-emerging sounds.

Dyson and Robinson (1987) echo Hodson (1980) in suggesting (No. 1, above) that patterns that affect 40% or more of relevant target words should be the highest priority. They suggest that a process should be considered to affect intelligibility (No. 2) if it applies to sounds that are frequent in the language (e.g., alveolar consonants, in English), it is an "idiosyncratic" (unusual) process, or it is frequent in the speech of unintelligible children. In addition, some processes have larger impacts on intelligibility than do others; for example, Klein and Flint (2006) found that final consonant deletion and stopping of fricatives generally tend to impair understanding more than does fronting of velars.

The remainder of the suggestions made by Dyson and Robinson (1987) (Nos. 3 to 5) reflect traditional views as well as those of more recent researchers, such as Rvachew (2005) and Rvachew and Nowak (2001), in suggesting that goals should be selected based upon the child's existing phonological knowledge of the sound class or structure (as evidenced by the fact that the pattern does not apply 100% of the time or that the class or structure or some features of it are preserved via a faithfulness constraint), the child's emerging articulatory ability to produce the sound or structure (stimulability), and the typical developmental order in the ambient language. Recall that others (especially Gierut et al., e.g., Gierut, 2001; Morrisette & Gierut, 2002) advocate the reverse—that in targeting more complex, less stimulable, later-developing sound classes or structures, the child's entire phonological system will be stimulated and the earlier, less complex targets will be reached without direct therapy. The solution to which approach is better may well depend upon child-specific factors, such as the source of the SSD (motor speech disorder, fluctuating hearing loss, limited implicit learning capability, etc.), the specific sound class or structure, or other factors.

Table 9-17 summarizes the relationships between some common processes and constraints, including the goals that might follow from each. Given the close reciprocal relationship between processes and constraints, the choice is not really whether to address either processes or constraints. Rather, processes can be reduced by targeting constraints. If the child is using cluster reduction, epenthesis, metathesis, and coalescence because of a constraint against clusters, all of these processes will diminish as his ability to produce clusters increases.

Many patterns that will be encountered can be described, at least partially, with respect to distinctive phonetic features: nonsonorant continuants (i.e., fricatives) are non-preferred (marked) and are therefore stopped (become [-continuant]); velar ([-anterior –coronal]) non-nasal noncontinuants (i.e., stops) are non-preferred, so they become [+anterior + coronal] (alveolar), and so on. However, many of these patterns are positional as well; they occur in a particular word or syllable position, such as in an onset, in a coda, in medial position, in a cluster, or in an unstressed syllable. Thus, it is important to always ask oneself what phonotactic factors need to be taken into account.

Additional contextual factors are more specific, depending upon the phonetic features of the surrounding sound segments. For example, noncontinuants may conform in place of articulation (i.e., harmonize) with other noncontinuants, as when alveolar stops become velar if there is a velar stop elsewhere in the word. Similarly, consonants may be voiced before vowels (because vowels are voiced in English) and so on. All of these factors must be included in the goals and objectives that we write. In some cases, the goal will be to introduce a new feature, such as the velar ([-anterior –coronal]) place of articulation, or a new combination of features, such as voiced fricatives ([+voice, +continuant, -sonorant]). In others, it will be to change the distribution of features, such that two different consonants can occur in the same word (i.e., there is not harmony), two consonants can occur in a row (a cluster), a voiced consonant can abut a voiceless one, etc.

Structural patterns—those that affect the structure of the syllable or the word—should also be identified and treated, of course. As noted in the previous chapter, the goal here is for a more mature structure to be produced. It may not be possible for both the structure and the segments to be correct initially. Thus, the goal for a child with no final consonants would be for her to produce final consonants in appropriate words, regardless of the featural accuracy of those consonants. Although the target word (or syllable or phrase, etc.) should always be modeled correctly, a production with the incorrect consonant would meet the objective (e.g., the child's production of [fut] instead of [fu] for "food" meets the objective of producing a final consonant, even though the voicing is not correct).

TABLE 9-17 Relationship Between Processes and Constraints and Their Respective Goals

Process: What Is the Child Doing (in Error)?	Process Goal: Stop It!	Constraint: What Is the Child Avoiding?	Constraint Goal: Do It!
Stopping	Reduce stopping from __% to __%	Fricatives	Increase fricatives from __% to __%
Gliding	Reduce gliding	Liquids	Increase liquids
Cluster reduction	Reduce CCR	Clusters	Increase CC
Final C deletion	Reduce FCD	Final C	Increase final C
Metathesis, movement	Reduce metathesis, movement	Varied distribution patterns in word	Increase varied distribution
Harmony, reduplication	Reduce harmony, reduplication	Varied C or V in word	Increase varied C or V
Coalescence	Reduce coalescence	Clusters	Increase CC
Syllable reduction	Reduce syllable reduction	Multiple syllables	Increase syllables

As noted above, the same goal may be expressed in a rules/processes framework (e.g., "Suzy will decrease final consonant deletion from 90% to 50%") or in a constraints framework (e.g., "Suzy will produce final consonants in appropriate words 50% of the time"). If the former wording is used, it is important to monitor whether some other inappropriate process is replacing the targeted process. For instance, is the child using epenthesis as a way of preserving (being faithful to) the final consonant without producing it in final position (e.g., saying [fudə] instead of [fu] for "food"), or omitting liquids in order to avoid gliding them, or something of that sort? "Keeping our eyes on the prize" involves focusing on what the child is not doing (what her constraints are) that we would like to see her do.

Specific Considerations

Generalization

The fact that we are working on patterns does not completely determine the manner in which the goals will be addressed. With respect to generalization, there are two primary approaches to take, as discussed in previous chapters:

1. A broad approach, focusing on the whole pattern. For example, we might use stimuli that target all fricatives together in order to increase production of a variety of fricatives—and thereby reduce stopping—in hopes that all of the specific fricatives that are in error (stopped) will be remediated as a group.
2. A narrow approach, focusing on one subpattern. For instance, we might select stimuli that target one specific fricative in order to increase production (and reduce stopping) of that particular fricative in the hopes that all of the other sounds in the class (i.e., all other fricatives) will be stimulated to change at the same time.

Both of these are valid approaches. The child's specific phonological and learning profiles will determine which is selected. For example, the first, broader approach might be more appropriate for a child with no "knowledge" of fricatives (i.e., no production or stimulability for this class in any contexts). Bombardment (i.e., intense exposure to many different fricatives) and elicitation of frication of any type might make the child aware of this class and stimulate the production of some frication. The productions might be incorrect initially. The nature of the frication that emerges would then in turn determine which specific fricatives might be targeted in a narrower approach. In this author's experience, some children bombarded with fricatives begin to produce [x]—a voiceless velar fricative not present in English—first, possibly due to its high level of auditory and tactile salience. Such children then become stimulable for [h] or [ʃ]—the farthest back voiceless fricatives in English. Others begin to produce [f], a highly visible fricative that is early developing in typically developing children. The choice of targets and intervention approaches will depend upon the child's specific profile and responses.

One Pattern at a Time Versus a Combination of Patterns

Another broad (= shallow) versus narrow (= deep) question that arises is whether to treat multiple error patterns at once or to treat one error pattern to mastery before addressing another. Again, one variation on the broad approach is Hodson's (e.g., 2006) "cycles" therapy, in which one set of patterns is addressed for a certain length of time. Then, one (or more) pattern is rotated out, regardless of the amount of progress the child has made. Hodson's claim is that this approach is more similar to typical developmental patterns, in which children make a small amount of progress in a certain area, then a similar amount in another area, and so on. It is unusual for a child to change from having no ability to produce a certain sound class or structure to mastering that skill set. Furthermore, if the SLP has selected a goal (or set of goals) that is, for reasons that were not obvious, not ideal for the child at this time, a cycles approach guarantees that a limited amount of time will be "wasted" on such an unfortunate choice of goals.

Another component of Hodson's (2006, among others) approach to highly unintelligible speech is based upon the idea of implicit learning. Each session includes a portion in which the client sits quietly—coloring, doing a puzzle, or some such task—listening to the SLP produce words that fit the targeted pattern at a slightly amplified volume. The idea is that intensive exposure may trigger change. In addition, exemplars (target words) are chosen carefully based on stimulability testing to ensure that the child can produce them accurately (with cueing, attention, etc.). Hodson states that by producing a small number of words correctly many times, auditory–kinesthetic connections are stimulated that will enhance self-monitoring in less structured, supported environments. Unfortunately, only case study–level research has been performed to support these theoretical assumptions. Furthermore, a retrospective study by Shriberg and Kwiatkowski (1990) indicated that this auditory bombardment approach is not associated with maximum progress.

Perception Versus Production; Contrast

A focus on sound classes and patterns does not preclude a contrast-based approach. Children whose patterns result in phoneme collapses (i.e., a lack of contrast between one class of sounds and another—liquids versus glides, affricates versus stops, etc.) may be unaware that these sound classes differ in communicatively important ways. Strategies originally proposed within minimal pairs approaches may be appropriate for such clients—discrimination or production activities using minimal pairs that highlight the contrasts that are being lost as a result of the child's production patterns. The factors that influence clinical choices in contrast therapy remain relevant to deciding which pairs should be contrasted—the target and the error, two sounds or sound classes that are both typically in error, that target and a maximally distinct sound? The additional choice to be made is whether specific sounds or broader classes of sounds will be targeted.

Change Pattern Versus Produce Sound Accurately

With the new perspective of speech sound errors provided by pattern analysis, a new intervention option emerges: Rather than having a goal that the client will produce every speech sound accurately, we may target simply that the deviant pattern will change in some way. As illustrated many times in this book (most recently via the case of T, who avoided vowel-final words and substituted [s] for many codas), children—especially those with SSDs—often demonstrate unexpected patterns. For example, a child who substituted fricatives for liquids (e.g., /ɹ/ → [ʃ], /l/ → [s]) would be highly unintelligible not only because of a loss of contrast but also because this pattern is so unusual. As a result, even adults accustomed to young children's speech errors would be unlikely to be able to decipher the child's words. A shift in this frication pattern to a pattern of gliding liquids would be a big improvement in this respect. In fact, this would represent a shift from a non-sonorant substitution for liquids to a sonorant one, because glides (like liquids) are sonorant, but fricatives are not. We would want to specify that the sonorant would be continuant to ensure that she would not shift from substituting fricatives for liquids to substituting nasals for liquids. Thus, the goal would be as follows: Child will produce a sonorant continuant consonant when the target is a liquid. The production of any glide or liquid but not any other consonant would constitute achieving this goal, because they are all sonorant continuants. Of course, because of implicit learning, the targets would always be produced accurately by the SLP. Gliding of liquids would never be modeled even though it would be accepted as an approximation.

Similarly, if a child who reduces all clusters can be taught to produce the correct number of consonants, even if they are not the correct consonants (e.g., liquids are glided and /s/ → [f], such that "slide" is produced as [fwaɪd]), his speech would become more intelligible. The goal would be as follows: Child will produce two consecutive consonants when the target is a cluster, regardless of phonetic accuracy.

Because of implicit learning, the correct model should always be provided, but phonetic approximations that match the structural goal would be accepted as meeting the objective. This type of consideration is especially important for children whose deviant speech patterns have been in place for lengthy periods of time, particularly if they are resistant to therapy.

Phonetic Versus Phonological Therapy

Most SLPs associate process analysis with "phonological" rather than "phonetic" therapy. Phonetic therapy is the traditional sort that focuses on articulation—explicitly addressing placement, manner of articulation, and corrections—and phonological therapy is concerned with communicative efficacy (i.e., contrast): Did the message get through or was the wrong word perceived as the result of production patterns? However, as noted previously, the existence of a pattern does not tell us whether the source of that pattern is motoric, cognitive–linguistic, or both. In addition, children may be more likely to use unusual phonological error patterns when trying to produce words that include sounds that they have neither produced nor attempted in the past (Leonard, Schwartz, Swanson, & Frome-Loeb, 1987). Therefore, there may be some benefit to focusing on stimulability for some period of time. Furthermore, as discussed in Chapter 7, some children may benefit from a combination of linguistic contrast therapy and motoric phonetic therapy (Saben & Ingham, 1991). Thus, the choice of phonetic versus phonological therapy approaches is not the rigid dichotomy that some may assume.

EXERCISE 9-3

Assessment and Intervention for Patterns

SUMMARY

A focus on patterns rather than on individual substitutions, omissions, distortions, additions, and movements yields much more efficient evaluation and intervention procedures. Generative rules highlight the features of consonants and vowels in great detail, but they are challenging to write, and they do not easily reveal generalizations about phonotactic patterns. Phonological process analysis is easier and more familiar for most speech-language pathologists, and many assessment and treatment tools associated with this perspective are available. However, the emphasis on what is being avoided that is provided by Optimality Theory can often lead to more general insights and to more focused goals.

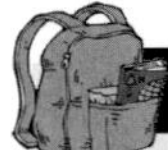

KEY TAKE-HOME MESSAGES

1. Addressing patterns is more effective than is focusing on individual sounds.
2. The presence of a pattern does not determine the cause of that pattern, which could be physiologic, sensory, due to motor programming/planning deficits, or linguistic–cognitive.
3. Process names may be misleading when they are too general (e.g., "fronting"); it is important to describe the specific nature and context of the difference between the target and the actual production.
4. Groups of processes may occur for a common reason, describable as a constraint.
5. Describing patterns as constraints rather than processes often makes the appropriate goals and strategies clearer.

CHAPTER 9

Phonological Patterns Review

Exercise 9-1

Multiple choice. Choose the best answer.

1. Within generative phonology, the "environment" refers to the:
   a. child's cultural context.
   b. child's linguistic context.
   c. articulatory position of the target sound.
   d. word position of the target sound.
2. Questions to be asked when writing generative phonological rules do not include:
   a. What is the faithful element?
   b. What is the environment?
   c. What is the target?
   d. What is the change?
3. 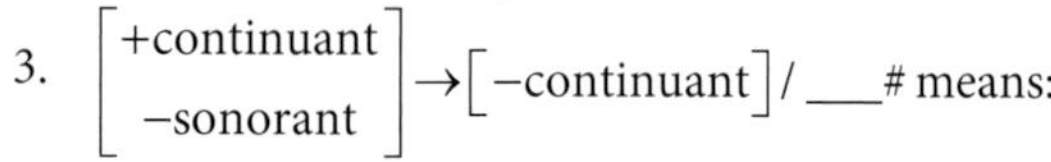
   a. fricatives are voiced in initial position.
   b. liquids are glided between vowels.
   c. fricatives are stopped in final position.
   d. stops are voiced in final position.
   e. none of the above.
4. $\begin{bmatrix} +\text{consonantal} \\ +\text{sonorant} \\ +\text{continuant} \\ +\text{coronal} \end{bmatrix} \rightarrow \begin{bmatrix} -\text{consonantal} \\ -\text{syllabic} \end{bmatrix} / \text{V}\_\text{V}$ means:
   a. fricatives are voiced in initial position.
   b. liquids are glided between vowels.
   c. fricatives are stopped in final position.
   d. stops are voiced in final position.
   e. none of the above.
5. $\begin{bmatrix} +\text{continuant} \\ -\text{sonorant} \end{bmatrix} \rightarrow \begin{bmatrix} +\text{consonantal} \\ +\text{sonorant} \\ +\text{continuant} \\ +\text{coronal} \end{bmatrix} / \#\_$ means:
   a. fricatives are voiced in initial position.
   b. liquids are glided between vowels.
   c. fricatives are stopped in final position.
   d. stops are voiced in final position.
   e. none of the above.
6. $\begin{bmatrix} -\text{continuant} \\ -\text{nasal} \end{bmatrix} \rightarrow [+\text{voice}] / \_\#$ means:
   a. fricatives are voiced in initial position.
   b. liquids are glided between vowels.
   c. fricatives are stopped in final position.
   d. stops are voiced in final position.
   e. none of the above.
7. Which of the following is NOT true in the theory of natural phonology?
   a. Processes are either suppressed totally or not at all.
   b. Processes are based on human physiologic limitations.
   c. The extent of suppression of a process depends on the language.
   d. Suppression of processes is sometimes context-specific.
8. If a child says [gʌk] for "duck," this is an example of:
   a. bidirectional assimilation.
   b. regressive harmony.
   c. feature coalescence.
   d. manner migration.

Exercise 9-2

A. *Essay questions.*

1. Some children demonstrate atypical processes or constraints that match neither universals nor the patterns of their own languages. Use information from this chapter, other chapters in this book, and other sources to speculate about other factors that may cause these patterns to occur.

B. *Multiple choice. Choose the best answer.*

1. Markedness constraints:
   a. are the same as substitution processes.
   b. are the same as phonotactic processes.
   c. represent the elements or structures that the child preserves.
   d. represent the elements or structures that the child avoids.
2. Faithfulness constraints:
   a. are the same as substitution processes.
   b. are the same as phonotactic processes.
   c. represent the elements or structures that the child preserves.
   d. represent the elements or structures that the child avoids.
3. "*CC#" refers to a:
   a. faithfulness constraint against epenthesis.
   b. markedness constraint against final clusters.
   c. universal distribution requirement.
   d. generative rule about obstruents.
4. According to Velleman and Vihman (2002):
   a. child constraint rankings vary by language.
   b. child constraint rankings reflect universals.
   c. syllables with vocalic nuclei are strongly preferred by most children.
   d. children may be faithful to frequency patterns in the language, to individual word forms, or to both.
   e. all of the above.
   f. none of the above.

Exercise 9-3

Case study questions.

A. Wally substitutes p/f, t/θ, t/s, t/ʃ, b/v, d/ð, d/z, d/ʒ in initial position. He omits /f, s/ from clusters in all word positions. His SLP is overwhelmed by the number of goals she will have to address. Isn't there a more efficient way to handle this? Describe Wally's errors in terms of error patterns. Write two pattern goals for Wally and justify them using information from this chapter or other sources.

B. Consider the following data from a hypothetical child named Connor, age 8;0:

Target	Production	Target	Production
1. haʊs	[faʊf]	26. tʃu	[fu]
2. tɹi	[ti]	27. bæθ	[bæf]
3. ˈwɪndo	[ˈwɪndo]	28. ɹɪŋ	[ɪn]
4. gʌm	[dʌm]	29. ˈmʌŋki	[ˈmʌŋki]
5. kʌp	[tʌp]	30. bəˈnænə	[ˈnænə]
6. naɪf	[naɪf]	31. ˈzɪpɚ	[ˈvɪpə]
7. spun	[fun]	32. ˈsɪzɚz	[ˈfɪvəv]
8. dʌk	[dʌk]	33. daɚk	[dak]
9. spɛl	[fɛʊ]	34. daɚt	[dat]
10. ˈwægən	[ˈwædən]	35. ˈfɪŋgɚ	[ˈfɪŋgə]
11. ˈʃʌvəl	[ˈfʌvəʊ]	36. θʌm	[fʌm]
12. plen	[fen]	37. ˈdʒʌmpɪŋ	[ˈvʌmpɪn]
13. ˈswɪmɪŋ	[ˈfɪnɪn]	38. pəˈdʒaməz	[ˈvaməv]
14. ˈwatʃɪz	[ˈwafɪv]	39. ˈwaʃɪŋ	[ˈwafɪn]
15. læmp	[jæmp]	40. ˈflaʊwɚz	[ˈfaʊwəv]
16. kaɚ	[ta]	41. bɹʌʃ	[bʌf]
17. blu	[fu]	42. dɹʌm	[fʌm]
18. ˈɹæbɪt	[ˈæbɪt]	43. fɹɔg	[fɔg]
19. tɹen	[fen]	44. gɹin	[fin]
20. got	[dʌt]	45. bəˈlunz	[jumv]
21. ˈfɪʃɪŋ	[ˈfɪfɪn]	46. ˈkɹaɪjɪŋ	[ˈfaɪjɪn]
22. tʃɛɚ	[fɛ]	47. kal	[taʊ]
23. ˈfɛðɚ	[ˈfɛvə]	48. slaɪd	[faɪd]
24. kʌm	[tʌm]	49. staɚz	[fav]
25. klin	[fin]	50. faɪv	[faɪv]

1. Phonological rules:
   a. List three rules in a phonological rule table for Connor.
   b. Write one of them formally, using phonetic features.
2. Phonological processes:
   a. List two substitution processes, with an example of each.
   b. List two phonotactic processes, with an example of each.
3. Phonological constraints:
   a. Write the two substitution processes as constraints: What feature combinations is Connor avoiding?
   b. Write the two phonotactic processes as constraints: What syllable or word structures is Connor avoiding?
4. Write two goals for Connor, each in two ways:
   a. as a process goal (decrease process use)
   b. as a constraint goal (increase use of avoided sound or structure).

Multiple choice. Choose the best answer.

1. Pattern intervention approaches to SSD:
   a. are only appropriate for children with linguistically based SSD.
   b. lead to more efficacious intervention.
   c. always proceed from most complex to less complex.
   d. always proceed from broad to narrow.
2. In Velleman's view, phonological constraints:
   a. are more directly related to appropriate goals.
   b. describe strategies used to stimulate certain sound classes or structures.
   c. are irrelevant after phonological systematization.
   d. have narrower explanatory value than phonological processes or rules.
3. The best assessment procedure for phonological processes:
   a. assesses a maximum number of processes.
   b. assesses a maximum number of words.
   c. depends on the specific situation.
   d. is based on a spontaneous speech sample.

References

Abraham, S. (1989). Using a phonological framework to describe speech errors of orally-trained, hearing-impaired school-agers. *The Journal of Speech and Hearing Disorders, 54*, 600–609.

Bankson, N. W., & Bernthal, J. E. (1990). *Bankson-Bernthal Test of Phonology*. Chicago: Riverside.

Barnes, E., Roberts, J., Long, S. H., Martin, G. E., Berni, M. C., Mandulak, K. C., et al. (2009). Phonological accuracy and intelligibility in connected speech of boys with Fragile X syndrome or Down syndrome. *Journal of Speech, Language, and Hearing Research, 52*, 1048–1061.

Bernhardt, B., & Stemberger, J. P. (1998). *Handbook of phonological development: From the perspective of constraint-based nonlinear phonology*. San Diego: Academic Press.

Chin, S., & Dinnsen, D. (1992). Consonant clusters in disordered speech: Constraints and correspondence patterns. *Journal of Child Language, 19*, 259–285.

Chomsky, N., & Halle, M. (1968). *The sound pattern of English*. New York, NY: Harper & Row.

Dinnsen, D. A. (2008). A typology of opacity effects in acquisition. In D. A. Dinnsen & J. A. Gierut (Eds.), *Optimailty theory, phonological acquisition, and disorders* (pp. 121–176). Oakville, CT: Equinox Publishing/DBBC.

Dinnsen, D. A., & Farris-Trimble, A. W. (2008). An unusual error pattern reconsidered. In D. A. Dinnsen & J. A. Gierut (Eds.), *Optimailty theory, phonological acquisition, and disorders* (pp. 177–204). Oakville, CT: Equinox Publishing/DBBC.

Donegan, P. J., & Stampe, D. (1979). The study of natural phonology. In D. A. Dinnsen (Ed.), *Current approaches to phonological theory* (pp. 126–173). Bloomington, IN: Indiana University Press.

Dyson, A. T., & Robinson, T. W. (1987). The effect of phonological analysis procedure on the selection of potential remediation targets. *Language, Speech, and Hearing Services in Schools, 18*, 364–377.

Eisenberg, S. L., & Hitchcock, E. R. (2010). Using standardized tests to inventory consonant and vowel production: A comparison of 11 tests of articulation and phonology. *Language, Speech and Hearing Services in Schools, 41*, 488–503.

Gierut, J. A. (2001). Complexity in phonological treatment: Clinical factors. *Language, Speech, and Hearing Services in Schools, 32*(4), 229–241.

Haelsig, P. C., & Madison, C. L. (1986). A study of phonological processes exhibited by 3-, 4-, and 5-year-old children. *Language, Speech and Hearing Services in Schools, 17*, 107–114.

Hodson, B. W. (1980). *The Assessment of Phonological Processes*. Danville, IL: Interstate.

Hodson, B. W. (2004). *Hodson Assessment of Phonological Patterns (HAPP-3)* (3rd ed.). East Moline, IL: LinguiSystems.

Hodson, B. W. (2011). Enhancing phonological patterns of young children with highly unintelligible speech. *The ASHA Leader*, 16–19.

Hodson, B. W., & Paden, E. P. (1991). *Targeting intelligible speech: A phonological approach to remediation* (2nd ed.). Austin, TX: Pro-Ed.

Klein, E. S., & Flint, C. B. (2006). Measurement of intelligibility in disordered speech. *Language, Speech, and Hearing Services in Schools, 37*, 191–199.

Leonard, L. B., & Brown, B. L. (1984). Nature and boundaries of phonologic categories: A case study of an unusual phonologic pattern in a language-impaired child. *The Journal of Speech and Hearing Disorders, 49*, 419–428.

Leonard, L. B., & McGregor, K. K. (1991). Unusual phonological patterns and their underlying representations: A case study. *Journal of Child Language, 18*(2), 261–272.

Leonard, L. B., Schwartz, R. G., Swanson, L. A., & Frome-Loeb, D. M. (1987). Some conditions that promote unusual phonological behavior in children. *Clinical Linguistics & Phonetics, 1*(1), 23–34.

McIntosh, & Dodd, B. (2008). Two-year-olds' phonological acquisition: Normative data. *International Journal of Speech-Language Pathology, 10*(6), 460–469.

Menn, L. (1978). Phonological units in beginning speech. In A. Bell & J. B. Hooper (Eds.), *Syllables and Segments* (pp. 157–171). Amsterdam, The Netherlands: North-Holland Publishing Co.

Menn, L., Schmidt, E., & Nicholas, B. (2013). Challenges to theories, charges to a model: The Linked-Attractor model of phonological development. In M. M. Vihman & T. Keren-Portnoy (Eds.), *The emergence of phonology: Whole-word approaches and cross-linguistic evidence* (pp. 460–502). Cambridge, UK: Cambridge University Press.

Morrisette, M. L., & Gierut, J. A. (2002). Lexical organization and phonological change in treatment. *Journal of Speech, Language, and Hearing Research, 45*(1), 143–159.

Pater, J. (2004). Bridging the gap between perception and production with minimally violable constraints. In R. Kager, J. Pater, & W. Zonneveld (Eds.), *Constraints in phonological development* (pp.219–244). Cambridge, UK: Cambridge University Press.

Roberts, J. E., Burchinal, M., & Footo, M. M. (1990). Phonological process decline from 2-1/2 to 8 years. *Journal of Communication Disorders, 23*, 205–217.

Roberts, J., Long, S. H., Malkin, C., Barnes, E., Skinner, M., Hennon, E. A., et al. (2005). A comparison of phonological skills of boys with Fragile X syndrome and Down syndrome. *Journal of Speech, Language, and Hearing Research, 48*, 980–995.

Rupela, V., Manjula, R., & Velleman, S. L. (2010). Phonological processes in Kannada-speaking adolescents with Down syndrome. *Clinical Linguistics and Phonetics, 24*(6), 431–450.

Rvachew, S. (2005). Stimulability and treatment success. *Topics in Language Disorders, 25*(3), 207–219.

Rvachew, S., & Nowak, M. (2001). The effect of target-selection strategy on phonological learning. *Journal of Speech, Language, and Hearing Research, 44*(3), 610–623.

Saben, C. B., & Ingham, R. J. (1991). The effects of minimal pairs treatment on the speech sound production of two children with phonological disorders. *Journal of Speech and Hearing Research, 34*, 1023–1040.

Shriberg, L. D., & Kwiatkowski, J. (1990). Self-monitoring and generalization in preschool speech-delayed children. *Language, Speech and Hearing Services in Schools, 21*, 157–170.

Smith, N. V. (1973). *The acquisition of phonology: A case study*. Cambridge, UK: Cambridge University Press.

Stampe, D. (1972). *A dissertation on natural phonology. (Doctoral dissertation)*, University of Chicago.

Stemberger, J. P., & Bernhardt, B. H. (1997). Optimality theory. In M. J. Ball & R. D. Kent (Eds.), *The new phonologies: Developments in clinical linguistics* (pp. 211–245). San Diego, CA: Singular.

Stoel-Gammon, C. (1996). On the acquisition of velars in English. In B. Bernhardt, J. Gilbert & D. Ingram (Eds.), *Proceedings of the UBC International Conference of Phonological Acquisition* (pp. 201–214). Somerville, MA: Cascadilla Press.

Stoel-Gammon, C. (2001). Down syndrome phonology: Development patterns and intervention strategies. *Down Syndrome Research and Practice, 7*(3), 93–100.

Tyler, A. A., Edwards, M. L., & Saxman, J. H. (1987). Clinical application of two phonologically based treatment procedures. *Journal of Speech and Hearing Disorders, 52*, 393–409.

Velleman, D. J. (2006). *How to prove it* (2nd ed.). Cambridge, UK: Cambridge University Press.

Velleman, S. L., & Vihman, M. M. (2002). The emergence of the marked unfaithful. In A. Carpenter, A. Coetzee, & P. De Lacy (Eds.), *University of Massachusetts Occasional Papers in Linguistics, 26: Papers in Optimality Theory II* (pp. 397–419). Amherst, MA: GLSA.

Vihman, M. M. (2014). *Phonological development: The first two years* (2nd ed.). Somerset, NJ: Blackwell-Wiley.

Vihman, M. M., & Velleman, S. L. (1989). Phonological reorganization: A case study. *Language and Speech, 32*, 149–170.

Vihman, M. M., & Velleman, S. L. (2000a). The construction of a first phonology. *Phonetica, 57*, 255–266.

Vihman, M. M., & Velleman, S. L. (2000b). Phonetics and the origins of phonology. In N. Burton-Roberts, P. Carr & G. Docherty (Eds.), *Conceptual and empirical foundations of phonology* (pp. 305–339). Oxford, UK: Oxford University Press.

Wolk, L., & Giesen, J. (2000). A phonological investigation of four siblings with childhood autism. *Journal of Communication Disorders, 33*, 371–389.

CHAPTER 10

Prosody

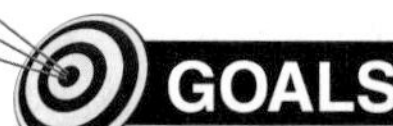

GOALS *of This Chapter*

1. Review key aspects of prosody, and describe their importance and their development in typically developing children.
2. Differentiate prosodic disability from dysprosody.
3. Identify aspects of prosody that are often impaired in children with specific diagnoses: Childhood Apraxia of Speech, autism spectrum disorders, cognitive impairments, and hearing loss.
4. Describe evaluation and intervention strategies for prosodic deficits.

After several years of therapy, Sammy's production of consonants is now accurate 90% of the time, and the school special education director feels Sammy is ready for discharge from therapy. Yet, her speech calls attention to itself because it is slow, choppy, monotone, and arrhythmic. In longer utterances, it is difficult for listeners to follow her train of thought. How can these deficits be characterized and documented? What intervention strategies are available to increase the age appropriateness of her prosody?

INTRODUCTION

Although some people may perceive prosody to be merely "frosting on the cake"—an interesting but nonessential aspect of speech—it actually is critical to successful oral communication. It's true that prosody has a strong affective impact; it conveys emotion and sociolinguistic information (e.g., the speaker's group membership, including geographic roots) in many subtle ways. We often are not even consciously aware of these. But the linguistic aspects of prosody also are key to successful communication. Intonation contours convey grammatical information (e.g., yes-or-no questions versus statements or wh- questions). They also impact intelligibility; utterances produced with a flattened fundamental frequency (i.e., a lack of pitch variation) are more difficult to understand (Laures & Weismer, 1999). Similarly, misapplied lexical stress can slow the listeners' processing of the utterance and decrease the likelihood they will recognize the target word (Goetry, Wade-Woolley, Kolinsky, & Mousty, 2006; van Rees, Ballard, McCabe, Macdonald-D'Silva and Arciuli, 2012). The placement of pauses within sentences (juncture; see Chapter 2) also affects listeners' comprehension (Wingfield, Lombardi, & Sokol, 1984). In short, it is highly likely that prosodic deficits have a significant negative impact on speakers' intelligibility (van Rees et al., 2012). As such, their inclusion in evaluation and treatment plans is vital.

PROSODIC DEVELOPMENT

Prosody is one of the first aspects of their native languages that infants discriminate and produce. This includes not only pitch contours but also the rhythm and the stress patterns of the language. Babies already recognize their own languages based on intonation alone at birth. As reviewed in Chapter 3, they gradually begin to discriminate the ambient language from others based on smaller and smaller units from clauses down to single words, using pitch contours, stress patterns, and pauses. Infant-directed speech (also known as motherese, baby talk, etc.) is an adaptation of adult–adult speech in which those characteristics, such as pitch contours, that are most likely to attract the infant's attention are highlighted. However, certain aspects of prosody, such as sarcasm, are also among the last aspects of phonology to be learned.

Development of Intonation and Tone

Production of language-appropriate intonation begins before meaningful speech. Falling pitch patterns predominate as early as 3 months of age. This is most likely for physiologic reasons (Kent & Bauer, 1985; Kent & Murray, 1982), although emotional factors may also have an impact (Snow, 2006). The child's frequency of falling versus rising pitch contours typically matches the ambient language late in the babbling period (Whalen, Levitt, & Wang, 1991). At 18 months, French infants show mostly rising contours, while those learning Japanese produce predominantly falling contours (Halle, Boysson-Bardies, & Vihman, 1991). In English-speaking children (at least), a wider range of pitch values is observed in falling contours, presumably because these occur earlier and are physiologically easier. However, their ranges decrease between 8 and 17 months and then increase again to the levels at which they will remain up to 4 years of age (Snow, 2001, 2006). This period from 8 to 17 months of age during which narrower pitch ranges are produced may be a reorganizational phase eventually resulting in higher levels of control of intonation (a typical U-shaped developmental curve).

At the age of 18 months is also when children use intonation to mark boundaries between utterances or parts of utterances. However, Branigan (1979) showed that when children first begin to produce two words in a row, they produce falling intonation in between them rather than linking them in one phrase contour. This suggests either that these productions are not yet formulated as single utterances or that the motor planning and control required to both produce particular words (as opposed to "random" babbles) and encapsulate them into a single prosodic contour is not yet present, or both. With respect to particular intonation contours, the ability to imitate rising pitch patterns (as in yes-or-no questions) lags behind that of falling pitch patterns (in English). Three-year-olds have more difficulty than do 5-year-olds imitating the intonation patterns in interrogatory (question) forms (Frome-Loeb & Allen, 1993). According to Snow (1998), 4-year-olds correctly imitate falling pitch, including rate of pitch change, in any sentence position. They also do well with rising contours in non–sentence-final positions (Grigos & Patel, 2007). Four-year-olds (but not 3-year-olds) also use lower pitch when they are told to talk more clearly or more like an adult (Redford & Gildersleeve-Neumann, 2009). However, they continue to make errors in producing rising contours at the ends of sentences, such as would occur in yes-or-no questions. Their control of the temporal articulatory differences between questions and statements is not mature until about 7 years of age; variability also decreases with age (Grigos & Patel, 2007).

The development of intonation appears to be independent of the development both of speech timing and of articulation (Snow, 2001, 2006).

In many of the world's languages, tone—the contrastive use of pitch at the word level—must be learned rather than intonation. In Cantonese, for example, there are six different tones that differentiate word meanings. Just as infants lose the ability to discriminate consonant and vowel contrasts to which they are not exposed (see Chapter 3), children learning English or French initially discriminate among these tones, but lose this ability by 9 months. Chinese children maintain these tone discrimination skills (Mattock & Burnham, 2006; Mattock, Molnar, Polka, & Burnham, 2008). Furthermore, most Chinese-learning children master the production of all language-specific tones by age 2. The easiest appears to be the highest tone; midtones and rising tones are more challenging for some children (Cheung & Abberton, 2000; So & Dodd, 1995). Among Cantonese children with SSD, tone appears to pose fewer problems than do consonants or vowels. Those with tone deficits typically find rising tones most challenging (Cheung & Abberton, 2000; So & Dodd, 1994), just as rising intonation can be more challenging than falling contours for typically developing children, as noted above.

Duration and Rhythm Including Pauses

Due to motoric immaturity, children speak more slowly than do adults, with their rates increasing over time. The speech of 3-year-olds is still significantly slower than that of 5-year-olds. Spontaneous speech is faster than is imitated speech but also much more variable (Walker, Archibald, Cherniak, & Fish, 1992). However, relative timing—the timing of certain aspects of speech versus others—is acquired long before absolute durations are adult-like. For example, by 18 months of age, the vowel durations of Japanese and French infants already reflect the relative durations of their native languages (Halle et al., 1991). Infants exposed to geminates (e.g., in Welsh or Finnish) produce longer medial consonants even in their babble as well as in their first words, differentiating long versus short segments although sometimes not in the appropriate words (Menn & Vihman, 2011). Furthermore, learners of Yucatecan Maya can master the long versus short vowel contrast in that language by the age of 2 (Archibald, 1996). At 4 years of age (but not at 3 years of age), youngsters are able to control their durations enough to vary their speech rate (i.e., their vowel durations) according to context (i.e., casual versus more formal speech) (Redford & Gildersleeve-Neumann, 2009). However, motor planning of the timing of phrases and sentences does not even approach adult-like efficiency until age 9. It continues to be more variable than adult phrase and sentence timing well into adolescence (Sadagopan & Smith, 2008).

As we have seen, two-word utterances are initially produced without a single prosodic contour (Branigan, 1979); sentence intonation comes with time. As children begin to combine words, they also demonstrate signs of the emergence of control of phrase-final lengthening, in which the last syllable of a phrase or sentence is protracted (Aoyama, Peters, & Winchester, 2010). By 18 months of age, Japanese children have learned not to use phrase-final lengthening, while French toddlers use it consistently (Halle et al., 1991). This developmental process may take several months, but by the time children are producing multiword sentences contained within a single utterance contour, usually sometime during the latter part of the second year of life, they are also correctly using phrase-final lengthening (Snow, 1994).

With respect to juncture, children know how to use pauses receptively to parse sentences into grammatical phrases (e.g., "Mommy and Daddy | went to the store") from early school age. In fact, Schreiber and Read (1980) demonstrated that 7-year-olds are far better at picking out phrasal nouns (e.g., "Mommy and Daddy," 91% of children) than at picking out subjects that consist of a single noun (e.g., "Mommy," 29% of children) from a sentence. The amount of "phonetic substance" in the single nouns also affected the subjects' success; they were far better at isolating words like "people, soap, elephants" than words like "he" and "we." Labelle (1973) similarly demonstrated that children comprehend lengthy sentences better when pauses are placed in syntactically appropriate locations than when pauses are either missing or misplaced.

The Development of Lexical and Phrasal Stress

The acquisition of word stress, like that of intonation, is a gradual process. Even though very young infants already prefer the predominant stress patterns of their own language (Segal & Kishon-Rabin, 2012), the production of language-appropriate stress patterns appears to be learned initially on a word-by-word basis. Only as the child's vocabulary grows does she abstract from her word knowledge to a more general understanding of this aspect of prosody.

Children learning French, a language with an invariant final-syllable stress pattern, are quite consistent and accurate by the time they have vocabularies of about 50 words (Vihman, Nakai, & De Paolis, 2006). Children learning English, a far more rhythmically complex language, may continue to mis-stress multisyllabic words or, even more commonly, to omit unstressed syllables, yielding forms like [ˈnænə] for "banana," [waʊn] for "around," and [ˈɛfʌn] for "elephant" up to the age of about 3. They are more likely to preserve final syllables and also syllables that occur within trochees (strong syllable + weak syllable, as in "CAmel") than those that occur within iambs (weak syllable + strong syllable, as in "giRAFFE;" Chiat & Roy, 2007; Gerken, 1994; Gerken & McGregor, 1998; Kehoe & Stoel-Gammon, 1997b; Schwartz & Goffman, 1995). This may be partly due to the fact that the vast majority (94%) of two-syllable English nouns are trochaic, while two-syllable English verbs tend to be iambic (69% to 76%) (van Rees et al., 2012). Initial weak syllables are 25 times more likely to be omitted from two-syllable words (e.g., "giraffe") and three times more likely to be omitted from initial position in three-syllable words (e.g., "banana") than are weak syllables later in the word (e.g., "monkey," "elephant") (Chiat & Roy, 2007). In typically developing English-learning children, omissions of weak syllables, especially in non-final position, are far more common than are stress shift errors in which all syllables are produced but with the wrong stress pattern (Kehoe & Stoel-Gammon, 1997a). Similarly, Fikkert (1994) found that both omission and stress shift errors are more likely to affect iambic (weak–strong) words than trochaic (strong–weak) words for children learning Dutch, a language with a similar rhythmic pattern to that of English.

Kehoe, Stoel-Gammon, and Buder (1995) reported that, although about 30% of their stress markings were inaccurate or indeterminate, children between 18 and 30 months did use all three parameters of English stress—duration, amplitude, and pitch—to differentiate strong versus weak syllables. Typically, the trochaic strong–weak stress pattern is mastered by age 3; the iambic pattern may still be developing at 7 years of age (Ballard, Djaja, Arciuli, James, & van Doorn, 2012). However, trochaic words may be produced by relying on early-established, more evenly stressed babbling patterns. In contrast, because the production of iambs requires more movement specificity, they may actually be more stable with more distinction between strong versus weak syllables (Goffman & Malin, 1999).

The stress pattern in a particular word may be influenced by the stress patterns of the words around it within a sentence. The preference for trochees in English-learning children noted above is seen at the sentence level as well (Gerken 1991; Gerken & McIntosh, 1993). However, children who omit weak syllables from phrases or sentences may leave "traces" (e.g., very brief pauses) that "mark" the deleted syllable. For instance, the child who produces "He kissed Lucinda" without the initial [lu] will nonetheless pause briefly between "kissed" and "Cinda" but will not pause between "kissed" and "Cindy" in the sentence "He kissed Cindy" (Carter, 1996; Carter & Gerken, 2004). Thus, as with phonological knowledge of phonemes (discussed in Chapter 7), children often know more about prosody than they are able to clearly demonstrate.

At the same time as these stress patterns normalize at about age 3, the durations of typically developing English-learning children's reduced vowels (such as [ə]) also become more adult-like instead of inappropriately long (Allen & Hawkins, 1980; Kent & Forner, 1980). By the time they master the less frequent iambic word stress patterns at about age 7, typically developing youngsters are also able to use stress to differentiate compound nouns versus phrases (as in the "WHITEhouse" where the president lives versus a simple "white HOUSE") (Clark, Gelman, & Lane, 1985, cited by Gerken & McGregor, 1998). Thus, different aspects of linguistic rhythmic ability appear to mature synchronously.

Given that stress patterns facilitate word recognition, it is not a surprise that stress processing skills are associated with lexicon size (Goetry, Wade-Woolley, Kolinsky, & Mousty, 2006). A larger vocabulary necessitates paying attention to stress differences that signal meaning. The period during which one can learn to attend to these cues lasts into preschool age at least. Although adult French monolinguals and those who learn other languages as adults have been reported to be "stress deaf" (Dupoux, Pallier, Sebastian, & Mehler, 1997; Dupoux, Peperkamp, & Sebastian-Galles, 2010), 4- to 5-year-old French children learning Dutch as a second language were nonetheless able to learn to pay attention to stress in the new language, even if they had not been doing so naturally. Stress processing abilities may also relate to later phonological awareness skills (Goetry, Wade-Woolley, Kolinsky, & Mousty, 2006; Wood, 2006).

Pragmatic Functions of Prosody

Although they are able to use prosody to understand speakers' emotions (negative like sadness versus positive like happiness) by the age of 5, French-speaking children up to the age of 9 will still rely on the situational context rather than prosody if the intonation doesn't match the context. Prosody conveying negative emotions influences their interpretations of situations more than does that conveying positive emotions (Aguert, Laval, Le Bigot, & Bernicot, 2010). In contrast, children understand sarcasm based on intonation only before they understand it based on context only, even when the context "strongly indicated a nonliteral interpretation" (Capelli, Nakagawa, & Madden, 1990, p. 1824). For example, 84% of the English-speaking third grade participants in the study by Capelli and colleagues (1990) perceived sarcasm when both intonation and context were provided; 69% did so when only intonation cued the irony; and only 34% detected the non-truthful nature of the communication when only context was provided to support that interpretation. This finding holds for French-learning children as well (Laval & Bert-Erboul, 2005). The difference between the findings about positive versus negative emotions as opposed to the findings about sarcasm may result from the more salient prosodic characteristics of sarcasm.

Summary

Although prosody is largely subconscious, it has important impacts on the communication of both information and emotion. Therefore, it is critical for successful human interaction. Infants recognize and prefer basic aspects of the prosody of their ambient languages, such as rhythm, very early. Infant-directed speech reflects these preferences. Some prosodic features are evident in children's vocalizations long before the first words are produced. However, other components of prosody, such as sarcasm, are very subtle and therefore learned quite late. As with other aspects of speech, language, and cognitive development, the process includes some periods of apparent regression as the child reorganizes and systematizes. For children learning English and most other western languages, intonation, lexical and phrasal stress, rhythm including pauses, and affective impacts of prosody must be mastered in order to comprehend and communicate in an adult-like manner.

EXERCISE 10-1

Prosodic Development

PROSODIC DISORDERS

There are two primary types of prosodic disorders, differentiated in Table 10-1—**dysprosody** and **prosodic disability**. Dysprosody, a phonetic disorder, is characterized by a physiologic inability to effectively use different levels of loudness, pitch, or duration. It may reflect a small range of muscular effort (e.g., poor breath support for anything other than very quiet speech) or an inability to grade actions so that only the extreme ends of the range can be used (e.g., very loud or very soft). It is pervasive and consistent and most likely to accompany dysarthria (Crystal, 1981).

Prosodic disability, on the other hand, occurs when prosodic features such as pitch, loudness, and duration are misused linguistically or paralinguistically. That is, the person does produce an appropriate range of loudnesses, pitches, and durations but not in the ways that are expected in her native language. For example, words may be mis-stressed, the person's pitch may rise or fall in inappropriate places in utterances, pauses may occur in locations that do not make grammatical sense, etc. Prosodic disability is most characteristic of apraxia, aphasia, and autism spectrum disorders (ASD) (Crystal, 1981).

Prosodic disability may reflect attempts to compensate for other aspects of a speech sound disorder. Suprasegmental effects are one possible source of contrast that children may seek to apply unconventionally if they are unable to add contrast to their systems in a more conventional manner. For example, Jaeger (1997) reports on an English-speaking child who was normally developing and who temporarily used word pitch as if English were a tone language. This author also worked with a child with a speech-language disorder who used fundamental frequencies ranging from 70 to 700 Hz in order to differentiate words that he couldn't differentiate

TABLE 10-1 **Types of Prosodic Disorders**

Dysprosody: Phonetic	Prosodic Disability: Phonological
Poor control of:	*Linguistic or pragmatic misuse of:*
pitch	intonation or tone
loudness	stress
duration	tempo (and stress)
rhythm	rhythmicality
silence	juncture

segmentally. For instance, a very high, sharply falling pitch pattern was used with [ʌbʌ] to request "open;" a flat contour with the same sequence of segments ([ʌbʌ]) meant "elephant." He undoubtedly borrowed the basic idea for this differentiation from English, as Americans do tend to use a falling pitch pattern when cueing a child to say "open" as a request; labels often are modeled somewhat more monotonically.

Another client of this author's, this one with Childhood Apraxia of Speech (CAS), used intonation (pitch, duration, and loudness) to modify his idiosyncratic words for "big" and "little." Both were pronounced [ˈmɑmə], but if this form meant "big," the syllables were prolonged and resonant with a lilting pitch pattern. "Little" was produced in a quiet monotone. Both productions were supplemented by appropriate hand gestures to enhance the contrast. Holly, another child with CAS, used [bijə], [bɛə], or [bɪʊ] to express a variety of [b]-initial words; she disambiguated "baby" by whispering (Velleman, 1994).

Summary

Disorders of prosody can be subcategorized into two types. The first is dysprosody, which often reflects low tone or muscle weakness, accompanies dysarthria, and is characterized by an inability to produce appropriate prosodic features in any context. The second, prosodic disability, comprises the inappropriate use of appropriate prosodic features and most often accompanies apraxia, aphasia, or ASD.

Prosodic Features Associated with Specific Disorders

Most children with SSD display age-appropriate prosody. However, prosodic disorders are associated with children from specific disorder groups. Some of these are described below.

Childhood Apraxia of Speech

Prosodic difficulties, primarily of the prosodic disability type, are a hallmark of CAS. For instance, Velleman and Shriberg (1999) found that children with SSDs persisted in weak syllable deletion up to the age of 6, while those with CAS persisted in weak syllable deletion into the teen years. Their deletion patterns were not atypical. However, their stress errors were both more frequent and more persistent than were those of typically developing children.

Shriberg and colleagues (e.g., Shriberg, Aram, & Kwiatkowski, 1997a, 1997b, 1997c) have characterized the prosody of children with CAS as excess equal stress. That is, these children fail to differentiate stressed versus unstressed syllables adequately, yielding the percept of syllables that are equally stressed, with unstressed syllables overstressed. Several studies have explored this phenomenon in more depth. Shriberg, Campbell, Karlsson, Brown, McSweeny, and colleagues (2003) studied the ratios of the durations of stressed versus unstressed syllables in children with CAS. The researchers found that these children's ratios were sometimes longer (i.e., stressed syllables were inappropriately prolonged) and sometimes shorter (i.e., unstressed syllables were inappropriately prolonged) in comparison to those of other children. In other words, the participants with CAS were not consistent in producing stressed syllables that were longer than unstressed syllables. Shriberg, Green, Campbell, McSweeny, and Scheer (2003) also found that children with CAS had more isochronous speech than did TD children; in other words, their speech was less variable with respect to duration. The stressed syllables that they produced were not consistently different from their unstressed syllables. This inappropriate sameness could be one cause of the robotic-sounding speech of many children with CAS. However, the pause durations of the children with CAS were not less variable. All three of these findings were confirmed by Velleman, Andrianopoulos, Boucher, Perkins, Averback, and colleagues (2009).

Choppy, "segregated" speech is another primary characteristic of CAS. This results in the perception that each syllable is produced individually, unconnected to the remaining syllables in the word or phrase. In fact, Maassen, Nijland, and Van Der Meulen (2001) have shown that children with CAS demonstrate less intersyllabic coarticulation than do those who are typically developing. Without these connections between syllables, speech does not flow smoothly.

Autism Spectrum Disorders

The pragmatic uses of prosody are a specific, consistent area of deficit in children with ASD (Wells & Peppe, 2003), reflecting prosodic disability. The use of prosody for interpersonal purposes includes using tone of voice to convey affect, such as whether or not one likes a certain food; chunking words as in "chocolate cake and cookies" versus "chocolate, cake, and cookies" to convey groupings; and stressing certain words for emphasis. Those with ASD have particular difficulty understanding intonational affect and emphatic stress and using these as well as chunking. Receptive and expressive prosody skills are related in this population, suggesting that expressive deficits may result, at least in part, from a lack of understanding of the functions of intonation and stress (Peppe, McCann, Gibbon, O'Hare, & Rutherford, 2007). In those with ASD but not those with specific language impairment (SLI), the ability to understand these prosodic functions is highly correlated with other language skills (McCann, Peppe, Gibbon, O'Hare, & Rutherford, 2007).

The prosody production deficits of children with ASD appear to reflect dysprosody at times as well as prosodic disability. Their challenges include difficulty controlling pitch and volume, poor vocal quality, increased pause durations (Zajac, Roberts, Hennon, Harris, Barnes, et al., 2006), and atypical patterns of stress and meter (Gerken & McGregor, 1998; Paul, Augustyn, Klin, & Volkmar, 2005; Wing, 1996). Atypical ranges of prosodic features (frequency, intonation contour, terminal fall, etc.) (Baltaxe, 1984; Baltaxe, Simmons, & Zee, 1984; Diehl, Watson, Bennetto, McDonough, & Gunlogson, 2009; Eisenmajer, Prior, Leekam, Wing, Gould, et al., 1996) and singsong intonation (Fay & Schuler, 1980) are also common. These prosodic differences are more prominent during spontaneous speech than in echoed speech (Wing, 1996). Notably, grammatical pauses are usually used appropriately (Thurber & Tager-Flusberg, 1993).

The fact that children with ASD have been noted to have difficulties with receptive as well as expressive prosody may partly account for their difficulties in understanding the pragmatics of conversational interactions (Peppe et al., 2007). Jarvinen-Pasley, Wallace, Ramus, Happe, and Heaton (2008) also found that children with ASD were better able to discriminate non-linguistic (i.e., musical) than linguistic pitch contours. However, contradictory findings were found for children with high-functioning autism, who were reported by Grossman, Bemis, Plesa Skwerer, and Tager-Flusberg (2010) to perform like peers on receptive tasks of lexical stress and affective prosody and to produce appropriate word stress, although their productions were atypically long.

Deficits in ASD also relate to pragmatic functions, such as producing contrastive stress in sentences. For example, they might fail to understand or produce the difference between "I didn't KNOW it was blue" (I suspected it but I wasn't sure) versus "I didn't know it was BLUE" (I thought it was a different color) (Baltaxe, 1984; Foreman, 2001). Children with ASD also misuse the grammatical functions of stress, such as by stressing function words instead of content words (Baltaxe & Simmons, 1985). Cleland (2010) goes so far as to suggest that prosody is impaired across the board in autism—not as a reflection of pragmatic deficits, but as a specific behavioral feature in its own right. She hypothesizes that due to "weak central coherence" (p. 17; a tendency to process different pieces or aspects of input individually), people with ASD cannot integrate multiple strands of information well, and prosodic information is a strand that they may ignore in preference for other cues to meaning.

Atypical rhythm is strongly associated with ASD. Even children with high-functioning ASD whose prosody is otherwise typical may produce abnormally long durations (Grossman et al., 2010; Shriberg, Paul, McSweeny, Klin, Cohen et al., 2001). Furthermore, Velleman and colleagues (2009) demonstrated that children with ASD as well as those with CAS are less likely to use phrase-final lengthening appropriately than are those who are typically developing.

Acoustic analyses of the speech of children with ASD have revealed wider ranges of pitch (Diehl et al., 2009), which tends to be lower during vowel prolongations but higher in connected speech tasks. There is a tendency for more tightly compressed formants due to high F1 values. With respect to rate and rhythm, they demonstrate decreased maximum phonation times, longer speech and pause durations, and production of fewer words per second in comparison to typically developing children. Some but not all of these features are shared with children with CAS (Velleman et al., 2009).

The use of excess equal stress, in which the differences between stressed and unstressed syllables are flattened yielding a robotic quality, is considered to be a primary characteristic of CAS (Shriberg, Aram, & Kwiatkowski, 1997c; Velleman & Shriberg, 1999). Despite the fact that children with high-functioning autism are unimpaired in receptive tasks of lexical stress (Grossman et al., 2010), Velleman and colleagues (2009) demonstrated a similar decrease in the production of the stressed–unstressed contrast in children with ASD.

Specific Language Impairment

It is less well known that "intonation difficulties may be present in children with language impairments who present with a range of different speech and language profiles, including children with and without accompanying speech output difficulties and pragmatic problems" (Wells & Peppe, 2003, p. 20). These most often reflect prosodic disability. For example, Cantonese children with SLI are not as competent at discriminating contrastive tones (which change word meanings) as are age-matched or vocabulary-matched peers (Wong, Ciocca, & Yung, 2009). With respect to English, Fisher, Plante, Vance, Gerken, and Glattke (2007) showed that preschool children (though not adults) with SLI are less able to use prosodic cues to help them understand sentences. Children with SLI also are less sensitive perceptually to the rhythms of languages (Weinert, 1992). These deficits may affect the ability to learn syntax. The placements of pauses within sentences help listeners parse the grammar of the sentence, because we tend to pause briefly (juncture) as well as lowering our pitch (phrase-final pitch declination; see Chapter 2) and extending the last syllable at the end of a phrase (phrase-final lengthening; see Chapter 2). These prosodic cues can help typically developing children learn new grammatical rules. Children with SLI, however, do not make use of such cues (Weinert, 1992).

In addition, stress patterns may affect the speech and the language production of children with SLI as well as those of children with SSD. McGregor and Leonard (1994), for instance, demonstrated that prosody and phonetic content (e.g., tense vowels or diphthongs) are more important factors than grammar in determining when children with SLI will omit function words. They were more likely to produce function words in object phrases (e.g., "the" in "feed the dog") than in subject phrases (e.g., "the" in "The dog ate") because phrase-initial position is a more vulnerable position prosodically. Even when they do produce weak syllables, those with SLI exhibit more motoric difficulty in doing so. Furthermore, their function words are more variable and less different from their content words than are those of children who are developing language more typically (Goffman, 2004). Bortolini and Leonard (1996) further showed that children who are better at producing iambic (weak–strong) words and phrases are more likely to produce grammatical morphemes (which tend to occur in just such prosodic contexts in English). In short, some of the morphologic errors produced by children with SLI have prosodic rather than (or perhaps as well as) grammatical sources.

de Bree, Wijnen, and Zonneveld (2006) explored the stress production of Dutch 3-year-olds who were at risk of dyslexia, a reading disorder that often accompanies SLI, in comparison to children with no risk factors. They found that those who had at least one family member with reading difficulties had more difficulty imitating irregular and non-Dutch stress patterns. Similarly, Goffman, Gerken, and Lucchesi (2007) found that children with SLI demonstrated somewhat more weak syllable deletion than did children who were typically developing. Their syllable deletion patterns were not atypical but immature. Chiat and Roy (2007) also reported that children with language impairments omit syllables more frequently than do children who are typically developing. Their participants usually demonstrated typical albeit delayed patterns of omission in terms of the word and stress positions that are most likely to favor syllable deletion/preservation. However, they did note two unusual tendencies: for trochaic words to lose a syllable (e.g., "ladder" pronounced as [jæd]) and for stressed syllables to be omitted by children with language impairments.

Cognitive Impairments

Children with cognitive impairments who often also have dysarthria (e.g., children with Down syndrome or Williams syndrome or with cerebral palsy resulting from perinatal anoxia) may demonstrate prosodic abnormalities. These most often fall into the "dysprosody" category. Due to low muscle tone, muscle weakness, or poor muscle innervation, they may understress all syllables, yielding **reduced equal stress** (Shriberg, Kwiatkowski, & Rasmussen, 1990). Other prosodic characteristics include slower speech and pauses in grammatically inappropriate places within sentences (e.g., in the middle of the subject phrase) (Thurber & Tager-Flusberg, 1993). These inappropriate pauses may reflect processing needs, such as word-finding difficulties, or motoric deficits, or both. Barnes, Roberts, Long, Martin, Berni and colleagues (2009) speculate that differences of prosody, including use of pauses in connected speech, may significantly impact intelligibility in persons with Fragile X syndrome or Down syndrome.

Hearing Loss

Children with hearing loss may also be hard to understand, partly due to prosodic differences. Speech duration and pitch contours are typically the areas of greatest concern in this respect (Monsen, 1978). Although these youngsters do differentiate between questions and statements, for example, they do so to a lesser extent than do children whose hearing is within normal limits (Allen & Arndorfer, 2000). Speech may also be staccato, without the pauses that help the listener parse the grammar of the sentence (Maassen, 1986).

Summary

Children with CAS are likely to display symptoms of prosodic disability, including inadequate differentiation of stressed versus unstressed syllables (excess equal stress) and segregated (choppy) speech. Those with SLI also demonstrate prosodic disability, both receptively and expressively. Their difficulty understanding prosodic cues, producing unstressed syllables and function words, and differentiating function versus content words impact their grammar skills, especially morphology. Children with ASD, like children with CAS, demonstrate excess equal stress and other rhythmic errors. Their prosodic disability, which is typically receptive as well as expressive, also encompasses difficulty expressing affect using intonation and emphatic stress. ASD is also associated with dysprosody, especially atypical ranges of many prosodic features, reflecting poor control of volume, pitch, pause durations, and meter. Cognitive deficits, such as those often associated with neurodevelopmental syndromes and cerebral palsy, may be accompanied by low tone, muscle weakness, and/or poor muscle innervation and, as a result, by dysarthria. This typically results in slow, low-volume speech with reduced equal stress and inappropriate pausing. Hearing loss results in decreased pitch ranges, reducing the impact of intonation for differentiating questions. Children with hearing deficits may also exhibit timing abnormalities.

In all of these cases, prosodic deficits have a significant impact on intelligibility and communicative effectiveness. In some cases, they impact comprehension as well.

ASSESSMENT

Perhaps because we begin learning it so early, prosody tends to be more intuitive and less easy to explicitly analyze than some other aspects of language. Thus, it has received less attention in both linguistics and in speech-language pathology than many other aspects of language.

Standardized Tests

Unfortunately, there are no prosody tests that have been normed on American children. The Preschool Repetition Test (Roy, Chiat, & Seeff-Gabriel, 2008) is a test developed in the United Kingdom that assesses young British children's ability to repeat real and nonsense words ranging from one to three syllables in length. The ultimate goal of the test is to predict which children are at higher risk for later language impairments, given that nonword repetition is correlated with SLI and reading difficulties. A norming study revealed that typically developing children performed better than did children who were referred for possible language impairment. All children had more difficulty with longer words and with syllables that were unstressed, especially those unstressed syllables that preceded a stressed syllable (Chiat & Roy, 2007).

Another British test, Profiling Elements of Prosodic Systems—Children (PEPS-C; Peppe and McCann, 2003; http://www.peps-c.com/peps-c-clinical-version-description.html), a standardized computer-based assessment tool, is appropriate for somewhat older children (at least 4 years of age) with prosodic deficits. It assesses four components of prosody:

- Turn end (indicating whether an utterance requires an answer [based on question intonation])
- Affect (indicating liking versus reservation [using intonation], in this test with respect to certain foods)

- Chunking (signaling prosodic phrase boundaries [differentiating compound words versus phrases])
- Focus (emphasizing one word in an utterance for contrastive accent) (Peppe et al., 2007, p. 1019)

Thus far, only limited norms are available, primarily for children learning Scottish English.

Most American SLPs will therefore use informal measures to assess this aspect of phonology in younger children. Assessment should include the components listed below.

Intonation

1. Comprehension of turn end can be assessed by asking a question in a statement format as is done on the PEPS-C test (Peppe & McCann, 2003). That is, apply rising intonation to an utterance that is grammatically in statement form, yielding a question such as "The truck won the race?" See if the child responds as if the utterance were a question or a statement. For production, note use of pitch to mark yes-or-no questions (rising pitch—e.g., "Is it Tuesday?" or "It's Tuesday?") versus statements and wh- questions (falling pitch—e.g., "It's Tuesday," "What day is it?").
2. Affect comprehension and production tasks might consist of an interchange such as the following between a child and an SLP holding a bear puppet, similar to the PEPS-C test (Peppe & McCann, 2003):

SLP: The bear says "strawberries" (with a "yummy" intonation pattern on the word "strawberries"). Does the bear like strawberries?

Child: Yes.

SLP: The bear says "raspberries" (with a "yucky" intonation pattern on the word "raspberries"). Does the bear like raspberries?

Child: No.

SLP: The bear doesn't like apples. What would he say?

Child: Apples (with "yucky" intonation pattern).

3. Comprehension of differently chunked phrases can be assessed by giving instructions such as "Point to the picture that shows 'cheese sandwich and milk'" versus "Point to the picture that shows 'cheese, sandwich, and milk,'" as is done on the PEPS-C test (Peppe & McCann, 2003). With respect to expressive use of chunking, note use of pauses in appropriate locations to demarcate grammatical units in sentences (e.g., "The pink giraffe | ate the green leaves | from my rose bush"). Also, pay attention to whether or not the child can use stress and pauses to differentiate compound words versus phrases. For example, "GREENhouses" are structures designed for growing plants. In contrast, "green HOUSES" are buildings that just happen to be green.
4. Comprehension of emphasis could be assessed using a dialogue such as the following, as is done on the PEPS-C test (Peppe & McCann, 2003) (possibly supplemented by picture choices):

SLP: When the mommy took everything out of her grocery bags, the girl said, "But I wanted APPLES and peaches." What did the mommy forget to buy?

Child: Apples.

SLP: At dinnertime, the girl said, "I like sauce on my RICE." What did the mommy do wrong?

Child: She put the sauce on something else.

Similarly, note the child's use of stress to indicate new or contrastive information (e.g., "I like VANILLA ice cream, not CHOCOLATE ice cream").

Assessments of prosody can be based on spontaneous language samples in play settings in which the SLP endeavors to elicit yes-or-no questions and (if the child produces long enough utterances) pauses between grammatical clauses. Differentiating compound words versus phrases may require the presence of carefully selected pictures or toys (a hotdog and a hot dog; a blackboard and a black board; a greenhouse and a green house; the Whitehouse and a white house; etc.). Objects or pictures depicting items that are the same except for one feature can help elicit contrastive stress (such as "Do you like the BLUE pony or the PINK pony?").

When reviewing these productions, listen for the use of each of the key prosody components—loudness, pitch, and duration (including duration of pauses)—both individually and in combination for stress. For each component, consider whether both the mean and the range are age appropriate. Listen for whether the child has control of *grading* within the range for that component. For example, can the child produce various levels of loudness or just "loud" versus "quiet," various levels of pitch, or just "high" versus "low?" Finally and most importantly, are these aspects of prosody used contrastively for pragmatic, grammatical, and affective functions?

Recall that this latter aspect of the assessment helps us differentiate dysprosody versus prosodic disability. If the child has poor ranges of pitch, loudness, or duration, or can only produce the endpoints of the range (e.g., loud versus quiet, not in between), dysarthria should be suspected. If he has the ability to produce the full range of all of these aspects, but he produces the wrong one at any given time (e.g., he mis-sequences) or cannot produce them upon request, a motor planning problem such as Childhood Apraxia of Speech may be more likely (Crystal, 1981).

Form 10-1 can be used to document prosodic ability versus disability. Indicate which of the prosodic components (columns) are used for the various linguistic functions (rows). The shaded areas represent prosodic components that are not typically used for a given prosodic function, although they might be, by a particular child.

Stress Patterns

Production of multisyllabic words is an important area to explore for older or less delayed children. The main question to be addressed is whether the child produces a variety of stress patterns or is limited due to phonological deficits

Form 10-1

Name: Age:
Date: Examiner:
Source of sample: Size of sample:

PROSODY COMPONENTS AND FUNCTIONS

Indicate which of the prosodic components (columns) are used for the various linguistic functions (rows). The shaded areas represent prosodic components that are not typically used for a given prosodic function but might be by a particular child.

	Pitch/ intonation	Loudness	Duration/ timing	Rhythm	Silence/ pause
Yes/no Q (pitch rise) vs. statement or wh- Q					
Word stress (trochaic vs. iambic)					
Pauses/ juncture					
Compound word vs. phrase					
Contrastive stress/ emphasis for new info					
Affect (emotion)					

to producing only a few. For example, a child might be segmentally accurate but be unable to produce words with non-trochaic (i.e., other than strong–weak) stress patterns. Form 10-2 is available to document the child's stress patterns using independent analysis.

On this form, examples of multisyllabic words produced by the child that exemplify various stress patterns should be listed. The example words given on the form are intended only to help the speech-language pathologist categorize the words the child has produced, regardless of whether or not the child's stress pattern matches the target stress pattern. (More examples are given in Appendix B.) The client shouldn't be required to repeat those particular words. In fact, even unintelligible words can be listed on this form. Sometimes it is the words with particular stress patterns that are the unintelligible ones because the child cannot control both a challenging stress pattern and challenging phonetics within the same word.

Form 10-2

Name: Age:
Date: Examiner:
Source of sample: Size of sample:
S: strong syllable W: weak syllable

STRESS PATTERNS: INDEPENDENT ANALYSIS

For each stress pattern, list words that the child produces with that pattern, *whether they are correct or not.* Examples in parentheses are for comparison/stress pattern recognition only. (See also examples in Appendix B.) The child should not necessarily be required to attempt these words. Include unintelligible words on this form.

TARGET STRESS PATTERN	—EXAMPLES — (from child)
SW (ex: ˈmonkey)	
WS (ex: giˈraffe)	
ˈSWˌS (ex: ˈteleˌphone)	
SWW/ˈSˌSW (ex: ˈhamburger)	
WSW (ex: spaˈghetti)	
WWS/ˌSWˈS (ex: ˌkangaˈroo)	
ˈSWˌSW (ex: ˈcaterˌpillar)	
WˈSWˌS/ ˌSˈSWW (rhiˈnoceros)	
WWSW/ ˌSWˈSW (disaˈppointed)	
OTHER 4 SYLL. (SWWS, WSWS, WSSW)	
5+ SYLLABLES	

Form 10-3

Name: Age:
Date: Examiner:
Source of sample: Size of sample:
S: strong syllable W: weak syllable

STRESS PATTERNS: RELATIONAL ANALYSIS

For each stress pattern, list words that the child attempts with that pattern, indicating whether the word is produced correctly, with weak syllable(s) omitted, with strong syllables omitted, or with other outputs (e.g., coalescence of two syllables into one). Examples in parentheses are for comparison/stress pattern recognition only.

TARGET STRESS PATTERN	Correct	W omitted	S omitted	Other
SW (ex: ˈmonkey)				
WS (ex: giˈraffe)				
ˈSWˌS (ex: ˈteleˌphone)				
SWW/ˈSˌSW (ex: ˈhamburger)				
WSW (ex: spaˈghetti)				
WWS/ˌSWˈS (ex: ˌkangaˈroo)				
ˈSWˌSW (ex: ˈcaterˌpillar)				
WˈSWˌS/ ˌSˈSWW (rhiˈnoceros)				
WWSW/ ˌSWˈSW (disaˈppointed)				
OTHER 4 SYLL. (SWWS, WSWS, WSSW)				
5+ SYLLABLES				

If a school-aged child attempts quite a few multisyllabic words but his or her productions of these fit only within the SW and SWSW categories, for example, this should be cause for concern. If some examples of WS, WSW, and similar patterns are found as well as earlier-developing trochaic patterns (such as SW and SWSW), then the child most likely does not have a deficit in stress pattern production. It is important to remember that the English language demonstrates a preference for trochaic (SW) words, so the proportion of iambic (WS) forms should not be expected to even approach 50%.

A second stress form (Form 10-3) facilitates relational analysis of stress patterns. For each stress pattern, the clinician should list words that the child attempts with that pattern, indicating whether the word is produced correctly, with weak syllable(s) omitted, with strong syllable(s) omitted, or with other outputs (e.g., coalescence of two syllables into one, stress on the wrong syllable). Once again, the examples in parentheses are intended to facilitate the speech-language pathologist's recognition of varied stress patterns only. The child should not necessarily be required to attempt these particular words. However, if necessary, pictures or objects with iambic names (baNAna, giRAFFe, spaGHEtti) or actions with iambic descriptions (aROUND, beFORE, beHIND; proTECT, preTEND, deFEND) can be incorporated into play or more structured activities in order to elicit words with a variety of stress patterns.

Summary

Unfortunately, standardized tests are not available for testing American English prosody. Informal probes and spontaneous speech samples can be used to determine whether the child is using all prosodic features (loudness, duration, pitch, rhythm, pauses) to achieve all prosodic functions (sentence forms, word stress, grammatical chunking, compound words versus phrases, emphasis, and affect).

TREATMENT

Prosody intervention can be quite successful (Hargrove, Roetzel, & Hoodin, 1989; van Rees et al., 2012). Despite this, prosody goals are often postponed until after segmental speech has been addressed for many years in therapy. This is a mistake for several reasons. First of all, prosody is one of the earliest respects in which children reflect characteristics of the ambient language. In this sense, it provides a foundation for the segmental aspects of speech that follow—a frame on which meaningful speech can be built. In addition, prosody has significant impacts on listener comprehension, but these impacts tend to be far less conscious than do other aspects of speech. We are far more likely to consciously notice a substitution error or a grammatical mistake than an instance of prosody being "off" even though the latter may result in misparsing and therefore misunderstanding the utterance. It may also have a much bigger effect on our judgment of and relationship with the speaker. Thus, prosodic deficits may have negative impacts on the speaker's ability to make friends and on how he is judged by others without any of the relevant communication partners being consciously aware of this.

Peppe and colleagues (2007) suggest that focusing on receptive prosody may improve the expressive prosodic skills of children with ASD. This type of intervention could have an important impact on their pragmatic skills as well: "Given the relevance of prosody to affective, nonlinguistic aspects of communication, increased awareness of the role of prosody could possibly lead to better social skills as well as improved communication" (pp. 1024–1025).

For children who demonstrate deficits in this area or who are at risk of doing so (e.g., CAS, ASD, hearing loss), prosody should be an early direct goal. When prosodic features are targeted, the precision of the segments within the words and sentences produced should not be the focus. Consonant and vowel approximations are acceptable—though the correct forms should always be modeled—as long as the intonation and stress patterns are correct.

Unfortunately, one of the reasons prosodic goals are often postponed is that few materials are available to address these objectives. Little research has been done on prosody treatment for children, and almost no commercialized materials exist to carry such treatment out. The suggestions below are based upon the limited research that is available, supplemented by the author's clinical experience with many children with CAS and/or ASD—diagnoses frequently associated with prosodic abnormalities.

Preschool Years

During the preschool years, intervention should focus on developing control of volume, duration/rate, pitch, and rhythm. Importantly, control does not constitute only the ability to achieve both ends of the range in each area but also to grade production of these features such that several steps on each continuum can be voluntarily reached. Because prosody is both associated with emotional content and with music, it is not difficult to develop play-based activities that incorporate prosody practice.

Pitch activities include songs, finger plays, and the use of different voices (for "daddy" versus "mommy" versus "baby," for large and small animals, vehicles, etc.) in pretend play. Volume control can be practiced by telling secrets or not waking the baby versus imitating a loud animal or object, pretending to yell, etc. Songs such as "B-I-N-G-O" and "John Jacob Jingleheimer Schmidt" (for those who can pronounce that name!) can also be used. "The Wheels on the Bus" is also easily adapted to emphasize either pitch or volume.

Duration and rhythm/stress pattern training can also include songs as well as finger plays, walking games ("Going on a Lion Hunt"), hand gestures or even body movements to accompany and mimic speech rhythms, and so forth. It's important not to encourage the child to produce marching-rhythm–like speech; this is not natural. It's what we are trying to prevent. The rhythms of speech, including stress patterns, are much more varied than are the beats of a drum or the repetitions babies produce during canonical babbling. However, for stress, one can use various objects or pictures to represent "loud" versus "quiet" (which are descriptions of stressed/unstressed that children will understand). For instance, one could use two different sizes of drums: one for the stressed syllables and one for the unstressed syllables, as illustrated in Figure 10-1.

Simple intonation and stress activities, such as those described in the "Assessment" section, can also be initiated. Those that are most likely to be accessible to young children include the use of prosody for affect (e.g., yummy versus

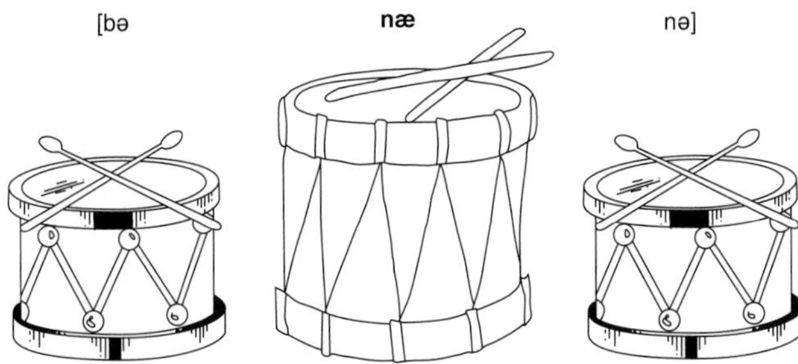

FIGURE 10-1. Example of lexical stress therapy activity.

yucky) and for emphasis (e.g., "I want the RED truck, not the BLUE truck"). Question versus statement intonation also should be able to be addressed with the preschool population as long as it's done within a play context.

School-Aged Children

As the child gains more and more metalinguistic awareness and more and more ability to read, prosody activities can become increasingly explicit within less play-based formats.

Backward Buildups

For school-aged children, the use of backward buildups (a.k.a. "back chaining") is very helpful for practicing appropriate prosody at the word, phrase, or sentence levels. Practicing a word or phrase "backward" is counterintuitive, but it makes sense when factors such as phrase-final lengthening (prolongation of the last syllable in a word or the last word in a phrase or sentence) and phrase-final declination (decreased pitch on the last syllable in a word or the last word in a phrase or sentence) are considered. If one were to practice a word such as "institution" from front to back, as instinct might dictate, practice would proceed as follows:

[ɪn] with phrase-final lengthening and phrase-final declination on [ɪn]

[ˌɪnstə] with phrase-final lengthening and phrase-final declination on [stə]

[ˌɪnstəˈtu] with phrase-final lengthening and phrase-final declination on [tu]

[ˌɪnstəˈtuʃən] with phrase-final lengthening and phrase-final declination on [ʃən]

The placement of the phrase-final prosody features changes as the speaker practices each part. Furthermore, for the first three pieces, those features are misplaced, each in a different way. In contrast, one can practice as follows:

[ʃən] with phrase-final lengthening and phrase-final declination on [ʃən]

[ˈtuʃən] with phrase-final lengthening and phrase-final declination on [ʃən]

[stəˈtuʃən] with phrase-final lengthening and phrase-final declination on [ʃən]

[ˌɪnstəˈtuʃən] with phrase-final lengthening and phrase-final declination on [ʃən]

In this case, the prosodic pattern of the word is both consistent and accurate throughout the task. Thus, there is a marked increase in prosodic naturalness that is gained by doing backward buildups. The same type of training can be used for sentences, again from "right to left." Frame-content (slot-and-filler) drills, in which the child learns to substitute a variety of words within a sentence frame, often involve varying the word in final position in the sentence (e.g., "Let's ____" or "That's my ____"). This is an excellent match for backward buildups; the new item is practiced first in isolation, then with more and more of the frame:

[hom]

[go hom]

[lɛts go hom]

Materials such as the Fokes Sentence Builder (Fokes, 1976) pictures are ideal for these activities when sentences are targeted. Note that each piece of the whole utterance should be practiced several times until it is smooth before additional material is added to the "front."

Motivating Sentence Frames

When selecting sentences for pattern practice, SLPs often forget that communication efficacy depends upon the triad: means, motive, and opportunity (Davis & Velleman, 2008). We focus on the means—the ability to accurately pronounce a grammatically correct sentence—forgetting that whenever possible, the goal should be an utterance that will be functional and motivating *for the client.* For example, "I want to go to the bathroom" is not at the top of most children's lists of messages that they want to convey, though it may be what their parents or teachers would like them to learn first. In fact, "I want ___" is not actually what children who are typically developing usually say when they want something. Yet, we spend many long hours in therapy drilling children on this sentence frame. Consider adding more natural frames to your pattern practice: "That's my ___," "Let's ___," and "More _____, please," and even "Gimme ___" and "I wanna ___" will help children with SSDs fit in better with their peers as well as be successful communicators.

Explicit Practice of Stress Patterns

As noted, trochaic (stress-initial) words are far more frequent in English than are iambic ones. However, there are many iambic words as well, even within early childhood vocabulary. Furthermore, phrases tend to be iambic (e.g., "the HORSE;" "is RUNning;" "up a TREE"). Therefore, a variety of stress patterns must be trained from an early age if the child's prosody is to approximate age appropriateness.

Word Stress

Many children are explicitly taught to count the number of syllables in a word as part of their phonological awareness training. If the child is not going to sound natural, we must *avoid* encouraging her to produce robotic speech—producing each syllable with equal loudness, duration, and pitch. Instead, encourage the child to produce natural stress patterns. Therefore, once the child has identified the number of syllables in the word, the next question should be "Which is the loudest part?" The syllables can be represented, for example, with small and larger blocks or even drums to represent unstressed and stressed syllables, as shown in Figure 10-1. Then the child can imitate the word with the appropriate stress pattern, using backward buildups as needed. Eventually, the child should be able to produce familiar multisyllabic words with the appropriate stress.

Ballard, Robin, McCabe, and McDonald (2010) demonstrated the success of a therapy approach for teaching word stress to a group of children with SSD. Their stimuli were written three- and four-syllable nonsense words with varying stress patterns ("e.g., SW: BAAteegoo; WS: baaTEEgoo" p. 1231), embedded in carrier phrases. They also incorporated the principles of motor learning into the intervention: complex, varied stimuli; high-intensity practice; random order of stimulus presentation within practice; and low-frequency knowledge of results feedback. The three 7- to 10-year-old participants, siblings who had CAS including difficulty with lexical stress, demonstrated improvement in their ability to control the three key parameters of stress: duration, loudness, and pitch. They did generalize to untreated nonsense words but unfortunately not to real words.

Although English stress patterns are quite complicated, there are rules that can be taught. For example, children can learn that nouns and adjectives tend to be trochaic (as in "PREsent" [ˈpɹɛzənt], "REcord" [ˈɹɛkɚd], and "FOREsight" [ˈfoɚˌsɑɪt]), while verbs are usually iambic (as in "preSENT" [pɹɪˈzɛnt], "reCORD" [ɹəˈkɔɚd], and "foreSEE" [ˌfoɚˈsi]).

Spelling patterns can also be helpful for teaching stress patterns in English. For example, two-syllable nouns ending with "-oin" or "-oon" are most likely to have stress on the final syllable; otherwise, disyllabic nouns usually have trochaic stress. Similarly, nouns beginning with "co-" or "ma-" are usually trochaic while those beginning with "be-" or "a-" are typically iambic. Disyllabic verbs ending with "-arge," "-inge," or "-udge" are equally likely to have first-syllable as second-syllable stress; other two-syllable verbs are most likely to have stress at the end (Arciuli & Cupples, 2006; Arciuli, Monaghan, & Seva, 2010). Children are likely to read most unfamiliar words with stress on the first syllable during the initial stages of literacy, but this tendency starts to decrease as early as age 7. At the same age, they show emerging signs of awareness that word endings are more useful for determining stress patterns when reading than are word beginnings (Arciuli et al., 2010). Typically developing 5- to 13-year-olds can learn to associate orthographic cues of this sort with the appropriate stress patterns, reading untrained nonsense words aloud with the correct stress pattern after as few as three to seven sessions of training on a different set of words. In this study, the children were explicitly told to pay attention to "long-short" (trochaic) versus "short-long" (iambic) words; in addition, the stimuli were presented in random order with high-intensity practice and low-frequency feedback (van Rees et al., 2012). Thus, it may be helpful to explicitly focus on stress patterns and their relationships to word endings when using the written language to help school-aged children learn stress patterns.

Recall that even clearer effects of word endings emerge when those word endings are morphologic suffixes. As discussed in Chapter 2, the impacts of suffixes on multisyllabic words often can be predicted based on the source language (German versus French versus Latin versus Greek) and on the stress pattern of the suffix itself. German morphemes like "-hood" typically have no impact (e.g., "CHILDhood"); French morphemes like "ique" pull the stress onto themselves (e.g., "unIQUE") as do some Greek trochaic morphemes such as "-atic" (e.g., "draMAtic"). Some Latin morphemes such "ity" are unstressed and therefore cause the preceding syllable of the word to be stressed (e.g., "creaTIvity"). There are exceptions to these rules, but an awareness of the patterns can nonetheless provide the student with a place to start when she is confronted with an unfamiliar word.

Phrasal Stress

Phrasal stress training is facilitated by the contrast provided by phrasal stress in English (which is lacking at the word level—"desert"/"dessert" is one of the very few word-stress minimal pairs in our language). As noted above, compound words have a trochaic SW stress pattern, while phrases have an iambic WS pattern. Many minimal pairs exist:

ˈhotˌdog (sausage) versus ˌhot ˈdog (warm pet)

ˈgreenˌhouse (plant-growing space) versus ˌgreen ˈhouse (abode of a certain color)

ˈblackˌboard (classroom wall) versus ˌblack ˈboard (dark plank)

The child can initially be asked to correctly match the spoken phrase (versus the corresponding compound word) with the intended meaning (e.g., a picture). Then she can correctly produce stress on the phrase to match the given meaning.

The production of iambic words may actually be facilitated by including them in phrases beginning with a stressed word, resulting in a trochaic phrase. For example, the child might be better able to produce the unstressed initial syllable of "banana" if it is preceded by a stressed word: "ONE baNAna." The stressed word can then be faded (whispered, then gestured, or thought but not pronounced) as she retains the unstressed initial syllable. As the child's productions of iambic words improve, her abilities can be challenged by including these words in more challenging phrases, such as phrases that begin with an unstressed word—"a baNAna"—and even phrases in which there are multiple unstressed syllables in a row—"EATing a baNAna" (Bernhardt, Stemberger, & Major, 2006).

Sentence Stress

Again, meaning can easily be used to differentiate sentence stress patterns. Pictures (e.g., those provided in the Fokes Sentence Builder, Fokes, 1976) may facilitate this. Initially, the child identifies the stressed word in a *heard* sentence. Next, she identifies which word should be stressed, given the meaning (e.g., "I don't like the white sweater. I want to wear my white *jacket*." versus "I want to wear my *pink* sweater"). If she is literate, she can read sentences with the correct stress pattern and then produce the correct stress in a drill, in a schema, and spontaneously. Repair activities are appropriate for this domain as well—training the child to use stress for clarification in response to listener confusion.

Wh- questions are an excellent tool for practicing sentence stress. Both the wh- words and the stress patterns can be trained simultaneously. For example, if the question is "who," the subject of the sentence should be stressed in the reply:

Q: "Who climbed the tree?"

A: "BONNIE climbed the tree" or "THE FISH climbed the tree," etc.

If the question is "where" or "what" or "when" the stress pattern in the sentence is adjusted accordingly:

Q: "What did Bonnie climb?"

A: "Bonnie climbed the TREE."

Q: "Where was the tree?"

A: "The tree was BESIDE THE LAKE."

For older children, a written paragraph is given. The child identifies the key words to be stressed, marks them, and then stresses them while reading aloud. Finally, generalization is practiced in scripted and then freer conversations.

Pitch

As with other intonation features, pitch can be highlighted in perception and production to enhance intelligibility and the typicality of the person's speech. The client can practice identifying and then producing whether the pitch is rising or falling in different types of utterances: rising for yes-or-no questions and tag questions and falling elsewhere. For literate children, question marks can assist as long as they know that the presence of a "wh" word typically "cancels out" the question mark—in other words, wh- questions have falling, not rising, pitch in English. It is important, too, to teach the child that pitch alone can successfully signal a yes-or-no question in a way that word order alone cannot (e.g., "You're leaving now?" would be instantly recognized as a question while "Are you leaving" produced without rising pitch at the end would be very confusing).

Again, activities can proceed from recognition to imitation to marking then reading sentences to controlled and finally free conversations.

Pauses

It has been this author's experience that many adolescents with low muscle tone and the resulting distortion errors (e.g., children with Down syndrome) remain unintelligible despite many years of speech-language therapy directed at precise production of consonants. In context, especially in longer utterances, maintaining accuracy in every word is simply not an option. Typically, they have a tendency to produce low-intensity, monostressed speech without syntactic pauses. Helping them properly use pauses to signal grammatical phrases (e.g., the subject noun phrase versus the predicate verb phrase) can markedly increase a child's intelligibility (Hargrove et al., 1989; Maassen, 1986), especially when combined with increased use of stress within sentences to highlight the key words in the sentence. With increased insight into the grammatical structure and the key words of the utterance, the listener can greatly compensate for a lack of consonantal clarity.

The process of training a client to use pauses to increase intelligibility should be quite familiar, given its resemblance to the above: identify pauses in heard sentences, mark pauses in written sentences, imitate sentences while maintaining the pauses, mark then read sentences with appropriate pauses, produce pauses in controlled conversation, produce pauses in conversation when asked to clarify, and finally produce proper pauses in free conversation. The use of sentences whose meanings change when pauses are misplaced (e.g., "I ate a donut | whole" versus "I ate | a donut hole;" "The police | shot | the man with the duck" versus "The police | shot the man | with the duck") can serve to illustrate the communicative value of accurate pausing.

EXERCISE 10-2

Prosody Assessment and Intervention

SUMMARY

Prosody is the first aspect of speech that infants detect and produce in their ambient languages. Perhaps as a result of this, prosody evokes emotional responses as well as semantic and grammatical responses as appropriate to its many varied functions in our and other languages.

Children with ASD, Williams syndrome, and other conditions respond more strongly to music than to speech, suggesting the potential usefulness of incorporating melody and rhythm into intervention (as in melodic intonation therapy). Yet, this realm of communication has received far less attention in our field than have most others. Assessment and treatment procedures for detecting, categorizing, and remediating prosodic differences and disorders are severely lacking. Despite the challenges, increasing a child's awareness and control of intonation can significantly improve his communicative effectiveness and naturalness. It's worth the effort!

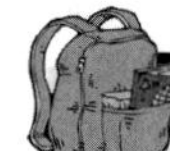

KEY TAKE-HOME MESSAGES

1. Prosody has important impacts not only on emotion and bonding but also on intelligibility. As such, prosody evaluation and intervention are important components of speech sound assessment and treatment.
2. The development of prosody is language specific; it spans infancy to late adolescence.
3. Specific prosodic deficits are associated with specific communication or other disorders.

CHAPTER 10
Prosody Review

Exercise 10-1

A. Multiple choice. Choose the best answer.

1. The earliest aspect of intonation that infants produce is:
   a. falling contour.
   b. rising contour.
   c. sentence contour.
   d. interrogatory contour.
2. Infant-directed speech includes:
   a. decreased pitch contours.
   b. decreased durations.
   c. decreased loudness.
   d. increased prosodic features.
3. Children's prosody begins to be language specific:
   a. in the teen years as sarcasm.
   b. during the late babbling period.
   c. with sentence contours on two-word utterances.
   d. at 12 months when infants mark utterance boundaries.
4. The latest aspect of prosody that young children master is:
   a. falling sentence contours.
   b. rising sentence contours.
   c. phrase-final lengthening.
   d. single utterance contours.
5. Syllables are most likely to be omitted from:
   a. iambic words.
   b. monosyllabic words.
   c. final position.
   d. stressed position.
6. Children learning English:
   a. master schwa before fuller vowels.
   b. master word stress by the time they have learned about 50 words.
   c. produce more omission errors than stress shift errors.
   d. use duration and amplitude but not pitch correctly by 30 months.
7. Children's prosodic abilities:
   a. are associated with lexicon size.
   b. may be associated with later phonological awareness.
   c. are facilitated by properly placed pauses.
   d. are better when negative rather than positive emotions are expressed.
   e. All of the above
   f. None of the above

B. Prosodic contrasts.

1. Use juncture marks (|) and stress marks (ˈ) to indicate two different ways to place juncture and/or stress within each headline (a to e) or sentence (f to g). Explain the difference in meaning between the two pronunciations of the utterance.
   a. Yellow Perch Decline To Be Studied
   b. Shark Attacks Puzzle Experts
   c. Hospital Fires Ten Foot Doctors
   d. Press Tours Ravaged City
   e. Eye Drops Off Shelf
   f. Drinking straws can be dangerous.
   g. Woman without her man is nothing.

Exercise 10-2

A. Essay questions.

1. After several years of therapy, Sammy's production of consonants is now accurate 90% of the time, and the school special education director feels Sammy is ready for discharge from therapy. Yet, her speech calls attention to itself because it is slow, choppy, monotone, and arrhythmic. In longer utterances, it is difficult for listeners to follow her train of thought. How can these deficits be characterized and documented? What intervention strategies are available to increase the age appropriateness of her prosody? Use information from this chapter and other sources to justify your response.

2. Consider the case of Kim, a child with Down syndrome (DS) who has been exposed equally to English and Cantonese from before birth. Review the information presented throughout this book (especially Chapters 3, 5, and 9 but also 4, 6, and 7) and in other sources (such as those cited herein) about the usual motor/motor speech, speech, cognitive, and hearing profiles of children with DS. Which of these factors could impact Kim's learning of the prosody of these two languages? What challenges could result from the prosodic differences between the two languages he's learning (as described in this chapter)? Given your answers to the previous questions and assuming that Kim's cognitive deficits are mild–moderate, what evaluation strategies would you use if he were 5 years old? 15 years old? What intervention strategies might be helpful if Kim were 5 years old? 15 years old??

B. *Multiple choice. Choose the best answer.*

1. Dysprosody is usually:
   a. linguistic.
   b. characteristic of apraxia.
   c. consistent.
   d. characteristic of autism.
2. Children with ASD typically do not make errors on:
   a. stress patterns.
   b. linguistic meter.
   c. receptive prosody.
   d. grammatical pauses.
3. Children with CAS typically do not demonstrate:
   a. reduced equal stress.
   b. excess equal stress.
   c. prolonged weak syllables.
   d. isochronous speech.
4. Children with SLI typically do not demonstrate:
   a. function word omissions predictable based on prosody.
   b. less prosodic contrast between content and function words.
   c. failure to use prosodic cues to identify phrase boundaries.
   d. atypical syllable deletion patterns.
5. Which of the following is not a recommended goal for prosody intervention?
   a. Grading of prosodic features
   b. Multi-modal input
   c. Equally stressed syllables
   d. Backward buildups

References

Aguert, M., Laval, V., Le Bigot, L., & Bernicot, J. (2010). Understanding expressive speech acts: The role of prosody and situational context in French-speaking 5- to 9-year-olds. *Journal of Speech, Language, and Hearing Research, 53*, 1629–1641.

Allen, G., & Arndorfer, P. M. (2000). Production of sentence-final intonation contours by hearing-impaired children. *Journal of Speech, Language, and Hearing Research, 43*, 441–455.

Allen, G. D., & Hawkins, S. (1980). Phonological rhythm: Definition and development. *Child Phonology, 1*, 227–256.

Aoyama, K., Peters, A. M., & Winchester, K. S. (2010). Phonological changes during the transition from one-word to productive word combination. *Journal of Child Language, 37*, 145–157.

Archibald, J. (1996). The acquisition of Yucatecan Maya prosody. In B. Bernhardt, J. Gilbert, & D. Ingram (Eds.), *Proceedings of the UBC International Conference on Phonological Acquisition* (pp. 99–112). Somerville, MA: Cascadilla Press.

Arciuli, J., & Cupples, L. (2006). The processing of lexical stress during visual word recognition: Typicality effects and orthographic correlates. *The Quarterly Journal of Experimental Psychology, 59*(5), 920–948.

Arciuli, J., Monaghan, P., & Seva, N. (2010). Learning to assign lexical stress during reading aloud: Corpus, behavioral, and computational investigations. *Journal of Memory and Language, 63*, 180–196.

Ballard, K. J., Djaja, D., Arciuli, J., James, D. G. H., & van Doorn, J. (2012). Developmental trajectory for production of prosody: Lexical stress contrastivity in children 3 to 7 years and adults. *Journal of Speech, Language, and Hearing Research*, Online 4/3/12. doi: 10.1044/1092-4388(2012/11-0257.

Ballard, K. J., Robin, D. A., McCabe, P., & McDonald, J. (2010). A treatment for dysprosody in Childhood Apraxia of Speech. *Journal of Speech, Language, and Hearing Research, 53*, 1227–1245.

Baltaxe, C. A. M. (1984). Use of contrastive stress in normal, aphasic, and autistic children. *Journal of Speech and Hearing Research, 27*, 97–105.

Baltaxe, C. A. M., & Simmons, J. Q. (1985). Prosodic development in normal and autistic children. In E. Schopler & G. B. Mesibov (Eds.), *Communication problems in autism* (pp. 95–125). New York, NY: Plenum.

Baltaxe, C. A. M., Simmons, J. Q., & Zee, E. (1984). Intonation patterns in normal, autistic and aphasic children. In A. Cohen & M. van de Broecke (Eds.), *Proceedings of the 10th International Congress of Phonetic Sciences* (pp. 713–718). Dordrecht, The Netherlands: Foris.

Barnes, E., Roberts, J., Long, S. H., Martin, G. E., Berni, M. C., Mandulak, K. C., & Sideris, J. (2009). Phonological accuracy and intelligibility in connected speech of boys with Fragile X syndrome or Down syndrome. *Journal of Speech, Language, and Hearing Research, 52*, 1048–1061.

Bernhardt, B. H., Stemberger, J. P., & Major, E. (2006). General and nonlinear phonological intervention perspectives for a child with a resistant phonological impairment. *International Journal of Speech-Language Pathology, 8*(3), 190–206.

Bortolini, U., & Leonard, L. (1996). Phonology and grammatical morphology in specific language impairment: Accounting for individual variation in English and Italian. *Applied Psycholinguistics, 17*(1), 85–104.

Branigan, G. (1979). Some reasons why successive single-word utterances are not. *Journal of Child Language, 6*(3), 411–421.

Capelli, C. A., Nakagawa, N., & Madden, C. M. (1990). How children understand sarcasm: The role of context and intonation. *Child Development, 61*(6), 1824–1841.

Carter, A. (1996). *An acoustic analysis of weak syllable omissions: Evidence for adult prosodic representations in young children's speech.* MA thesis, University of Arizona.

Carter, A., & Gerken, L. (2004). Do children's omissions leave traces? *Journal of Child Language, 31*(3), 561–586.

Cheung, P., & Abberton, E. (2000). Patterns of phonological disability in Cantonese-speaking children in Hong Kong. *International Journal of Language and Communication Disorders, 35*(4), 451–473.

Chiat, S., & Roy, P. (2007). The Preschool Repetition Test: An evaluation of performance in typically developing and clinically referred children. *Journal of Speech, Language, and Hearing Research, 50*, 429–443.

Clark, E. V., Gelman, S. A., & Lane, N. M. (1985). Compound nouns and category structure in young children. *Child Development, 56*(1), 84–94.

Cleland, J. (2010). *Speech and prosody in developmental disorders: Autism and Down's [sic] syndrome.* (Doctoral dissertation), Queen Margaret University.

Crystal, D. (1981). *Clinical linguistics.* Vienna, Austria: Springer-Verlag.

Davis, B. L., & Velleman, S. L. (2008). Establishing a basic speech repertoire without using NSOME: Means, motive, and opportunity. *Seminars in Speech and Language, 29*(4), 312–319.

de Bree, E., Wijnen, F., & Zonneveld, W. (2006). Word stress production in three-year-old children at risk of dyslexia. *Journal of Research in Reading, 29*(3), 304–317.

Diehl, J. J., Watson, D., Bennetto, L., McDonough, J., & Gunlogson, C. (2009). An acoustic analysis of prosody in high-functioning autism. *Applied Psycholinguistics, 30,* 385–404.

Dupoux, E., Pallier, C., Sebastian, N., & Mehler, J. (1997). A destressing "deafness" in French? *Journal of Memory and Language, 36*(3), 406–421.

Dupoux, E., Peperkamp, S., & Sebastian-Galles, N. (2010). Limits on bilingualism revisited: Stress "deafness" in simultaneous French–Spanish bilinguals. *Cognition, 114,* 266–275.

Eisenmajer, R., Prior, M., Leekam, S., Wing, L., Gould, J., Welham, M., & Ong, B. (1996). Comparison of clinical symptoms in autism and Asperger's disorder. *Journal of the American Academy of Child & Adolescent Psychiatry, 35*(11), 1523-1531. http://www.sciencedirect.com/science/article/pii/S0890856709664145

Fay, W., & Schuler, A. L. (1980). *Emerging language in autistic children.* Baltimore, MD: University Park Press.

Fikkert, P. (1994). *On the acquisition of prosodic structure.* Dordrecht, The Netherlands: Holland Institute of Generative Linguistics.

Fisher, J., Plante, E., Vance, R., Gerken, L. A., & Glattke, T. J. (2007). Do children and adults with language impairment recognize prosodic cues? *Journal of Speech, Language, and Hearing Research, 50,* 746–758.

Fokes, J. (1976). *Fokes Sentence Builder.* Boston, MA: Teaching Resources Corporation.

Foreman, C. G. (2001). *The use of contrastive focus by high-functioning children with autism.* (Doctoral Dissertation), UCLA, Los Angeles.

Frome-Loeb, D., & Allen, G. D. (1993). Preschoolers' imitation of intonation contours. *Journal of Speech and Hearing Research, 36,* 4–13.

Gerken, L. (1991). The metrical basis for children's subjectless sentences. *Journal of Memory and Language, 30*(4), 431–451.

Gerken, L. A. (1994). A metrical template account of children's weak syllable omissions from multisyllabic words. *Journal of Child Language, 21,* 565–584.

Gerken, L. A., & McGregor, K. K. (1998). An overview of prosody and its role in normal and disordered child language. *American Journal of Speech-Language Pathology, 7*(2), 38–48.

Gerken, L., & McIntosh, B. (1993). Interplay of function morphemes and prosody in early language. *Developmental Psychology, 29*(3), 448–457.

Goetry, V., Wade-Woolley, L., Kolinsky, R., & Mousty, P. (2006). The role of stress processing abilities in the development of bilingual reading. *Journal of Research in Reading, 29*(3), 349–362.

Goffman, L. (2004). Kinematic differentiation of prosodic categories in normal and disordered language development. *Journal of Speech, Language, and Hearing Research, 47,* 1088–1102.

Goffman, L., Gerken, L. A., & Lucchesi, J. (2007). Relations between segmental and motor variability in prosodically complex nonword sequences. *Journal of Speech, Language, and Hearing Research, 50,* 444–458.

Goffman, L., & Malin, C. (1999). Metrical effects on speech movements in children and adults. *Journal of Speech, Language, and Hearing Research, 42,* 1003–1015.

Grigos, M. I., & Patel, R. (2007). Articulator movement associated with the development of prosodic control in children. *Journal of Speech, Language, and Hearing Research, 50,* 119–130.

Grossman, R. B., Bemis, R., Plesa Skwerer, D., & Tager-Flusberg, H. (2010). Lexical and affective prosody in children with high-functioning autism. *Journal of Speech, Language, and Hearing Research, 53,* 778–793.

Halle, P., Boysson-Bardies, B. D., & Vihman, M. M. (1991). Beginnings of prosodic organization: Intonation and duration patterns of disyllables produced by French and Japanese infants. *Language and Speech, 34,* 299–318.

Hargrove, P. M., Roetzel, K., & Hoodin, R. B. (1989). Modifying the prosody of a language-impaired child. *Language, Speech, and Hearing Services in Schools, 20,* 245–258.

Jaeger, J. J. (1997). How to say "Grandma" and "Grandpa": A case study in early phonological development. *First Language, 17*(1), 1–29.

Jarvinen-Pasley, A., Wallace, G. L., Ramus, F., Happe, F., & Heaton, P. (2008). Enhanced perceptual processing of speech in autism. *Developmental Science, 11*(1), 109–121.

Kehoe, M., & Stoel-Gammon, C. (1997a). The acquisition of prosodic structure: An investigation of current accounts of children's prosodic development. *Language, 73*(1), 113–144.

Kehoe, M., & Stoel-Gammon, C. (1997b). Truncation patterns in English-speaking children's word productions. *Journal of Speech, Language, and Hearing Research, 40*(3), 526–541.

Kehoe, M., Stoel-Gammon, C., & Buder, E. H. (1995). Acoustic correlates of stress in young children's speech. *Journal of Speech and Hearing Research, 38*(2), 338–350.

Kent, R. D., & Bauer, H. R. (1985). Vocalizations of one-year-olds. *Journal of Child Language, 12,* 491–526.

Kent, R. D., & Forner, L. L. (1980). Speech segment durations in sentence recitations by children and adults. *Journal of Phonetics, 8,* 157–168.

Kent, R. D., & Murray, A. D. (1982). Acoustic features of infant vocalic utterances at 3, 6, and 9 months. *Journal of the Acoustical Society of America, 72*(2), 353–365.

Labelle, J. L. (1973). Sentence comprehension in two age groups of children as related to pause position or the absence of pauses. *Journal of Speech and Hearing Research, 16,* 231–237.

Laures, J. S., & Weismer, G. (1999). The effects of a flattened fundamental frequency on intelligibility at the sentence level. *Journal of Speech, Language, and Hearing Research, 42,* 1148–1156.

Laval, V., & Bert-Erboul, A. (2005). French-speaking children's understanding of sarcasm: The role of intonation and context. *Journal of Speech, Language, and Hearing Research, 48,* 610–620.

Maassen, B. (1986). Marking word boundaries to improve the intelligibility of the speech of the deaf. *Journal of Speech and Hearing Research, 29,* 227–230.

Maassen, B., Nijland, L., & Van Der Meulen, S. (2001). Coarticulation within and between syllables by children with developmental apraxia of speech. *Clinical Linguistics and Phonetics, 15*(1&2), 145–150.

Mattock, K., & Burnham, D. (2006). Chinese and English infants' tone perception: Evidence for perceptual reorganization. *Infancy, 10*(3), 241–265.

Mattock, K., Molnar, M., Polka, L., & Burnham, D. (2008). The developmental course of lexical tone perception in the first year of life. *Cognition, 106,* 1367–1381.

McCann, J., Peppe, S., Gibbon, F. E., O'Hare, A., & Rutherford, M. (2007). Prosody and its relationship to language in school-aged children with high-functioning autism. *International Journal of Language and Communication Disorders, 42*(6), 682–702.

McGregor, K. K., & Leonard, L. B. (1994). Subject pronoun and article omissions in the speech of children with specific language impairment: A phonological interpretation. *Journal of Speech and Hearing Research, 37*(1), 171–181.

Menn, L., & Vihman, M. M. (2011). Features in child phonology: Inherent, emergent, or artefacts of analysis? In N. Clements & R. Ridouane (Eds.), *Where do phonological features come from? Cognitive, physical and developmental bases of distinctive speech categories.* Amsterdam, The Netherlands: John Benjamins.

Monsen, R. B. (1978). Toward measuring how well hearing-impaired children speak. *Journal of Speech and Hearing Research, 21*(2), 197–219.

Paul, R., Augustyn, A., Klin, A., & Volkmar, F. R. (2005). Perception and production of prosody by speakers with Autism Spectrum Disorders. *Journal of Autism and Developmental Disorders, 35*(2), 205–220.

Peppe, S., & McCann, J. (2003). Assessing intonation and prosody in children with atypical language development: The PEPS-C test and the revised version. *Clinical Linguistics and Phonetics, 17*(4–5), 345–354.

Peppe, S., McCann, J., Gibbon, F., O'Hare, A., & Rutherford, M. (2007). Receptive and expressive prosodic ability in children with High-Functioning Autism. *Journal of Speech, Language, and Hearing Research, 50*, 1015–1028.

Redford, M. A., & Gildersleeve-Neumann, C. (2009). The development of distinct speaking styles in preschool children. *Journal of Speech, Language, and Hearing Research, 52*,1434–1448.

Roy, P., Chiat, S., & Seeff-Gabriel, B. (2008). *Early Repetition Battery (ERB)*. London, United Kingdom: Pearson Education, Inc.

Sadagopan, N., & Smith, A. (2008). Developmental changes in the effects of utterance length and complexity on speech movement variability. *Journal of Speech, Language, and Hearing Research, 51*(5), 1138–1151.

Schreiber, P., & Read, C. (1980). Why short subjects are harder to find than long ones. In E. Wanner & L. R. Gleitman (Eds.), *Language acquisition: The state of the art* (pp. 78–101). New York, NY: Cambridge University Press.

Schwartz, R. G., & Goffman, L. (1995). Metrical patterns of words and production accuracy. *Journal of Speech and Hearing Research, 38*(4), 876–888.

Segal, O., & Kishon-Rabin. (2012). Evidence for language-specific influence on the preference of stress patterns in infants learning an iambic language (Hebrew). *Journal of Speech, Language, and Hearing Research, 55*, 1329–1341.

Shriberg, L. D., Aram, D. M., & Kwiatkowski, J. (1997a). Developmental Apraxia of Speech: I. Descriptive and theoretical perspectives. *Journal of Speech, Language, and Hearing Research, 40*(2), 273–285.

Shriberg, L. D., Aram, D. M., & Kwiatkowski, J. (1997b). Developmental apraxia of speech: II. Toward a diagnostic marker. *Journal of Speech, Language, and Hearing Research, 40*(2), 286–312.

Shriberg, L. D., Aram, D. M., & Kwiatkowski, J. (1997c). Developmental apraxia of speech: III. A subtype marked by inappropriate stress. *Journal of Speech, Language, and Hearing Research, 40*(2), 313–337.

Shriberg, L. D., Campbell, T. F., Karlsson, H. B., Brown, R. L., McSweeny, J. L., & Nadler, C. J. (2003). A diagnostic marker for childhood apraxia of speech: The lexical stress ratio. *Clinical Linguistics and Phonetics, 17*(7), 549–574.

Shriberg, L. D., Green, J. R., Campbell, T. F., McSweeny, J. L., & Scheer, A. R. (2003). A diagnostic marker for childhood apraxia of speech: The coefficient of variation ratio. *Clinical Linguistics and Phonetics, 17*(7), 575–595.

Shriberg, L. D., Kwiatkowski, J., & Rasmussen, C. (1990). *Prosody—Voice Screening Profile*. Tucson, AZ: Communication Skill Builders, Inc.

Shriberg, L. D., Paul, R., McSweeny, J. L., Klin, A., Cohen, D. J., & Volkmar, F. R. (2001). Speech and prosody characteristics of adolescents and adults with high-functioning autism and Asperger syndrome. *Journal of Speech, Language, and Hearing Research, 44*(5), 1097–1115.

Snow, D. (1994). Phrase-final syllable lengthening and intonation in early child speech. *Journal of Speech and Hearing Research, 37*(4), 831–840.

Snow, D. (1998). Children's imitations of intonation contours: Are rising tones more difficult than falling tones? *Journal of Speech, Language, and Hearing Research, 41*, 576–587.

Snow, D. (2001). Imitation of intonation contours by children with normal and disordered language development. *Clinical Linguistics & Phonetics, 15*, 567–584.

Snow, D. (2006). Regression and reorganization of intonation between 6 and 23 months. *Child Development, 77*(2), 281–296.

So, L. K. H., & Dodd, B. (1994). Phonologically disordered Cantonese-speaking children. *Clinical Linguistics & Phonetics, 8*, 235–255.

So, L. K. H., & Dodd, B. (1995). The acquisition of phonology by Cantonese-speaking children. *Journal of Child Language, 22*, 473–495.

Thurber, C., & Tager-Flusberg, H. (1993). Pauses in the narratives produced by autistic, mentally retarded and normal children as an index of cognitive demand. *Journal of Autism and Developmental Disorders, 23*, 309–322.

van Rees, L. J., Ballard, K. J., McCabe, P., Macdonald-D'Silva, A. G., & Arciuli, J. (2012). Training production of lexical stress in typically developing children using orthographically biased stimuli and principles of motor learning. *American Journal of Speech-Language Pathology, 21*, 197–206.

Velleman, S. L. (1994). The interaction of phonetics and phonology in developmental verbal dyspraxia: Two case studies. *Clinics in Communication Disorders, 4*(1), 67–78.

Velleman, S. L. (2009, March 6). *Assessment and Treatment of Childhood Apraxia of Speech*. Paper presented at the Ohio Speech-Language-Hearing Association, Columbus, OH.

Velleman, S. L., Andrianopoulos, M. V., Boucher, M., Perkins, J., Averback, K. E., Currier, A., . . . Van Emmerik, R. (2009). Motor speech disorders in children with autism. In R. Paul & P. Flipsen (Eds.), *Speech sound disorders in children: In honor of Lawrence D. Shriberg* (pp. 141–180). San Diego, CA: Plural.

Velleman, S. L., & Shriberg, L. D. (1999). Metrical analysis of the speech of children with suspected developmental apraxia of speech and inappropriate stress. *Journal of Speech, Language, and Hearing Research, 42*(6), 1444–1460.

Vihman, M. M., Nakai, S., & De Paolis, R. (2006). Getting the rhythm right: A cross-linguistic study of segmental duration in babbling and first words. In L. Goldstein, D. H. Whalen & C. Best (Eds.), *Papers in laboratory phonology 8: Varieties of phonological competence*. Berlin/New York: Mouton de Gruyter.

Walker, J. F., Archibald, L. M. D., Cherniak, S. R., & Fish, V. G. (1992). Articulation rate in 3- and 5-year-old children. *Journal of Speech and Hearing Research, 35*, 4–13.

Weinert, S. (1992). Deficits in acquiring language structure: The importance of using prosodic cues. *Applied Cognitive Psychology, 6*(6), 545–571.

Wells, B., & Peppe, S. (2003). Intonation abilities of children with speech and language impairments. *Journal of Speech, Language, and Hearing Research, 46*(1), 5–20.

Whalen, D. H., Levitt, A. G., & Wang, Q. (1991). Intonational differences between the reduplicative babbling of French- and English-learning infants. *Journal of Child Language, 18*, 501–516.

Wing, L. (1996). Autistic spectrum disorders. *British Medical Journal, 312*, 327–328.

Wingfield, A., Lombardi, L., & Sokol, S. (1984). Prosodic features and the intelligibility of accelerated speech: Syntactic versus periodic segmentation. *Journal of Speech and Hearing Research, 27*, 128–134.

Wong, A. M.-Y., Ciocca, V., & Yung, S. (2009). The perception of lexical tone contrasts in Cantonese children with and without Specific Language Impairment (SLI). *Journal of Speech, Language, and Hearing Research, 52*, 1493–1509.

Wood, C. (2006). Metrical stress sensitivity in young children and its relationship to phonological awareness and reading. *Journal of Research in Reading, 29*(3), 270–287.

Zajac, D. J., Roberts, J. E., Hennon, E. A., Harris, A. A., Barnes, E. F., & Misenheimer, J. L. (2006). Articulation rate and vowel space characteristics of young males with Fragile X syndrome: Preliminary acoustic findings. *Journal of Speech, Language, and Hearing Research, 49*, 1147–1155.

APPENDIX B

Examples of Stress Patterns

SW

cookie
bottle
monkey
apple
window
wagon
chicken
zipper
scissors
yellow
vacuum
matches
shovel
pencil
carrot
orange
Santa
Christmas
basket
candle
crayons
feather
after
early
every

WS

Many verbs (forget, pretend, etc.)
giraffe
balloon
around
canteen
maroon
TV
macaque
kaboom
baboon
raccoon
canoe
cassette
shampoo
Japan
motel
Vermont
above
before
behind
between

ŚWS̀ /SWW

telephone
elephant
cowboy hat
music box
envelope
valentine
gasoline
hospital
ambulance
astronaut
pillowcase
tablecloth
magazine (dialectal)
photograph
ambulance
dinosaur
evergreen
library
medicine
calendar
cucumber
temperature
vegetable
alphabet
hamburger

S̀WŚ/WWS

violin
understand
chimpanzee
kangaroo
tangerine
engineer

WŚWS̀/WŚWW/S̀ŚWW

thermometer
aquarium
speedometer
extinguisher
binoculars
librarian
material
harmonica
rhinoceros
asparagus
experiment
historian
biologist
comedian
custodian
peripheral
astronomy

cartographer
capitulate

WSW/WŚS̀

announcement
assignment
vacation
papaya
pajamas
potato
banana
tomato
spaghetti
umbrella
prescription
computer
eraser
tuxedo
mechanic
musician
detective
director
reporter
cartoonist
designer
bewildered
embarrassed
excited
endangered
terrific
burrito
fajitas
lasagna

ŚWS̀W

television
watercolors
secretary
radiator
elevator
caterpillar
supermarket
cauliflower
calculator
motorcycle
dictionary
peanut butter
alligator
watermelon

S̀WŚW/WWSW

macaroni
ravioli
perspiration
readjustment
disappointed
horizontal
satisfactory

S̀WŚWW

cafeteria
auditorium
hippopotamus
condominium

ŚS̀

Any "spondee" (e.g., hot dog, blackboard, baseball)

WŚWS̀W

refrigerator
contaminated
electrifying

GLOSSARY

7q11.23 Duplication syndrome (Dup7) A genetically based neurodevelopmental syndrome characterized by social anxiety; motor speech, speech, and language deficits.

A

accidental gap A sound (or other element) that would be expected in a phonetic (or other) repertoire in a certain language, based upon the features being used by that language, but that is not present.

achondroplasia A genetic disorder in which cartilage is not appropriately converted to bone.

across-class generalization Transfer of learning from one category (e.g., one type of consonant) to another; a type of response generalization.

advanced tongue root Positioning of the tongue in a more forward position; sometimes used to distinguish tense vowels (advanced) from lax vowels (not advanced).

afferent neuron Neuron carrying a signal toward the central nervous system (e.g., a sensory neuron).

allophone A non-contrastive variant of a phoneme (e.g., [tʰ] as an allophone of /t/).

Angelman syndrome A rare neurodevelopmental syndrome resulting in cognitive delays and severe/profound speech deficits.

anoxia Lack of oxygen to the brain (severe hypoxia).

anterior Front or forward.

apparent regression A change in behavior that mimics an earlier stage but is in fact a sign of systematization or reorganization and therefore of the emergence of more mature behavior.

articulation disorder A deficit in the production of speech sounds; usually used in reference to a mild, isolated difficulty (e.g., a lisp or an imprecise /ɹ/ in the absence of any other errors).

articulation test Standardized, norm-referenced evaluation tool designed to assess children's productions of consonants (and sometimes consonant clusters and/or vowels), usually by single-word naming of pictures.

aspiration *Phonetics*: a burst of air that is perceptible due to a "long lag" voice-onset time such that voicing begins after the release of the consonant closure. *Medicine*: entry of liquid or food particles into the lungs due to inadequate protection of the airway during feeding/eating.

assessment Comprehensive evaluation to develop a thorough profile of a child's strengths and weaknesses in a particular area of functioning.

assimilation A production change resulting in two adjacent sounds or syllables becoming more alike (such as a vowel being nasalized before a nasal consonant).

associative learning Learning that two events or types of events consistently occur together or in sequence.

athetoid cerebral palsy A type of motor disorder due to a cerebral malformation or injury resulting in slow, writhing movements and fluctuating muscle tone.

auditory processing disorder (APD) A deficit in the ability to analyze and interpret auditory signals received by the ear and transmitted to the brain.

B

babbling ratio The percentage of a child's babble syllables that are of CV form (the number of CV syllables divided by the total number of syllables produced).

baby talk The manner in which adults address infants, included exaggerated prosody. Also known as "motherese," "infant-directed speech," "child-directed speech."

ballistic syllable Syllable in which the consonant and vowel share place of articulation, thereby reducing the motor complexity of the syllable. See also "CV association," "consonant–vowel assimilation."

basal ganglia A set of subcortical nuclei with strong interconnections to many other portions of the brain; primarily responsible for control and regulation of actions.

bidirectional harmony A production change in which segments both before and after the triggering segment are changed to be more like the triggering segment.

bilirubin The product of the body's elimination of aged red blood cells.

biting reflex Mouth closing in response to light touch on the gums.

blocked practice Focusing on a single target/a single goal until it has been mastered. Compare to "random practice."

body (of a syllable) The onset plus the nucleus of a syllable.

bound morpheme A morpheme that only occurs in combination with other morphemes (e.g., -s, -ed, pre-, -ly).

brainstem A posterior part of the brain that connects to the spinal cord.

broncho-pulmonary dysplasia A respiratory disorder affecting premature infants due to a lack of surfactant (a liquid that coats the inside of the lungs to help keep them open).

C

C:V ratio The proportion of consonants versus vowels in a child's babbling (number of consonants used divided by number of vowels used). Also known as "closant curve."

canonical babble Babble (prelinguistic vocalization) composed of syllables that include both true consonants and fully resonant vowels. Includes reduplicated babbling and variegated babbling. Compare to "marginal babble."

categorical perception Abrupt perceptual differentiation between speech sound categories (e.g., consonants sound voiced or voiceless, not in between).

central pattern generator Neuronal circuit that synchronizes oscillation as in sucking and babble.

cerebellum A grooved structure connected to the bottom of the brain with the primary functions of coordination and timing of movements.

cerebral palsy A set of motor disorders due to a cerebral malformation or injury.

challenge point The point at which a task taxes the client just enough for maximal learning without decreasing motivation.

child-directed speech The manner in which adults address infants, included exaggerated prosody. See also "baby talk," "motherese," "infant-directed speech."

Childhood Apraxia of Speech (CAS) A neurologically based motor speech disorder characterized by deficits in motor programming and planning.

chromosomal translocation Movement of some genetic material (a whole chromosome or part of a chromosome) from its typical location to another location.

chronological mismatch A type of disorder characterized by uneven development such that the child's overall profile is not typical of any age, although each component may appear to be delayed rather than disordered.

cleft palate An opening in the palate due to incomplete closure during embryonic development.

closant A prelinguistic consonant-like sound that lacks the complete closure of a true consonant.

closed syllable Syllable ending with a consonant (regardless of onset).

cluster reduction Omission of one or more consonants from a cluster.

coalescence Merger of two consonants into one including some features of each (e.g., the cluster sw- pronounced as [f], preserving the continuance of the /s/ and the labiality of the /w/) or of two syllables into one (e.g., /bəˈnænə/ pronounced as [ˈbænə], retaining the consonant from the first syllable and the vowel from the second).

cochlear implant Device surgically implanted to carry out the functions of the inner ear, transmitting sound to the brain.

coda Syllable-final consonant.

code switching Mixing languages within one utterance by bilinguals or mixing dialects by bidialectal speakers.

cognitive–linguistic impairment/disorder Disorder characterized by incomplete or inaccurate learning of the rules or patterns of language, possibly reflecting deficits in implicit learning. See "phonological disorder."

columella The tissue in between the nares, connecting the tip of the nose to the philtrum.

communicative grunt The deliberate production of a grunt-like vocalization to communicate that a task is difficult (e.g., grunting right before opening a heavy door).

communicative intent Motivation to transmit some meaning to another person, by whatever means (vocal, gestural, etc.).

co-morbidity Medical symptom or deficit that co-occurs with another symptom or deficit.

compartmentalization A bilingual learner's use of two languages in separate contexts (e.g., using German in school and Spanish at home).

complementary distribution Allophones occurring in different contexts (e.g., [o] occurring before a non-nasal consonant, [õ] occurring before a nasal consonant).

consonant diversity Measure of variety of consonants in a child's babble: the number of different consonants (i.e., the number of consonant types) divided by the total number of consonants produced (i.e., the number of consonant tokens).

consonantal Having the articulatory characteristics of a consonant.

consonant–vowel assimilation A change to a consonant or a vowel, or both, that results in the two being more similar (e.g., a consonant becoming rounded before a round vowel). See CV associations.

constant practice Repeatedly practicing the same target in the same context. Compare to "variable practice."

constraint A tendency to avoid certain features, segments, or structures (markedness constraint) or to preserve certain features, segments, or structures (faithfulness constraint) or to use certain strategies to make a word more pronounceable (faithfulness constraint).

constraint hierarchy, constraint ranking Prioritization for honoring constraints (e.g., a child's highest-ranked constraint is "preserve /s/" but "avoid clusters" is also high ranked, so the child cannot avoid sn- by deleting [s]. Therefore, she migrates the [s], saying [nos] for "snow" instead of [no] for "snow.").

continuant Consonant feature referring to the ongoing flow of air through the mouth (as for fricatives).

continuous feedback Information about achievement provided for 100% of responses.

contrastive analysis Comparison of the phonologies of two languages in order to determine which elements or structures will be challenging for a speaker of one of the languages learning the other.

core syllable Most basic consonant + vowel syllable shape, most common in the languages of the world, in babble, and in early words; also called "canonical syllable."

core vocabulary A therapy approach focusing on the recognizable (if not accurate) production of key words to increase communicative effectiveness for young/severe children.

corner vowels The vowels at the extreme corners of the vowel triangle, [i], [ɑ], [u].

coronal Produced with the front portion of the tongue on the palate (dental, alveolar, palatal).

criterion referenced For the purposes of comparing a person's performance at a given time with the same person's performance at another time (i.e., not intended for comparing one person's performance with that of other people).

critical difference An articulatory or acoustic difference that signals a phonemic contrast (e.g., amount of voicing is a critical difference between voiced and voiceless consonants).

CV association A change to a consonant or a vowel, or both, that results in the two being more similar (e.g., a consonant becoming rounded before a round vowel). See "consonant–vowel assimilation."

cycles An intervention strategy in which a small set of exemplars is trained for a certain period of time, then the goal is shifted regardless of progress.

D

dark [l] /l/ produced with the tongue bunched toward the velum, yielding a vocalic-sounding liquid.

declarative memory The explicit, conscious learning of facts, word meanings, etc. Compare to "implicit learning."

default Least marked; most commonly used; used unless conditions mandate otherwise.

deictic gesture Hand or arm movement indicating a location (e.g., pointing, reaching).

de Lange syndrome Genetically based neurodevelopmental syndrome resulting in severe cognitive deficits, social-pragmatic challenges, and physical differences, including craniofacial anomalies.

delay (speech delay) Condition in which behavior/performance is similar to that of a typically developing younger child.

delayed feedback Response that does not occur until about five seconds after the client's attempt.

delayed release Description of a consonant that is stopped then released slowly in a fricative, as an affricate.

deviant process An error pattern that is atypical in child development or a pattern that is unusual in the languages of the world; also called an "atypical" or "marked" process.

diagnosis A label referring to a speech, language, or other condition applied in a particular case based on a comprehensive profile of strengths, weaknesses, and symptoms.

dialect A variation of a language spoken by a group delineated by geography, ethnicity, age, culture, or other factors.

difference (linguistic difference) Pattern of linguistic behavior reflecting exposure to and/or learning of a non-mainstream dialect or language or of more than one dialect or language.

discourse An amount of oral communication longer than a sentence; an oral speech act, ranging in length from a greeting ritual to a full speech or interview.

disorder (speech sound disorder) A condition in which speech performance is either (a) atypical, that is, the child produces elements, structures, or patterns that are not seen in typical children, regardless of age or (b) uneven, such that some behaviors or skill sets are at different age expectation levels with respect to each other. See also "speech sound disorder," "phonological disorder," "functional phonological disorder," "chronological mismatch."

distinctive feature Characteristic of speech sounds that differentiates them from each other in a given language (e.g., voicing distinguishes /t/ from /d/).

distributed practice Either training sessions or practice of a particular target/practice on a particular goal are spread out in time, separated either by time without therapy or by therapy time devoted to some other target/goal.

distributional probability The likelihood (frequency) that elements, structures, or events will occur simultaneously or sequentially. See also "phonotactic probability," "co-occurrence," "distribution requirement."

distribution requirement Restriction on positions or combinations in which segments or structures may occur (e.g., [ŋ] cannot occur in initial position in English).

disyllabic Composed of two syllables.

DIVA The "directions into velocities of articulators" model of speech production, focusing on sensory-motor interactions especially feedforward and feedback processes critical for motor programming and planning.

dorsal Produced with the back (dorsum) of the tongue.

Down syndrome (DS) A genetically based neurodevelopmental syndrome characterized by low muscle tone, mild-to-moderate cognitive deficits, and speech-language deficits.

drill Repeated production of a task out of context with an explicit non-social reward (e.g., tokens).

drill play Repeated production of a task in which a game is used to reward this behavior.

Duchenne dystrophy A form of muscular dystrophy characterized by muscle degeneration; occurs primarily in males.

duration *Phonetics*: the length, in time, of a linguistic unit. *Intervention*: the length, in time, of a therapy session.

dynamic assessment The systematic identification of levels of performance in response to varying levels and types of cueing and other support during a therapy task.

dynamic systems theory A model in which development is seen as ever-changing and self-organizing, with a focus on the emergence of collaborative systems of motor, perceptual, and cognitive functions and the external factors that facilitate or impede them.

dynamic temporal and tactile cueing (DTTC) A therapy approach focusing on the type and timing of modeling that is provided.

dysarthria A condition characterized by deficits in respiration, phonation, articulation, resonance, and/or prosody as a result of damage or difference in a variety of neuromotor systems.

E

ear training Intervention method focused on training the child to differentiate a target sound. Also known as "identification training."

ease of perception The tendency in languages for the set of sounds in the language to be not only objectively easily perceptible but also different enough from each other that the listener can consistently tell which sound is intended by the speaker.

ease of production The tendency in languages for the set of sounds in the language to be not only objectively easy to produce but also different enough from each other that the speaker can consistently produce them distinctively.

emergentism The view that language is learned in functional communication contexts using more general human cognitive abilities (such as implicit learning). Compare to nativism.

environment The context in which a segment or structure occurs (e.g., in final position, before a high vowel).

epenthesis Addition (insertion) of a sound or sequence of sounds to a word form (e.g., schwa added between the consonants in a cluster to make it easier to produce).

episodic memory Conscious memory of specific experiences as whole events.

error-free learning An approach to intervention in which objectives are only selected if the child is able to produce the target correctly in some context in order to minimize the number of errors and avoid allowing practice of incorrect forms.

excess equal stress Reduced differentiation of stressed versus unstressed syllables in the word, with all syllables receiving more equal levels of duration and loudness than appropriate.

exemplar Target word or syllable.

expressive learning style Formulaic learning style resulting in higher proportion of phrases (e.g., "I love you", "pick you up") learned as wholes and higher proportion of verb use as well as less distinct articulation.

F

faithfulness constraint A tendency to preserve certain features, segments, or structures or to use certain strategies to make a word more pronounceable.

familial dysautonomia A genetic neurodevelopmental syndrome affecting the nerve cells in the central nervous system.

fast speech rules Patterns found in casual speech.

feedback Internal (e.g., proprioception) or external (e.g., SLP) responses indicating outcomes of behavior. External feedback is also known as "reinforcement."

feedback conditions Schedules, frequency, and types of reinforcement.

feedforward Sensory-motor planning processes.

FOXP2 A chromosomal translocation resulting in cognitive differences, craniofacial anomalies, and motor speech deficits.

Fragile X syndrome A genetic neurodevelopmental syndrome resulting in mild-to-moderate impairments in cognition, speech, and language; attention and social-pragmatic symptoms are common. More common in males.

free morpheme A morpheme (unit of meaning) that can stand on its own as a word (but may also combine with other morphemes, such as "berry").

free nerve ending Type of sensory receptor.

free variation Allophones occurring in the same contexts as each other (with no meaning change).

frequency *Acoustics:* pitch (fundamental frequency). *Implicit learning*: how often an element, structure, or word occurs in the ambient language. *Intervention*: how often therapy sessions occur (e.g., once a week).

frontal lobe Portion of the brain at the front of the cerebral cortex primarily responsible for planning (with respect to both motor control and behavior).

fronting Production of a consonant sound (typically, a velar) more anteriorly (typically, at the alveolar ridge) than expected in adult speech.

frozen form Pronunciation of a word that does not change when the child's system changes, so it is not consistent with the child's other productions. See "phonological idiom."

functional load The amount of contrast provided by a sound or structure within a language.

functional phonological disorder A condition in which speech performance is either (a) atypical, that is, the child produces elements, structures, or patterns that are not seen in typical children, regardless of age, or (b) uneven, such that some behaviors or skill sets are at different age expectation levels with respect to each other. See also "speech sound disorder," "phonological disorder," "disorder," "chronological mismatch."

fundamental frequency Pitch.

G

galactosemia A genetic disorder that interferes with the body's ability to use a kind of sugar (galactose) to produce energy, with impacts on intellectual and speech development.

geminate Speech sound with double or triple length.

generalization Application of learning to new material or new contexts.

generative phonological rule A linguistic change or tendency that is consistent (within all languages, within all speakers of a language, or within one person's speech) described with a focus on the distinctive features involved (e.g., a continuant sound [such as a fricative] that becomes noncontinuant [such as a stop]). See also "phonological rule," "pattern," "process," "constraint."

gestural phonology A model of speech production that focuses on the overall articulatory plan for a given word rather than on individual segments.

glottalization Production of a consonant with partial closure of the glottis (either dialectal or in error).

Golgi tendon organ A sensory receptor that detects changes in muscle tension.

H

harmony A change resulting in two consonants or two vowels that are separated by some other segment(s) becoming more alike. See also "assimilation."

harmony/assimilation pattern See harmony, assimilation.

heavy syllable Syllable with a diphthong and/or a coda (final consonant or cluster).

heterorganic Containing consonants from different places of articulation (said of clusters; opposite of homorganic).

hiatus The occurrence of two vowels in a row, either within a word or between two words.

high-amplitude sucking An experimental procedure measuring an infant's sucking rate to determine whether or not an acoustic change has been detected.

hippocampus A ridge of gray matter on the floor of the lateral ventricles of the brain, with important roles in memory and the limbic system.

homonymic clash Potential confusion resulting from words becoming homonyms as a result of phonological changes within a language.

homonymy The presence of words that sound the same but have different meanings (such as "reed" and "read").

homorganic Produced in the same (or similar) place of articulation.

I

iambic With an unstressed first syllable and stress on the second syllable.

identification The process of determining whether a communication problem may exist in order to decide whether or not further evaluation is warranted. See "screening."

idiolect Individual style of speaking, including accent, vocabulary, grammar, etc.

implicational universal A tendency for the presence of one element or structure in a language or in the languages of the world to imply the presence of another element or structure (e.g., if a language has [k] it most likely also has [t]).

implicit learning Learning based on distributional probabilities that is unconscious and automatic. See also "procedural learning;" contrast "declarative memory."

inconsistency Difference in production from one time to the next or in a different context. See "variability."

independent analysis Assessment of a child's productions without reference to the target words (e.g., determining which consonants the child produces in any context, regardless of whether they are the target consonants in those contexts or not).

Index of Phonetic Complexity Measure of phonetic and phonotactic maturity.

infant-directed speech (IDS) The manner in which adults address infants, included exaggerated prosody. See also "baby talk," "motherese," "child-directed speech."

inherent relative duration The relative length in time of a segment in comparison to other segments (e.g., vowels are always longer than consonants regardless of the speaker's rate of speech).

intensity *Acoustics*: loudness. *Intervention:* number of repetitions of target per session.

interference Error resulting from the influence of one language on another. See "transfer."

interincisal distance The distance between the upper and lower teeth when the child opens his or her mouth as far as possible with the tongue tip on the upper teeth.

intervocalic position Between two vowels.

intonation The combination of the rise and fall of the fundamental frequency with the increases and decreases in duration and intensity that ties together and adds meaning to a phrase or sentence. See also "prosody," "intonation contour," "prosodic contour," "pitch contour," "phrase-final lengthening," and "phrase-final declination."

J

jargon Sequences of variegated syllables that have the intonation contours of the ambient language.

juncture Linguistic pause.

K

knowledge of performance Feedback focused on whether or not the task was performed correctly (e.g., Was the tongue in the correct position?).

knowledge of results Feedback focused on whether the performance of the task was successful (e.g., Did the listener understand the message?).

L

language specificity Occurring in a specific language, that is, not universal.

Laurence-Moon-Biedl syndrome A genetic disorder that may result in vision difficulties, obesity, learning challenges, physical differences, delayed motor skills, and speech deficits.

lexical Related to vocabulary.

light syllable Syllable with a single/simple vowel and no coda.

Lindamood LiPS program Intervention program focused on matching articulatory characteristics of sounds with letter names and letter sounds.

lingual frenulum Membrane connecting the underside of the tongue to the floor of the mouth.

M

maintenance Continuing to use new-found knowledge or skills for a period of time (e.g., a month) after therapy has ceased; retention.

mandibular Of or relating to the lower jaw.

manner of articulation The way in which a sound is produced, especially the amount of closure (e.g., tight closure for stops, shaping of the airflow only for glides).

Marfan syndrome A genetic syndrome affecting vision, the heart, and the skeleton.

marginal babble Rhythmic babble composed of closants and vocants that lack the timing of more mature consonants and vowels. Compare to "canonical babbling."

marked Occurring but rarely (said of linguistic elements, structures, or patterns); may apply to linguistic universals, specific languages, or individuals' phonological systems.

markedness constraint A restriction on which elements, structures, or patterns will occur universally, within a particular language, or within a particular person's linguistic system.

massed practice Many training sessions or many trials of the same target many times in a short amount of time.

maxillary Of or relating to the upper jaw.

McGurk effect An illusion that occurs when a person is shown a movie clip in which the audio and the video don't match phonetically, so the person has to integrate the visual and the auditory input (e.g., the video is of a person saying [gɑ], but the audio is of the same person saying [bɑ]; the listener perceives [dɑ]).

mean babble level (MBL) Measure of consonant maturity and variety in babble.

Metaphon A therapy method involving using real-world contrasts (e.g., short-long) to teach phonemic contrasts.

metathesis The interchange of elements within a word (e.g., saying [pʌk] for "cup").

migration Movement of an element (usually a sound) within a word (e.g., saying [neɪks] for "snake").

minimal pair A pair of words that differ by a single phoneme (e.g., [ˈmuvi] "movie" and [ˈmudi] "moody").

minimal pairs therapy Intervention focused on the communicative function of phonemes via examples of words whose meanings change if one phoneme is substituted for another.

mirror neuron Motor neuron that fires when a person observes someone else performing a motor action that the first person knows how to do.

mixed speech sound disorder A disorder with symptoms from at least two disorder types: cognitive–linguistic, motor speech, articulatory.

monosyllabic One syllable.

morpheme Unit of meaning.

motherese The manner in which adults address infants, included exaggerated prosody. See also "baby talk," "infant-directed speech," "child-directed speech."

motor plan A set of signals sent to the muscles to achieve a particular action.

motor program An abstract set of motor commands ready to be adapted to a particular task, based upon experience carrying out similar tasks in the past.

mucosal receptor A sensory receptor that detects changes in muscle tension.

multiple oppositions therapy A therapy approach in which multiple phoneme collapses are treated together.

multisyllabic Having three or more syllables.

muscle spindle A sensory fiber embedded in a muscle to detect position, velocity, and motion of the muscle.

muscle tone Readiness for action of a muscle at rest.

muscular dystrophy A genetic syndrome impacting the production of protein for creating healthy muscle, resulting in progressive weakness and muscle mass loss.

myelinate To cover with insulating material (myelin) that speeds the transmission of nerve impulses.

N

nasal With the velum lowered to allow air to flow through the nasal cavity.

nativism Theory of language acquisition based upon assumption that linguistic knowledge is innate, with the child's task being to select among the options given by linguistic universals.

natural class Set of speech sounds that share certain distinctive features (e.g., voiced stops, front vowels). See also "sound class," "class."

natural phonological process A physiologically motivated speech pattern. See "phonological process," "natural process."

natural phonology A model of phonology based on the premise that all phonological patterns have their basis in human physiologic limitations on speech production.

natural process A physiologically motivated speech pattern described with a focus on the outcome—that is, the nature of the final production (e.g., the phonological process name "stopping" is used to indicate that some non-stop consonant has been produced as a stop). See "phonological process," "natural phonological process."

negative evidence Lack of evidence as a source of learning (e.g., understanding that "We donated the church the money" is ungrammatical because one has never heard anyone say that).

neighborhood density The number of minimal pairs ("neighbors") a word has; a word with high neighborhood density is more typical of the language than a word with low density.

neocortical Relating to the mammalian cerebral cortex.

neutralized Lacking contrast in a particular context (e.g., /t/ and /d/ are both pronounced as [ɾ] in between two vowels when the first one is stressed, in English).

non-functioning Lacking communicative effectiveness (said of a phonological system).

Noonan syndrome A genetic syndrome associated with a variety of physical effects, including oral–facial anomalies.

nucleus The heart of a syllable, usually a vowel, that carries most of the pitch and loudness information.

O

onset The first consonant or set of consonants in a syllable or a word.

open bite Upper teeth that protrude enough beyond the lowers to hide the tops of the lower teeth. See "overbite."

open syllable Syllable without a final consonant or cluster (regardless of onset).

overbite Upper teeth that protrude enough beyond the lowers to hide the tops of the lower teeth. See "open bite."

P

palatalization Inappropriately producing a consonant in a palatal place of articulation.

paralinguistic Related to language but not strictly linguistic (e.g., tone of voice).

partially neutralized Lacking contrast in a particular context (e.g., /t/ and /d/ are both pronounced as [ɾ] in between two vowels when the first one is stressed, in English).

pattern, phonological pattern A phonetic or phonotactic change or tendency that is consistent (within all languages, within all speakers of a language, or within one person's speech). See "rule," "process," "constraint."

percent consonants correct-revised A procedure for estimating the severity of a speech deficit developed and revised by Shriberg and colleagues; PCC-R.

performance The client's behavior during a therapy session.

philtrum The vertical groove between the upper lip and the nose.

phoneme A speech sound with a contrastive function in a particular language; a speech sound that changes word meanings in a particular language.

phonemic repertoire The set of phonemes in a particular language or a particular person's linguistic system.

phone Speech sound (whether it has a contrastive function or not).

phonetic Relating to speech sounds.

phonetically consistent form Vocalization associated with a certain event, person, thing, etc., but not based on a true word.

phonetic contingency Responding to a child's vocalization by producing an utterance or word that is similar with respect to the sounds or sound structures (e.g., the infant says [dɑ] and the adult says "dolly").

phonetic feature Phonetic (articulatory or acoustic) characteristic of speech sounds (e.g., for consonants, place, manner and voicing; for vowels, height, backness, tenseness, and rounding). See also "distinctive feature."

phonetic repertoire The set of speech sounds in a particular language or produced by a particular person (whether correct or not).

phonetic universal A tendency relating to speech sounds that is shared by most languages.

phonological analysis procedures Non-standardized, non-normed procedures for analyzing children's speech.

phonological awareness The ability to consciously reflect upon (e.g., discuss) speech sounds and their written representations (e.g., letters). Compare to "phonological knowledge."

phonological idiom Word production pattern that is not consistent with the child's production of other words. See "frozen form."

phonological knowledge Subconscious information about the sounds in a word (as evidenced, e.g., by a child who omits final nasal consonants but nonetheless nasalizes the vowels that come before them; he is acting based upon the presence of the nasals even though he doesn't produce them). Compare to "phonological awareness."

phonological loop Short-term memory of acoustic information about heard speech.

phonological mean length of utterance (PMLU) A measure of the phonetic maturity and variety in a child's meaningful speech.

phonological pattern A phonetic or phonotactic change or tendency that is consistent (within all languages, within all speakers of a language, or within one person's speech). See "rule," "process," "constraint."

phonological process A linguistic change or tendency that is consistent (within all languages, within all speakers of a language, or within one person's speech) described with a focus on the outcome—that is, the nature of the final production (e.g., the phonological process name "stopping" is used to indicate that some non-stop consonant has been produced as a stop). See also "rule," "pattern," "constraint."

phonological process test Standardized, norm-referenced evaluation tool designed to assess children's error patterns, often by single-word naming of pictures.

phonological rule A linguistic change or tendency that is consistent (within all languages, within all speakers of a language, or within one person's speech) described with a focus on the distinctive features involved (e.g., a continuant sound [such as a fricative] that becomes noncontinuant [such as a stop]). See also "pattern," "process," "constraint."

phonologically conditioned Impacted by the phonetic/phonological context (said of a morpheme; e.g., the morpheme "in" is pronounced as [ɪm] before a labial consonant).

phonology A child's or a language's phones, phonemes, allophones, syllable and word shapes, the production and perception of these, and the patterning of these in rules, processes, or constraints.

phonotactic constraint A tendency to avoid certain syllable or word structures (markedness constraint) or to preserve certain syllable or word structures (faithfulness constraint) or to use certain strategies to make a word more pronounceable (faithfulness constraint).

phonotactic probability The frequency at which two sounds occur as a sequence in a given language.

phonotactic repertoire The set of syllable and word shapes in a particular language or produced by a particular person.

phrase-final lengthening An increase in the duration of the final syllable in a phrase or sentence.

phrase-final pitch declination A decrease in the pitch of the final syllable in a phrase or sentence.

phrase-level effect A pattern (rule, process, constraint) that applies at the level of the phrase (i.e., across words) (e.g., [dɪdʒu] for "did you").

pitch contour The rise and fall of the fundamental frequency that ties together and adds meaning to a phrase or sentence. Compare to "intonation contour," "prosodic contour."

place of articulation Position of the primary articulator involved in producing a sound (e.g., the place of articulation for [ŋ] is "velar" because the dorsum of the tongue is raised to the velar region).

play therapy A flexible child-centered intervention approach in which the SLP models, elicits, and provides social reinforcement for speech and language production in a naturalistic context.

positive evidence Learning based on direct observation of a speech event.

practice conditions The context in which a target behavior is repeated in order to improve performance.

Prader-Willi syndrome A genetic syndrome characterized by low tone, nutrition issues, and intellectual and learning disabilities.

prepractice Preparing a child for a task (e.g., by giving instructions, demonstrating the use of materials).

prevoiced Voicing begins before consonant release; not a typical voicing option in English.

procedural learning Learning based on distributional probabilities that is unconscious and automatic. See "implicit learning;" compare "declarative memory."

process A linguistic change or tendency that is consistent (within all languages, within all speakers of a language, or within one person's speech) described with a focus on the outcome—that is, the nature of the final production (e.g., the phonological process name "stopping" is used to indicate that some non-stop consonant has been produced as a stop). See also "rule," "pattern," "constraint," "phonological process."

process test A standardized normative assessment with the purpose of identifying phonological processes.

progressive harmony The influence of a sound earlier in the word on a sound later in the word with the result that the two sounds are pronounced more similarly; also called "perseveratory harmony." Compare to "regressive harmony."

PROMPT Intervention program focused on using dynamic tactile cues to facilitate speech production.

proprioception Sensations of movement and orientation in space that are based upon internal stimuli.

prosody The combination of the rise and fall of the fundamental frequency with increases and decreases in duration and intensity that ties together and adds meaning to a phrase or sentence. See "suprasegmental patterns," "prosodic contour." Compare to "pitch contour," "phrase-final lengthening," and "phrase-final declination."

protoword Vocalization associated with a certain event, person, thing, etc., but not based on a true word.

pure tone average The mean of a person's hearing threshold levels at 500, 1,000, 2,000, and 4,000 Hz, in decibels.

R

random practice Therapy approach in which trials of various different targets are intermixed throughout the session. Compare "blocked practice."

rapid syllable transition treatment (ReST) A therapy approach in which carefully selected nonsense words are used as exemplars and principles of motor learning are applied.

reduplicated babbling Babble (prelinguistic vocalization) composed of repetitions of syllables that include both true consonants and fully resonant vowels (e.g., [bɑbɑbɑbɑ]); a type of canonical babble. Compare to "variegated babbling."

reduplication Production with repeated syllables (e.g., [bɑbɑ] for "bottle.")

recurrent otitis media Chronic ear infections.

referential gesture Body movement used to label an object.

referential learning An analytical learning style resulting in a preponderance of nouns, learned singly (not in phrases). Also known as "analytical learning."

reflexive vocalization Involuntary sound (sigh, burp, etc.); vegetative sound.

register A language style used in a particular context or for a particular purpose (e.g., banking register, baby talk register).

regressive harmony The influence of a sound later in the word on a sound earlier in the word with the result that the two sounds are pronounced more similarly; also called "anticipatory harmony." Compare to "progressive harmony."

reinforcement Response to a behavior that is intended to increase the frequency of that behavior; one type of "feedback."

relational analysis Comparison of a child's production to the adult target; evaluation of the correctness of the child's productions.

repair strategies *Linguistics*: patterns preferred in a given language for making words easier to pronounce; faithfulness constraints (e.g., cluster reduction is preferred over epenthesis in English but the opposite applies in Japanese). *Intervention*: a speaker's manners of clarifying when not understood (e.g., rephrasing, emphasizing key words, slowed speech).

response generalization Transfer of skills from one target to another; includes within-in class generalization and across-class generalization.

resyllabification The coda of a word in a phrase used as the onset of the next word in order to avoid vowel-initial words (e.g., [pʊ tɪ tɑn] for "put it on").

retention Continuing to use new-found knowledge or skills for a period of time (e.g., a month) after therapy has ceased; maintenance.

Rett syndrome A degenerative genetic neurologic syndrome that results in decreasing function including hand use, communication, and learning.

rhotic vowel A vowel comprised of or impacted by the liquid /ɹ/ sound (e.g., [ɚ], [ɔɪɚ]); an "r-colored vowel."

rhyme *Phonotactics*: the nucleus plus the coda (if any) of a syllable. *Literacy*: the occurrence of a shared nucleus + coda (e.g., "cat" and "fat" rhyme because they have the same nucleus + coda combination).

rooting reflex A subconscious movement that includes turning the head, opening the mouth, and sucking and/or swallowing movements in response to light touch to the mouth area.

rounding Producing a sound with lip-rounding under the influence of a nearby round vowel (e.g., producing the [s] in "Sue" with slightly rounded lips because [u] is round).

rule governed Systematic; based on consistent patterns.

rule A linguistic change or tendency that is consistent (within all languages, within all speakers of a language, or within one person's speech) described with a focus on the distinctive features involved (e.g., a continuant sound [such as a fricative] that becomes noncontinuant [such as a stop]). See "pattern," "process," "constraint."

S

salience Easy detectability.

sensorineural Of the inner ear or the auditory nerve; a type of hearing loss.

semantic contingency Responding to a child's vocalization by producing a word that is related to the child's meaning or interest.

sequential bilingual A person who masters most of one language before beginning to learn another.

simultaneous bilingual A person who learns two languages at the same time.

socioeconomic status A measure of family financial and educational level.

SODA analysis Assessment of a child's speech errors: subsitutions, omissions, and distortions.

somatosensory Sensory information about touch, temperature, and body position from the skin and the internal organs.

sonority A measure of the openness of the oral cavity or the amount of energy produced for a given sound.

sonority hierarchy A ranking of speech sounds based upon relative openness/amount of energy.

sonorous Characterized by a high level of sonority.

Sotos syndrome A genetic disorder characterized by growth differences as well as movement and learning disabilities.

sound class A set of speech sounds that share certain distinctive features (e.g., voiced stops, front vowels). See also "natural class."

specific language impairment (SLI) A developmental language disorder that occurs in the absence of other cognitive/learning deficits.

speech screening A procedure for rapidly determining whether further evaluation of a child's speech is warranted. See "identification."

spina bifida A neural tube defect caused by incomplete development of the spinal cord during embryonic development.

spinal muscular atrophy A genetic disorder characterized by a loss of motor neurons that results in muscular weakness and a loss of motor control. See "Werdnig-Hoffman disease."

static assessment Evaluation based upon testing in one manner and in one context. Compare "dynamic assessment."

stimulable Able to be produced with cues or other supports.

stimulus generalization The transfer of knowledge or skills from one set of stimulating conditions to another.

stopping Producing a continuant sound (usually a fricative) as a noncontinuant sound (a stop).

stress Emphasis; increased intensity, duration, and pitch on a particular syllable or word.

strident Characterized by a relatively loud fricative sound.

strong Stressed (said of a syllable).

submucous cleft An opening in the palate, due to incomplete closure during embryonic development, that is covered by membrane.

sucking reflex Involuntary rhythmic mouth movements triggered by touch on the palate.

supraglottal Produced with a constriction above the glottis (i.e., an oral constriction); oral.

suprasegmental pattern The combination of the rise and fall of the fundamental frequency with increases and decreases in duration and intensity that ties together and adds meaning to a phrase or sentence. See also "prosody," "prosodic contour." Compare to "intonation contour," "pitch contour," "phrase-final lengthening," and "phrase-final declination."

suppression The act of overcoming or reducing the frequency of a pattern that results in non–adult-like productions.

surface representation The actual form of a word as it is produced or heard (i.e., the allophones).

syllabic Vowel-like; carrying the prosodic features of the syllable.

syllabic consonant A consonant that plays the role of the nucleus of the syllable, that is, that has a vowel-like function.

syllable A basic unit of speech production composed of at least a vowel; often with one or more consonants.

symptom complex A set of frequently co-occurring characteristics associated with a medical condition or other diagnosis, not all of which need to be present for a diagnosis and which may change over time; syndrome. Compare "unitary disorder."

syndrome A set of frequently co-occurring characteristics associated with a medical condition or other diagnosis, not all of which need to be present for a diagnosis and which may change over time; symptom complex. Compare "unitary disorder."

systematic gap A sound class that does not occur in the inventory of a given language or person (e.g., English does not have uvular consonants).

T

Tay-Sachs disease A degenerative genetic disorder that results in muscle weakness, decreased motor control, seizures, sensory deficits, intellectual disabilities, and other symptoms.

template A preferred production pattern resulting in the child selecting words that fit the pattern or adapting other words to fit the pattern.

temporal lobe Portion of the cerebral cortex important for auditory processing.

thalamus A neurologic structure between the cerebral cortex and the midbrain that is a relay station for sensory and motor signals.

tone *Physiology*: a muscle's readiness for action when it is at rest; muscle tone. *Prosody*: the use of pitch to differentiate words.

token-to-token variability Inconsistent production of a syllable or word when repeated in a series (as in alternate motion rates or sequential motion rates, i.e., diadochokinesis). Common in CAS. See also "inconsistency."

training broad Therapy approach in which varied exemplars from a category are addressed until criterion is reached; a type of variable practice.

training narrow Therapy approach with massed practice on a few exemplars until criterion is reached.

transfer error Error resulting from the influence of one language on another. See "interference."

transition Movement of the articulators from one configuration to the next (e.g., from a consonant into a vowel).

trochaic Having a strong-weak (stressed-unstressed) stress pattern.

true consonant A supraglottal, non-glide consonant (not [ʔ], [h], [w], [j]).

U

underbite Lower teeth protruding beyond the upper teeth.

underlying representation The mental (conceptual, phonemic) representation of a word.

unitary disorder Condition or disorder with a single, unchanging list of symptoms that must all be present for a diagnosis to be made. Compare "symptom complex," "syndrome."

universality Occurrence in all (or almost all) languages of the world or in all (or almost all) typically developing children. See "phonetic universal."

unmarked Preferred or common (universally, in a particular language, or in a particular person's phonological system). Compare to "marked."

uvula Structure composed of tissue, glands, and muscle fibers that dangles from the back of the soft palate.

V

variability Difference in production from one time to the next or in a different context. See "inconsistency." Compare to "variety."

variable practice Intervention using a variety of exemplars, contexts, or even goals within the same session. Compare to "constant practice."

variable feedback Therapy approach in which responses to the child's production attempts are provided less than 100% of the time, "randomly." Compare to "continuous feedback."

variegated babbling Prelinguistic vocalizations in which different consonants and vowels occur within the same vocalization; a type of canonical babbling. Compare to "reduplicated babbling."

variety Functional use of a set of different elements or forms. Compare to "variability" and "inconsistency."

vegetative sounds Involuntary sounds (sighs, burps, etc.); reflexive vocalizations.

velocardial facial syndrome (VCF) A genetic disorder resulting in cleft palate, motor speech disorders, and nonverbal intelligence deficits; also called "22q.11 syndrome."

velopharyngeal insufficiency Inability to completely raise the velum in order to close off airflow to the nasal cavity, resulting in hypernasality; VPI.

visual-spatial sketch pad The component of working memory responsible for retaining visual-spatial information.

vocal play Exploration of the sounds that can be made with the mouth, including squeals, grunts, clicks, and the like.

vocant A vowel-like sound that is not fully resonant; that is, the mouth is not fully open.

voiced Produced with vibration of the vocal folds.

voiceless aspirated With a "long lag" between the release of the consonant and onset of voicing, so that the aspiration can be heard.

voiceless unaspirated With consonant release and the onset of voicing at about the same time, so that aspiration is not heard; referred to as "voiced" by English speakers.

voicing Use of the vocal folds during segment production.

volubility A measure of the frequency of vocalization.

vowel formants Resonances resulting from configuration of the vocal tract, especially the articulators.

vowel triangle The three "corner" vowels, [i], [ɑ], [u].

W

weak Unstressed (said of syllables).

Werdnig-Hoffman disease A severe form of spinal muscular atrophy characterized by a loss of motor neurons that results in muscular weakness, a loss of motor control, developmental deficits, and swallowing and breathing difficulties.

within-class generalization Transfer of learning from one goal in a category to another within the same category (e.g., from one type of fricative to another); a type of response generalization.

Williams syndrome Neurodevelopmental syndrome caused by deletion of genes at 7q11.23, resulting in cognitive deficits, low muscle tone, and cardiac abnormalities.

Word Complexity Measure (WCM) Measure of the phonetic and phonotactic maturity of a child's early words.

word recipe A child's preferred production pattern.

working memory The ability to hold information in short-term memory while mentally manipulating that information.

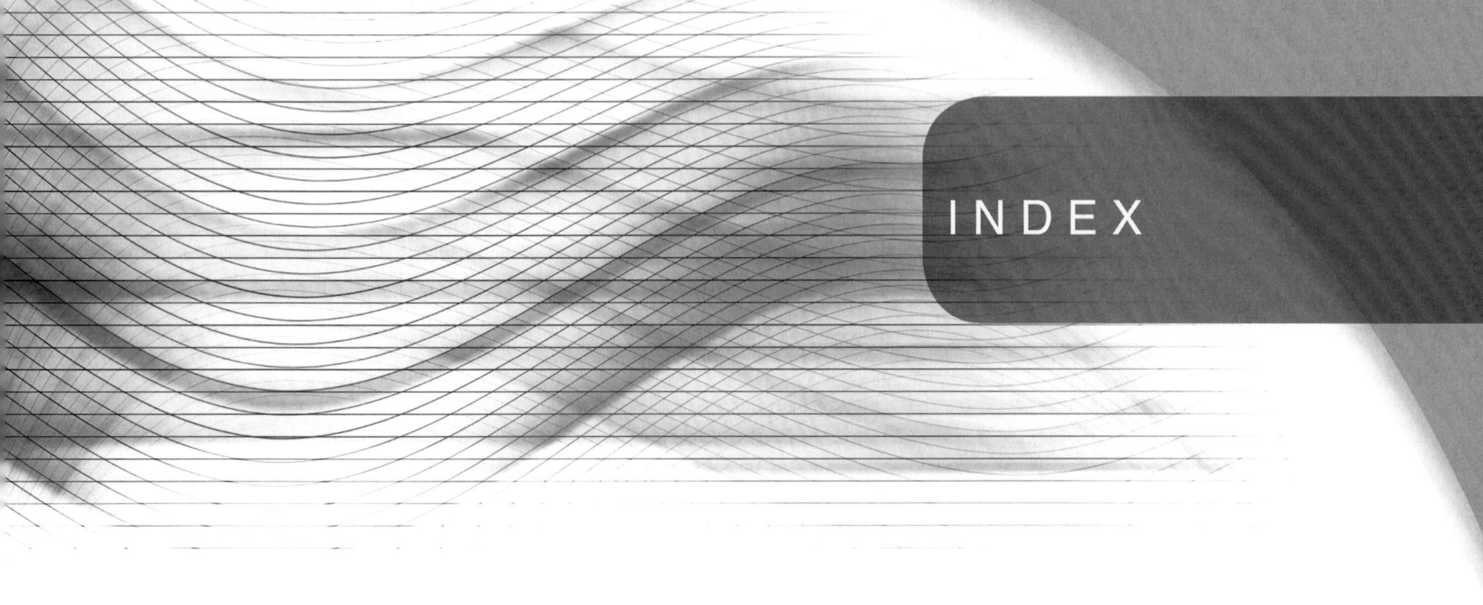

INDEX

***Note:* Page numbers followed by "f" indicate figure; those followed by "t" indicate table.**

R

T

U

V

W